Intelligent and Biosensors

Edited by

Vernon S. Somerset

Intelligent and Biosensors
Edited by Vernon S. Somerset

This is a reprint of the book published in 2010 by Intech

Republished by InTech
Janeza Trdine 9, 51000 Rijeka, Croatia

Technical Editor Teodora Smiljanic

Cover Designer Dino Smrekar

Additional hard copies can be obtained from orders@intechopen.com

Intelligent and Biosensors, Edited by Vernon S. Somerset
p. cm.
ISBN 978-953-7619-58-9

For EU product safety concerns:
IN TECH d.o.o., Prolaz Marije Krucifikse Kozulić 3, 51000 Rijeka, Croatia,
info@intechopen.com or visit our website at intechopen.com.

Preface

The term intelligent sensor (or smart sensor) has been used in the sensor industry to describe sensors that provide not only measurements, but also functionality to specific measurements. There are three characteristics that define an intelligent sensor: i) firstly, it contains a sensing element that measures one or more physical parameter; ii) secondly, it has a computational element that analyses the measurements made by the sensing element; iii) thirdly, it contains a communication interface enabling interaction with the outside world in order to exchange information with other components in a larger system. Furthermore, intelligent sensors allow networks of sensors to connect to each other, locally or around the globe in order to accomplish specific tasks. The use of intelligent sensors have revolutionised the way in which we gather data from the world around us, also how we extract useful information from that data, and the manner in which we use the newly obtained information for various operations and decision making.

The field of Electrochemical sensors have shown that various methods can be employed in transducer modification in order to produce analytical probes that can be applied for the analysis of clinical, industrial, food and environmental samples. One specific type of electrochemical sensor that has received serious research attention over several decades is the Biosensor. A Biosensor can be defined as a compact analytical device containing biological material that is closely associated with a physico-chemical transducer, to produce either discrete or continuous digital electronic signals that are proportional to a single analyte or a related group of analytes. In this book the particular emphasis is on biosensors for the detection of organophosphorous and carbamate pesticide compounds. These pesticide compounds are known for their toxic effects due to their ability to irreversibly modify the catalytic serine residue in acetylcholinesterases (AChE) and subsequent inhibition of the AChE effectively prevents nerve transmission by blocking the breakdown of the transmitter choline.

This book is an attempt to highlight the current research in the field of Intelligent and Biosensors, thereby describing state-of-the-art techniques in the field and emerging new technologies, also showcasing some examples and applications.

The focus of the first eight chapters is on Intelligent Sensors. In Chapter 1 we are introduced to the work of Chen and co-workers on the design of a smart jacket and a power supply for neonatal monitoring with wearable sensors. This work has shown how it is possible to improve the comfort and quality of life for the child by elimination of the adhesive electrodes and by the elimination of wires. In Chapter 2, we are introduced to a comprehensive survey of signal processing, feature extraction/selection and classification methods used to provide the readers with guidelines on design *brain-computer interfaces (BCIs)*. This work by Al-Ani and Trad have shown that the exploration of new methods in BCI design would be strongly driven by new properties that will have to be taken into consideration in the real future applications of *BCIs*. In Chapter 3, Sashima and Kurumatani proposes some views of what a mobile sensor fusion platform can contribute to the field and two types of fusion architecture, e.g. "mobile sensing architecture" and "stable sensing architecture" are described with a prototype platform of the mobile sensing architecture introduced. In Chapter 4, the focus is on the assessment of the biomineralization capacity of polyamidoamine (PAMAM) dendrimers amino- and carboxylic-terminated immobilized on solid supports. This work by Stancu is aimed as the first attempt of investigation of biomaterials-induced biomineralization through the label-free Surface Plasmon Resonance Imaging (SPRi). In Chapter 5, the work of Rangelova and co-workers discusses the use of soft computing techniques for modelling the inputoutput dependency of a dopamine biosensor that takes into account the simultaneous influence of pH and temperature over the output current. In Chapter 6, Gargiulo and co-workers describes a long term, wearable personal monitoring system that is wireless, low power and uses convenient dry electrodes. The use of this system for electrocardiogram (ECG) and athlete monitoring has also been demonstrated. In Chapter 7, the work by De Silva and co-workers presents a framework to transfer the natural gestural behaviours of a human agent to a robot through a robust imitation algorithm. The novelty of their proposed algorithm is the use of symbolic postures to generate the gestural behaviours of a robot without using any training data or trained model. The idea behind using symbolic postures is that a robot is flexibly able to generate its own motion. In Chapter 8, the author Bae focuses our attention on a newly designed sensor or structure of an *in-vitro* giant magnetoresistance (GMR) biosensor with a specially designed magnetic shield layer (MSL). The physical sensing characteristics of the in-vitro GMR biosensor with an immobilized single FNSA are also discussed to explore its feasibility to a single molecular based disease diagnostic biosensor system.

The work in the following chapters focus on Biosensors for the detection of various analytes. In Chapter 9, Somerset and co-workers describe the application of a mercaptobenzothiazole-on-gold biosensor system for the analysis of organosphosphorous and carbamate pesticide compounds. The aim of this work was to improve the detection limit of these insecticides with an AChE biosensor, applied to various water miscible organic solvents. In Chapter 10, the work of Cortina-Puig and co-workers focuses on AChE biosensors as a rapid and simple alternative method for the detection of organophosphorous insecticides. They indicate that such sensors should be small, cheap, simple to handle and able to provide reliable information in realtime with or without minimum sample preparation. In Chapter 11, the work of Stoytcheva highlights the fact that the analytical potential of electrochemical biosensors for the detection of organophosphorous insecticides is obvious, despite the fact that they still demonstrate limited application in the quantification of real samples. In Chapter 12, Srivastava and co-workers focus our attention on the first continuous, electrochemical biosensor for real-time, rapid measurement of Neuropathy Target Esterase (NEST (or NTE) esterase activity. The biosensor was fabricated by coimmobilizing NEST protein and tyrosinase enzyme on an electrode using the layer by layer assembly approach. In Chapter 13, the work of Nien and co-workers showcase two systems. In the first system, a poly(3,4-ethylenedioxythiophene) (PEDOT) modified electrode was used as a matrix to entrap glucose oxidase and was integrated in a flow system for sensing chip applications. In the second system, the proposed electrode fabricated by multilayer structures successfully works as a glucose biosensor in the oxygen-independence solution, and the anode of the biofuel cell operates not only on glucose solution but also on real blood of human beings. In Chapter 14, Budai discuss the fabrication of single- and multibarrel carbon fiber (CF) microelectrodes, the covalent modifications of the carbon surface as well as the applications of CF microelectrodes in recording spikes from neurons, electrochemical or biosensor signals from various tissues. This chapter further discuss the novel use of CF microelectrodes as oxygen detectors usable *in vitro* and *in vivo* applications. In Chapter 15, the work of Reshetilov and co-workers focuses on microbial biosensors and showcase that the properties of microbial sensors are in many respects analogous to the properties of enzyme biosensors. In Chapter 16, the work of Mateo-Martí and Pradier focuses on DNA biosensors with specific attention on a new artificial nucleic acid, PNA, as a highly specific probe. They also provide an overview of some surface analysis techniques that have been successfully applied to the detection of PNA-DNA hybridisation. In Chapter 17, the work of Yakhno and co-workers demonstrate the unique use of an uncoated quartz resonator in the diagnostics of multi-component liquids without detection of their content. This is a new type of analytical instrument, based on non-linear non-equilibrium processes in drying drops, so called selforganization. The main feature of this approach is that phase transitions in drying drops were registered and used as the informative parameter. In Chapter 18, Konuk and co-workers introduce and ALAD (δ-Aminolevulinic Acid Dehydratase) biosensor and indicates that the expression of ALAD activity gives us a clear indication of the severity of the effect of Pb pollution along the pollution gradient. In Chapter 19, the work of Vidic focuses on a bioelectronic nose based on olfactory receptors indicating that the development of sensor technology incorporating natural olfactory receptors provides the basis for a bioelectronic nose mimicking the animal olfactory system. Such devices can be used for qualitative and quantitative identification and monitoring of a spectrum of odorants with much higher selectivity and sensibility than the present electronic devices.

It is envisaged that this book will provide valuable reference and learning material to other researchers, scientists and postgraduate students in the field. The references at the end of each chapter serve as valuable entry points to further reading on the various topics discussed and should provide guidance to those interested in moving forward in the field of Intelligent and Biosensors.

My sincere gratitude is expressed to the contributing authors for their hard work, time and effort in preparing the different chapters, because without their dedication this book would not have been possible.

Editor

Vernon S. Somerset
Cape Town,
South Africa

Contents

1

Intelligent Design for Neonatal Monitoring with Wearable Sensors

Wei Chen[1], Sibrecht Bouwstra[1], Sidarto Bambang Oetomo[1,2] and Loe Feijs[1]
[1]*Department of Industrial Design, Eindhoven University of Technology,*
[2]*Department of Neonatology, Máxima Medical Center, Veldhoven,*
The Netherlands

1. Introduction

Neonatal monitoring refers to the monitoring of vital physiological parameters of premature infants, full term infants that are critically ill, and a combination thereof. Babies that are born after a pregnancy lasting 37 weeks or less are typically considered premature. Critically ill neonates are a special group of patients that consist of premature infants who may suffer from diseases that are mainly caused by immaturity of their organs, and full term infants, who become severely ill during or immediately after birth. In particular, these premature infants can weigh as little as 500g with a size of a palm and are highly vulnerable to external disturbances. Critically ill newborn infants are normally admitted to a Neonatal Intensive Care Unit (NICU) for treatment by neonatologists and specialized nurses.

Continuous health monitoring for the neonates provides crucial parameters for early detection of in adverted events (such as cessation of breathing, heart rhythm disturbances and drop in blood oxygen saturation), and possible complications (such as seizures). Immediate action based on this detection increases survival rates and positively supports further development of the neonates. Advances in medical treatments over the last decades resulted in a significant increase of survival. As a result, neonates born after 25 weeks of pregnancy can survive with adequate medical care and appropriate medical care in NICU (Costeloe et al., 2000). Encouraged by this success NICUs are populated by a large proportion of infants, born after very short gestational age. Survival and long-term health prospects strongly depend on medical care and reliable and comfortable health-status monitoring systems.

In the last decades several important treatment modalities emerged that had a substantial impact on the mortality of prematurely born infants. However there is a concomitant increase of neurobehavioral problems on long-term follow-up (Perlman, 2001; Hack & Fanaroff, 1999; Chapieski & Evankovitch, 1997). Follow-up studies indicate that preterm infants show more developmental delay compared to their full-term peers. More than 50% of them show deficits in their further development, such as visual-motor integration problems, motor impairments, speech and language delay, behavioral, attention, and learning problems (Marlow et al. 2007). Medical conditions including chronic lung disease, apnea and bradycardia, transient thyroid dysfunction, jaundice and nutritional deficiencies, are potential contributing factors. In addition infants in a busy NICU are often exposed to stressful environmental conditions. Examples are the attachment to multiple monitoring devices and intravenous lines, high noise levels and bright light (Perlman, 2003). A concept of interactions in the developing neonatal brain with maternal separation and exposure to pain and stress is illustrated in Fig. 1, according to Anand and Scalzo (Anand & Scalzo, 2000). These negative stimuli can interfere with the normal growth and development of the neonates and hamper the parent-child interaction (Als et al., 2003). Thus, it is essential to develop comfortable care solutions for NICU and follow-up.

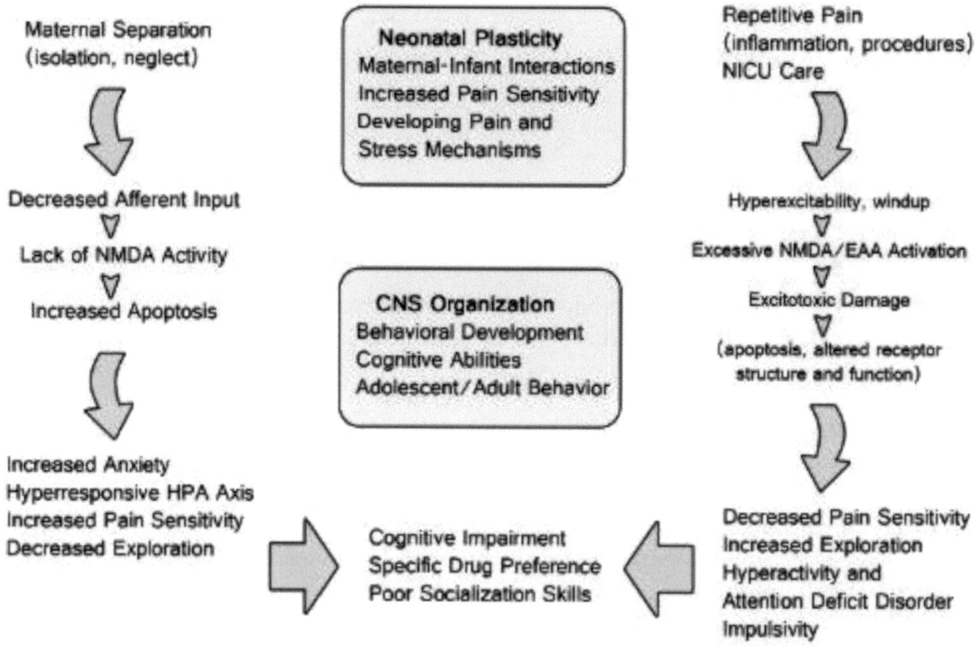

Fig. 1. Schematic diagram of the effects of neonatal pain and maternal separation in the neonate on brain plasticity and long term effects on subsequent brain development and behaviour

Vital parameters of clinical relevance for neonatal monitoring include body temperature, electrocardiogram (ECG), respiration, and blood oxygen saturation (Als, 1986; Polin & Fox, 1992). Presently, body temperature is monitored with adhesive thermistors; ECG and respiration are obtained by adhesive skin electrodes. The oxygen saturation of the blood is monitored by a pulse oximeter with the sensor applied on the foot or palm of the neonate (Murković et al. 2003). Placement of these adhesive sensors and the presence of all the wires lead to discomfort and even painful stimuli when the electrodes have to be removed. Preterm infants, in particular the ones with an immature central nervous system, are highly sensitive for external stimuli such as noise, bright light, and pain. As the survival rate of neonates has increased significantly in the last decades (de Kleine et al., 2007), the quality of life of NICU graduates becomes an important issue as well. Alternative, non-invasive monitoring of vital physiological functions is a pressing need to provide convenient care and hence, may lead to improved developmental outcome of the neonates.

Recent advances in sensor technologies (Yang, 2006; Van Langenhove, 2007; Murković et al., 2003) and wireless communication technologies (Goldsmith, 2005) enable the creation of a new generation of healthcare monitoring systems with wearable electronics and photonics (Tao, 2005; Aarts & Encarnação, 2006).

The Eindhoven University of Technology (TU/e) in the Netherlands has started a 10-year project on non-invasive perinatal monitoring in cooperation with the Máxima Medical Centre (MMC) in Veldhoven, the Netherlands. The goal of this collaboration is to improve the healthcare of the pregnant woman, and her child before, during, and after delivery. In the work on neonatal monitoring, we aim to integrate a multidisciplinary network of sensor technology, medical clinics and signal processing into revolutionary neonatal monitoring solutions (Chen et al., 2010b). The design skills needed range from medical science, human factors, material knowledge, smart textiles and form-giving to circuit design, user research, power management, signal processing and software engineering. Some intelligent designs have been developed covering different aspects of on non-invasive neonatal monitoring with wearable sensors, such as vital signs monitoring (Bouwstra et al, 2009; Chen, et al., 2010a; Chen, et al., 2010c), data transmission (Chen et al, 2009a), and power supply (Chen et al, 2008; Chen et al, 2009b). In this chapter, we present the design work of a smart jacket integrated with textile sensors and a power supply based on contactless energy transfer for neonatal monitoring.

The chapter is structured as follows. Section 2 explains the design process and design requirements. Section 3 describes the smart jacket design. Section 4 presents the wireless power supply design. Both section 3 and section 4 consist of the design concept, prototype implementation, and clinical testing or experimental results. Section 5 concludes the chapter.

2. Design process and design requirements

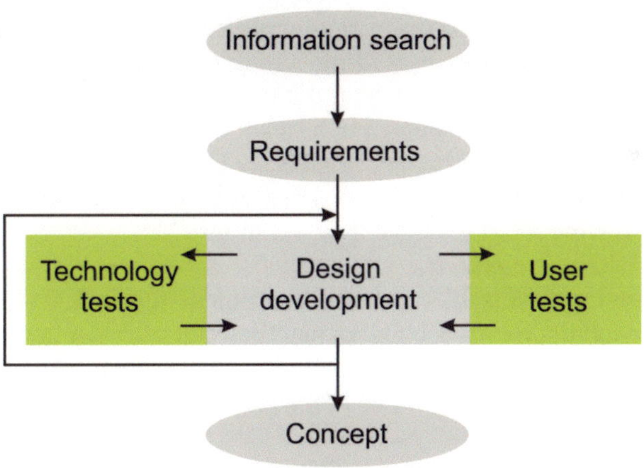

Fig. 2. Design process model

Methodologies from the field of Industrial Design are applied in the design process, which involves a unique integration of knowledge from medical science, design, and sensor technology. Fig. 2 shows the design process. The iterative process begins with an information search that includes user research involving doctors and nurses at MMC in Veldhoven and gathering of information on neonatal monitoring, smart textiles, power supply, etc.. Requirements were derived from the information search, forming a base for brainstorm sessions which resulted in ideas about technological challenges, functionality issues within NICU as well as form and senses. The ideas are then placed in a morphological diagram and combined to several initial concepts. Design choices are made through an iterative process in which proof of technology and user feedbacks provide clues for further development. The three aspects 'Technology, User Focus and Design', are strongly interwoven along the process.

With consideration of both user aspects and technical functions, the design should meet the following requirements:

- support the vital health monitoring functions
- be safe to use in the NICU environment
- be scalable to include more monitoring functions and local signal processing
- support continuous monitoring when the baby is inside the incubator or during Kangaroo mother care
- gain the feeling of trust by the parents and the medical staff through an attractive design
- be non-intrusive and avoid disturbance of the baby and avoid causes of stress
- provide appropriate feedback which is also interpretable for parents and hospital staff on whether the system's components are correctly functioning
- non-washable parts must be easy to remove
- look friendly, playful and familiar

3. Smart jacket design for neonatal monitoring

3.1 Design concept

The vision of the Neonatal Smart Jacket is a wearable unobtrusive continuous monitoring system realized by sensor networks and wireless communication, suitable for monitoring neonates inside the incubator and outside the incubator during Kangaroo mother care. The Neonatal Smart Jacket aims for providing reliable health monitoring as well as a comfortable clinical environment for neonatal care and parent-child interaction. The first step towards the Smart Jacket is the design of a jacket that:

1. contains the integration of conductive textiles for ECG monitoring,
2. forms a platform for future research, in which wireless communication, power supply and sensors are developed,
3. obtains a sense of trust by parents.

The concept of Diversity Textile Electrode Measurement (DTEM) is applied for the smart jacket design. The neonate wears a baby jacket that contains six conductive patches that sense biopotential signals at different positions to perform diversity measurements. Depending on the way the baby lies or is held, there are always patches that are in close contact with the skin because of pressure. When one sensor becomes loose from the skin, another sensor can provide a better signal. The system continuously measures which leads of the suit have superior contact and chooses the strongest signal for further processing. The concept offers a solution for skin contact, without jeopardizing comfort by tightness. It might also solve the problem of searching optimal electrode positions in the jacket, which varies per baby.

3.2 Prototype

A prototype jacket as shown in Fig. 3 was built according to the design requirements. The jacket is open at the front and has an open structure fabric on the back and hat, with the purpose of skin-on-skin contact, phototherapy and medical observation. The hat contains eye-protection and leaves room for future sensors. The aesthetics are designed to appear as regular baby clothing. The color combination of white and green with colorful happy animal heads is chosen because it is unisex while looking cheerful and clean.

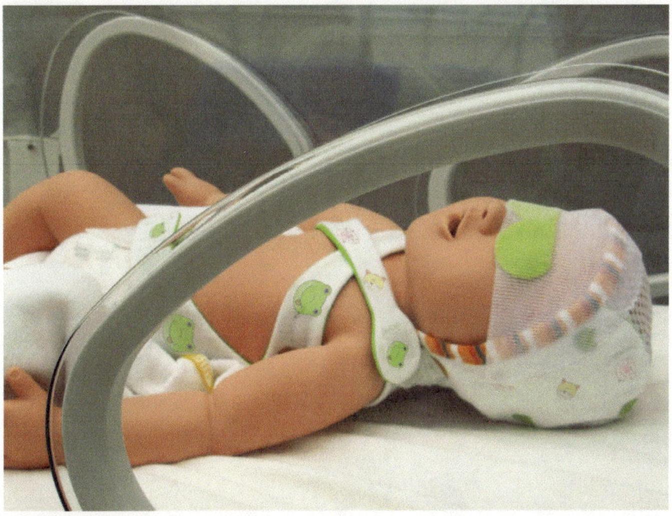

Fig. 3. Prototype smart jacket

The prototype is designed to have a stress-less dressing process as shown in Fig. 4: (1) the baby is laid down on the open jacket, (2) the lower belt is closed, (3) the hat is put on, and (4) finally the chest straps are closed.

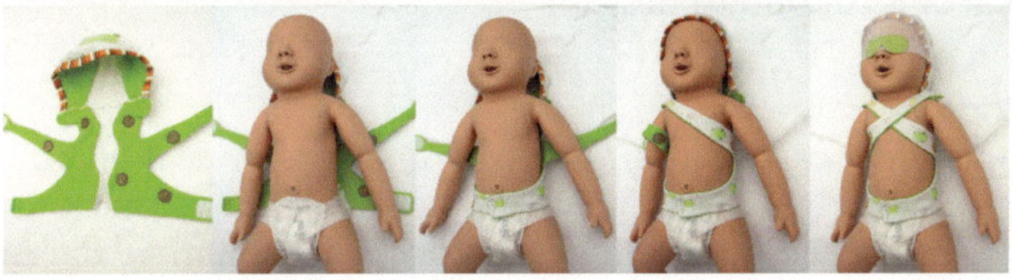

Fig. 4. Stress-less dressing process

Fig. 5 demonstrates the test patches with different versions of silver and gold textile electrodes and a blanket with large silver electrodes. The silver textile electrodes consist of silver plated nylons produced by Shieldex®. Construction details can be seen in Fig. 6. Three layers (1) of cotton are used and on the middle layer (2) the circuit is sewn with Shieldex® silver plated yarn. On the first layer the electrode is sewn, stitching through the circuit on the middle layer (3). The electrode's connection to the monitor is realized by carbon wires obtained from regular disposable gel electrodes: the end of the carbon wires are stripped and sewn onto the circuit on the middle layer (4). (Carbon wire is a good alternative to metal buttons which are often applied, because it avoids the less stable soft-hard connection). Finally the third cotton layer for isolation is sewn to the others (5).

The gold printed electrodes consist of a thin smooth fiber with a metal print developed by TNO at Eindhoven, the Netherlands. The gold test patches are created in a similar way to the silver test patches, however in future application the circuit and electrode can be printed in one piece.

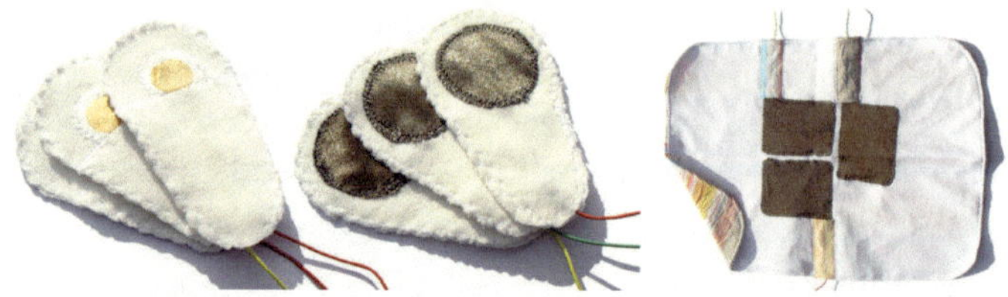

Fig. 5. Test patches and blanket

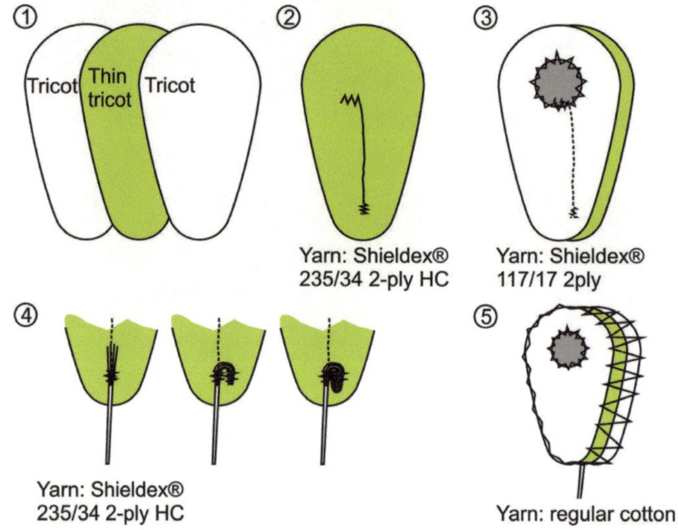

Fig. 6. Construction of textile electrodes

3.3 Clinical testing

Several experiments were carried out, ranging from experiments on adults as alternative subjects to neonates in the NICU at the MMC Veldhoven, the Netherlands. The goals are comparisons between the various textile electrodes, verification of their functioning on a neonate and verification of the DTEM concept. Finally, a wearability test of the jacket was performed.

An analysis of risks was performed before applying the prototypes to the NICU. Together with clinical physicists, a hospital hygiene and infection expert, and a neonatologist, the safety of the monitoring system and hygiene and allergy risks were analyzed. Precautions such as disinfection and allergy tests were taken. The ethical commission of the MMC Veldhoven approved the experiments.

First, we tested the quality of the ECG signals obtained by textile electrodes varying in material and size and gel electrodes (3M™ 2282E) are qualitatively compared. Fig. 7 shows the test setup. The electrodes were tested with two subjects: one neonate of 30 weeks and 5 days and one of 31 weeks and 6 days, both admitted in the NICU Veldhoven. The ECG is sensed by three textile electrodes in regular configuration and the data is acquired with a GE Heathcare Solar® 8000M. The unprocessed digital data of derivation II was obtained from a network and imported and filtered in MATLAB. A notch, high pass and low pass filter are applied to remove the 50 Hz and higher harmonics, DC (direct current) component and high frequency noise.

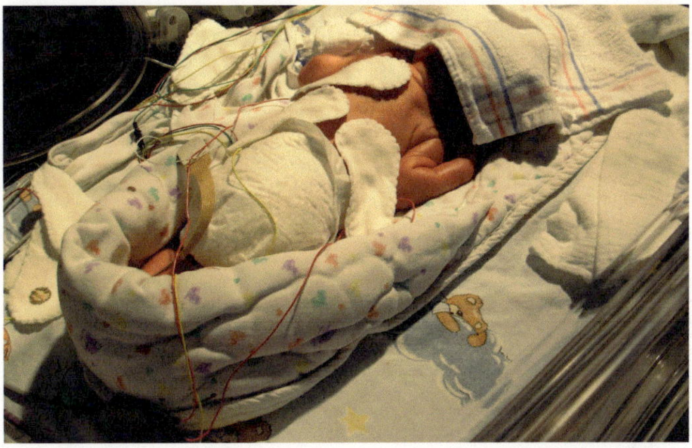

Fig. 7. Test setup

From Fig. 8 we can see that the quality of ECG obtained by the golden printed textile electrodes is good and the QRS complex can be seen clearly. The ECG curve in Fig. 8 is representative for the ECG quality by gold electrodes when the baby lies still.

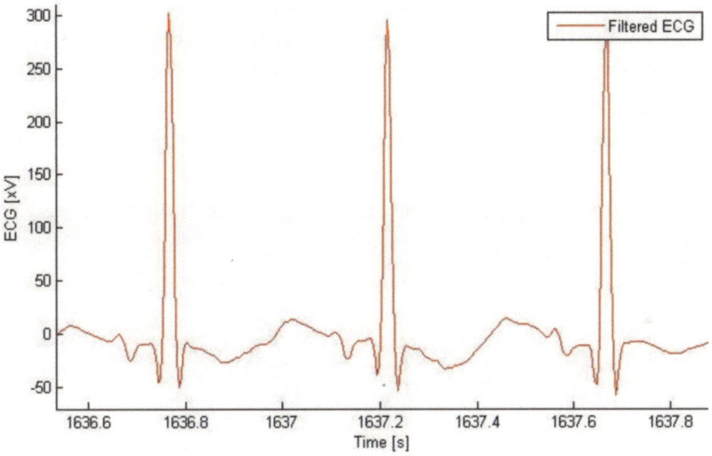

Fig. 8. Gold printed electrodes D=15mm

Secondly, we carried out tests to find out whether the concept of DTEM (Diversity Textile Electrode Measurement, see section 3.1) can improve the signal quality. The ECG obtained by large silver textile electrodes in a blanket where the neonate lies on, is compared to the ECG obtained by large silver patches held on the back. By this way, the effect of pressure by body weight can be investigated. From Fig. 9 we can see that the quality of ECG obtained by the silver textile electrodes is good and the QRS complex can be seen clearly as well. The shape of the ECG complex looks different from Fig. 8, because the heart is monitored from another angle.

Apart from reliable technology, the success of the Smart Jacket largely depends on the wearable comfort of the jacket. Tightness is desirable for sensor contact, although it might be in conflict with wearable comfort. Therefore, extra caution is taken by performing a

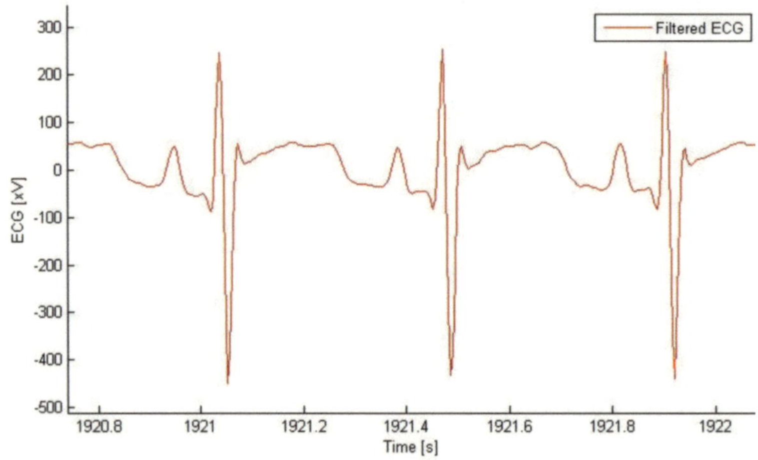

Fig. 9. Silver Shieldex®, 50mmx60mm, blanket

wearability test in an early design stage. Fig. 10 shows a stable neonate of 34 weeks being dressed in the first prototype of the Smart Jacket while being filmed. Compared to the stress that was caused when undressing the regular premature baby clothing, the dressing process of the Smart Jacket was very calm. The dressing time is about one minute. The model needs to be more adjustable in size due to large variations in proportions and range of dimensions: in the NICU neonates can grow from 500g to 2000g and body proportions vary especially when caused by medical conditions. The straps need to be improved for comfort in the next design iteration.

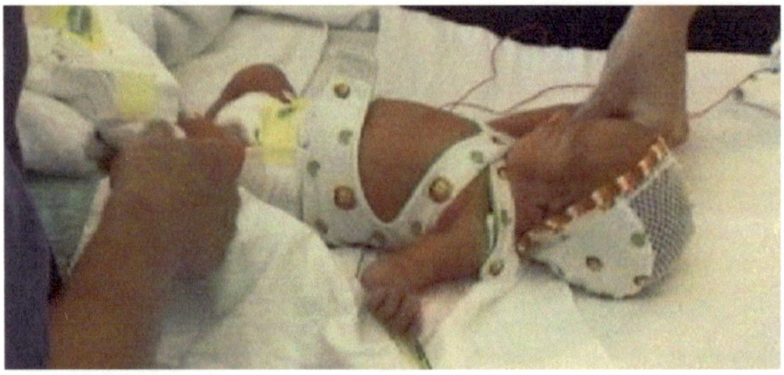

Fig. 10. Wearability test with the first prototype

3.4 Discussion and improvements

Due to the nature of conductive textiles, the quality of the ECG signal obtained with textile electrodes cannot exceed the gel electrodes: they are 'dry' electrodes with relatively loose skin contact and have a flexible structure that causes artifacts. However, the specific application of ECG monitoring neonates offers new design opportunities:

- A premature has smoother skin, which results in better skin contact
- The premature moves relatively little, which results in less movement artifacts
- The premature always lies or is being held, which offers continuous pressure, which leads to better skin contact

Two textile electrode designs turn out very promising: (1) large (±D=40mm) silver plated textile electrodes and (2) small (±D=15mm) gold printed electrodes. Both have different strengths and weaknesses. Large silver electrodes offer a stable ECG signal with low noise under the condition that pressure is applied. The silver seems hypoallergenic and does not change properties considerably after a few washing cycles.

The small gold printed electrodes, obtain a stable ECG signal with low noise, under the condition that pressure is applied in the beginning; once skin contact is established, little pressure is required. The gold print however is not hypoallergenic and looses conductivity after washing, due to corrosion of the metal layer beneath the gold. Although the silver electrodes could be applied without much adjustment, the gold prints are worth further development. They require less space due to higher conductivity, have a smoother surface that leads to better skin contact, are less flexible which leads to less artifacts and are seamless which leads to more comfort.

The monitoring of a neonate's ECG by diversity measurements realized by textile electrodes in the jacket definitely is a useful idea. Through experimental verification it is found that the quality of the ECG signal improves significantly due to a neonate's own body weight and is comparable to the quality of ECG signal obtained by gel electrodes.

Based on interviews with parents and medical staff, the conclusion can be drawn that the user groups are positive about the first results. They especially appreciate the freedom of movement, the aesthetic design, stress-less dressing process and integrated eye-protection. Improvements has been made on the design and a new version of the smart jacket has been developed as shown in Fig. 11.

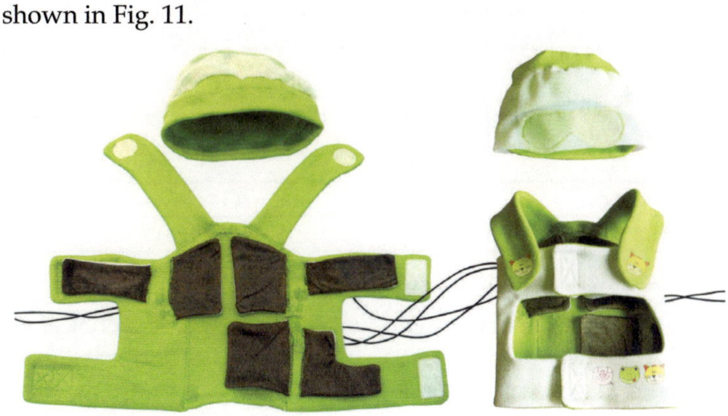

Fig. 11. New version of the smart jacket

The new version contains an extremely stretchable fabric that likely ensures adjustability to different sizes and proportions. The hat is kept separate for the same reasons. Furthermore, the straps are designed to prevent tightness around the neck. Large silver textile electrodes are applied in the new version. They are connected only on one of the four sides, in order to allow stretch of the jacket without stretch of the electrode itself. The medical staff and parents embrace the latest version of the smart jacket. At present this prototype is ready for further clinical testing within the MMC Veldhoven. The development of the Smart Jacket will be continued, initially by further development of the ECG sensors, wireless transmission and an adjustable size for different patients which enable clinical reliability tests.

4. Power supply design for neonatal monitoring

4.1 Design concept

A key question for health monitoring with wearable sensors is how to obtain reliable electrical power for the sensors, signal amplifiers, filters and transmitters. The deployment of new sensing and monitoring devices for non-invasive healthcare and clinical applications requires design of the new power supplies. The power supply should be either long lasting or easy to recharge during usage (Tao, 2005) to perform near-real-time continuous monitoring. The need to minimize maintenance and replacement costs of batteries drives the development of innovative power solutions, encompassing energy scavenging (i.e. energy harvesting) technologies that exploit renewable and ambient sources of energy, such as solar energy, energy harvested from body heat and movement (Paradiso, 2005; Qin, 2008), and wireless power supplies (Catrysse, 2004; Ma, 2007).

Fundamental physiological parameters that should be continuously monitored during neonatal care are electrocardiogram (ECG), respiration, oxygen saturation of the blood (O2-Sat), and body temperature. The amount of power required by different health monitoring sensors and processors is important for designing the power supply. We summarize the power consumption of monitoring and processing in Table 1. Based on the information of power consumption, our power supply should be able to deliver 150-200 mW for the health monitoring functions and more power is needed when charging batteries.

Function	Power Consumption
Data transmission	about 50 mW
ECG Read-out amplifier for textile sensors	about 1 mW
body temperature sensors	50 mW
SpO2 sensors	45 mW
Respiration sensors	below 1mW

Table 1. Power consumption for monitoring and processing

With the above design requirements in mind, we come up with a technical solution and the concept of "PowerBoy", which uses contactless power and a rechargeable battery embedded in a plush toy for neonatal care. We propose to apply inductive energy transfer for the power supply due to its wireless feature and scalability. Inductive energy transfer will be employed for continuous power supply and for charging the battery when a neonate is lying inside the incubator. The rechargeable battery is used for energy storage and continuous power supply when the neonate is outside of incubator during Kangaroo mother care.

Fig. 12 shows an overview of the proposed system. In the system, a primary rectangular spiral winding, labelled S_A, is placed underneath a 60 mm thick incubator mattress. The primary winding forms part of a series resonant circuit driven by a half-bridge inverter and a power supply. The PowerBoy plush toy is equipped with, amongst other things, a secondary hexagon spiral winding, denoted S_B.

When the PowerBoy toy is placed on the mattress above the primary winding, the magnetic field is "picked-up" and an inductive link is formed. Power is then transferred from the primary winding to the secondary winding through their mutual inductance. A rectifier

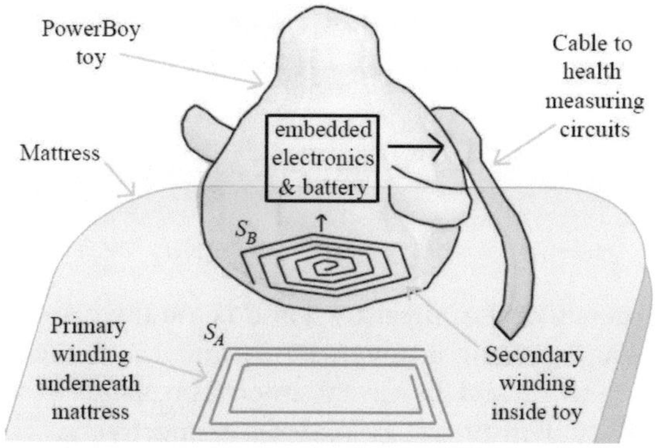

Fig. 12. An overview of the PowerBoy system

circuit and power converter charges a battery inside the toy, and supplies the monitoring equipment with power via a power cable, inside the toy's fluffy tail. When the baby and the PowerBoy toy are lifted up from the incubator, the inductive link is broken. The circuitry inside the toy detects this, and switches on the battery for powering the monitoring equipment. As the baby is laying down in the incubator again, and the PowerBoy toy placed in its correct position, inductive power is again restored and used for monitoring health parameters as well as charging the battery.

The power supply design focuses on the contactless energy transfer system as well as the primary and secondary windings that generate the magnetic fields. Afterwards, the mutual inductances are calculated and the power transfer equations solved to transfer the required amount of power. The magnetic field intensities are also estimated and discussed, as well as the battery charging circuitry.

4.2 System design

4.2.1 Principle of contactless energy transfer

Contactless Energy Transfer (CET) is the process in which elec¬trical energy is transferred between two or more electrical devices through inductive coupling as opposed to energy supply through conventional "plug and socket" connectors. The main method through which energy is transferred in the system is by magnetic fields and the mutual inductance between their primary and secondary coils (Sonntag, 2008). The CET system employs primary and secondary series resonance. This increases the efficiency. Fig. 13 shows a simplified schematic diagram of the CET circuit, which consists of two coils, forming a loosely coupled transformer. The primary coil generates a magnetic field, which is partly picked up by the secondary coil. The primary circuit and secondary circuit are separated by an air gap (incubator mattress).

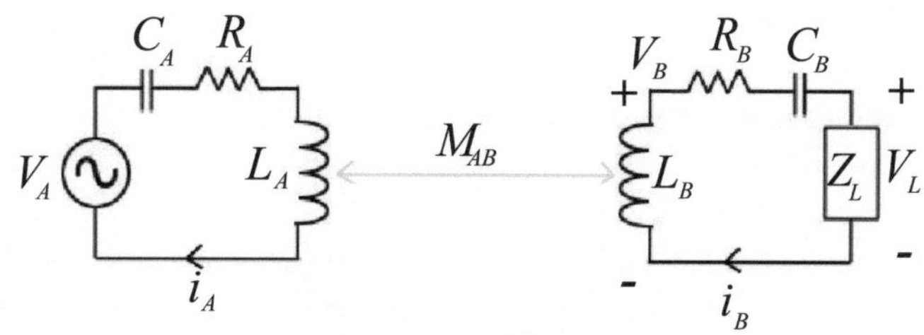

Fig. 13. Principle of inductive contactless energy transfer

In this way, power can be transferred wirelessly. Assuming steady-state sinusoidal voltages and currents, the inductive link from Fig. 13 can be described mathematically by the following formulae:

$$V_A = j\omega L_A i_A + i_A / j\omega C_A + R_A i_A - j\omega M_{AB} i_B \,, \tag{1}$$

$$j\omega M_{AB} i_A = j\omega L_B i_B + i_B / j\omega C_B + R_B i_B + Z_L i_B \,. \tag{2}$$

Here, ω is the radial frequency of the current. V_A and i_A are the primary voltage and current, respectively. The secondary current is given as i_B, and the induced secondary winding voltage is V_B. R_A and L_A, and R_B and L_B are the internal resistances and self inductances of the primary and secondary windings, S_A and S_B, respectively. The mutual inductance between the primary and secondary winding is denoted as M_{AB}. C_A and C_B are the primary and secondary resonance capacitors, respectively. Z_L represents the secondary equivalent load impedance and V_L the voltage over the load.

4.2.2 Primary and secondary windings

The primary and secondary CET windings play a vital role in determining the power transfer capability of the system. The size of the secondary winding is chosen so that it can fit into the bottom of the PowerBoy toy. A two layer hexagon spiral winding with a radius of 40 mm is used. The primary coil is a rectangular spiral winding with 120 mm length and 100 mm width. The primary and secondary windings are shown in Fig. 14 (a) and (b). Table 2 summarizes their physical dimensions and electrical properties.

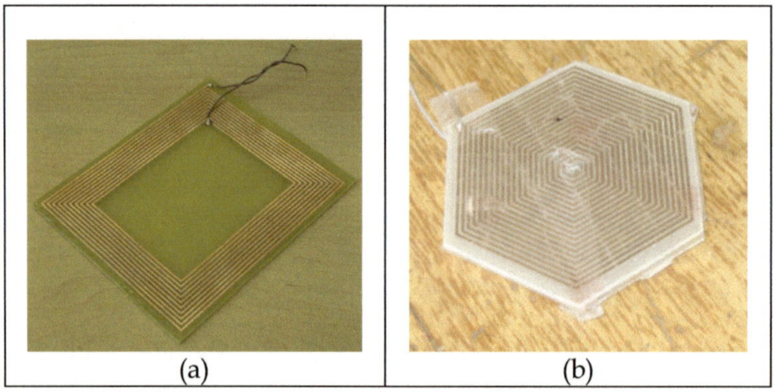

(a) (b)

Fig. 14. (a) Primary rectangular spiral winding, and (b) secondary hexagon spiral winding

4.2.3 Mutual inductance values & calculated power transfer

The mutual inductance between the primary and secondary windings, as shown in equations (1) and (2), is vital in calculating the secondary windings' induced voltage and the power transfer capability of the system. Using finite element analysis software (Maxwell 3D version 11, Ansoft Corporation) the primary and secondary windings are simulated using a three-dimensional environment. The mutual inductance between the windings is estimated using the magneto-static solution type. Fig. 15 shows a three-dimensional image of the mutual inductance results. The results show a maximum mutual inductance of 1.32 μH when the secondary winding is centred directly above the primary winding, i.e. the best-

Parameter	Primary Winding Value	Secondary Winding Value
Dimensions	100 mm x 120 mm	40 mm radius
Turns per layer	10 turns	19 turns
Layers	1	2
Thickness	100 μm	100 μm
Track width	1 mm	1 mm
Track spacing	1 mm	0.5 mm
Inductance	17.5 μH	34.56 μH
Resistance (DC)	2.48 Ω	3.34 Ω
Resistance (2.5 MHz)	3.47 Ω	8.80 Ω

Table 2. Physical dimensions & electrical properties of the primary and secondary windings

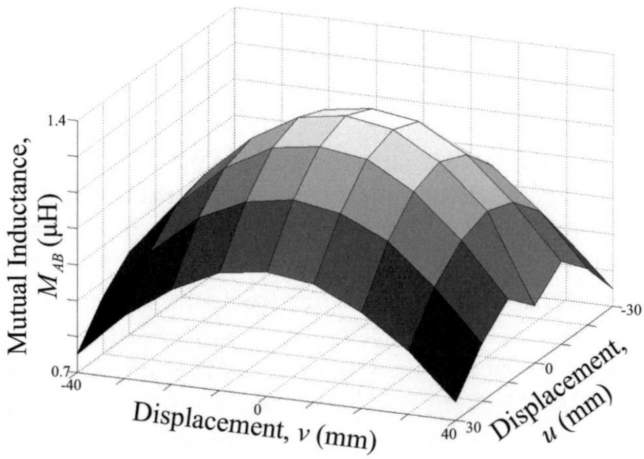

Fig. 15. A three-dimensional image of the mutual inductance results

case secondary winding and the preferred PowerBoy toy placement. The worst-case mutual inductance occurs when the secondary winding is placed close to the corners of the primary winding. At these positions, the mutual inductance is approximately 0.75 μH. This is the furthest distance the PowerBoy toy may be placed from the primary winding, to still operate normally.

The CET system should be able to power a 840 mW equivalent load impedance. This takes into account the 200 mW for the health monitoring systems, and 500 mW (100 mA @ 5 V) for charging the battery. An extra 20 % is added to compensate for any unforeseen losses. The power transfer equations are solved in equation (1) and (2) by making sure that the system can power the maximum load at the worst-case winding placement, so that it will guarantee normal operation and transfer of power for the system, at any toy position within the primary winding area. Table 3 shows the calculated primary currents, secondary currents and load voltages, for the worst-case and best-case toy placements, for three different power transfer scenarios. Firstly, for a fully charged battery, only 200 mW load power is required for the health monitoring systems. Secondly, for a partially charged battery, 450 mW is required (i.e. 200 mW health monitoring system + 250 mW for half the battery charging power). Thirdly, for a completely discharged battery, the full 700 mW is transferred. From

Table 3, it can be seen that for a certain load power, the best-case PowerBoy toy placement has a higher induced voltage than the worst-case placement.

Load power value	Best PowerBoy toy placement	Worst PowerBoy toy placement
200 mW	i_A = 1.53 A (peak) i_B = 13 mA (peak) V_L = 31.1 V (peak)	i_A = 1.53 A (peak) i_B = 23 mA (peak) V_L = 17.5 V (peak)
450 mW	i_A = 1.42 A (peak) i_B = 31 mA (peak) V_L = 29 V (peak)	i_A = 1.42 A (peak) i_B = 57 mA (peak) V_L = 16 V (peak)
700 mW	i_A = 1.29 A (peak) i_B = 54 mA (peak) V_L = 25.9V (peak)	i_A = 1.27 A (peak) i_B = 100 mA (peak) V_L = 13.8 V (peak)

Table 3. Power transfer results for different winding placements and load power

4.2.4 Magnetic field values

The magnetic fields created by the currents circulating in the primary and secondary windings are estimated using finite element analysis software (Maxwell 3D version 11, Ansoft Corporation) and solving the fields using the magneto-static solution type. According to (ICNRP, 1998), the exposure to time-varying magnetic field values at a frequency of 2.4576 MHz (the optimum operating frequency for the proposed system) is safe for general public exposure, at approximately 0.3 A/m (RMS) and less. The results from the magnetic field estimation show that the magnetic field produced by the primary winding has a maximum value of 4.2 A/m on the surface of the mattress. The magnetic field intensity reaches a value of 0.3 A/m at a radius of approximately 155 mm from the centre of the winding. The magnetic field from the secondary winding is mostly contained inside the PowerBoy toy and is negligible outside the toy. Thus, for safety reasons, it is advisable to place the baby at least 155 mm away from the centre of the primary winding.

4.2.5 Battery charging circuit

The battery charging circuit comprises of a rechargeable 2400 mAh 3.6 V NiMH battery and a battery charging circuit. The battery charging current is limited 100 mA. A fully discharged battery will thus take approximately 24 hours to charge. The battery has the ability to power the 200 mW health monitoring circuits for approximately 40 hours.

4.3 Prototype

A prototype was built to demonstrate the performance of the proposed power supply. The users of the power supply will be hospital staff (e.g. doctors, nurses and technicians) working at NICUs in hospitals, as well as parents and the neonates under monitoring. Therefore, we take the aspects of aesthetics and user friendliness into our design. The PowerBoy power supply system consists of a PowerBoy toy, a PowerBoy house and a soft sheet as shown in Fig. 16. In this subsection, the details of the electronics in the prototype are presented.

The prototype is implemented modularly, and contains eight major sub-systems as shown in the block diagram in Fig. 17. Here the black arrows indicate the flow of power, while the grey arrows show magnetic fields.

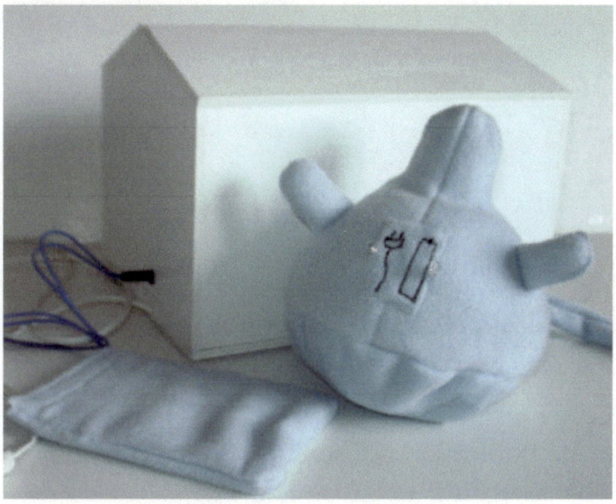

Fig. 16. The PowerBoy system, consisting of a toy, a house and a soft sheet

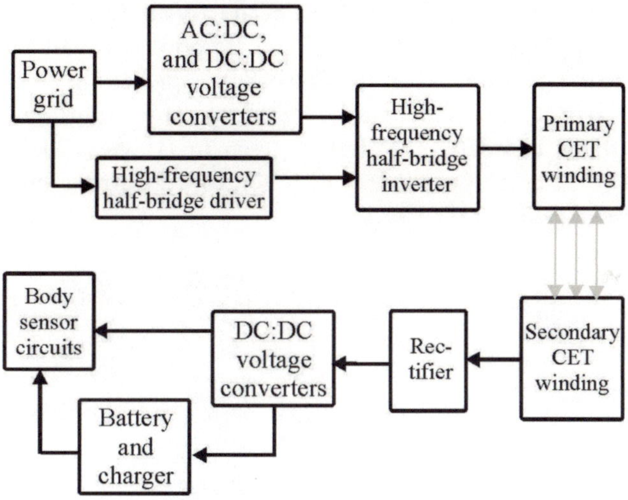

Fig. 17. Block diagram of CET power supply

Firstly, integrated into the PowerBoy house, is the circuitry used to generate the required voltages and signals used in the contactless energy transfer system. This includes three AC-to-DC power converters, for converting the 230 V, 50 Hz mains voltage into +9V, -9V and 24V (DC), respectively. Additionally, it contains a DC-to-DC converter which generated a 3.3 V (DC), a 2.4576 MHz oscillator (XO53B-2.4576M) a half-bridge inverter (using two IRF510 N-channel MOSFETS) and a high-frequency MOSFET driver, based on the designs in (Sonntag, 2008). This house encloses the PCBs of the drive circuit and the power supply box. Fig. 18 gives a top view of the drive circuits in the PowerBoy housing. In this manner the system can become portable.

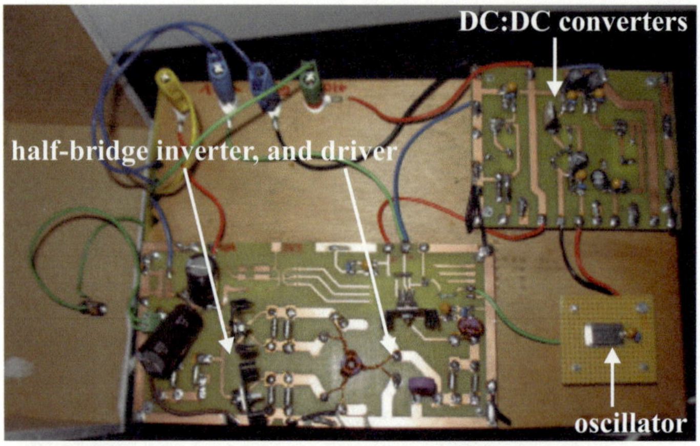

Fig. 18. Top view of the drive circuit in the PowerBoy house

Secondly, is the PowerBoy toy as shown in Fig. 19 (a): Integrated into the toy is the secondary winding (on the bottom). Additionally, it contains the rectifier circuit, a voltage converter and the battery charging circuits. The PowerBoy is designed to be a friendly companion for the neonates and is made from soft materials which are stitched together, to make a spherical-shaped toy. A process of participatory de-sign was followed for the formgiving and material choosing. On the chest of the toy are two LEDs which indi-cate the status of the power supply and the battery. When CET power is available, the left LED next to the power-plug icon lights up. When the PowerBoy is picked up and the battery is used, the right side LED next to the battery icon lights up. The battery charg-ing circuitry as shown in Fig. 19 (b) is based on the design given in (Hayles, 2008) and consists of a programmed PIC17C711 microprocessor and a controlled current source using a LM317 voltage regulator and a BC548 transistor.

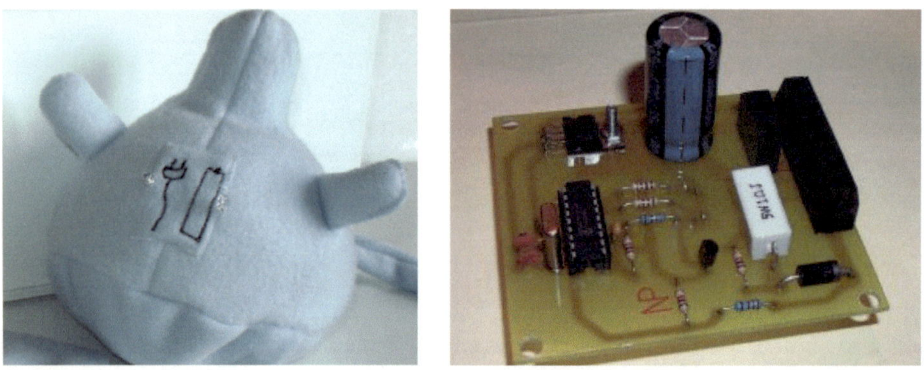

(a) (b)

Fig. 19. (a) PowerBoy toy and (b) battery charging circuit

Thirdly, the primary winding is integrated into a soft material pocket called the soft sheet. This sheet softens the hard edges of the PCB containing the primary winding. It does not come in to contact with the baby but it feels and looks friendlier when inter-acting with it. This sheet is positioned underneath the mattress.

Instead of an additional technical device in the incubator, PowerBoy is an attractive alternative with its baby-friendly appearance. Parents will appreciate this design, and may experience some relief of tension.

4.4 Experimental results

To verify the power transfer calculations and results, several power transfer experiments are preformed. Fig. 20 draws the implemented circuits for the prototype and experiments. Here, T_1 and T_2 are the two MOSFETS used in the half-bridge inverter, and V_{AA} is its input voltage. The final output voltage- and current to the neonatal health monitoring system is V_O and I_O, respectively.

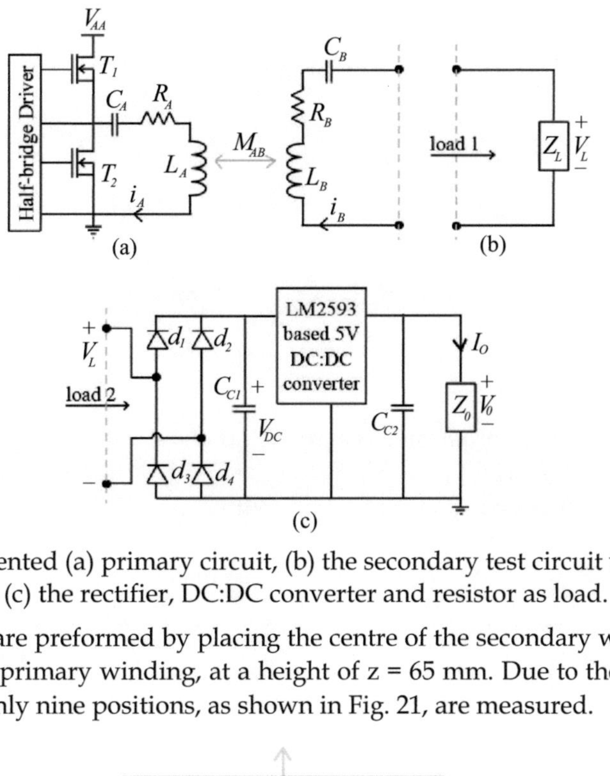

Fig. 20. The implemented (a) primary circuit, (b) the secondary test circuit with only a resistor as load, and (c) the rectifier, DC:DC converter and resistor as load.

The measurements are preformed by placing the centre of the secondary winding at discrete positions above the primary winding, at a height of z = 65 mm. Due to the symmetry in the primary winding, only nine positions, as shown in Fig. 21, are measured.

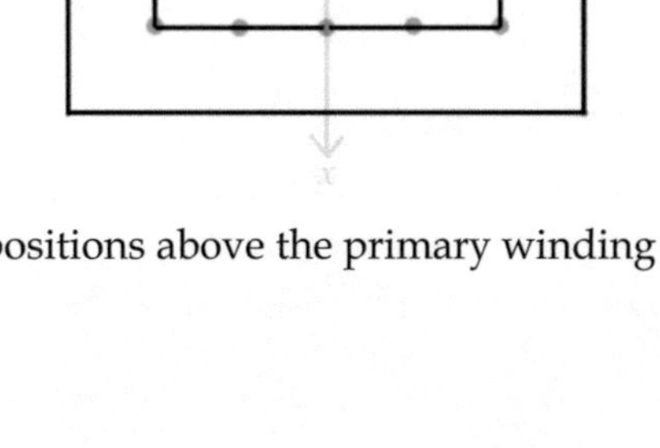

Fig. 21. The measurement positions above the primary winding

Firstly, the system is implemented with the primary circuit (a) and secondary circuit (b) as shown in Fig. 20. The peak secondary load voltage, V_L, is measured for a no-load situation ($Z_L \to \infty$). The primary current of 1.28 A (peak) is achieved by driving the half-bridge inverted with a voltage of, V_{AA} = 23.5 V. Fig. 22 illustrates a graph with a clear peak at the centre. This confirms the mutual inductance maximum at this point. The maximum secondary induced voltage is 26.5 V (peak) and the minimum is 13.78 V (peak).

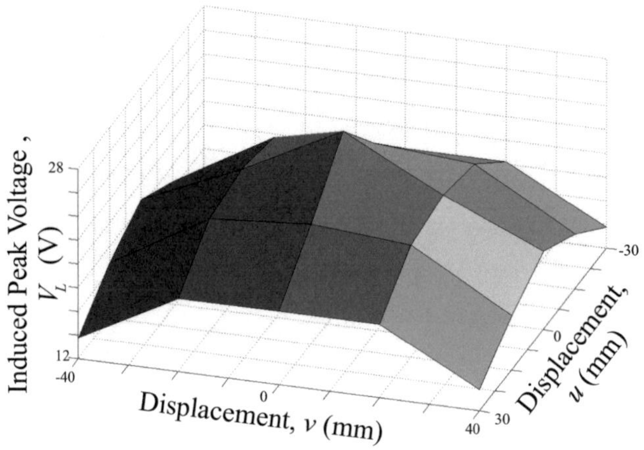

Fig. 22. The peak induced voltage

Secondly, the primary current, secondary current, and load voltage is measured using a load resistance of Z_L = 85.8 Ω. This corresponds to an 840 mW power transfer at the worst-case secondary winding placement (P_{33} on Fig. 21). With V_{AA} = 23.5 V, the results are shown in Table 4. From Table 4, we can see that at the worst-case secondary winding placement, the system is capable of transferring the needed 840 mW at approximately 12 V (peak).

Secondary winding position	**Primary winding current i_A (peak)**	**Secondary winding current i_B (peak)**	**Load voltage V_L (peak)**	**Load power P_L**
P_{11}	1.08 A	185 mA	16.55 V	1.53 W
P_{12}	1.08 A	184 mA	16.0 V	1.47 W
P_{13}	1.25 A	156 mA	13.7 V	1.07 W
P_{21}	1.10 A	185 mA	16.0 V	1.48 W
P_{22}	1.15 A	177 mA	15.5 V	1.37 W
P_{23}	1.25 A	176 mA	13.5 V	1.19 W
P_{31}	1.22 A	180 mA	14.0 V	1.26 W
P_{32}	1.22 A	180 mA	13.5 V	1.22 W
P_{33}	1.16 A	150 mA	11.7 V	878 mW

Table 4. Experimental results of 840 mW power transfer

Thirdly, experiments are conducted with the implementation of the secondary circuit (c) as shown in Fig. 20. Simulating a fully charged battery (a battery charger is not drawing any current), a load power of 200 mW is required. With an expected load voltage, V_O = 5 V (DC), an equivalent load resistance of 125 Ω (126 Ω implemented) is used. The expected load current is I_O = 39.7 mA. With V_{AA} = 23.5 V, the primary and secondary winding currents, the rectifier voltage, V_{DC}, and the load voltage V_O, are measured. Table 5 shows that the load voltage of 5 V, and consequently 200 mW load power, was maintained at all the measuring positions.

Secondary winding position	**Primary winding current i_A (peak)**	**Secondary winding current i_B (peak)**	**Rectifier Voltage V_{DC} (DC)**	**Load Voltage V_O (DC)**
P_{11}	1.30 A	48 mA	17.6 V	5 V
P_{12}	1.32 A	48 mA	16.7 V	5 V
P_{13}	1.26 A	55 mA	12.5 V	5 V
P_{21}	1.28 A	50 mA	16 V	5 V
P_{22}	1.26 A	50 mA	15 V	5 V
P_{23}	1.28 A	58 mA	11.7 V	5 V
P_{31}	1.28 A	52 mA	13.3 V	5 V
P_{32}	1.28 A	50 mA	12.5 V	5V
P_{33}	1.30 A	59 mA	9.6 V	5 V

Table 5. Experimental results of power transfer under the condition of fully charged battery

Fourthly, simulating a completely drained battery, a load power of 700 mW is required (200 mW for the health monitoring circuits and 500 mW for the battery charging). The equivalent load resistor of 35.7 Ω (36.1 Ω implemented) is used. The expected load current is I_O = 139 mA). With V_{AA} = 23.5 V, the primary and secondary winding currents, the rectifier voltage, V_{DC}, and the load voltage V_O, are measured. Table 6 shows the results.

Secondary winding position	**Primary winding current i_A (peak)**	**Secondary winding current i_B (peak)**	**Rectifier Voltage V_{DC} (DC)**	**Load Voltage V_O (DC)**
P_{11}	1.10 A	158 mA	14 V	5 V
P_{12}	1.13 A	160 mA	13.5 V	5 V
P_{13}	1.17 A	184 mA	9.9 V	5 V
P_{21}	1.14 A	170 mA	12.2 V	5 V
P_{22}	1.14 A	170 mA	12.2 V	5 V
P_{23}	1.18 A	194 mA	8.8 V	5 V
P_{31}	1.17 A	182 mA	10.4 V	5 V
P_{32}	1.18 A	190 mA	10 V	5 V
P_{33}	1.18 A	200 mA	6.7 V	5 V

Table 6. Experimental Results Of Power Transfer under the condition of completely drained battery

These results show that the load voltage of 5 V, and consequently 700 mW load power, was maintained at all the measuring positions. The system is thus capable of charging a completely discharged battery, while providing 200 mW of power to the neonatal health monitoring circuit, and still maintaining a 5 V (DC) output voltage.

4.5 Discussion

The proposed power supply satisfies the requirements of neonatal monitoring and provides continuous power when the neonate is inside the incubator or during Kangaroo mother care. The PowerBoy prototype was designed and implemented to demonstrate the performance of the power supply and the possibilities for aesthetic features. Experimental results showed that the prototype transfers approximately 840 mW of power. To evaluate the PowerBoy concept with user feedback, we had meetings with the group leader of the NICU at MMC, Prof. dr. Sidarto Bambang Oetomo and the head of the NICU nurses, Astrid Osagiator. They were enthusiastic about the concept and prototype. Further improvements and clinical verification will be conducted at MMC to integrate the power supply into the non-invasive neonatal monitoring systems.

New development of CET has the potential to enable automatic location detection and power switching, consequently, automatic power management with less magnetic fields can be foreseen for neonatal monitoring when the baby is at different locations inside the incubator.

Due to the amount of energy consumption of current sensor technologies, it is not yet feasible to harvest enough power from the NICU environment. Further development on sensors and components with low power consumption could bring opportunities for energy harvesting technologies to support neonatal monitoring.

5. Conclusion

In this chapter we presented the design of a smart jacket and the design of a power supply for neonatal monitoring with wearable sensors. These are examples of what can be done now, in the first decade of the new millennium. In this section we put these examples in a larger perspective, from both a technological and a societal viewpoint.

The technology demonstrated in this chapter shows how it is possible to improve the comfort and quality of life for the child by elimination of the adhesive electrodes and by the elimination of wires. In fact, the elimination of wires goes in steps, the first of which is the decision to transfer signals via radio rather than by wired transmission. In order to make this happen, the amplifiers and filters must move from the remote monitoring area into the body area which introduces the need for energy to power the amplifiers, filters and radio transmitters. This, in turn, introduces the need for local energy, either through new wires, batteries or by wireless energy transmission. Therefore the second step is to eliminate this local energy problem, which is precisely what the PowerBoy system does. Bringing the amplifiers and the filters closer to the body will give an additional advantage, which is not fully exploited yet in the current version of the smart jacket. The advantage will be that all the electric interference picked up by the traditional long leads is strongly reduced. Still, precautions will be needed to prevent the newly introduced power-supply and radio-transmission carriers from inducing new artifacts, notably in the pre-amplifier stages. For the time being, some care is thus needed with pulse and amplitude based modulation techniques. On the long term, ultra-low power transmission techniques will take care of this potential problem. Another concern is the question whether the newly introduced high-frequency fields could be harmful for the child. It is advisable to stay on the safe side, which is why the PowerBoy is a separate toy and the child is outside of the field. This is a good solution now. In ten years from now, low power radio and low power photoplethysmography (PPG) sensors could well be available, allowing for full integration of all electronics into the jacket itself. The introduction of textile electrodes is another technological step, which has introduced a new problem. The problem is the signal quality, since the signal is weaker and more sensitive to movement artifacts. An alternative technology would be capacitive electrodes, but these have similar problems. Of course proper placement of the electrodes helps, as shown in the smart jacket design for neonatal monitoring. Multi-modal signal processing will be the way ahead. For example, combining movement sensors, ECG sensors and PPG sensors gives extra information which can be used to automatically distinguish artifacts from genuine heart rate abnormalities.

Taking a societal viewpoint, the smart jacket and power system fit into the ambient intelligence approach. The sensors could become invisible and important monitoring tasks taken over by computers which could become invisible as well. In general, the societal debate about ambient intelligence in health care has hardly begun. In the Netherlands, the report issued by the Rathenau Institute (Schuurman et al., 2007) is one of the examples of the beginning debate. A European perspective can be found in the paper by Duquenoy and Whitehouse (Duquenoy & Whitehouse, 2006) who explain ambient intelligence as combining developments in information and communication technologies with notions of 'pervasive' and 'ubiquitous' computing, and describing an intelligent environment operating in the background in an invisible and non-intrusive way. Several communities have different views, but doubtlessly problems such as information overload and conflict of governmental and/or commercial interests with private interests will arise. For prematurely born infants, monitoring of vital functions while raising the comfort level is a medical necessity. Gradually it will become possible, however, to transfer the solutions developed for critically ill children towards the larger potential buyer groups (parents of the healthy newborns). These solutions could become modern versions of the old FM audio baby monitors and the present-day baby cams. But is it necessary that parents are reading more and more bodily parameters of their child? Is it wise to collect such data in computers with the possibility that more and more parties get hold of the data? These are not technological questions, but topics for political, social, organizational, economic, legal, regulatory, and ethical debate.

6. References

Aarts, E. H. L. & Encarnação, J. L. (Eds.). (2006). *True Visions the Emergence of Ambient Intelligence,* Springer-Verlag, Berlin, Heidelberg.

Als, H.; Lawhon, G.; Brown, E.; Gibes, R.; Duffy, H.; Mcanulty, G. B. & Blickman, J. G. (1986). Individualized behavioral and environmental care for the very low birth weight preterm infant at high risk for bronchopulmonary dysplasia: Neonatal intensive care unit and developmental outcome. *Pediatrics*, Vol. 78, No. 6, 1986, pp. 1123-1132.

Als, H; Gilkerson, L.; Duffy, F. H.; Mcanulty, G. B.; Buehler, D. M.; Vandenberg, K.; Sweet N.; Sell, E.; Parad, R. B.; Ringer, S. A.; Butler, S. C.; Blickman, J. G. & Jones, K. J. (2003). A three-center, randomized, controlled trial of individualized developmental care for very low birth weight preterm infants: medical, neurodevelopmental, parenting and caregiving Effects. *Journal of Developmental and Behavioral Pediatrics,* Vol. 24, 2003, pp. 399-408.

Anand, K. J. S. & Scalzo, F. M. (2000). Can adverse neonatal experiences alter brain development and subsequent behaviour?. *Biology of the Neonate,* Vol. 77, No. 2, Feb. 2000, pp. 69-82.

Bouwstra, S.; Chen, W.; Feijs, L. M. G. & Bambang Oetomo, S. (2009). Smart jacket design for neonatal monitoring with wearable sensors, *Proceedings of Body Sensor Networks (BSN 2009)*, pp. 162 – 167, Berkeley, USA, June 2009.

Catrysse, M.; Hermans B. & Puers, R. (2004). An inductive power system with integrated bi-directional data-transmission. *Sensors and Actuators A: Physical,* Vol. 115, No. 2-3, 21 September 2004, pp. 221-229.

Chapieski, M. L. & Evankovitch, K. D. (1997). Behavioral effects of prematurity. *Semin. Perinatol.,* Vol. 21, 1997, pp. 221-239.

Chen, W.; Sonntag, C. L. W.; Boesten, F.; Bambang Oetomo, S. & Feijs, L. M. G. (2008). A power supply design of body sensor networks for health monitoring of neonates, *Proceedings of the Fourth International Conference on Intelligent Sensors, Sensor Networks and Information Processing (ISSNIP 2008)*, pp.255-260, Sydney, Australia, Dec. 2008.

Chen, W.; Nguyen S. T.; Coops, R.; Bambang Oetomo, S. & Feijs, L. M. G. (2009a). Wireless transmission design for health monitoring at neonatal intensive care units, *submitted to the 2nd international symposium on applied sciences in biomedical and communication technologies (ISABEL 2009),* Bratislava, Slovak Republic, Nov. 2009.

Chen, W.; Sonntag, C. L. W.; Boesten, F.; Bambang Oetomo, S. & Feijs, L. M. G. (2009b). A design of power supply for neonatal monitoring with wearable sensors. *Journal of Ambient Intelligence and Smart Environments-Special Issue on Wearable Sensors,* Vol.1, No. 2, 2009, pp. 185 – 196, IOS press.

Chen, W.; Ayoola, I. B. I.; Bambang Oetomo, S. & Feijs, L. M. G. (2010a). Non-invasive blood oxygen saturation monitoring for neonates using reflectance pulse oximeter, *submitted to Design, Automation and Test in Europe - Conference and Exhibition 2010 (DATE 2010),* Dresden, Germany, March 2010.

Chen, W.; Bambang Oetomo, S. & Feijs, L. M. G. (2010b). Neonatal monitoring – current practice and future trends. *Handbook of Research on Developments in e-Health and Telemedicine: Technological and Social Perspectives,* IGI Global, to be published in 2010.

Chen, W.; Dols, S.; Bambang Oetomo, S. & Feijs, L. M. G. (2010c). Monitoring body temperature of a newborn baby", *to be submitted to the Eighth Annual IEEE International Conference on Pervasive Computing and Communications (PerCom 2010),* Mannheim, Germany, March 2010.

Costeloe, K.; Hennessy, E.; Gibson, A. T.; Marlow, N. & Wilkinson, A. R. (2000). The EPICure study: Outcome to discharge from hospital for infants born at the threshold of viability. *Pediatrics*, Vol. 106, No. 4, 2000, pp. 659-671.

de Kleine, M. J.; den Ouden, A. L.; Kollée, L. A.; Ilsen, A.; van Wassenaer, A. G.; Brand R. & Verloove -Vanhorick, S.P. (2007). Lower mortality but higher neonatal morbidity over a decade in very preterm infants. *Paediatr Perinat Epidemiol*, Vol. 21, No. 1, 2007, pp. 15-25.

Duquenoy, P. & Whitehouse, D. (2006). A 21st century ethical debate: pursuing perspectives on ambient intelligence. IFIP International Federation for Information Processing, the Information Society: Emerging Landscapes, Vol. 195, 2006, pp 293-314, Springer Boston.

Goldsmith, A. (2005). *Wireless Communications*, Cambridge University Press.

Hack, M. & Fanaroff, A. A. (1999). Outcomes of children of extremely low birth weight and gestational age in the 1990's. *Early Hum Dev.*, Vol. 53, 1999, pp. 193-218.

Hayles, P. (2008). Intelligent NiCd battery charger. [Online], Retrieved 2008. Available: http://www.angelfire.com/electronic/hayles/charge1.html.

International Commission on Non-Ionizing Radiation Protection (ICNRP) (1998). Guidelines for limiting exposure to time-varying electric, magnetic, and electromagnetic fields (up to 300 GHz). *Health Physics Society*, Vol. 74, No. 4, pp. 494-522, April 1998.

Ma, G.; Yan, G. & He, X. (2007). Power transmission for gastrointestinal microsystems using inductive coupling. *Physiol. Meas.*, Vol. 28, 2007, pp. N9–N18.

Marlow, N.; Hennessy, E. M.; Bracewell, M. A. & Wolke, D. (2007). Motor and executive function at 6 years of age after extremely preterm birth. *Pediatrics*, Vol. 120, No. 4, 2007, pp. 793-804.

Murković, I.; Steinberg, M. D. & Murković, B. (2003). Sensors in neonatal monitoring: Current practice and future trends. *Technology and Health Care*, Vol. 11, IOS Press, 2003, pp. 399–412.

Paradiso, J. A. & Starner, T. (2005). Energy scavenging for mobile and wireless electronics. *IEEE Pervasive Comput.*, Vol. 4, No. 1, 2005, pp. 18–27.

Perlman, J. M. (2001). Neurobehavioral deficits in premature graduates of intensive care - Potential medical and environmental risks factors. *Pediatrics*, Vol. 108, No. 6, 2001, pp. 1339-1348.

Perlman, J. M. (2003). The genesis of cognitive and behavioural deficits in premature graduates of intensive care. *Minerva Pediatr.*, Vol. 55, 2003, pp. 89-101.

Polin, R. A. & Fox, W. W. (Eds.). (1992). *Fetal and Neonatal Physiology*, W. B. Saunders Company.

Qin, Y.; Wang, X. & Wang, Z. L. (2008). Microfibre–nanowire hybrid structure for energy scavenging. *Nature*, Vol. 451, 14 Feb. 2008, pp. 809 - 813.

Schuurman, J.; El-Hadidy, F.; Krom, A. & Walhout B. (2007). Ambient Intelligence. Toekomst van de zorg of zorg van de toekomst? Rathenau Instituut, Den Haag:

Sonntag, C. L. W.; Lomonova, E. A. & Duarte, J. L. (2008). Power transfer stabilization of the three-phase contactless energy transfer desktop by means of coil commutation, *Proceedings of the 4th IEEE Young Researchers Symposium in Electrical Engineering (YRS 2008)*, pp. 1-6, Eindhoven, the Netherlands, February 2008.

Tao, X. M. (Ed.). (2005). *Wearable Electronics and Photonics,* CRC press, Woodhead Publishing Ltd., England.

Van Langenhove, L. (Ed.). (2007). *Smart Textiles for Medicine and Healthcare: Materials, Systems and Applications,* CRC press, Woodhead Publishing Ltd., England.

Yang, G. Z. (Ed.). (2006). *Body Sensor Networks,* Springer-Verlag London Limited.

2

Signal Processing and Classification Approaches for Brain-computer Interface

Tarik Al-ani[1,2] and Dalila Trad[1,3]
[1]*LISV-UVSQ, 10-12 Av de l'Europe, 78140 Velizy*
[2]*Department of Informatics, ESIEE-Paris, Cité Descartes-BP 99 93162 Noisy-Le-Grand*
[3]*UTIC-ESSTT, University of TUNIS 5, avenue Taha Hussein, B.P. 56 Bab Menara 1008- Tunis*
[1,2]*France*
[3]*Tunisia*

1. Introduction

Research on *brain-computer interface* (*BCI*) systems began in the 1970s at the University of California Los Angeles (UCLA) (Vidal, 1973; 1977). The author gave in his papers the expression "Brain Computer Interface" which is the term currently used in literature.

A *BCI* system is a direct communication pathway between a brain and an external artificial device. *BCI* systems were aimed at assisting, augmenting or repairing *human cognitive* or *sensory-motor functions*.

The *BCI* systems (*BCIs*) allow control of an artificial device based on the features extracted from voluntary electric, magnetic, or other physical manifestations of brain activity collected from epi- or subdurally from the cortex or from the scalp or in invasive electrophysiological manner, i.e. brain signals recorded intracortically with single electrode or multi-electrode arrays (Dornhege et al., 2007). There is a variety of non-invasive techniques for measuring brain activity. These non-invasive techniques include, the *electroencephalography* (*EEG*), *magnetoencephalography* (*MEG*), *positron emission tomography* (*PET*), *functional magnetic resonance imaging* (*fMRI*), and *optical imaging*. However, for technical, time resolution, real-time, and price constraints, only *EEG* monitoring and related techniques are employed in the *BCI* community. For more details refer to (Wolpaw et al., 2002; Mason et al., 2007; Dobkin, 2007). The neuronal electrical activity contain a broad band frequency, so the monitored brain signals are filtered and denoised to extract the relevant information (see section 3) and finally this information is decoded (see section 6) and commuted into device commands by *synchronous control* or more efficiently by *self-paced* or *asynchronous control* in order to detect whether a user is intending something or not (see chapter 7 in (Dornhege et al., 2007) for details), Fig. 1. For some specific *BCI* tasks, raw brain signal serves as stimulus as well as a control interface feedback.

The direct *BCIs* can be seen as a new means of communication that may be used to allow tetraplegic or individuals with severe motor or neuromuscular diseases (e.g. Amyotrophic lateral sclerosis (*ALS*), brainstem stroke, brain or spinal cord injury, cerebral palsy, muscular

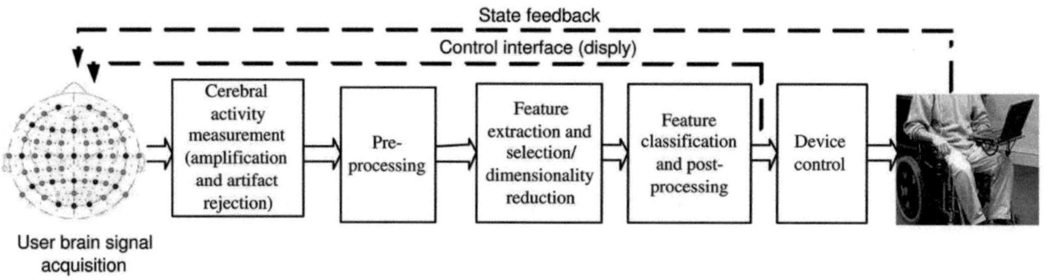

Fig. 1. Basic *BCI* layout.

dystrophies, multiple sclerosis) to have effective control over artificial devices or external environment in order to increase or improve their communication qualities or their independence. Recent studies have demonstrated correlations between *EEG* signals and actual or imagined movements and between *EEG* signals and mental tasks (Keirn & Aunon, 1990; Lang et al., 1996; Pfurtscheller et al., 1997; Anderson et al., 1998; Altenmüller & Gerloff, 1999; McFarland et al., 2000; Wessberg et al., 2000; Pfurtscheller et al., 2000b; Nicolelis, 2001; Pfurtscheller et al., 2003). The *BCIs* can be used also in therapeutic applications by neurofeedback for rehabilitation or functional recovery (Birbaumer & Cohen, 2007; Dobkin, 2007; Birbaumer et al., 1999; Dornhege et al., 2007).

The *BCI* is a communication system that does not require any peripheral muscular activity. It has been shown by (Pfurtscheller & Aranibar, 1977; Pfurtscheller, 1999c; Neuper & Pfurtscheller, 1999a) that the imagination of either a left or right hand movement results in an amplitude attenuation (*event-related desynchronization* (*ERD*) of μ (8-13Hz) and central β (13-30Hz) rhythms at the contra-lateral sensori-motor representation area and, in an amplitude increase (*event-related synchronization* (*ERS*) within the γ band (30-40Hz) at the ipsi-lateral hemishpere. The event related (de)synchronisation(*ERD*, *ERS*) (Pfurtscheller et al., 1999a), see Fig. 2 and Fig. 3.

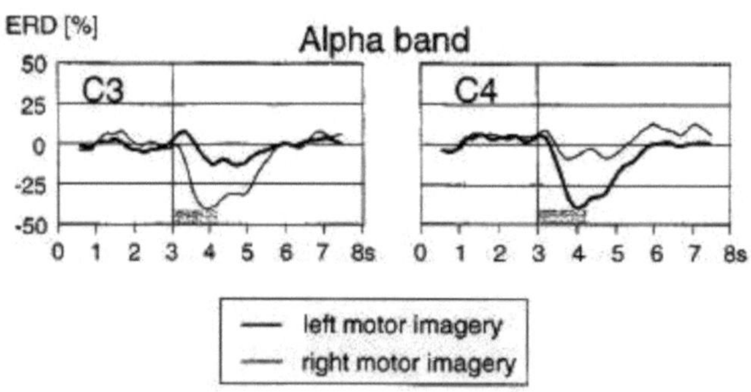

Fig. 2. Grand average *ERD* curves recorded during motor imagery from the left (C3) and right sensorimotor cortex (C4) (the electrodes C3 and C4 are placed according to the International 10-20 system). The ERD time courses were calculated for the selected bands in the alpha range for 16 subjects. Positive and negative deflections, with respect to baseline (second 0.5 to 2.5), represent a band power increase (*ERD*) and decrease (*ERD*), respectively. The gray bar indicates the time period of cue presentation (i.e. the imagination starts at second 3). Figure from (Pfurtscheller et al., 2000a) which is modified from (Neuper & Pfurtscheller, 1999a).

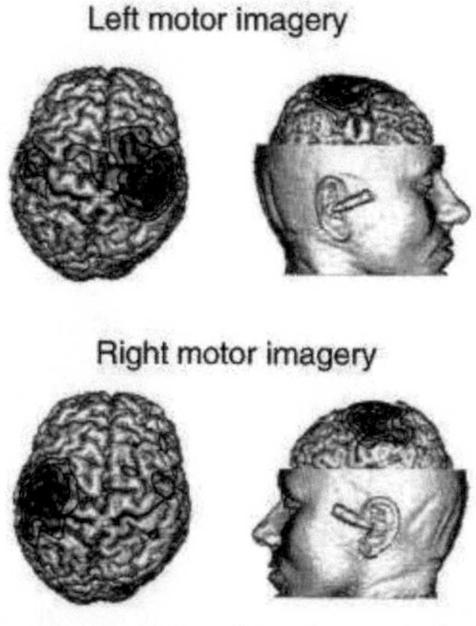

Fig. 3. ERD maps for a single subject calculated for the cortical surface of a realistic head model. Figure from (Pfurtscheller et al., 2000a) which is modified from (Neuper & Pfurtscheller, 1999a).

The direct *BCIs* can also be seen as a new means to extend communication for healthy subjects in many fields such as multimedia communication, control of robots, virtual reality and video games (Thomas, 1977; Friedman et al., 2004; Bell et al., 2008; Lécuyer et al., 2008). There are in general two types of *BCI* systems: *endogenous tasks* and *exogenous tasks* based systems (Dornhege et al., 2007).

The *endogenous tasks BCI* systems, which are based on spontaneous activity, use brain signals that do not depend on external stimuli and that can be influenced by concentrating on a specific mental task. In order to obtain an efficient task recognition system, several concentration trials of human are, in general, realized. The concentration constraint is a very tiring mental task especially for disabled subjects who might have difficulties in acquiring voluntary control over their brain activity and it must be reduced in order to obtain an efficient task recognition system.

The *exogenous tasks BCI* systems, which are based on evoked activity, use brain signals that do depend on external stimuli. Particularly interesting are systems based either on the *P300* or on *SSVEPs* (see section 2). Advantages of these potentials are that they are relatively well understood from a neurophysiologic point of view and that they can be evoked robustly across different subjects. Moreover, feedback training is not necessary in these systems, as theses potentials appear "automatically" whenever subjects concentrate onto one out of several stimuli presented in random order (Hoffman et al., 2008). Note that the material presented in this chapter is strongly biased towards *sensorimotor* (Changes in brain rhythms (μ, β, and γ)) and *P300* electrophysiological activities using *EEG* records.

In order to improve the performance of the *BCI* system design, it is necessary to use a good method of *signal processing* to allow easier extraction of physiological characteristics and also to use a good *classifier* adapted to the specificities of the *BCI* system. This chapter presents a compact guide to different *signal processing* techniques that have received more attention in *BCIs*. We introduce then some selected feature extraction and *classification* approaches in the context of *BCI* systems. A more exhaustive and excellent surveys on *signal processing* and *classification* algorithms may be found in the papers (Bashashati et al., 2007; Lotte et al., 2007). Then this chapter describes the application of two *classification* approaches, *hidden Markov models* (HMMs) and *support vector machines* (*SVM*), in the context of *exogenous tasks BCI* systems based on *P300 evoked potential*. The chapter ends with a global conclusions and perspectives.

The methods presented in sections 3.3, 4, 5 and 6 are based on the statistical results given in the comprehensive survey of 96 *BCI* designs using electrical signal recordings published prior to January 2006 by (Bashashati et al., 2007). Among these methods, we give here only a brief descriptions of the most applied methods. They are introduced here without referencing all the published papers for the 96 *BCI* designs. The reader may refer to the paper (Bashashati et al., 2007) to find a rich bibliographical work. However, we give only the original references corresponding to each proposed method.

2. Electrophysiological control activities in *BCIs*

Current *BCI* systems fall into seven main categories, based on the neuromechanisms and recording technology they use to generate control signals (Bashashati et al., 2007). The following list give a short descriptions of these electrophysiological activities used in *BCI* designs. This list is borrowed and adapted (with the authorization of authors) from the paper (Bashashati et al., 2007). We omitted the references of the different approaches given in this list. Many of these references are given in (Bashashati et al., 2007).

- ***Sensorimotor activity*** *BCI* designs that use sensorimotor activity as the neural source of control can be divided into three sub-categories:
  - ***Changes in brain rhythms*** (μ, β, *and* γ)

    μ rhythms in the range of 8-12 Hz and β rhythms in the range of 13-30 Hz both originate in the sensorimotor cortex and are displayed when a person is not engaged in processing sensorimotor inputs or in producing motor outputs. They are mostly prominent in frontal and parietal locations. A voluntary movement results in a circumscribed desynchronization in the μ and lower β bands. This desynchronization is called *event-related desynchronization* (*ERD*) (Pfurtscheller & Aranibar, 1977; Pfurtscheller, 1999c; Neuper & Pfurtscheller, 1999a) and begins in the contralateral rolandic region about 2 s prior to the onset of a movement and becomes bilaterally symmetrical immediately before execution of movement. After a voluntary movement, the power in the brain rhythms increases. This phenomenon, called *event-related synchronization* (*ERS*), is dominant over the contralateral sensorimotor area and reaches a maximum around 600 ms after movement offset. γ rhythm is a high-frequency rhythm in the *EEG*. Upon the occurrence of a movement, the amplitude of γ rhythm in the range of 30-40 Hz increases. Gamma γ are usually more prominent in the primary sensory area.
  - ***Movement-related potentials (MRPs)***

    MRPs are low-frequency potentials that start about 1-1.5 s before a movement. They have bilateral distribution and present maximum amplitude at the vertex. Close to the movement, they become contralaterally preponderant.
  - ***Other sensorimotor activities***

    The sensorimotor activities that do not belong to any of the preceding categories are categorized as other sensorimotor activities. These activities are usually not restricted to a particular frequency band or scalp location and usually cover different frequency ranges. An example would be features extracted from an *EEG* signal filtered to frequencies below 30 Hz. Such a range covers different *eventrelated potentials* (*ERPs*) but no specific neuromechanism is used.

- ***Slow cortical potentials (SCPs)***
  Slow cortical potentials (*SCPs*) are slow voltage shifts in the *EEG* occurring in the frequency range 1-2 Hz. Negative SCPs correspond to a general decrease in cortical excitability. Positive *SCPs* correspond to a general increase in cortical excitability. Through feedback training subjects can learn to voluntarily control their *SCPs* (Birbaumer et al., 1999; 2000; Hinterberger et al., 2003; 2004; Bostanov, 2004).
- ***P300 Evoked potential***
  Infrequent or particularly significant auditory, visual, or somatosensory stimuli, when interspersed with frequent or routine stimuli, typically evoke in the *EEG* over the parietal cortex a positive peak at about 300 ms after the stimulus is received. This peak is called *P300*.
- ***Visual evoked potentials (VEPs)***
  VEPs are small changes in the ongoing brain signal. They are generated in response to a visual stimulus such as flashing lights and their properties depend on the type of the visual stimulus. These potentials are more prominent in the occipital area. If a visual stimulus is presented repetitively at a rate of 5-6 Hz or greater, a continuous oscillatory electrical response is elicited in the visual pathways. Such a response is termed steady-state visual evoked potentials (*SSVEP*). The distinction between *VEP* and *SSVEP* depends on the repetition rate of the stimulation.
- ***Response to mental tasks***
  BCI systems based on non-movement mental tasks assume that different mental tasks (e.g., solving a multiplication problem, imagining a 3D object, and mental counting) lead to distinct, task-specific distributions of *EEG* frequency patterns over the scalp.
- ***Activity of neural cells (ANC)***
  It has been shown that the firing rates of neurons in the motor cortex are increased when movements are executed in the preferred direction of neurons. Once the movements are away from the preferred direction of neurons, the firing rate is decreased.
- ***Multiple neuromechanisms (MNs)***
  BCI systems based on multiple neuromechanisms use a combination of two or more of the above mentioned neuromechanisms.

3. Signal pre-processing methods in *BCIs*

To extract *features* (see section 4), it is necessary to pre-process first the data. Three steps are necessary to achieve this goal: *Referencing*, *Temporal filtering* and *signal enhancement*.

3.1 Referencing

(Hagemann et al., 2001) have stated that the differences between results of different studies are partly due to the differences in referencing. In the case of *EEG* recordings from the cortex or from the scalp, these recordings are obtained using, in general, different electrodes on different positions. Since the brain activity voltage measured by a given electrode is a relative measure, the measurement may be compared to another reference brain voltage situated on another site. This results in a combination of brain activity at the given electrode, brain activity at the reference site and noise. Because of this, the reference site should be chosen such that the brain activity at that site is almost zero. Typically, the nose, mastoids and earlobes are used (Dien, 1998). In general, there are three referencing methods

- *Common reference*
  The common reference technique is widely used in *BCIs*. This method uses one common reference for all electrodes. In general, the site of this reference is situated at large distance from all electrodes. The activity at the reference site influences all measurements equally, and differences between electrode measurements still contain all information needed.
- *Average reference*
  The average reference subtracts the average of the activity at all electrodes from the measurements. This method is based on the principle that the activity at the whole head at every moment sums up to zero. Therefore, the average of all activity represents an estimate of the activity at the reference site. Subtracting this average produces in principle a dereferenced solution. However, the relatively low density of the electrodes and the fact that the lower part of the head is not taken into account, bring some practical problems along (Dien, 1998).
- *Current source density (CSD)*
  The current source density (*CSD*) is used in many *BCIs*. It is "the rate of change of current flowing into and through the scalp" (Weber, 2001). This quantity can be derived from *EEG* data, and it may be interpreted as the potential difference between an electrode and a weighted average of their surrounding electrodes. The *CSD* can be estimated by computing the *laplacian*. The *laplacian* computes the sum of the differences between an electrode and its neighbours. A problem with this estimation is that it is actually only valid when the electrodes are in a two dimensional plane and equally distant.

3.2 Temporal filtering in *BCIs*

The brain signals are naturally contaminated by many internal and external noises. They can be removed using simple filters. The relevant information in *BCIs* is found in the frequencies below 30Hz. Therefore, all noise with higher frequencies (e.g. noise from the electrical net has a fixed frequency of 50Hz or 60 Hz) can be removed using *FIR low pass filter*. Specific frequency bands may also be selected using FIR bandpass filters.

3.3 Signal enhancement methods in *BCI* designs

The choice of a suitable enhancement technique is dependent on several factors such as the recording technology, number of electrodes, and neuromechanism of the *BCI* (Bashashati et al., 2007). Among seventeen pre-processing methods given by (Bashashati et al., 2007), we describe here briefly only six methods which are the most applied in *BCI* designs:

- *Spatial filters - Referencing methods*
  The proper selection of a spatial filter for any *BCI* is determined by the location and extent of the selected brain control signal and of the various sources of *EEG* or *non-EEG* noise.
  - *Common average referencing (CAR)*
    Common-average or "reference-free" recording has been suggested as a solution to the problem of the reference electrode (Offner, 1950; lehmann & Skrandies, 1984; Stanny, 1989). Common-average referencing involves recording in bipolar fashion from a number of electrodes, all referred to a single site. One then calculates the

grand mean *EEG* waveform, by averaging across electrodes, and subtracts the result pointwise from the *EEG* recorded at each electrode. Activity recorded by the reference electrode is theoretically of equal magnitude in the mean and individualelectrode waveforms. Consequently, the effect of the reference electrode should be eliminated from each recording electrode's output when the common-average waveform is subtracted (Stanny, 1989).

- ***Surface Laplacian (SL)***
  The *SL* is defined as the 2nd order spatial derivative of the surface potential. Due to its intrinsic spatial high-pass filtering characteristics, the SL can reduce the volume conduction effect by enhancing the high-frequency spatial components, therefore can achieve higher spatial resolution than surface potentials.

- ***Principal component analysis (PCA)***
  The *PCA* (Pearson, 1901) is a linear mapping that transforms a number of possibly correlated variables into a smaller number of uncorrelated variables called principal components. The first principal component accounts for as much of the variability in the data as possible, and each succeeding component accounts for as much of the remaining variability as possible. Depending on the field of application, it is also named the discrete *Karhunen-Loève transform* (*KLT*), the *Hotelling transform* or *proper orthogonal decomposition* (*POD*). The *PCA* reveals the internal structure of the data in a way which best explains the variance in the data. If a multivariate dataset is visualised as a set of coordinates in a high-dimensional data space (1 axis per variable), *ICA* supplies the user with a lower-dimensional representation.
- ***Independent component analysis (ICA)***
  The more important *artefacts* in *BCIs* are generated by muscles and eyes blink (Gupta & Singh, 1996). Classical automatic methods for removing such artefacts can be classified into *rejection* methods and *subtraction* methods.
  - ***Rejection*** methods consist of discarding contaminated EEG, based on either automatic or visual detection can be used in the *BCI* applications framework. Their success crucially depends on the quality of the detection.
  - ***Subtraction*** methods are based on the assumption that the contaminated EEG is a linear combination of an original *EEG* and other independent *artefact* signals generated by the muscles and eyes blink. The original *EEG* is hence recovered by either subtracting separately recorded *artefact*-related signals from the measured *EEG*, using appropriate weights or by applying recent approaches for *artefacts rejection*: such as *independent component analysis* (*ICA*) (Common, 1994; Hyvärinen & Oja, 2000), *peak elimination* (Nakamura et al., 1996), *neural network* (Urszula et al., 1999) and *fixed bandpass FIR filter* based approach (Gupta & Singh, 1996).

  The *ICA* (Common, 1994; Hyvärinen & Oja, 2000) is the more used technique. It is a computational method for separating a multivariate signal into additive subcomponents supposing the mutual statistical independence of the non-Gaussian source signals. It is a special case of *blind source separation* (*BSS*). *ICA* is particularly efficient when the *EEG* and the *artefacts* have comparable amplitudes. For more details about their advantages, their limitations and their applications for the removal of eyes activity artefacts, refer to (Jung et al., 1998; 2000).
- ***Common spatial patterns (CSP)***
  The *CSP* (Koles, 1991; Müller-Gerking et al., 1999) is a technique used to find the common projection matrix that decomposes the different classes of single trial *EEG*

datasets, and more specifically to find spatial structures of event-related (de)synchronization (*ERD/ERS*) in a *EEG* context. Such matrix maximizes the differences between the classes. (Guger et al., 2000) demonstrated the efficiency of the *CSP* method for real-time *EEG* analysis and concluded that only parameters that must be adjusted for the *CSP* are the time segment for the calculation of the *CSP* and, during on-line processing, the time window for the calculation of the variances. But the selection of these parameters is not very crucial. An advantage of the *CSP* method is that it does not require a priori selection of subject-specific frequency bands, as necessary for bandpower or frequency estimation methods (Pfurtscheller et al., 1996; McFarland et al., 1997b).

- The CSP method is very sensitive to artefacts. A single trial containing, for example, a movement artifact can cause severe changes in the *CSP* (Müller-Gerking et al., 1999). The reason is the sample covariance (nonrobust estimate), which is used to estimate the covariance for the calculation of the spatial filters. However, during on-line operation of the *BCI*, the spatial filters perform a weighted spatial averaging of the *EEG*, and this reduces the influence of artefacts (Guger et al., 2000).
- in some applications, many electrodes are needed, (e.g. more than 18 (Ramoser et al., 2000), which necessitates costly hardware.
- since the CSP method detects spatial patterns in the EEG, any change in the electrode positions may render the improvements in the *classification* accuracy gained by this method useless. Therefore, this method requires almost identical electrode positions for all trials and sessions which may be difficult to accomplish (Ramoser et al., 2000). (Guger et al., 2000) recommended not to apply the electrodes anew after setting up a new *CSP* for the following feedback sessions. For long-term implications to analyze the *EEG* in real time, *EEG* data of several sessions can be used for the calculation of the *CSP*. This allows the generation of a more robust filter in order to overcome the mentioned problems.

- ***Common spatial subspace decomposition (CSSD)***
  The *CSSD* can extract signal components specific to one condition from multiple *MEG/EEG* data sets of multiple task conditions. Signal matrices or covariance matrices are decomposed using spatial factors common to multiple conditions. The spatial factors and corresponding spatial filters are then dissociated into specific and common parts, according to the common spatial subspace which exists among the data sets. Finally, the specific signal components are extracted using the corresponding spatial filters and spatial factors. (Wang et al., 1999).
- ***Frequency normalization (Freq-Norm)***
  (Bashashati et al., 2005).
- Other methods are given by (Bashashati et al., 2007).

The study of (Bashashati et al., 2007) showed that

- signal pre-processing algorithms have been used for *EEG*-based *BCIs* and the *ANC*-based *BCIs*, but no signal enhancement algorithms have been applied on *electrocorticogram* (*ECoG*)-based *BCIs*. Only *PCA* has been used in both groups, and
- *spatial filtering* including *referencing* (*CAR* and *SL*) methods and *CSP* are among the most used techniques that have become increasingly popular in *EEG*-based *BCIs*.

Fig.4 shows the statistical results of the study realised by (Bashashati et al., 2007) concerning *pre-processing* methods in *BCI* designs. (Bashashati et al., 2007) concluded that 96 *BCI* designs that employ signal enhancement techniques before extracting the features from the signal, 32% use surface Laplacian (*SL*), 22% use either principal component analysis (*PCA*) or independent component analysis (*ICA*), 14% use common spatial patterns (*CSP*) and 11% use common average referencing (*CAR*) techniques.

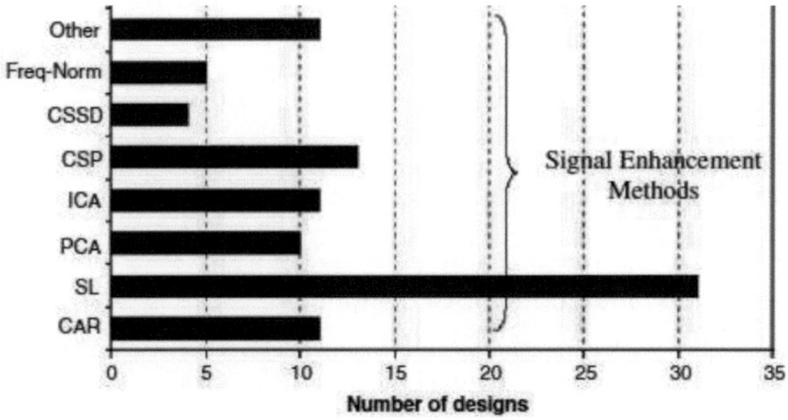

Fig. 4. Signal enhancement methods in *BCI* designs. Figure modified from (Bashashati et al., 2007) with authorisation.

In the following, we give a breif description of the two most used methods: *Spatial filters* and *Common spatial patterns*.

3.3.1 Spatial filters: (SL) and (CAR)

(McFarland et al., 1997a) showed that the variability of the *EEG* or *non-EEG* noise sources within the different *BCI* designs and even within individuals make difficult the application of the spatial filters. For *BCIs* that use the μ and β rhythms, the *SL* and *CAR* methods are superior to the ear reference method. However, it was shown that the reference method (*CAR, bipolar, large Laplacian, small Laplacian,* and *referenced to the ear* (McFarland et al., 1997a)) had minor influence on the *classification* accuracy (Ramoser et al., 2000). Fast and continuous feedback can also enhance the performance of the system (Guger et al., 2001; Neuper et al., 1999b). In the following, we introduce only the principles of the *CSP* given in (Guger et al., 2000).

3.3.2 Common spatial patterns (CSP)

As described by (Guger et al., 2000), the *CSP* method uses the covariance to design *common spatial patterns* and is based on the simultaneous diagonalisation of two covariance matrices (Fukunaga, 1972). The decomposition (or filtering) of the *EEG* leads to new time series, which are optimal for the discrimination of two populations (or classes). The patterns are designed such that the signal resulting from the *EEG* filtering with the *CSP* has maximum variance for population and minimum variance for the second population and vice versa. In this way, the difference between the first and second populations is maximized, and the only information contained in these patterns is where the variance of the *EEG* varies most when comparing two conditions.

Given *N* channels of *EEG* for each trial **X** of population 1 and population 2, the *CSP* method gives an *NxN* projection matrix according to (Koles, 1991; Müller-Gerking et al., 1999; Ramoser et al., 2000; Guger et al., 2000). This matrix is a set of subject-specific spatial patterns, which reflect the specific activation of cortical areas during hand movement imagination. With the projection matrix **W**, the decomposition of a trial **X** is described by

$$\mathbf{Z} = \mathbf{W}\mathbf{X}. \quad (1)$$

This mapping projects the variance of **X** onto the rows of **Z** and results in new time series. The columns of $\mathbf{W}^{-1}$ are a set of *CSPs* and can be considered as time-invariant *EEG* source distributions. After interpolation, the patterns can be displayed as topographical maps.
By construction, the variance for population 1 is largest in the first row of **Z** and decreases with the increasing number of the subsequent rows. The opposite is the case for a trial with population 2.

4. Feature extraction methods in BCI designs

This section describes briefly the common *BCI* features extraction methods. Concerning the design of a *BCI* system, some critical properties of these features must be considered (Lotte et al., 2007):

- noise and outliers: the brain signals (e.g. *EEGs*) have a poor signal-to-noise ratio;
- high dimensionality: in *BCI* systems, feature vectors are often of high dimensionality. Several features are generally extracted from several channels and from several time segments before being concatenated into a single feature vector;
- time information: *BCI* features should contain time information as brain activity patterns are generally related to specific time variations of *EEG*;
- the brain signals are non-stationary in nature;
- the brain signals are non-linear in nature;
- non sufficient training sets: training process is time consuming and demanding for the subjects.

There are many methods used in *BCI*, depending of the type of the *BCI* systems. In the following we describe some main and specific methods. More exhaustive details are given by (Bashashati et al., 2007). The feature extraction methods described here are: *Band powers* (*BP*), *Cross-correlation between* EEG *band powers*, *frequency representation* (*FR*), *time-frequency representation* (*TFR*), *Hjorth parameters*, *parametric modelling*, *inverse model* and specific techniques used for *P300* and *VEP* such as *Peak picking* (*PP*) and *Slow cortical potentials calculation* (*SCPs*).

4.1 Band powers (BP)

The features may be extracted from the *EEG* signals by estimating the power distribution of the *EEG* in predefined frequency bands. (Pfurtscheller et al., 1997) used the *band powers* (*BP*) and demonstrated that for each subject, different frequency components in the α and β band were found which provided best discrimination between left and right hand movement imagination. These frequency bands varied between 9 and 14 Hz and between 18 and 26 Hz.

4.2 Cross-correlation between EEG band powers

In the case of *EEG* measurements the cross-correlation coefficients between the *EEG* activity may be calculated to obtain some information from comparing different locations and different frequency bands (Farwell & Donchin, 1988; Musha et al., 1997; Bayliss & Ballard, 1999; 2000a;b; Wang et al., 2004a;b).

4.3 Frequency representation (FR)

Frequency representation (*FR*) features have been widely used in signal processing because of their ease of application, computational speed and direct interpretation of the results (Wolpaw et al., 2000; Blankertz et al., 2006). Specifically, about one-third of *BCI* designs have used *power-spectral density* (*PSD*) features (Bashashati et al., 2007).

4.4 Time-frequency representation (TFR)

Due to the non-linearity and non-stationarity nature of the *EEG* signal, the classical methods based on *Fourier transform* (*FT*) are, in general, not efficient for feature extraction because the obtained features do not provide any time domain information, i.e. these features do not analyze the time-varying spectral content of the signals.

Time-frequency methods decompose the *EEGs* into a series of frequency bands, and the instantaneous power is represented by the envelop of oscillatory activity, which forms the spatial patterns for a given electrode montage at a time-frequency grid (Millán & Mouriño, 2003; Wang et al., 2004a).

Wavelet-based feature extraction algorithms (Qin & He, 2005; Xu & Song, 2008; Haibin et al., 2008) necessitate the choice of a particular wavelet called *mother wavelet* in order to extract useful information. This choice of an appropriate *mother wavelet* may be simplified by the prior knowledge of the physiological activity in the brain.

(Huang et al., 1998) proposed a more fairly recent technique called the *Empirical Mode Decomposition* (*EMD*) was proposed for nonlinear and non-stationary time series data. The (*EMD*) is a data driven approach (i.e. one does not need to define a *mother wavelet* beforehand) that can be used to decompose adaptively a signal into a finite well-defined high frequency and low frequency components, which are known as intrinsic mode functions (*IMFs*) or modes. They consider signals at their local oscillations, but they are not necessarily considered in the sense of Fourier harmonics. Their extraction is non-linear, but their recombination for exact reconstruction of the signal is linear. We think that this approach might be useful in *BCI* design.

4.5 Hjorth parameters

(Hjorth, 1970) has described three parameters that characterize the temporal dynamics of *EEG* signal, ($X(t)$), of length N in terms of *amplitude, time scale* and *complexity*. The parameters are measured in the time domain, as opposed to the other features, which are measured in the frequency domain. It has been shown that these parameters are capable of discriminating between different mental states (Vourkas et al., 2000). The parameters are:

- *Activity*: a measure of the mean power of the signal (variance of X ($VAR(X)$)). It is measured as the standard deviation.

$$Activity(X(t)) = VAR(X(t)) = \frac{\sum_{n=1}^{N}(X(n) - \overline{X})^2}{N}, \tag{2}$$

where $\overline{X}$ denotes the mean of X.

- *Mobility*: represents the mean frequency in the signal. The mobility can be computed as the ratio of the standard deviation of the slope and the standard deviation of the amplitude.

$$Mobility(X(t)) = \sqrt{\frac{Activity(\frac{dX(t)}{dt})}{Activity(X(t))}} = \sqrt{\frac{VAR(\frac{dX(t)}{dt})}{VAR(X(t))}}. \quad (3)$$

- *Complexity*: tries to capture the deviation from the sine wave. It is expressed as the number of standard slopes actually seen in the signal during the average time required for one standard amplitude, as given by the mobility.

$$Complexity(X(t)) = \frac{Mobility(\frac{dX(t)}{dt})}{Mobility(X(t))}. \quad (4)$$

These parameters are mainly used as features for the *classification* of motor imagery (Obermeier et al., 2001; Boostani & Moradi, 2004; Lee & Choi, 2003; Pfurtscheller & Neuper, 2001).

4.6 Parametric modelling

In *statistics*, a *parametric model* or *parametric family* or *finite-dimensional model* refers to a family of distributions which can be described using a finite number of parameters. These parameters are usually collected together to form a single k-dimensional parameter vector $\Theta = (\theta_1, \theta_2, ..., \theta_k)$. In *system theory, parametric model* assume that the time series under analysis to be the output of a given linear mathematical model. They require an a priori choice of the structure and order of the signal generation mechanism model.
Among the more used parametric modelling in *BCIs* are the *autoregressive parameters (AR)* and their variants such as *multivariate AR parameters (MVAR), AR parameters with exogenous input (ARMAX)* and *Adaptive AR parameters (AAR)* (Anderson & Sijercic, 1996; Schlogl et al., 1997; Anderson et al., 1998; Roberts & Penny, 2000; Burke et al., 2005; Vidaurre et al., 2007).
AR methods assume that a signal $X(t)$, measured at time t, can be modeled as a weighted sum of the values of this signal at previous time steps, to which we can add a noise term E_t (generally a *Gaussian white noise*):

$$X(t) = a_1X(t-1) + a_2X(t-2) + ... + a_pX(t-p) + E_t, \quad (5)$$

where the weights a_i are the *autoregressive parameters* which are generally used as features for *BCI*. *AAR* assume that the weights a_i can vary over time. It seems that (*AAR*) parameters would give better results than (*AR*) parameters for motor imagery *classification* (Schlögl et al., 1997; Pfurtscheller et al., 1998), whereas they would give worse results for the *classification* of cognitive tasks such as mental computations, mental rotation of a geometric figure, etc. (Huan & Palaniappan, 2004a; Huan & Palaniappan, 2004b). It should be noted that it is possible to derive a frequential information from the a_i coefficients (McFarland & Wolpaw, 2005).

4.7 Inverse model

Inverse models have shown to be promising feature extraction algorithms (Qin et al., 2004; Grave et al., 2005; Wentrup et al., 2005; Congedo et al., 2006). Such models are able to compute the activity in the whole brain volume, only using *EEG* and a head model that generally represents the brain as a set of *volume elements* (*voxels*). The activity thus calculated in some relevant brain regions or *voxels* may be used as efficient features for *BCI* systems.

4.8 specific techniques

4.8.1 Peak picking (PP)

Peak picking (*PP*) method detects a specific pattern based on its peak value in a region associated with a specific cognitive component. It is used specifically for the evoked potential *P300* (or *P3*)-based *BCI* system (Meinicke et al., 2003; Garrett et al., 2003; Bayliss et al., 2004; Bayliss & Inverso, 2005; Salimi Khorshidi et al., 2007; Hoffman et al., 2008), Fig.5.

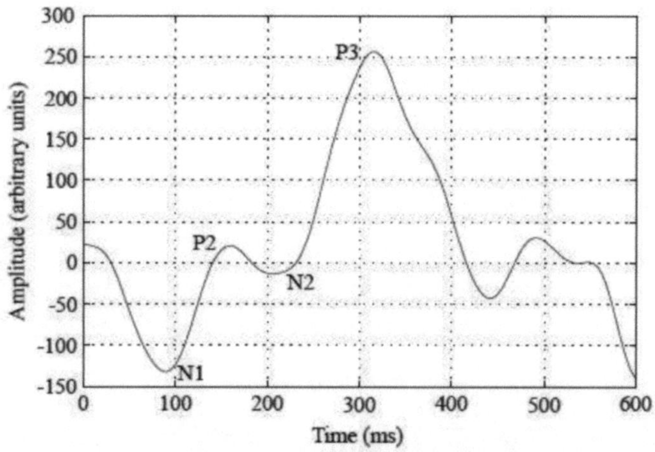

Fig. 5. Typical P300 wave. From (Hoffman et al., 2008).

PP is a simple algorithm to recognize a *P300* component using the difference between the minimum and maximum amplitude in a trial. A trial with a prototypical evoked potential *P300* component contains a large peak from 300-400 ms and *PP* recognizes the *P300* signal when the amplitude difference is greater than or equal to a specified voltage difference between the minimum, $min(x)$, and maximum, $max(x)$, voltage points within a specified time window, where x is a vector which represents the data for a single *P300* response. For recognition, the time window with the best results may be between three and six hundred milliseconds citepbayliss04.

4.8.2 Slow cortical potentials (SCPs) calculation methods

The *SCPs* amplitudes are extracted on-line from the regular electroencephalogram, filtered, corrected for eye movement artefacts and fed back to the patient with visual, auditory or tactile feedback (Birbaumer et al., 1999; 2000; Hinterberger et al., 2004). The *TFR* methods are also used to extract the features of the *SCPs* (Hinterberger et al., 2003; Bostanov, 2004). Fig.6 shows the statistical results of the study realised by (Bashashati et al., 2007) concerning *feature extraction* methods in *BCI* designs. (Bashashati et al., 2007) concluded that 41% of the *BCIs* are based on the sensorimotor activity use *PSD* features, 16% rely on parametric modelling of the data, 13% use *TFR* methods and 6% do not employ any feature extraction methods. 74% of the *SCP*-based *BCI* designs calculate SCP signals using low-pass filtering methods, and 64% of the *VEP*-based *BCIs* use *power-spectral* features at specific frequencies. 26% of the *BCIs* based on *P300* calculate the *PP*; 22% use *TFR*-based methods, 22% use no feature extraction method, and 15% use cross-correlation with a specific template. 41% of the *BCI* designs that use mental tasks to control a *BCI* use *power spectral* features and 37% use *parametric modelling* of the input signal. As most of the *BCI* designs that are based on neural

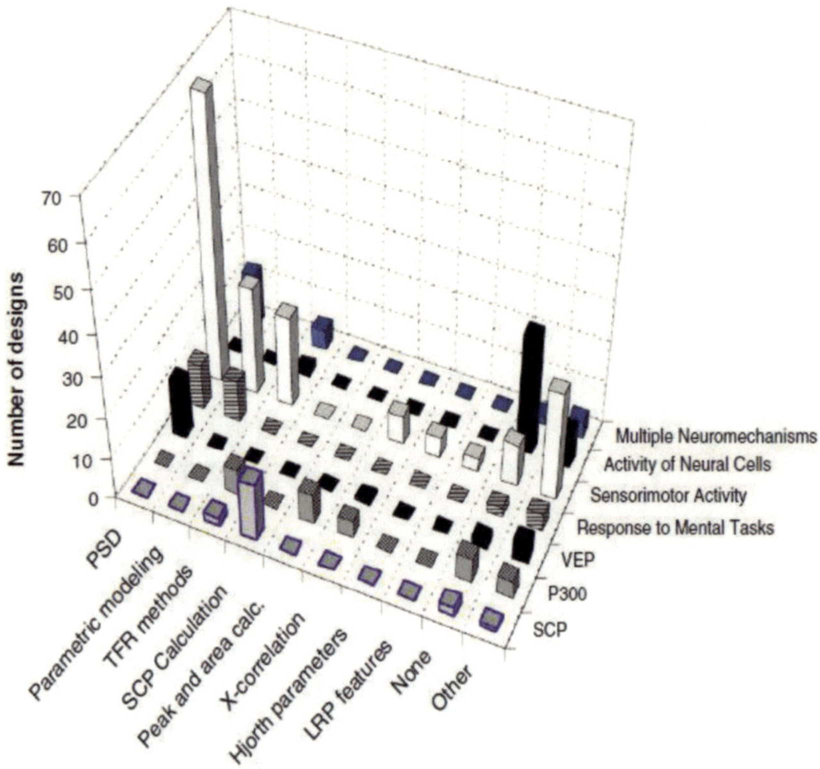

Fig. 6. Feature extraction methods in *BCI* designs based on sensorimotor activity, VEP, P300, SCP, response to mental tasks, activity of neural cells, and multiple neuromechanisms. Taken from (Bashashati et al., 2007).

cortical recordings mainly try to model the direct relationship between the neural cortical recordings and movements, they do not use a feature-extraction algorithm. 45% of the *BCI* designs that are based on multiple neuromechanisms rely on power-spectral features, 17% use parametric modelling, and 17% use *TFR* methods.

5. Feature selection and dimensionality reduction methods in BCI designs

In *BCI* applications, several features are generally extracted from several brain activity channels (several electrodes in the case of *EEG* measurements) and from several time segments (or sessions), before being concatenated into a single feature vector. Hence, the *BCIs* are often affected by a problem known as *curse of dimensionality* (Bellman, 1961). It was demonstrated that the amount of data needed to properly describe the different classes increases exponentially with the dimensionality of the feature vectors (Friedman, 1997; Jain, 2000).

(Flotzinger et al., 1994) and (Pfurtscheller & Guger, 1999b) have shown that when feature selection is used, the *classification* accuracy is better than when all the features are used. If the number of training data is small relatively to the number of features, the *classification* algorithm which will use these features and data will very likely give bad results. It is recommended to use at least 5 to 10 times more training data per class than the number of features (Jain & Chandrasekaran, 1982; Raudys & Jain, 1991). Unfortunately this cannot be applied in all *BCI* systems as generally the dimensionality is high and the training set small. Among fourteen feature selection and dimensionality reduction methods in *BCI* designs given by (Bashashati et al., 2007), we give here briefly the definitions of only three methods which are the most applied in *BCI* designs:

- ***Genetic algorithm (GA)***
  A *Genetic algorithm* (*GA*) (Goldberg, 1989; Flotzinger et al., 1994) is a search technique used in computing to find exact or approximate solutions to optimization and search problems. Genetic algorithms are categorized as global search heuristics. They are a particular class of *evolutionary algorithms* (*EA*) that use techniques inspired by evolutionary biology such as inheritance, mutation, selection, and crossover. These algorithms are based on a sequence of generations whereby the population in each generation produces the next while trying to optimize some *fitness criterion* (Brill, 1992), such as maximum ability to classify the training set in the *classification* stage. Each member of the current population is assigned a binay-valued chromosome of length n (for an n-dimensional *classification* problem), whereby the value of each bit within the chromosome defines whether this feature is to be used for *classification* or not. A chromosome 11 11 1 ...1 , therefore, means that all parameters are to be used for evaluation of the member's fitness and a chromosome 10100 ... 0 means that only the first and third parameters are to be used. The accuracy which can be achieved using a specific chromosome is calculated using a *clustering algorithm* such as *k-nearest-neighbour classifier* (*K-NN*) or any other *clustering algorithm*. For *k-nearest-neighbour classification* the k nearest data vectors are found for a new input vector which is then classified to the label to which the majority of these k data vectors belong. For more details, refer to (Flotzinger et al., 1994; Brill, 1992).
- ***Principal component analysis (PCA)***
  Principal component analysis (*PCA*) may be used in *pre-processing* stage of *BCI* designs (see section 3.3). *PCA* may also be used as a dimensionality reduction technique in terms of capturing the variance of the data, and it accounts for correlation among variable. It gives lower-dimensional representations of the data which better generalize to data independent of the training set than using the entire dimensionality of the observation space (Scholkopf, 1999). The *PCA* transforms a set of m variables into another set of $k \leq m$ uncorrelated variables, maintaining as many of the variance of original data as possible (Moghaddam, 2002).
- ***Distinctive sensitive learning vector quantization (DSLVQ)***
  The influence of distinctive features on the distance function in the standard *learning vector quantisation* (*LVQ*) (Kohonen, 1990) is equal. The *Distinction Sensitive* (*DS*) algorithm (*DSLVQ*) (Flotzinger et al., 1994) employs an *adaptive weighted distance function* where the influence of features which frequently contribute to misclassifications is reduced while the influence of features which are shown to be very significant for proper *classification* is increased. For the *weighted distance function* of *DSLVQ* a *global weights vector* w is used which stores the distinctiveness, i.e. the *relevance*, of every single feature. This weights vector is adapted interactively along with the codebook. The distance function used may be the *Euclidean distance*, or any other *weighted distance functions*. (Flotzinger et al., 1994) proposed the following *Euclidean distance* between two feature vectors x and y:

$$DSdist(x,y,w) = \sqrt{\sum_{i=1}^{N}(w_i(x_i - y_i))^2}. \tag{6}$$

The weights vector w can be seen as a scaling transformation from the original feature space into a *DS*-feature space. This transformation increases distances for very distinctive features and decreases distances for common features. Despite the usage of a *weighted distance function*, the codebook learning for *DSLVQ* is the same as for the *LVQ3* algorithm. Additionally, the weights vector w must be updated with every learning iteration. Learning weights and codebook settings in parallel facilitate a quick approximation of these related parameters. For more details, refer to (Flotzinger et al., 1994).

Fig. 7 shows the statistical results of the study realised by (Bashashati et al., 2007) concerning *feature selection* and *dimensionality reduction* methods in *BCI* designs. (Bashashati et al., 2007) concluded that thirty-eight of the reported *BCI* designs employ feature selection and dimensionality reduction algorithms; 26% of these 38 designs use *genetic algorithms* (*GA*), 24% use *distinctive sensitive learning vector quantization* (*DSLVQ*), and 13% use PCA.

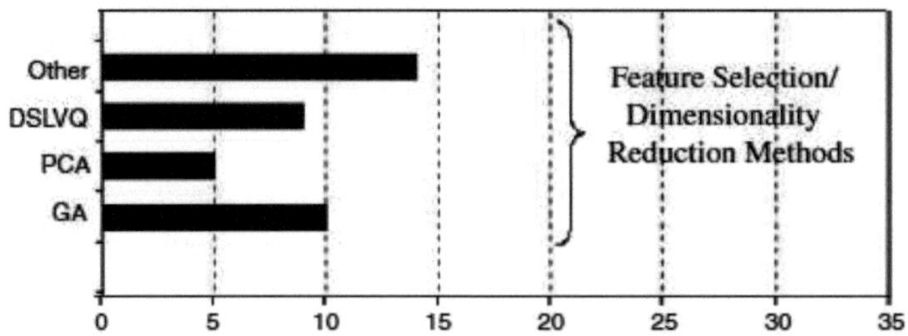

Fig. 7. Feature selection and dimensionality reduction methods in *BCI* designs. Figure modified from (Bashashati et al., 2007) with authorisation.

6. Classification in BCIs

Brain activity patterns are considered as dynamic stochastic processes due both to biological and to technical factors. Biologically, they change due to user fatigue and attention, due to disease progression, and with the process of training. Technically, they change due to amplifier noises, ambient noises, and the variation of electrode impedances (Wolpaw et al., 2002). Therefore, the time course of the generated time series signals (e.g. *EEG*) should be taken into account during feature extraction (Wolpaw et al., 2002). To use this temporal information, three main approaches have been proposed (Lotte et al., 2007):

- concatenation of features from different time segments: extracting features from several time segments and concatenating them into a single feature vector (Pfurtscheller et al., 1997; Haselsteiner & Pfurtscheller, 2000);
- combination of *classifications* at different time segments: it consists in performing the feature extraction and *classification* steps on several time segments and then combining the results of the different *classifiers* (Penny & Roberts, 1999; Lemm et al., 2004);
- dynamic *classification*: it consists in extracting features from several time segments to build a temporal sequence of feature vectors. This sequence can be classified using a dynamic *classifier* (Haselsteiner & Pfurtscheller, 2000; Obermeier et al., 2001).

The first approach is the most widely used despite that the obtained feature vectors are often of high dimensionality.

6.1 Classifier selection criteria

In order to choose the most appropriate *classifier* for a given set of features, the properties of the available *classifiers* must be chosen according to the following four *classifier* taxonomy and two main problems in *BCI* design as described by (Lotte et al., 2007):

6.1.1 Classifier taxonomy

- ***Generative or Informative classifier - Discriminative classifier***
  Generative classifiers, e.g., *Bayes quadratic,* learn the class models. To classify a feature vector, generative *classifiers* compute the likelihood of each class and choose the most likely. Discriminative ones, e.g., *support vector machines* (*SVM*), only learn the way of discriminating the classes or the class membership in order to classify a feature vector directly (Ng & Jordan, 2002; Rubinstein & Hastie, 1997);
- ***Static classifier - Dynamic classifier***
  static classifiers, e.g., *multilayer perceptrons* (*MP*), cannot take into account temporal information during *classification* as they classify a single feature vector. In contrast, *dynamic classifiers* such as *hidden Markov model* (*HMM*) (Rabiner, 1989), *FIR filters-multilayer perceptrons* (*FIR-MLP*) (Haselsteiner & Pfurtscheller, 2000) and *Tree-based neural network* (*TBNN*) (Ivanova et al., 1995), can classify a sequence of feature vectors and thus catch temporal dynamics.
- ***Stable classifier - Unstable classifier***
  Stable classifiers, e.g., *linear discriminant analysis* (*LDA*), have a low complexity (or capacity (Vapnik, 1995; 1999)). They are said to be *stable* as small variations in the training set do not considerably affect their performance. In contrast, *unstable classifiers,* e.g., *multilayer perceptron,* have a high complexity. As for them, small variations of the training set may lead to important changes in performance (Breiman, 1998).
- ***Regularized classifier***
  Regularization consists in carefully controlling the complexity of a *classifier* in order to prevent *overtraining*. Regularization helps limit (a) the influence of *outliers* and strong *noise,* (b) the *complexity* of the *classifier* and (c) the *raggedness* of the decision surface (Müller et al., 2003). A *regularized classifier* has good *generalization* performances and is more robust with respect to outliers (Duda, 2001; Jain, 2000) (see section 6.1.2).

6.1.2 Main classification problems in BCI research

While performing a pattern recognition task, *classifiers* may be facing two main problems related to the feature properties. These problems are: the *curse-of-dimensionality* and the *bias-variance tradeoff.* The first problem is discussed in section 5. The second problem is a general one where three inherent errors may occur.

Independently of the applications of the *classification,* this stage consists in association of the true *class* label c^* corresponding to a feature vector x using a mapping (or a *model* f that may be learnt from a training set T. Let f^* the optimal unknown theoretical mapping that has generated the labels. If the *mean square error* (*MSE*) is considered to evaluate the inherent classification errors, then these errors can be decomposed into three terms (Breiman, 1998; Friedman, 1997):

$$
\begin{aligned}
MSE &= E[(c^* - f(x))^2] \\
&= E[(c^* - f^*(x) + f^*(x) - E[f(x)] + E[f(x)] - f(x))^2] \\
&= E[(c^* - f^*(x))^2] + E[(f^*(x) - E[(f(x)]^2)] + E[(E[(f(x)] - f(x))^2] \\
&= noise^2 + bias(f(x))^2 + variance(f(x)),
\end{aligned} \tag{7}
$$

where the expectation is with respect to the distribution over c^* and the introduced term $E[f(x)]$ is the mean value of the estimated class label. These three terms describe three possible sources of inherent *classification* error:

- ***noise***: represents the irreducible noise within the system;
- ***bias***: represents a systematic error which is the divergence between the estimated mapping (i.e. the estimated class label) and the best mapping (i.e. the true class label). This term depends strongly on the classification method that has been chosen to obtain f (*linear, quadratic, . . .*);
- ***variance***: reflects the sensitivity to the used training set T.

The only terms that may be minimised are the *bias* and the *variance* terms. *Simple classifiers* (e.g. *linear classifiers*) have a high *bias* but low *variance* whereas more *complex classifiers* (e.g. *polynomial classifiers*) have a low *bias* but a high *variance*. To select the *optimal model complexity*, we must solve this *bias-variance dilemma* (Geman et al., 1992).

Actually, *stable classifiers* tend to have a high *bias* and a low *variance*, whereas the inverse is true for *unstable classifiers*. This can explain why *simple classifiers* sometimes outperform more complex ones. A low *variance* can be a solution to cope with the stochastic nature of brain signals. In the presence of strong noise and *outliers*, even linear systems can fail. One way of overcoming this problem is to use techniques, known as *stabilization techniques*. These techniques can be used to reduce the *variance*, e.g. *combination of classifiers* (Breiman, 1998) and *regularisation* techniques (Duda, 2001; Jain, 2000).

The *nonlinear classifiers* have more number of parameters than those in the *linear classifiers*. In addition, these parameters must be chosen appropriately. However, when there are large amounts and limited knowledge of data, *nonlinear classifiers* are better suited in finding the potentially more complex structure in the data. In particular, when the source of the data to be classified is not well known, using methods that are good at finding nonlinear transformation of the data is suggested. In these cases, *kernel*-based and *neural-networks* based methods can be used to determine the transformations. *Kernel*-based classifiers are classification methods that apply a linear classification in some appropriate (*kernel*) feature space. Thus, all the beneficial properties of linear classification are maintained, but at the same time, the overall classification is nonlinear. Examples of such *kernel*-based classification methods are *support vector machines* (*SVMs*) (Vapnik, 1999) and *kernel Fisher discriminant* (*KFD*) (Müller et al., 2003).

Better performances might also be achieved by using *group* (*committee*) of *classifiers* rather than using a single *classifier* but only a few *BCI* designs have employed such an approach in classifying features and achieved performance improvements (Millan et al., 2000; Peters et al., 2001; Varsta et al., 2000; Millan et al., 2002).

6.2 Classifiers used in BCI research

There are many categories of *classification* algorithms used to design *BCIs*. Among the more used *Classifiers* in the *BCI* community are: *linear discriminant classifiers (LDC), neural networks (NN), nonlinear Bayesian classifiers (NBC), nearest neighbours classifiers (NNC)* and *combinations of classifiers*. As a *linear discriminant classifiers (LDC)*, we introduce in this section only the *linear discriminant analysis (LDA)* and *support vector machines (SVMs)*, and as *nonlinear Bayesian classifiers (NBC)*, we introduce in this section only the *hidden Markov models (HMMs)*. For an extensive description and tutorials on these and other approaches, refer to (Lotte et al., 2007; Bashashati et al., 2007; Hung et al., 2005).

6.2.1 linear discriminant classifiers (LDC)

LDC are the most popular in *BCI* design. Two main kinds of *LDC* have been used for *BCI* design, namely, *linear discriminant analysis* (*LDA*) and *support vector machine* (*SVM*).

6.2.1.1 Linear discriminant analysis (LDA)

LDA or *Fisher's LDA* has been used with success in many of *BCIs* such as motor imagery based *BCI* (Pfurtscheller, 1999c), P300 applications (Bostanov, 2004; Hoffman et al., 2008), multiclass (Garrett et al., 2003) or asynchronous (Scherer et al., 2004) *BCI*. It has a very low computational requirement and it is simple to use and generally provides good results.
The idea of *LDA* (Fukunaga, 1990; Duda, 2001) is to find a *weight vector* **w** so that two projected *clusters* c_1 and c_2 of N_1 and N_2 training feature vectors $\{x_1, x_2,..., x_{N_1}\}$ and $\{x_1, x_2,..., x_{N_2}\}$ on **w** can be well separated from each other by *hyperplanes* while keeping small *variance* of each *cluster*. This can be done by maximizing the so-called *Fisher's criterion*. *LDA* assumes normal distribution of the data, with equal covariance matrix for both classes. The separating *hyperplane* is obtained by seeking the projection that maximizes the distance between the two classes' means and minimizes the between variance (Fukunaga, 1990).

$$J(\mathbf{w}) = \frac{\mathbf{w}^T S_b \mathbf{w}}{\mathbf{w} S_{\mathbf{w}} \mathbf{w}}, \tag{8}$$

with respect to w, where S_b is the *between-class variance matrix*:

$$S_b = (m_{c_1} - m_{c_2})(m_{c_1} - m_{c_2})^T, \tag{9}$$

and S_w is the *within-class variance matrix*:

$$S_w = \sum_{x \in c_1} (x - m_{c_1})(x - m_{c_1})^T + \sum_{x \in c_2} (x - m_{c_2})(x - m_{c_2})^T, \tag{10}$$

where m_{c1} and m_{c2} are the cluster mean of classes c_1 and c_2 respectively.
The optimal *weight vector* **w** is the eigenverctor corresponding to the largest eigenvalue of $S_w^{-1} S_b$. Once this vector is obtained using the training data x_i is obtained by means of the training data, the classification then may be done by projecting the *test feature vectors* on it, and then the projected *test feature vectors* may be classified by employing a clustering rule such as *k-nearest-neighbor* decision rule.
In the case of *multiclass* separation problem (c_i, $i > 2$), several hyperplanes are used. The strategy generally used in this case is the *one versus the rest* (*OVR*) (Schlögl et al., 2005) which separate each class from all the others. This technique is suitable for the on-line *BCIs* because it has a very low computational requirement. It is simple to use and generally provides good results. The main drawback of LDA is its *linearity* that can provide poor results on complex nonlinear *EEG* data (Garcia et al., 2003). A *regularized Fisher's LDA* (*RFLDA*) has also been

used in the field of *BCI* (Blankertz et al., 2002; Müller et al., 2004) and give better results for *BCI* than the non-regularized version (Blankertz et al., 2002; Müller et al., 2004).

6.2.1.2 Support vector machine (SVM)

The generalization of the pattern recognition or regression results obtained from a limited sample constitutes the essential stake of the artificial training (machine learning). It is known that the only minimization of the empirical risk (the error of training) does not guarantee a weak error on a corpus of test. Thus the techniques of regularization, used since the years 1960, allow to carrying out a compromise between the capacity of the model to be learned (related to its complexity) and its aptitude to be generalized. From the point of view conceptual, the concept of structural risk introduced by Vladimir Vapnik into the years 1990 (Vapnik, 1995; Cortes & Vapnik, 1995; Vapnik, 1999) gives a bound of the error of test according to the error of training and of the complexity of the model. *Support vector machine (SVM)* have been applied in various domains for classification and regression.
In the following, we will outline briefly the idea of *SVM* for *binary classification* and then how this method can be applied to solve *multi-class classification* problems.

- ***Binary classification SVM***
  Support vector machines were originally designed for binary classification (Cortes & Vapnik, 1995). The main idea of this approach is to construct a *hyperplane* in order to separate two classes ($ci \in \{-1, 1\}$ or $ci \in \{0, 1\}$) so that the margin (Friedman, 1996) (the distance between the *hyperplane* and the nearest point(s) of each classes) is maximal and with minimal error. The theoretical principle of the *SVM* comprises two fundamental steps:
  1. Make a nonlinear mapping Φ of the feature vectors from *input space* towards another space (*redescription space*) of higher dimension provided with a scalar product (*Hilbert space*), Fig. 8.

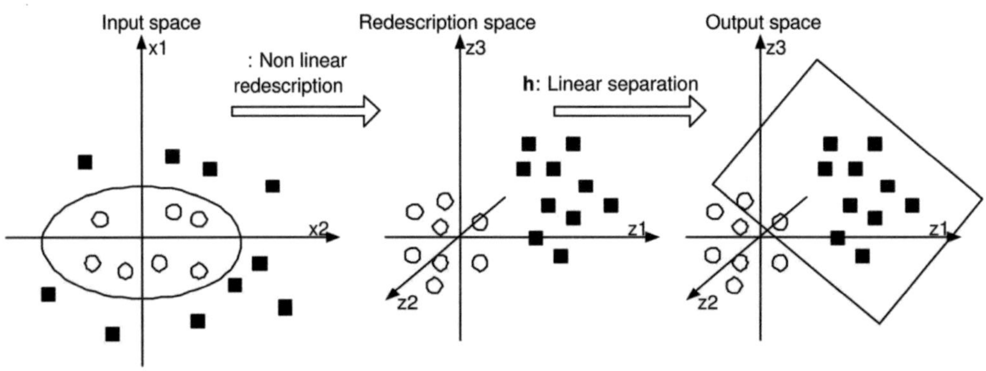

Fig. 8. The idea of the *SVM*: transform a nonlinear problem of separation in the *representation space* into a linear problem of separation in a *redescription space* of higher dimension.

  2. Construct an optimal *hyperplane* allowing an optimal linear separation in this *redescription* space.

  The interest of this mapping is that in the *redescription space* the pattern recognition can prove easy task: intuitively, more the dimension of the *redescription space* is hight; more the probability of being able to find a *hyperplane* separating between the *feature vectors* is high, Fig. 9.

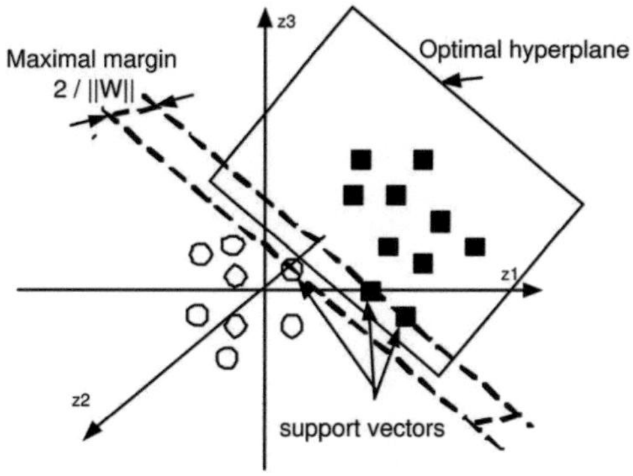

Fig. 9. Linear mapping: the optimal separating *hyperplane* is that which maximizes the margin in the *redescription space*.

From the mathematical point of view, the nonlinear mapping ($\Phi : \mathbb{R}^2 \rightarrow \mathbb{R}^n$) is realized via a *Kernel function* (*Hilbert-Schmidt Kernel*) easy to calculate. In practice, some families of Kernel functions are known and it is allocated to the user of *SVM* to carry out test to determine that which is appropriate for its application (it is a question of translating the maximum a priori knowledge of which one lays out on the studied problem and the data). Fig. 10 shows a non-linear separation example.

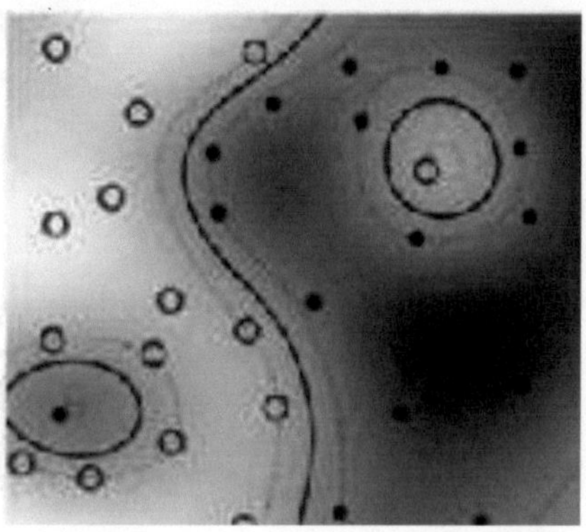

Fig. 10. *Non-linear mapping*: a complex shape. Figure from Schölkopf & Smola (2002).

Let **x** denote a vector drawn from the *input space*, assumed to be of dimension N_0 and let $\{\Phi_j(\mathbf{x})\}$, j = 1, 2, ..., N_1 denote a set of *nonlinear transformations* from the *input space* to the *redescription space*, where N_1 is the dimension of the *redescription space*. Given such a set of *nonlinear transformations*, we may define a *hyperplane* acting as the *decision surface* which is computed in the *redescription space* in terms of the *linear weights* of the machine as follows:

$$\sum_{j=0}^{N_1} \mathbf{w}_j \Phi_j(\mathbf{x}) = 0, \tag{11}$$

where $\mathbf{w} = \{\mathbf{w}_0, \mathbf{w}_1, ..., \mathbf{w}_{N_1}\}$ denotes a set of *linear weights* connecting the *redescription space* to the *output space*. And it is assumed that $\Phi_0(\mathbf{x}) = 1$ for all **x**, so that $\mathbf{w}_0$ denotes the bias. Define the vector $\Phi(\mathbf{x}) = [\Phi_0(\mathbf{x}), \Phi_1(\mathbf{x}), ..., \Phi_{N_1}(\mathbf{x})]^T$, then we can rewrite the *decision surface* in the compact form:

$$\mathbf{w}^T\Phi(\mathbf{x}) = 0. \tag{12}$$

Given the *training feature vectors*, $\Phi(\mathbf{x}_i)$ corresponds to the *input pattern* $\mathbf{x}_i$, and the corresponding desired response d_i, i = 1, 2, ...,N_0, which is either 1 or -1 (or, 0 or 1), it has been shown that (Haykin, 1994) the *optimal weight vector* **w** can be expressed as

$$\mathbf{w} = \sum_{i=1}^{N_0} \alpha_i d_i \Phi(\mathbf{x}_i), \tag{13}$$

where $\{\alpha_i\}$, i = 1, 2, ..., N_0 is the *optimal Lagrange multipliers* resulted from maximizing the *subject function*

$$Q(\alpha) = \sum_{i=1}^{N_0} \alpha_i - \frac{1}{2}\sum_{i=1}^{N_0}\sum_{j=1}^{N_0} \alpha_i\alpha_j d_i d_j \Phi^T(\mathbf{x}_i)\Phi(\mathbf{x}_j), \tag{14}$$

subject to the constraints
(1) $\sum_{i=1}^{N_0} \alpha_i d_i = 0$, and
(2) $0 \le \alpha_i \le C$,
where C is a user-specified constant which may be considered as *regulation parameter*. Substituting equation (13) into (12), we obtain the *optimal hyperplane*

$$\sum_{i=1}^{N_0} \alpha_i d_i \Phi^T(\mathbf{x}_i)\Phi(\mathbf{x}) = 0, \tag{15}$$

which will be used for linearly separating the *testing data*, i.e. for any testing sample **x**, if

$$\sum_{i=1}^{N_0} \alpha_i d_i \Phi^T(\mathbf{x}_i)\Phi(\mathbf{x}) \ge 0, \tag{16}$$

then **x** is classified into the subset having the training response d_i = 1, otherwise it is classified into the other subset with d_i = –1 (or 0). The user may choose the *radial basis function* (*RBF*) in defining the *inner product kernel* $K(\mathbf{x}, \mathbf{x}_i) = \Phi^T(\mathbf{x}_i)\Phi(\mathbf{x})$.
According to equation (16), once the number of nonzero Lagrange multipliers, α_i, is determined, the number of *radial basis functions* and their centers are determined automatically. This differs from the design of the conventional neural network, such as the *back-propagation neural network* or *radial-basis function network* (Haykin, 1994), where the numbers of hidden layers or of hidden neuron are usually determined heuristically. The *kernel* generally used in *BCI* research is the *Gaussian* or *radial basis function* (*RBF*) kernel:

$$K(\mathbf{x}, \mathbf{x_i}) = exp(-\frac{\|\mathbf{x} - \mathbf{x_i}\|^2}{2\sigma^2}). \tag{17}$$

In this case, the *SVM* is known as *Gaussian SVM* or *RBF SVM* (Burges, 1998; Bennett & Campbell, 2000; Garrett et al., 2003; Kaper et al., 2004).
This classifier has been applied, with success, to a relatively large number of *BCIs* problems (Blankertz et al., 2002; Garrett et al., 2003; Rakotomamonjy et al., 2005; Helmy et al., 2008; Trad et al., 2009).

- Multiclass SVM (M-SVM)
  To solve a given multiclass problem it is preferable to use a combination of several *binary SVM classifiers* and a decision strategy to decide the class of the input pattern. The most popular methods to achieve this goal are: *one-versus-all* method using *Winner-Takes- All* strategy (*WTA-SVM); One-Versus-One* method implemented by *Max-Wins Voting* (*MWV-SVM*) (Duan et al., 2007); *Decision Directed Acyclic Graph* (*DAGSVM*) (Platt et al., 2000); and *error correcting codes* (Dietterich & Bakiri, 1995).

6.2.2 Nonlinear Bayesian Classifiers (NBC)

This section introduces one Bayesian classifier used for *BCI*: *hidden Markov models* (*HMMs*). This Classifier produces *nonlinear decision boundaries*. Furthermore, they are *generative*, which enables them to perform more efficient rejection of uncertain samples than *discriminative classifiers*. As brain signals used to drive *BCI* have specific time courses, *HMM* have been applied to the classification of temporal sequences of *BCI* features or even raw *EEG* (Obermeier et al., 2000; 2001; Cincotti et al., 2003; Schlogl et al., 2005; Helmy et al., 2008; Trad et al., 2009).

HMMs are very efficient nonlinear techniques used for the classification of time series (Rabiner, 1989). *HMMs* have been widely applied in automatic speech recognition and now being applied to many fields, e.g. signal processing, pattern recognition, modelling and control. Their use necessitates two stages: a *training stage* where the stochastic process models are estimated through extensive observation corpus and decoding or *detection stage* where the model may be used off/on-line to obtain the likelihoods of the given testing sequence evaluated by each model.

In its conventional definition, a *HMM* is defined by the following compact notation to indicate the complete parameter set of the model $\lambda = (\Pi,\mathbf{A},\mathbf{B})$, where Π, $\mathbf{A}$ and $\mathbf{B}$ are the initial state distribution vector, matrix of state transition probabilities and the set of the observation probability distribution in each state, respectively: $\Pi = [\pi_1,\pi_2, ...,\pi_N]$, with $\pi_i = P(q_1 = s_i)$, $\mathbf{A} = [a_{ij}]$, with $a_{ij} = P(q_{t+1} = s_j \mid q_t = s_i)$, $1 \le i, j \le N$, s_i, s_j 2 S, $S = \{s_1, s_2, ..., s_N\}$, $t \in \{1, 2, ...,T\}$. The observation at time (or index) t, $\mathbf{O}_t$, is considered in this paper as continuous $\mathbf{O}_t \in \mathbb{R}^K$. For a continuous observation (*CHMMs* case), the state conditional probability of the observation $b_i(\mathbf{O}_t)$ may be defined by a finite mixture of any log-concave or *elliptically symmetric probability density function* (*pdf*), e.g. *Gaussian pdf*, with *state conditional observation mean vector* ¯ᵢ and *state conditional observation covariance matrix* Σ_i. In this paper we consider only a single *Gaussian pdf*, so $\mathbf{B}$ may be defined as $\mathbf{B} = \{ ¯_i, \Sigma_i\}$, $i = 1, 2, ..., N$. At each instant of time t, the model is in one of the states i, $1 \le i \le N$. It outputs $\mathbf{O}_t$ according to a *density function* $b_i(\mathbf{O}_t)$ and then jumps to state j, $1 \le j \le N$ with probability a_{ij}. The *state transition matrix* defines the structure of the *HMM* (Rabiner, 1989). The model λ may be obtained off-line by a given training procedure. In practice, given the observation sequence $O_l = \{\mathbf{O}_1,\mathbf{O}_2, ...,\mathbf{O}_T\}$, $1 \le l \le L$ and a model λ, the *HMMs* need three fundamental problems to be solved

1. How to calculate the likelihood $P(O_l \mid \lambda)$? The solution to this problem provides a scoren of how O_l belongs to λ.
2. How to determine the most likely state sequence that corresponds to O_l? The solution to this problem provides the sequence of the hidden states corresponding to the given observation sequence O_l.
3. How to adjust the model λ in order to maximize $P(O_l \mid \lambda)$? This is the problem of estimating the model parameters given a corpus of training observations sequences.

Problems 1 and 2 are solved in the decoding or detection stage using the forward or the *Viterbi algorithms* (Rabiner, 1989), while problem 3 is solved during the training phase using either a conventional algorithm such as the Baum-Welch algorithm (Rabiner, 1989) or another optimization based algorithm such as the simulated annealing based algorithm (Alani & Hamam, 2010).

7. Hidden Markov models and support vector machines approaches applied to P300-based Brain-Computer interface - a comparative study

This section reports on our contribution to investigate the use of *Hidden Markov Models* (*HMMs*) and *Support Vector Machines* (*SVMs*) approaches for tasks classification in *P300*-based Brain-Computer Interface (*BCI*) system. These approaches are applied to electroencephalogram (*EEG*) data sets of the École Polytechnique Fédérale de Laussane - *BCI* Groupe. These data are issued from five disabled subjects and four able-bodied subjects. For each subject, the *HMMs* and *SVM* are trained on different sets. Each set represents a specific *P300 potential evoked* task and contains multiple sequences (issued from different trials) of *EEG* records. For each task, the *HMMs* and the *SVM* that have been built take into account the variability of *EEGs* during different trials. Based on *Bayesian Inference Criterion* (*BIC*) (Schwarz, 1978), the proposed *HMM* training algorithm is able to select the optimal number of states corresponding to each task. This scheme makes the training procedure independent of the initialization problem and the a priori knowledge of the optimal number of *HMM*-related states needed in the training algorithm. The *SVM* is trained by introducing the different sets at the same time. We report training procedures and testing results for the *HMMs* and the *SVM* then we compare the performance of the two approaches on the same testing data sets. We also present promising preliminary comparative results based on the two classification approaches with correct classification rates for all subjects.

7.1 Problem definition

It has been shown by (Hoffman et al., 2008) that evoked potential (*P300*) in *EEG* data due to different images (tasks) appearing randomly on a computer screen in face of the subject may be efficiently used for exogenous mental task recognition. In Hoffman's work, extensions of *LDA* have been employed for pattern recognition. In our work we investigate the use of *HMMs* and *SVM* to classify the same *P300* based tasks defined in (Hoffman et al., 2008) and using tasks data given in (Hoffman et al., 2009).

7.2 Data structure and feature extraction

For the clarity of the following sections, this section introduce briefly the experimental setup and the data given by Hoffman et al. (Hoffman et al., 2008), (Hoffman et al., 2009) that we adopted in our work.

7.3 Hoffman's experimental setup

In the experimental setup given by Hoffman et al., the users used a laptop screen displaying randomly six images (a television, a telephone, a lamp, a door, a window, and a radio), Fig. 11. Subjects were asked to count silently how often a prescribed image was flashed. The six images (Tasks) were displayed on the screen and a warning tone was issued.

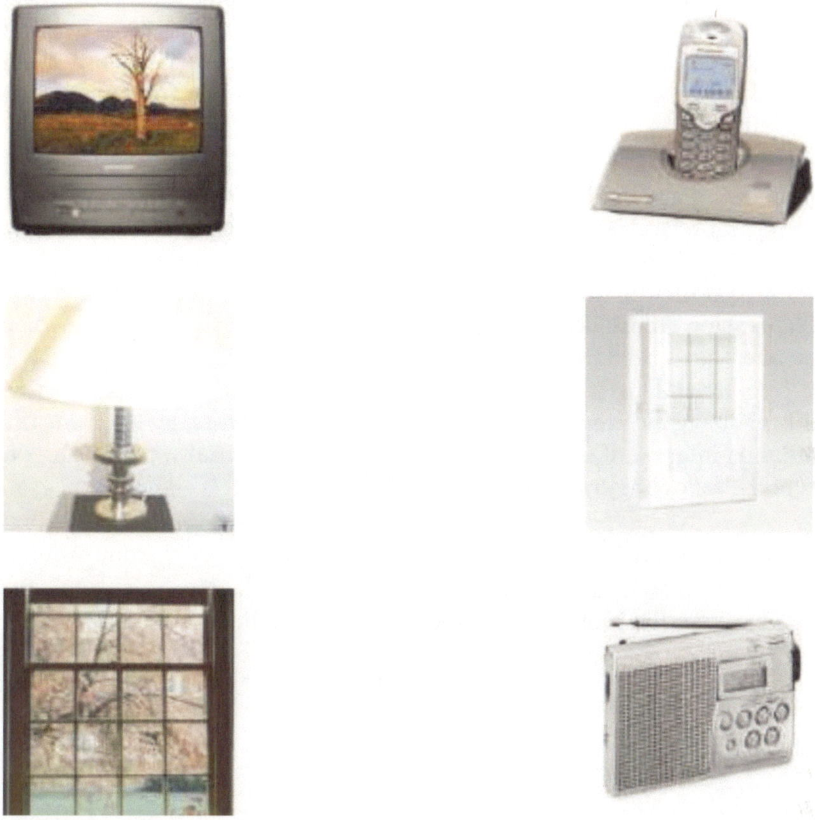

Fig. 11. The display used for evoking the *P300*. One image was flashed at a time (Hoffman et al., 2008), (Hoffman et al., 2009).

These images were selected in order to control some electrical appliances based on the *BCI* system. Each image flashed during 100 ms followed by a period of 300 ms of non flashing. The sampling rate of *EEG* was 2048 Hz using 32 electrodes according to the 10-20 international system.

7.3.1 Subjects

The recorded data given by Hoffman et al. (Hoffman et al., 2009) and used in our work are issued from five disabled subjects (subjects 1 to 5) and four able-bodied subjects (subjects 6 to 9). The disabled subjects were all wheelchair-bound but had varying communication and limb muscle control abilities. Subjects 1 and 2 were able to perform simple, slow movements with their arms and hands but they were unable to control other extremities. Spoken communication with subjects 1 and 2 was possible, although both subjects suffered from mild dysarthria. Subject 3 was able to perform restricted movements with his left hand but was unable to move his arms or other extremities. Spoken communication with subject 3 was impossible. However the patient was able to answer yes/no questions with eye blinks. Subject 4 had very little control over arm and hand movements. Spoken communication was possible with subject 4, although a mild dysarthria existed. Subject 5 was only able to perform extremely slow and relatively uncontrolled movements with hands and arms. Due to a severe hypophony and large fluctuations in the level of alertness, communication with subject 5 was very difficult, thus this subject was not taken into account by Hoffman at al. (Hoffman et al., 2008), (Hoffman et al., 2009). Subjects 6 to 9 were normal persons (all male, age 30 to 32). None of subjects 6 to 9 had known neurological deficits. In this study we use the data from all subjects.

7.3.2 Preprocessing and feature extraction

The data were preprocessed (referencing, bandpass-filtering, downsampling, and artefacts rejection). The *EEG* was downsampled from 2048 Hz to 32 Hz by selecting each 64th sample from the bandpass-filtered data. For each subject, the data were obtained during four sessions. One session comprised on average 810 trials, and the whole data for one subject consisted on average of 3240 trials. One trial duration takes 1000 *ms*. Single trials of duration 1000 *ms* were extracted from the data. Single trials started at stimulus onset, i.e. at the beginning of the intensification of an image, and ended 1000 *ms* after stimulus onset. Due to the Inter-stimulus interval of 400 ms, the last 600 ms of each trial were overlapped with the first 600 ms of the following trial.

7.3.3 Electrode selection

Hoffman et al. (Hoffman et al., 2008), (Hoffman et al., 2009) proved that the configuration with 8 electrodes gives the best result for the studying data Fig. 12.

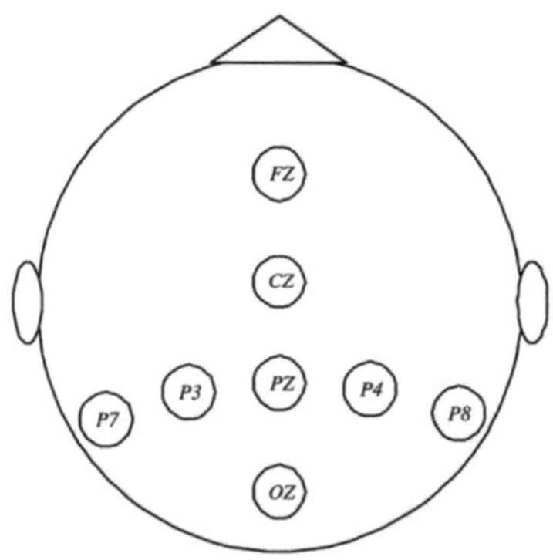

Fig. 12. The best configuration with 8 electrodes given by Hoffman et al. (Hoffman et al., 2008), (Hoffman et al., 2009).

7.3.4 Feature vectors construction

The samples from the selected electrodes were concatenated to obtain matrices of feature vectors. Each matrix is composed of N_e lines and N_t columns, where N_e denotes the number of electrodes and N_t denotes the number of temporal samples (feature vectors) in one trial. Due to the trial duration of 1000 *ms* and the downsampling to 32 *Hz* in (Hoffman et al., 2008) and (Hoffman et al., 2009), N_t is always taken equal to 32. In this work, we consider only matrices of dimension 8 × 32, i.e. each matrix O contains a sequence of 32 feature vectors $O = \{\mathbf{O}_1, \mathbf{O}_2, ..., \mathbf{O}_{32}\}$, $\mathbf{O}_t \in \mathbb{R}^K$, $K = 8$. For the purpose of our *HMMs* or *SVM* training and testing schemes, we divided the set of all matrices corresponding to each subject into two parts: training set and testing set. Each set contains six subsets of multiple observation sequences (feature matrices $\{O_1, O_2, ..., O_L\}$, $L \geq 1$), one subset for each image (Task) issued from different trials. Fig. 13 summarizes the training and data structures used in this work

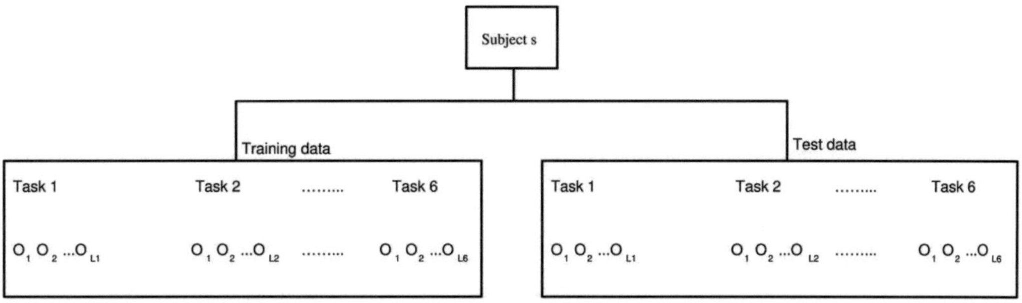

Fig. 13. Structures of the training and testing data sets for subject s, $1 \leq s \leq 8$. There are six subsets of multiple observation sequences (feature matrices $\{O_1, O_2, ...,O_L\}$, $L \geq 1$), one subset for each image (Task). Each matrix is of dimension 8 ×32.

7.4 Method

In this section, we give the *HMM* and *SVM* training schemes and their implementations in the context of our work.

7.5 *HMM* training algorithm

Given a set of L training data sequences $\{O_1, O_2, ..., O_L\}$, $O_l = \{\mathbf{O}_1,\mathbf{O}_2, ...,\mathbf{O}_{T_l}\}$, $1 \leq l \leq L$ issued from one of Z classes of stochastic processes p_z, $z \in 1, 2, 3, ..., Z$. The problem of the training in our work is to build Z *HMMs* for each process p_z.

We consider that each *HMM* contains an optimal state number N_{opt} of internal states to be determined automatically between N_{min} and N_{max}. In order to determine N_{opt}, we developed an optimal state number selection algorithm based on the Bayesian Inference Criterion. This algorithm constructs a number of *HMMs* with different number of states between *Nmin* and *Nmax* given by the user. For every state number, each iteration is initialized by the most appropriate model using data clustering, and by the rejection of the least linked state or the rejection of the least probable state of the previous iteration. Consequently, every training iteration begins by a more precise model. After constructing these *HMMs*, the algorithm selects the optimal *HMM* with the number of states that maximize the *BIC*.

Given N_{min} and N_{max}, the algorithm may be summarized as follows:

1. Initialization (clustering): estimate the initial *HMM* λ_0 with N_{max} states using k-mean clustering algorithm.
2. While $N \geq N_{min}$, do:
   a. run a training algorithm such a Baum-Welch algorithm (used in this work) until some convergence criterion is satisfied
   b. calculate and save the selection criterion, $BIC(N)$, of the current model

$$BIC(N) = \log P(O|\lambda_N) - \frac{F_N}{2}\log(T_t).$$

F_N is the total number of free parameters of the current estimated *HMM* (λ_N) and T_t be the total number of observations in all training observation sequences, i.e. $T_t = \sum_{l=1}^{L} T_l$

c. determine the number of zeros in each line of the state transition matrix, *A*.

d. select the best initialization method for the next *HMM* according to the following criterion:

   i. if all the lines of *A* contain zeros, then make a clustering of the observation data.

   ii. if all the lines of *A* don't contain zeros but only some lines, then find and reject the state with minimal connections to other states.

   iii. else, calculate the least probable state and reject it.

e. obtain a reduced model $\overline{\lambda}$

f. Fixe $N \leftarrow N - 1$ and λ_N $\overline{\lambda}$ and go to step 2

In this work we consider only a single *Gaussian pdf*, so **B** may be defined as **B** = {$\overline{\ }_i$, Σ_i}, i = 1, 2, ...,N. In this case F_N is calculated by

$$F_N = N(N-1) + N[K + (K(K+1))/2] + (N-1),$$

where $\mathbf{O}_t \in \mathbb{R}^K$. In our case, we used $N_{min} = 2$ and $N_{max} = 4$. These values were chosen in order to not constraint the clustering algorithm because the number of feature vectors is always equal to 32 (see section 7.2). The training and testing data sets for each subject described in section 7.2 were used for the following training and testing schemes:

7.5.1 Training scheme

Using the above algorithm, the goal of this scheme is to construct, for each subject, six *HMMs*: *HMM*1, *HMM*2, .., *HMM*6 corresponding to six images (Tasks). Each *HMM* is constructed with either 2 states, 3 states or 4 states. The training data sequences for all subjects $s, 1 \le s \le 8$ and for the six images, all collected from different trials (see section 7.2), are given by the set {*Tr_s_I*}, $1 \le s \le 8$, $1 \le I \le 6$, where .*Tr*. and .*I*. denote training and image (or task) number respectively.

7.5.2 Off-line testing scheme

Our task is to classify six given testing feature sequences into class I, $1 \le I \le 6$. In order to make off-line (or on-line detection in future work) of these sequences, a stochastic dynamic programming based (*Viterbi decoding algorithm*) (Rabiner, 1989) has been used. This algorithm gives at the same time the solution to problems 1 and 2 of *HMMs* discussed in section 6.2.2. In this case, the likelihoods of the data sequence are compared with respect to all six built *HMMs*. The selected *HMM* (i.e. task) is the model that maximize the likelihood. The testing data sequences for all subjects $s, 1 \le s \le 8$ and for the six images, all collected from six trials (Hoffman et al., 2008), (Hoffman et al., 2009), are given by the set {*Te_s_I*}, $1 \le s \le 8$, $1 \le I \le 6$, where *Te* and *I* denote testing and image (or task) number respectively. Fig 14 show the training and testing schemes for one subject and for six images.

7.5.3 Multiclass SVM (M-SVM)

In our work, we used a modified version of the *multiclass SVM* (*M-SVM*). The *M-SVM* method adopted in this work is the *one-versus-all*. This method is done by winner takes-all

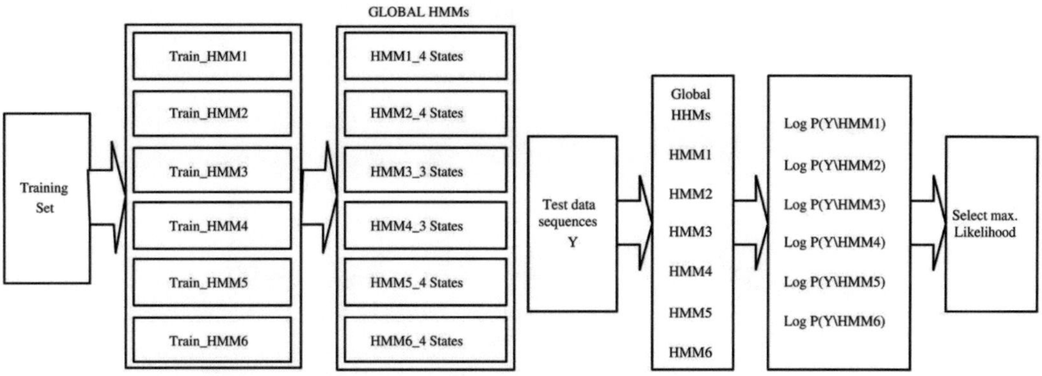

Fig. 14. Left: Training scheme for one subject and for six images. Right: Testing scheme for one subject given one or more task-related sequences.

combination strategy (Friedman, 1996), the outputs of the *binary one-vs-all classifiers* are compared and the most probable output among the other ones is chosen. The ith *SVM* is trained with all of the examples in the ith class with positive labels, and the rest with negative labels. An optimal hyperplane is constructed to separate N/M positive examples from $N(M - 1)/M$ negative examples where M is the number of *SVMs* and N is the number of the training examples used to construct an *SVM* for a given class. The same training and testing data structures, described in sections 7.2, 7.5.1 and 7.5.2, were used for *SVM* training and testing. To train or to test the *SVM* for a one subject, a number of $6 \times L$ training or testing feature matrices for all 6 tasks corresponding to this subject were concatenated and fed together to the *M-SVM* algorithm.

7.6 Results

The performance of *BCI* depends on different evaluation parameters. Among these evaluation parameters of interest in this work is the classification accuracy. This section reports experimental evaluations of the classification accuracy based on the testing scheme introduced in section 7.5.2. Using 60 testing feature matrices for all tasks corresponding to each subject (10 feature matrices for each task), the obtained classification results give the highest percentages of classification rates for the two applied approaches *SVM* and *HMMs*. The highest classification percent rates for all subjects are shown in the diagonals of the confusion matrices given in Table 1, see (Appendix). To conclude on the obtained results, we consider the case of comparison between the one of the more severely disabled subject, i.e. subject 3 (late-stage *amyotrophic lateral sclerosis*) and one of the able-bodied subjects, i.e subject 6 (subject had no known neurological deficits). Fig. 15 show the *HMMs-SVM* based comparative result for subject 3 and for subject 6. Fig. 15 and Table 1 show that the overall classification percent rates give a satisfactory and promising results for all the disabled subjects compared to the able-bodied ones. Fig. 16 show the *HMMs-SVM* based comparative results of the means and standard deviations of all the tasks generated by all subjects.

Fig. 16 show that

- In both the *HMMs* and the *SVM* cases, the means and the standard deviations of the classification percent rates in the disabled subjects are approximately the same or slightly higher than those in the able-bodied.

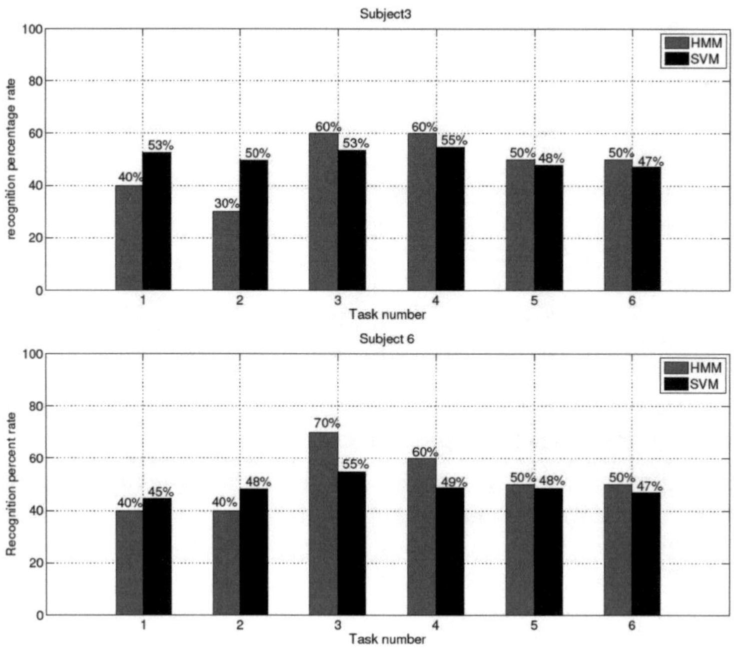

Fig. 15. Classification percent rates versus task number for subject 3 (top): late-stage amyotrophic lateral sclerosis and for subject 6 (down): subject had no known neurological deficits.

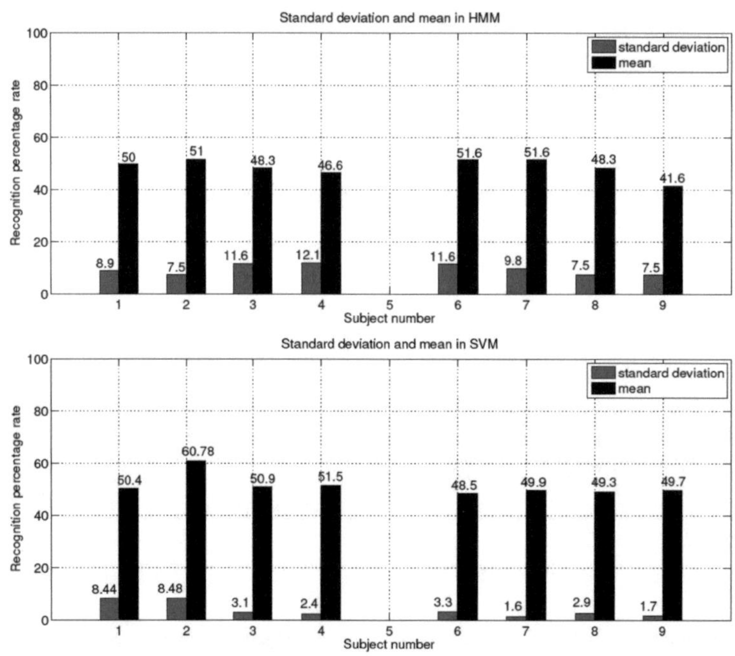

Fig. 16. Means and standard deviations of the classification percent rates in all tasks versus subject number (top: *HMMs* case, down: *SVM* case).

- In both the *HMMs* and the *SVM* cases, the means of the classification percent rates for the disabled subjects (except subject 2) as well as for the able-bodied subjects (except subject 9) are approximately uniformly distributed.
- The standard deviations of the classification percent rates for all subjects in the *SVM* case are less than or equal to those in the *HMMs* case.

These results give a way to study the ability of the different persons to learn the different *P300*-based *BCI* tasks.

8. Conclusions

This chapter have introduced a comprehensive survey of *signal processing, feature extraction/ selection* and *classification* methods used to provide the readers with guidelines on design *brain-computer interfaces* (*BCIs*). Based on the results given by (Bashashati et al., 2007) and (Lotte et al., 2007), this chapter shows which method have received more attention by the *BCI* community prior to 2006. However, other existing methods, not currently applied in *BCI* design, could be explored. The exploration of new methods would be strongly driven by the new properties that will have to be taken into consideration in the real future applications of *BCIs*.
As a contribution to the *classification* methods, a *Hidden Markov Models* (*HMMs*) and *support vector machines* (*SVM*) approaches for task *classification* in *P300*-based *BCI* system is presented. In the *HMMs* case, we proposed a training algorithm which is able to select automatically the optimal number of *HMM*-related states corresponding to each set of *EEG* training records. In the *SVM* case, we applied a *multiclass SVM* based on the *one-versus-all* method. The *confusion matrices* give a correct classification rates for the able-bodied subjects as well as for the disabled subjects. The comparative results demonstrate that the two approaches are promising. If the *HMMs* are not constructed correctly or the training data set is not sufficient, the *HMM* approach gives in this case a low classification rates. In such cases, a hybrid *HMM-SVM* may be employed, where the *HMM* is used as a *dynamic classifier* and the *SVM* is used as a good *discriminative classifier* by considering all the training examples in the training data set and train all the task-related models simultaneously. The authors are currently working on extending this work to include off-line and on-line training and classification schemes by using this strategy. The information transfer rate (bit rate) will be taken into account to include both accuracy and speed of a *BCI* system.

9. Acknowledgments

The authors would like to thank Dr. U. Hoffman and the EPFL-Brain-Computer team for the data and the software given in (Hoffman et al., 2008) that they were used in this work. The authors would like also to thank Dr. A. Bashashati for his authorization to use or modify some figures given in the paper (Bashashati et al., 2007) to illustrate some sections given in this chapter.

10. References

Anderson, C.W. & Sijercic, Z. (1996). Classication of EEG signals from four subjects during five mental tasks. In Solving Engineering Problems with Neural Networks.

Proceedings of the International Conference on Engineering Applications of Neural Networks (EANN.96).

Anderson, C.W.; Stolz, E. A. & Shamsunder, S. (1998). Multivariate autoregressive models for classification of spontaneous electroencephalographic signals during mental tasks. *IEEE Trans Biomed Eng*, 45, pp. 277-286.

Altenmüller, E. O.; Gerloff, C. (1999). Psychophysiology and the EEG. In: *Niedermeyer E, Lopes da Silva FH*, editors. Electroencephalography: basic principles, clinical applications and related fields, 4th ed. Baltimore, MD: Williams and Wilkins, pp. 637-655.

Al-ani, T. & Hamam, Y. (2010). A low Complexity Simulated Annealing Approach For Training Hidden Markov Models. *Int. J. of Operational Research (IJOR)*, (Accepted for publication), Vol. 8, No. 3.

Bayliss, J. D. & Ballard, D. H. (1999). Single trial P300 recognition in a virtual environment. *Proc. Int. ICSC Symp. on Soft Computing in Biomedicine*, (Genova, Italy).

Bayliss, J. D. & Ballard, D. H. (2000a). Recognizing evoked potentials in a virtual environment. *Advances in Neural Information Processing Systems*, Vol 12, ed S A Solla, T K Leen and K R Müller (Cambridge, MA: MIT Press), pp. 3-9.

Bayliss, J. D. & Ballard, D. H. (2000b). A virtual reality testbed for brain-computer interface research *IEEE Trans. on Rehabilitation Engineering*, Vol. 8, pp. 188-190.

Bayliss, J. D.; Inverso, S. A. & Tentler, A. (2004). Changing the P300 Brain-Computer Interface. *Journal of CyberPsychology & Behavior*, Vol. 7, No.6, pp.694-704.

Bayliss, J. D. & Inverso, S. A. (2005). Automatic Error Correction Using P3 Response Verification for a Brain-Computer Interface. *Proc. 11th International Conference on Human- Computer Interaction*, July 22-27, Las Vegas, NV. Mahwah: Lawrence Relbaum Associates.

Bashashati, A.;Ward R. K. & Birch, G. E. (2005). A new design of the asynchronous brainŰ - computer interface using the knowledge of the path of features. *Proc. 2nd IEEE-EMBS Conf. on Neural Engineering*, (Arlington, VA), pp. 101-104.

Bashashati, A.; Fatourechi, M.;Ward R. K. & Birch, G. E. (2007). A survey of signal processing algorithms in brain-computer interfaces based on electrical brain signals, *J. Neural Eng.*, June, Vol. 4, No. 2, pp. R32-R57.

Bellman, R. (1961). Adaptive Control Processes: A Guided Tour. Princeton University Press, New Jersey.

Bell, C. J.; Shenoy, P.; Chalodhorn, R. & Rao, R. P. N. (2008). Control of a humanoid robot by a noninvasive brainŰcomputer interface in humans, *J. Neural Eng.* 5, pp. 214-220.

Bennett, K. P. & Campbell, C. (2000). Support vector machines: hype or hallelujah?, *ACM SIGKDD Explor. Newslett.*, pp. 21-13.

Birbaumer, N.; Flor, H.; Ghanayim, N.; Hinterberger, T.; Iverson, I.; Taub, E.; Kotchoubey, B.; Kubler, A. &. Perelmouter, J. (1999). A spelling device for the paralyzed, *Nature*, Vol.398, No. 6725, pp. 297-298.

Birbaumer, N.; Kübler, A.; Ghanayim, N.; Hinterberger, T.; Perelmouter, J.; Kaiser, J.; Iversen, I.; Kotchoubey, B.; Neumann, N. & Flor, H. (2000). The thought translation device (TTD) for completely paralyzed patients. *IEEE Trans. Rehab. Eng.*, Vol. 8, No. 2, pp. 190-192.

Birbaumerl, N. & Cohen, L. G. (2007). Brain-computer interfaces: communication and restoration of movement in paralysis. *The journal of Physiology*, Vol. 579, No. 3, pp. 637-642.

Blankertz B; Curio, G. & Müller, K. R. (2002). Classifying single trial EEG: towards brain computer interfacing. *Adv. Neural Inf. Process. Syst. (NIPS 01)*, Vol. 14, 157-164.

Blankertz, B.; Dornhege, G.; Krauledat, M.; Müller, K. R.; Kunzmann, V.; Losch, F. & Curio, G. (2006). The Berlin brain-computer interface: EEG-based communication without subject training. *IEEE Trans. on Rehabilitation Engineering*, Vol. 14, No. 2., pp. 147-152.

Boostani, R. & Moradi, M. H. (2004). A new approach in the BCI research based on fractal dimension as feature and adaboost as classifier. *Journal of Neural Engineering*, Vol. 1, No. 4, pp. 212-217.

Bostanov, V. (2004). BCI competition 2003-data sets ib and IIb: feature extraction from eventrelated brain potentials with the continuous wavelet transform and the t-value scalogram. *IEEE Trans. Biomed. Eng.*, Vol. 51, pp. 1057-1061.

Breiman, L. (1998). Arcing classifiers. *Ann. Stat.*, Vol. 26, pp. 801-849.

Brill, F.Z.; Brown, D.E. & Martin, W.N. (1992). Fast Genetic Selection of Features for Neural Network Classsers. *IEEE Transactions on Neural Networks*, Vol. 3, pp. 324-328.

Burges, C. J. C. (1998). A tutorial on support vector machines for pattern recognition. *Knowl. Discov. Data Min.*, Vol. 2, pp. 121-167.

Burke, D. P.; Kelly, S. P.; deChazal, P.; Reilly, R. B. & Finucane, C. (2005). A parametric feature extraction and classification strategy for brain-computer interfacing. *IEEE Trans. On Rehabilitation Engineering*, Vol. 13, No. 1.

Cincotti, F.; Scipione, A.; Tiniperi, A.; Mattia, D.; Marciani, M. G.; Millán J. del R; Salinari, S.; Bianchi, L. & Babiloni, F. (2003). Comparison of different feature classifiers for brain computer interfaces. *Proc. 1st Int. IEEE EMBS Conf. on Neural Engineering*.

Comon, P. (1994). Independent Component Analysis: a new concept?. *Signal Processing, Elsevier*, Vol. 36, No. 3, pp. 287-314.

Congedo, M.; Lotte, F. & Lécuyer, A. (2006). Classification of movement intention by spatially filtered electromagnetic inverse solutions. *Physics in Medicine and Biology*, Vol. 51, No. 8, pp. 1971-1989.

Cortes, C. & Vapnik, V. (1995). Support vector networks. Machine Learning. *Machine Learning*, Vol. 20, pp. 273-297.

Dien, J. (1998). Issues in the application of the average reference: Review, critiques, and recommendations. Behavior Research Methods. *Instruments, & Computers*, Vol. 30, No. 1, pp. 34-43.

Dietterich, T. & Bakiri, G. (1995). Solving multiclass learning problems via error-correcting output codes. *Journal of Artificial Intelligence Research*, Vol. 2, pp. 263-286.

Dobkin B. H. (2007). Brain-computer interface technology as a tool to augment plasticity and outcomes for neurological rehabilitation, *Journal of physiology*, vol. 579, No. 3, pp. 637-642.

Dornhege, G.; Millán, J. del R.; Hinterberger, T.; McFarland, D. J.; Müller, K-R; Sejnowski, T. J. (2007). An introduction to brain computer interfacing. In: *Towards. Brain-Computer Interfacing*, MIT Press, Cambridge.

Duda, R. O.; Hart, P. E. & Stork, D. G. (2001). Pattern Recognition. *2nd. ed. (New York: Wiley-Interscience).*

Duan, K-B.; Rajapakse, J.C. & Nguyen, M.F. (2007). One-versus-one and one-versus-all multiclass SVM-RFE for gene selection in cancer classification. In: *EvoBIO*, pp. 228-234.

Farwell, L. A. & Donchin, E. (1988). Talking off the top of your head: Towards a mental prosthesis utilizing event-related brain potentials Electroencephalogr. *Clin. Neurophysiol.*, Vol. 80 510-523.

Flotzinger, D.; Pregenzer, M. & Pfurtscheller, G. (1994). Feature selection with distinction sensitive learning vector quantisation and genetic algorithms. *Proc. IEEE Int. Conf. on Neural Networks*, (Orlando, FL), pp. 3448-3451

Friedman, J. H. (1996). Another approach to polychotomous classification. *Technical report*, Department of Statistics, Stanford University.

Friedman, J. H. K. (1997). On bias, variance, 0/1-loss, and the curse-of-dimensionality. *Data Min. Knowl. Discov.*, Vol. 1, pp. 55-77.

Friedman, D.; Slater, M.; Steed, A.; Leeb, R.; Pfurtscheller, G. & Guger, C. (2004). Using a brain-computer-interface in a highly immersive virtual reality. In *IEEE VR Workshop*.

Fukunaga, K. (1972). In: *Introduction to Statistical Pattern Recognition*, Oxford, UK., Clarendon.

Fukunaga, K. (1990). Statistical Pattern Recognition. *2nd edn (New York: Academic).*

Garcia, G.; Ebrahimi, T. & Vesin, J. M. (2003). Support vector EEG classification in the Fourier and time-frequency correlation domains. *Proc. 1st IEEE-EMBS Conf. on Neural Engineering*, Capri Island, Italy, pp. 591-594.

Garrett, D.; Peterson, D. A.; Anderson, C. W. & nd Thaut, M. H. (2003). Comparison of linear, nonlinear, and feature selection methods for EEG signal classification. *IEEE Trans. On Rehabilitation Engineering*, Vol. 11, pp. 141-144.

Geman, S.; Bienenstock, E. & Doursat, R. (1992). Neural Networks and the Bias/Variance Dilemma. *Neural Computation*, Vol. 4, pp. 1-58.

Goldberg, D.E. (1989). Genetic Algorithms in Search, Optimization. and Machine Learning. *Addison-Wesley.*

Grave de Peralta Menendez, Gonzalez Andino, R.; S.; Perez L.,; Ferrez, P. & Millán, J. (2005). Non-invasive estimation of local field potentials for neuroprosthesis control. *Cognitive Processing*, Special Issue on Motor Planning in Humans and Neuroprosthesis Control.

Gupta, S. & Singh, H. (1996) Preprocessing EEG signals for direct human-system interface. Intelligence and Systems. *IEEE International Joint Symposia on*, pp. 32-37.

Guger, C.; Ramoser, H. & Pfurtscheller G. (2000). Real-Time EEG Analysis with Subject-Specific Spatial Patterns for a Brain-Computer Interface (BCI). *IEEE Trans. on rehabilitation engineering*, Vol. 8, No. 4, pp. 447-456.

Guger, C.; Schlögl, A.; Neuper, C.; Walterspacher, D.; Strein, T. & Pfurtscheller, G. (2001). Rapid prototyping of an EEG-based brain-computer interface (BCI). *IEEE Trans. Rehab. Eng.*, Vol. 9, No. 1, pp. 49-58.

Hagemann, D.; Naumann, E. & Thayer, J.F. (2001). The quest for the EEG reference revisited: A glance from brain asymmetry research. *Psychophysiology*, Vol. 38, 847-857.

Haibin, Z; Xu, W. & Hong, W. (2008). Brain-computer interface design using relative wavelet energy. *The 2nd International Conference on Control and Decision*, pp. 3558-3561, 2-4 July.

Haselsteiner, E. & Pfurtscheller, G. (2000). Using time-dependant neural networks for EEG classification. *IEEE Trans. on Rehabilitation Engineering*, Vol. 8, pp. 457-463.

Haykin, S. (1994). Neural Network: A Comprehensive Foundation. *New York: Macmillan College Publishing Company*.

Helmy, S.; Al-ani, T.; Hamam, Y. & El-madbouly, E. (2008). P300 Based Brain-Computer Interface Using Hidden Markov Models. *ISSNIP 2008*, Sydney, 15-18 Dec.

Hinterberger, T.; Kubler, A.; Kaiser, J.; Neumann, N. & Birbaumer, N. (2003). A brain-computer interface (BCI) for the locked-in: comparison of different EEG classifications for the thought translation device. *Electroencephalogr. Clin. Neurophysiol.* Vol. 114, pp. 416-25.

Hinterberger, T.;Weiskopf, N.; Veit, R.;Wilhelm, B.; Betta, E. & Birbaumer, N. (2004). An EEGDriven Brain-Computer Interface Combined With Functional Magnetic Resonance Imaging (fMRI). *IEEE Transactions On Biomedical Engineering*, June, Vol. 51, No. 6.

Hjorth, B. (1970). EEG analysis based on time domain properties. *Electroencephalography and Clinical Neurophysiology*, Vol. 29, No. 3, pp. 306-310.

Hoffmann, U.; Vesin, J.-M.; Ebrahimi, T. & Diserens K. (2008). An efficient P300-based braincomputer interface for disabled subjects, *Journal of Neuroscience Methods*, Vol. 167, No. 1, pp. 115-125.

Hoffmann, U.; Vesin, J.-M.; Ebrahimi, T. & Diserens K. (2009). An efficient P300- based brain-computer interface for disabled subjects. Available from URL: http://mmspl.epfl.ch/page33712.html. Visited on September, 10, 2009.

Huan, N.-J. & Palaniappan, R. (2004a). Classification of mental tasks using fixed and adaptive autoregressive models of EEG signals. In: *IEMBS .04. 26th Annual International Conference of the IEEE Engineering in Medicine and Biology Society*, pp. 1-5.

Huang, N. E.; Shen, Z.; Long, S. R.; Wu, M. C.; Shih, H. H.; Zheng, Q.; Yen, N. C.; Tung, C. C. & Liu, H. H. (1998). The empirical mode decomposition and the Hilbert spectrum for nonlinear and non-stationary time series analysis. *Proceedings of the Royal Society*, Vol. 454, pp. 903-995.

Huan, N.-J. & Palaniappan, R. (2004b). Neural network classification of autoregressive features from electroencephalogram signals for brain-computer interface design. *J. Neural Eng.*, Vol. 1, pp. 142-150.

Hung, C-I.; Lee, P-L.; Wu, Y-T.; Yeh, T-C. & Hsieh, J-C. (2005). Recognition of Motor Imagery Electroencephalography Using Independent Component Analysis and Machine Classifiers. *Annals of Biomedical Engineering*, Vol. 33, No. 8, pp. 1053-1070.

Hyvärinen, A. & Oja, E. (2000). Independent Component Analysis: A Tutorial. *Neural Networks*, Vol. 13, No. 4-5. , pp. 411-430.

Ivanova, I.; Pfurtscheller, G. & Andrew, C. (1995). AI-based classification of single-trial EEG data. *Proc. 17th Annual Int. Conf. of the IEEE Engineering in Medicine and Biology Society*, (Montreal, Canada), pp. 703704.

Jain, A. K. & Chandrasekaran, B. (1982). Dimensionality and sample size considerations in pattern recognition practice. In: *Handbook of Statistics*, Vol. 2, pp. 835-855.

Jain, A. K.; Duin, R. P.W. & Mao, J. (2000). Statistical pattern recognition: a review. *IEEE Trans. Pattern Anal. Mach. Intell.*, Vol. 22, pp. 4-37.

Jung, T-P.; Humphries, C., Lee, T-W., Makeig, S.; McKeown, M. J.; Iragui, V. & Sejnowski T. J. (1998). Removing electroencephalographic artefacts: comparison between ICA and PCA. *Neural Networks Signal Processing*, Vol. III, pp. 63-72.

Jung, T-P.; Makeig, S.; Westerfieldad, M.; Townsendad, J.; Courchesnead, E. & Sejnowski T. J. (2000). Removal of eye activity artefacts from visual event-related potentials in normal and clinical subjects. *Clinical Neurophysiology*, Vol. 111, pp. 1745-1758.

Kaper, M.; Meinicke, P.; Grossekathoefer, U.; Lingner, T. & Ritter, H. (2004). BCI competition 2003-data set iib: support vector machines for the p300 speller paradigm. *IEEE Trans. Biomed. Eng.*, Vol. 51, pp. 1073-1076.

Keirn, ZA. & Aunon, JI. (1990). A new mode of communication between man and his surroundings. *IEEE Trans Biomed Eng*, 37, pp. 1209-1214.

Kohonen, T. (1990). The Self-Organizing Map. *Proc. IEEE.* Vol. 78, No. 9, pp. 1161-1180.

Koles, Z. J. (1991). The quantitative extraction and topographic mapping of the abnormal components in the clinical EEG, *Electroenceph. Clin. Neurophysiol.*, Vol. 79, pp. 440-447.

Lang, W.; Cheyne, D.; Hollinger, P.; Gerschlager, W. & Lindinger, G. (1996). Electric and magnetic fields of the brain accompanying internal simulation of movement, *Cogn Brain Res*, 3, pp. 125-129.

Lehmann, E. & Skrandies,W. (1984). Spatial Analysis of Evoked Potentials in Man - A Review. *Progress in Neurobiology*, Vol. 23, pp. 227-250.

Lee, H. & Choi, S. (2003). PCA+HMM+SVM for EEG pattern classification. In: Proceedings of the Seventh International Symposium on Signal Processing and Its Applications.

Lemm, S.; Schafer, C. & Curio, G. (2004). BCI competition 2003-data set iii: probabilistic modelling of sensorimotor mu rhythms for classification of imaginary hand movements. *IEEE Trans. Biomed. Eng.*, Vol. 51, pp. 1077-1080.

Lécuyer A.; Lotte, F.; Reilly, R. B.; Leeb, R.; Hirose, M.; Slater, M. (2008). Brain-Computer Interfaces, Virtual Reality, and Videogames. *IEEE Computer*, Vol. 41, No. 10, pp.66-72.

Lotte, F.; Congedo, M.; Lécuyer, A.; Lamarcheand, F. & Arnaldi, B. (2007). A review of classification algorithms for EEG-based brain-computer interfaces. *J. Neural Eng.*, 4, pp. R1-R13.

Mason, S; Bashashati, A.; Fatourechi, M.; Navarro, K. & Birch, G. (2007). A comprehensive survey of brain interface technology designs, *Annals of Biomedical Engineering*, Vol. 35, No. 2, pp. 137-169.

Meinicke, P.; Kaper, M.; Hoppe, F.; Heumann, M., & Ritter, H. (2003). Improving Transfer Rates in Brain Computer Interfacing: a Case Study. In: *Advances in Neural*

Information Processing Systems, Cambridge, MA, 15, Eds.: Suzanna Becker and Sebastian Thrun and Klaus Obermayer, MIT Press.

McFarland, D. J.; McCane, L. M.; David, S. V. &Wolpaw, J. R. (1997a). Spatial filter selection for EEG-based communication Electroencep. *Clin. Neurophysiol.*, Vol. 103, pp. 386-394.

McFarland, D. J.; Lefkowicz, A. T. & Wolpaw, J. R. (1997b). Design and operation of an EEGbased brain-computer interface (BCI) with digital signal processing technology. *Behav. Res. Meth. Instrum. Comput.*, Vol. 29, pp. 337-345.

McFarland D. J.; Miner L. A.; Vaughan T. M. & Wolpaw J. R. (2000). Mu and beta rhythm topographies during motor imagery and actual movement. Brain Topogr, 3, pp. 177- 186.

McFarland, D. J. &Wolpaw, J. R. (2005). Sensorimotor rhythm-based brain-computer interface (BCI): feature selection by regression improves performance. *IEEE Trans. on Rehabilitation Engineering*, Vol. 13, No. 3, pp. 372-379.

Millan, J.; Mourino, J.; Cincotti, F.; Varsta, M.; Heikkonen, J.; Topani, F.; Marciani, M. G.; Kaski, K. & Babiloni, F. (2000). Neural networks for robust classification of mental tasks. *Proc. 22nd Annual Int. Conf. of the IEEE Engineering in Medicine and Biology Society*, (Chicago, IL), pp. 1380-1382.

Millan, J.; Mourino, J.; Franze, M.; Cincotti, F.; Varsta, M.; Heikkonen, J. & Babiloni, F. (2002). A local neural classifier for the recognition of EEG patterns associated to mental tasks. *IEEE Trans. Neural Netw.*, Vol. 13 pp. 678-686.

Millán J. R. & Mouriño, J. (2003). Asynchronous BCI and local neural classifiers: an overview of the adaptive brain interface project. *IEEE Trans. on Rehabilitation Engineering*, Vol. 11 159-61.

Moghaddam, B. (2002).Principal Manifolds and Probabilistic Subspaces for Visual Recognition. *IEEE Trans. Patern Analysis and Machine Intelligence*, Vol. 24, No. 6, pp. 780-788.

Müller-Gerking, J.; Pfurtscheller, G. & Flyvbjerg, H. (1999). Designing optimal spatial filters for single-trial EEG classification in a movement task. *Clinical Neurophysiology*, Vol. 110, No. 5, pp.787-798.

Müller, K. R.; Anderson, C.W. & Birch, G. E. (2003). Linear and nonlinear methods for brain-computer interfaces. *IEEE Trans. on Rehabilitation Engineering*, Vol. 11, pp. 165-169.

Musha, T.; Terasaki, Y.; Haque, H.A. & Ivanitsky, G.A. (1997). Feature extraction from EEGs associated with emotions. *Artificial Life and Robotics*, Vol. 1, No. 1, pp. 15-19.

Müller, K. R.; Krauledat, M.; Dornhege, G.; Curio, G. & Blankertz, B. (2004). Machine learning techniques for brain-computer interfaces. *Biomed. Technol.*, Vol. 49, pp. 11-22.

Nakamura, A.; Sugi T.; Ikeda, A.; Kakigi, R. & Shibasaki, H. (1996). Clinical application of automatic integrative interpretation of awake background EEG: quantitative interpretation, report making, and detection of artefacts and reduced vigilance level. *Electroenceph. Clin. Neurophysiol.*, Vol. 98, pp. 103-112.

Neuper, C. & Pfurtscheller, G. (1999a). Motor imagery and ERD Related Desyncronization, *Handbook of Electroencepalography and Clinical Neurophysiology*, (Revised Edition), pp. 303-525, Vol. 6, Elsevier, Amsterdam.

Neuper, C.; Schlögl, A. & Pfurtscheller, G. (1999b). Enhancement of left-right sensorimotor EEG differences during feedback-regulated motor imagery. *J. Clin. Neurophysiol.*, Vol. 16, pp. 373-382.

Ng, A. Y. & Jordan, M. I. (2002). On generative versus discriminative classifiers: a comparison of logistic regression and naive Bayes. *Neural Information Processing Systems, Ng, A.Y., and Jordan, M.*

Nicolelis, M.A.L. (2001). Actions from Thoughts. In: *Nature*, Vol. 409, January 18, pp. 403-407.

Obermaier, B.; Neuper, C., Guger, C. & Pfurtscheller, G. (2000). Information transfer rate in a five-classes brain-computer interface. *IEEE Trans. Neural Syst. Rehabil. Eng.*, Vol. 9, pp. 283-288.

Obermeier, B.; Guger, C.; Neuper, C. & Pfurtscheller, G. (2001). Hidden markov models for online classification of single trial EEG. *Pattern recognition letters*, pp. 1299-1309.

Offner, F.F. (1950). The EEG as Potential Mapping: The Value of the Average Monopolar Reference. *Electroencephalography and Clinical Neurophysiology*, VoI. 2, pp. 215-216.

Pearson, K. (1901). On Lines and Planes of Closest Fit to Systems of Points in Space. *Philosophical Magazine* Vol. 2, No. 6, pp. 559- 572.

Penny, W. D. & Roberts, S. J. (1999). EEG-based communication via dynamic neural network models. *Proc. Int. Joint Conf. on Neural Networks.*

Peters, B. O.; Pfurtscheller, G. & Flyvbjerg, H. (2001). Automatic differentiation of multichannel EEG signals. *IEEE Trans. Biomed. Eng.*, Vol. 48, pp. 111-116.

Pfurtscheller, G.; Kalcher J.; Neuper, C.; Flotzinger D & Pregenzer, M. (1996). On-line EEG classification during externally-paced hand movements using a neural network-based classifier. *Electroenceph. Clin. Neurophysiol.*, Vol. 99, pp. 416-425.

Pfurtscheller, G.; Neuper, C.; Flotzinger D & Pregenzer, M. (1997). EEG-based discrimination between imagination of right and left hand movement, *Electroenceph clin Neurophysiol*, 103, pp. 642-651.

Pfurtscheller, G. & Aranibar, A. (1977). Event related cortical desynchronization detected by power measurements of scalp EEG. *Electroenceph Clin Neurophysiol*, Vol. 42, pp. 817-826.

Pfurtscheller, G.; Neuper, C.; Schlogl, A. & Lugger, K. (1998). Separability of EEG signals recorded during right and left motor imagery using adaptive autoregressive parameters. *IEEE Trans. on Rehabilitation Engineering*, Vol. 6, pp. 316-325.

Pfurtscheller, G.; Neuper C.; Ramoserb H. & Müller-Gerking J. (1999a). Visually guided´lmotor imagery activates sensorimotor areas in humans. *Neuroscience Letters*, Vol. 269, No. 3, pp. 153-156.

Pfurtscheller, G. & Guger, C. (1999b). Brain-computer communication system: EEG-based control of hand orthesis in a tetraplegic patient. *Acta Chir. Austriaca*, Vol. 31 23-25.

Pfurtscheller, G. (1999c). EEG Event-related Desynchronisation (ERD) and Event-related Synchronisation (ERS). In *Niedermeyer*, pp. 958-967, E., Lopes da Silva, F.H. (Eds.), *Electroencephalography. Basic Principles, Clinical Applications, and Related Fields*, forth ed., Williams and Wilkins, Baltimore.

Pfurtscheller, G.; Neuper, C.; Guger, C.; Harkam, W.; Ramoser, H.; Schlogl, A.; Obermaier, B. & Pregenzer, M. (2000a). Current trends in Graz brain-computer interface (BCI) research. *IEEE Trans. on Rehabilitation Engineering*, Vol. 8, No. 2, pp. 216-219.

Pfurtscheller, G.; Guger, C.; Müller, G.; Krausz, G. & Neuper, C. (2000b). Brain oscillations control hand orthosis in a tetraplegic, *Neurosci. Lett.*, Vol.292, pp. 211-214.

Pfurtscheller, G. & Neuper, C. (2001). Motor imagery and direct brain-computer communication. *proceedings of the IEEE*, Vol. 89, No. 7, pp. 1123-1134.

Pfurtscheller, G.; Müller, G. R. ; Pfurtscheller, J.; Gerner, H. J. & Rupp, R. (2003). `Thought' - control of functional electrical stimulation to restore hand grasp in a patient with tetraplegia. *Neuroscience Letters*, V. 351, Issue 1, 6 November, pp. 33-36.

Platt, J.; Cristanini, N. & Shawe-Taylor, J. (2000) . Large margin DAGs for multiclass classification. *Advances in Neural Information Processing Systems*, Vol. 12, pp. 543-557, MIT Press.

Qin, L.; Ding, L. & He, B. (2004). Motor imagery classification by means of source analysis for brain computer interface applications. *Journal of Neural Engineering*, Vol. 1, No. 3, pp. 135-141.

Qin, L. & He, B. (2005). A wavelet-based time-frequency analysis approach for classification of motor imagery for brain-computer interface applications. *J. Neural Eng.*, Vol. 2, pp. 65-72.

Rabiner, L. R. (1989). A tutorial on hidden Markov models and selected applications in speech recognition. *Proc. IEEE*, Vol. 77, pp. 257-286.

Raudys, S. J. & Jain, A. K. (1991). Small sample size effects in statistical pattern recognition: Recommendations for practitioners. *IEEE Transactions on Pattern Analysis and Machine Intelligence*, Vol. 13, No. 3, pp. 252-264,.

Rakotomamonjy, A.; Guigue, V.; Mallet, G. & Alvarado, V. (2005). Ensemble of SVMs for improving brain computer interface p300 speller performances. *Int. Conf. on Artificial Neural Networks*.

Ramoser, H.; Müller-Gerking, J. & Pfurtscheller, G. (2000). Optimal spatial filtering of singletrial EEG during imagined hand movement. *IEEE Trans. Rehab. Eng.*, Vol. 8, pp. 441-446.

Roberts, S. J. & Penny,W. D. (2000). Real-time brain-computer interfacing: a preliminary study using Bayesian learning. *Med Biol Eng Comput.*, Jan, Vol. 38, No. 1, pp. 56-61.

Rubinstein, Y. D. & Hastie, T. (1997). Discriminative versus informative learning. In: *Proceedings of the Third International Conference on Knowledge Discovery and Data Mining*, pp. 49-53.

Salimi Khorshidi, G., Jaafari, A., Motie Nasrabadi, A., Hashemi Golpayegani, M. (2007). Modifying the Classic Peak Picking Technique Using a Fuzzy Multi Agent to Have an Accurate P300-based BCI. *EUSFLAT Conf.* (2) pp. 143-147.

Schwarz, G. (1978). Estimating the dimension of a model. *Ann. Statist.*, Vol. 6, No. 2, pp. 461-464.

Schlögl, A.; Flotzinger, D. & Pfurtscheller, G. (1997). Adaptive autoregressive modelling used for single-trial EEG classification. *Biomed. Technik*, Vol. 42, pp. 162-167.

Scherer, R.; Müller, G. R.; Neuper, C.; Graimann, B. & Pfurtscheller, G. (2004). An asynchronously controlled EEG-based virtual keyboard: improvement of the spelling rate. *IEEE Trans. Biomed. Eng.*, Vol. 51, pp. 979-984.

Schlögl, A.; Lee, F.; Bischof, H. & Pfurtscheller, G. (2005). Characterization of four-class motor imagery EEG data for the BCI-competition. *J. Neural Eng.*, Vol. 2, pp. L14-L22.

Scholkopf, B.; Mika, S.; Burges, C. J. C.; Knirsch, P.; müller, K. R.; Ratsch, G. & Smola., A. J. (1999). Input space versus feature space in kernel-based methods. *IEEE Trans. Neural Networks*, Vol. 10, No. 5, pp. 1000-1017.

Schölkopf, B. & Smolan A. J. (2002). Learning with kernels. *The MIT Press.*

Schlogl, Lugger, A.; K. & Pfurtscheller, G. (1997). Using adaptive autoregressive parameters for a brain-computer-interface experiment. In: *Proceedings 19th International Conference IEEE/EMBS*, pp. 1533-1535.

Solhjoo, S., Nasrabadi, A. M. & Golpayegani, M. R. H. (2005). Classification of chaotic signals using HMM classifiers: EEG-based mental task classification. *Proc. European Signal Processing Conference.*

Stanny, R. R. (1989). Mapping the event related Potentials of the brain: Theoretical issues, Technical considerations and computer programs. *Naval aerospace Medical Research Laboratory, Naval Air Station*, Pensacola, Florida 32506-5700.

Sun, S.; Lan, M. & Lu, Y. (2008). Adaptive EEG signal classification using stochastic approximation methods. *Proceedings of the 33rd IEEE International Conference on Acoustics, Speech, and Signal Processing (ICASSP)*, pp. 413-416.

Thomas C. (1977). Firefox, New York, NY: *Holt, Rinehart and Winston.*

Trad, D.; Helmy, S.; Al-ani, T.; Delaplace, S. (2009). Hidden Markov Models and Support Vector Machines applied to P300 Based Brain-Computer Interface - a Comparative study. *ICTA 09*, Hammamet, 7-9 Mai.

Urszula, S. T.; Urszula, M-k & Kozik, A. (1999). Blinking Artefact Recognition in EEG Signal Using Artificial Neural Network. In: *Fourth Conference Neural networks and Their Applications*, Czestochowa.

Vapnik, V. N. (1995). The nature off Statistical Learning Theory. *Springer-Verlag.*

Vapnik, V. N. (1999). An overview of statistical learning theory. *IEEE Trans. Neural Netw.*, Vol. 10, pp. 988-999.

Varsta, M.; Heikkonen, J.; Millan, J. D. R. & Mourino, J. (2000). Evaluating the performance of three feature sets for brain-computer interfaces with an early stopping MLP commitee. *Int. Conf. on Pattern Recognition*, (Barcelona, Spain), pp. 907-910.

Vidal, J. J. (1973), Toward direct brain-computer communication. In: *Annual Review of Biophysics and Bioengineering*, L. J. Mullins (Ed.), Annual Reviews, Inc., Palo Alto, Vol. 2, pp. 157-80.

Vidal, J. J. (1977), Real-time detection of brain events in EEG. In: *Proceedings of the IEEE*, May 1977, Vol. 65, No. 5, pp.633-641.

Vidaurre, C.; Schlögl, A.; Cabeza, R.; Scherer, R. & Pfurtscheller G. (2007). Study of On-Line Adaptive Discriminant Analysis for EEG-Based Brain Computer Interfaces. *IEEE Transactions On Biomedical Engineering*, Vol. 54, No. 3, March, pp. 550-556.

Vourkas, M.; Papadourakis, G. & Micheloyannis, S. (2000). Use of ann and hjorth parameters in mental-task discrimination. In: *First International Conference on Advances in Medical Signal and Information Processing*, pp. 327-332.

Wang, Y.; Berg, P. & Scherg, M. (1999). Common spatial subspace decomposition applied to analysis of brain responses under multiple task conditions: a simulation study. *IEEE Trans. Biomed. Eng.*, Vol. 110, Issue 4, pp. 604-614.

Wang, T.; Deng, J. & He, B. (2004a). Classifying EEG-based motor imagery tasks by means of time-frequency synthesized spatial patterns. *Clin. Neurophysiol.*, Vol. 115 2744-2753.

Wang, T.; Deng, J. & He, B. (2004b). Classification of motor imagery EEG patterns and their topographic representation. *Proc. 26th Annual Int. Conf. of the IEEE Engineering in Medicine and Biology Society*, (San Francisco, CA), pp. 4359-4362.

Weber, D.L. (2001) Scalp current density and source current modelling. http://dnl.ucsf.edu/users/dweber/dweber_docs/eeg_scd.html. Visited on September, 10, 2009.

Wessberg, J.; Stambaugh, C. R.; Kralik, J. D.; Beck, P. D.; Laubach, M.; Chapin, J. K.; Kim, J.; Biggs, S. J.; Srinivasan, M. A. & Nicolelis, M. A. (2000). Real-time prediction of hand trajectory by ensembles of cortical neurons in primates, *Nature*, 16 Nov, Vol. 408, pp. 361-365.

Wentrup, M. G.; Gramann, K.;Wascher, E. & Buss, M. (2005). Eeg source localization for brain-computer-interfaces. In: *2nd International IEEE EMBS Conference on Neural Engineering*, pp. 128-131.

Wolpaw, J. R.; McFarland, D. J. & Vaughan, T. M. (2000). Brain-computer interfaces for communication and control, *IEEE Trans. on Rehabilitation Engineering*, June, Vol. 8, No. 2, pp. 222-226.

Wolpaw, J. R.; Birbaumer, N.; McFarland, D. J.; Pfurtscheller, G. & Vaughan, T. M. (2002). Brain-computer interfaces for communication and control, *Clin. Neurophysiol*, 113, pp. 767-91.

Xu, B-G. & Song, A-G. (2008). Pattern recognition of motor imagery EEG using wavelet transform. *J. Biomedical Science and Engineering*, Vol. 1, pp. 64-67.

11. Appendix

Subj./Task	Taskl	Task2	Task3	Task4	Task5	Task6	Taskl	Task2	Task3	Task4	Task5	Task6
1/1	**50**	0	10	10	20	10	**66**	6	6	6	3	13
1/2	10	**40**	10	30	10	0	21	**47**	8	6	3	15
1/3	0	10	**50**	0	20	20	128	3	**49**	6	3	11
1/4	0	0	10	**60**	20	10	23	8	7	**45**	3	14
1/5	0	0	10	30	**60**	0	31	4	4	6	**43**	12
1/6	0	0	10	30	20	**40**	28	3	9	6	2	**52**
2/1	**60**	20	10	10	0	0	**58**	7	8	8	10	9
2/2	30	**50**	10	10	0	0	9	**48**	11	8	14	10
2/3	0	0	**50**	30	20	0	9	9	**55**	8	11	8
2/4	30	10	0	**60**	0	0	6	5	6	**72**	6	5
2/5	30	20	10	0	**40**	0	7	6	7	6	**67**	7
2/6	30	10	0	0	10	**50**	8	7	7	5	8	**65**
3/1	**40**	10	10	20	20	0	**53**	10	6	15	8	8
3/2	0	**30**	20	20	20	10	11	**50**	8	15	7	9
3/3	0	0	**60**	20	10	10	11	11	**53**	10	7	8
3/4	0	0	20	**60**	20	0	13	10	10	**55**	5	7
3/5	0	10	10	20	**50**	10	13	7	8	15	**48**	9
3/6	0	0	10	10	30	**50**	21	6	5	15	6	**47**
4/1	**30**	20.00	10	10	10	20	**51**	9	6	7	12	15
4/2	20	**60**	0	0	0	20	8	**51**	10	8	12	11
4/3	0	30	**40**	0	10	20	12	12	**52**	7	9	8
4/4	0	30	0	**40**	20	10	7	8	7	**48**	10	20
4/5	0	20	0	0	**60**	20	10	7	8	7	**55**	13
4/6	20	20	0	10	0	**50**	5	8	10	10	13	**53**
5/1 - 5/6	-	-	-	-	-	-	-	-	-	-	-	-
6/1	**40**	0	30	20	10	0	**45**	27	10	7	9	2
6/2	0	**40**	10	10	10	30	11	**48**	12	11	11	7
6/3	20	0	**70**	10	0	0	10	4	**55**	10	13	8
6/4	10	0	20	**60**	10	0	10	8	13	**49**	11	9
6/5	0	0	10	20	**20**	20	68	13	19	7	**48**	5
6/6	0	0	20	20	10	**50**	11	4	7	10	21	**47**
7/1	**40**	0	0	20	10	30	**49**	10	9	10	10	12
7/2	0	**50**	0	30	20	0	7	**51**	11	11	7	13
7/3	0	0	**70**	30	0	0	9	12	**51**	10	8	10
7/4	0	40	10	**50**	0	0	11	11	10	**48**	10	10
7/5	0	0	10	20	**50**	20	9	12	10	9	**49**	11
7/6	10	0	0	30	10	**50**	11	8	9	8	12	**52**
8/1	**60**	10	0	0	30	0	**54**	9	11	7	9	10
8/2	20	**40**	0	10	20	10	14	**47**	12	9	9	9
8/3	20	0	**50**	0	30	0	10	4	**49**	13	12	12
8/4	20	0	0	**40**	30	10	13	4	17	**49**	10	7
8/5	20	10	10	0	**50**	10	13	7	10	9	**50**	11
8/6	10	10	0	0	30	**50**	12	8	13	8	13	**46**
9/1	**40**	10	20	0	20	10	**51**	10	6	9	15	9
9/2	0	**30**	20	10	20	20	12	**48**	9	10	11	10
9/3	0	10	**50**	0	10	30	9	8	**52**	13	12	6
9/4	0	0	20	**40**	30	10	8	11	10	**49**	16	6
9/5	0	10	30	10	**40**	10	9	12	9	9	**51**	10
9/6	10	10	20	0	10	**50**	10	8	8	10	16	**48**

Table 1. Confusion matrices for the eight subjects and the six tasks (subject 5 is not taken into account). Left: *HMMs*-based, right: *M-SVM*-based. All the values are rounded to make the text readable.

3

Toward Mobile Sensor Fusion Platform for Context-Aware Services

Akio Sashima, Takeshi Ikeda, and Koichi Kurumatani
National Institute of Advanced Industrial Science and Technology / CREST, JST
Japan

1. Introduction

To recognize a context of a user, it is important to know a physical condition of the user and a status of his/her surrounding environment. For example, to maintain a healthcare condition of an elderly person, his/her care workers require monitoring not only his/her physiological conditions but also physical statuses of his/her surroundings, such as room temperatures. However, most approaches to the context recognition have been focusing on either environmental-centric recognition or user-centric recognition.

In ubiquitous computing researches, most approaches have focused on environment-centric recognition mechanism; they specifically examine how to recognize user's activities by sensors embedded in an environment (Garlan et al., 2002; Roman et al., 2001). The recognition includes location of the users. On the other hand, in research fields of wearable mobile computing, most approaches have focused on user-centric recognition mechanism; they specifically examine activity recognition by using sensors worn by the users, such as wristwatch-type accelerometers (Van Laerhoven et al., 2008; Clarkson et al., 2000). Hence, context-aware systems that use both wearable body sensors and environmental sensors have been few.

In this study, we specifically address context-aware services by using both wearable body sensors and surrounding wireless sensor networks, and propose a concept of *mobile sensor fusion platform*. Mobile sensor fusion platform is a new concept of a mobile service platform coordinating mobile phones and wireless sensor devices, such as wearable body sensors and environmental sensor networks. It will provide the following facilities to recognize user's contexts: 1) communicating with wearable body sensors and surrounding wireless sensor devices via mobile phone, 2) analyzing and fusing the sensed data by cooperating with sensor middleware, which manages sensed data on a remote server and 3) providing context-aware services for users by using mobile phones, such as remote monitoring of physiological status. In this chapter, we propose our vision of mobile sensor fusion platform. First, we describe services, requirements, and two types of the fusion architecture: "mobile sensing architecture" and "stable sensing architecture." Then, we propose a prototype platform, called CONSORTS-S (Sashima et al., 2008), of the mobile sensing architecture. As an exemplar service of the platform, we show a mobile healthcare service being aware of user's physical conditions such as heartbeat, posture, and movement based on analysis of physiological signals (e.g., electrocardiograph, thermometer, and 3-axis accelerometer). The service can be also aware of environmental status (e.g., temperature).

Then, an indoor temperature monitoring system, an example of the sensor fusion and analysis based on stable sensing architecture, is described. Finally, we discuss possibilities and future work of the platform.

2. Related work

In ubiquitous computing studies, a few works specifically address the context-awareness of mobile users. For example, Solar (Chen & Kotz, 2002) is a platform for context-aware mobile applications. Although the work provides a sophisticated programming model to access local resources seamlessly, no application using sensor devices has been shown.
Some services for mobile users have been studied in mobile computing for many years. However, studies examining the use of everyday mobile phones with sensor technologies are few. Several studies in the field of ubiquitous computing have been undertaken to detect a user's contexts using sensor devices embedded in mobile phones (Lester et al., 2006; Kawahara et al., 2007). In addition, various kinds of services on top of the mobile phone infrastructure have drawn attention from researches and applications. A typical service is providing healthcare service by using mobile phones (Leijdekkers & Gay, 2006; Oliver & Flores-Mangas, 2006). Contrasted against these studies, our work specifically examines the cooperative architecture that comprises independent components, such as wireless sensors, mobile sensor routers, mobile phones, and sensor middleware.
Recently, the concepts of people-centric sensing (Campbell et al., 2006; Miluzzo et al., 2008) and community sensing (Krause et al., 2008) were proposed. People-centric sensing is designed to realize large-scale, general-purpose sensor networks for the general public (e.g. consumers). Community sensing offers mechanisms for sharing data from privately held sensors, such as GPS devices. Although our platform shares similar concepts related to personal information devices (e.g. mobile phone) as sensor nodes, we specifically address supporting users to access the sensed data derived from surrounding wireless sensor networks and provide personalize services based on the data. To motivate such a concept, we present an implementation of healthcare services using commercially available mobile phones.

3. Mobile sensor fusion platform for context-aware services

3.1 Service scenarios

In this study, we have been developing applications to maintain and promote one's health condition by monitoring both environmental information (e.g., room temperature) and physiological information (e.g., heartbeat, posture and skin temperature) from surrounding sensors. As such services of mobile sensor fusion platform, we have considered the following application scenarios.

Mobile and remote healthcare service for elderly people: In this scenario, the service system detects and prevents health troubles of elderly person caused by improper room temperature, such as heatstroke. The users wear physiological sensors and carry mobile phones. The service system always monitors a user's health conditions (e.g., heartbeat, posture, and locomotion) based on the sensed data. In addition, the mobile phone communicates with environmental sensors to monitor environmental conditions (e.g., room temperature). If it detects the conditions are harmful for users, it notifies them.

Self-monitoring service on physical exercise: When a person is doing physical exercise, such as aerobics, running, and sports, it is important to monitor his/her physical conditions for effective and safe trainings. In this scenario, service users wear physiological sensors and carry mobile phones. The service system analyzes a user's health conditions (e.g., heartbeat and locomotion) based on the sensed data. In addition, the mobile phone communicates with environmental sensors to monitor environmental conditions (e.g., air pollution level and temperature). If it detects the conditions are harmful for users, it notifies them.

Remote health monitoring service in emergency situation: When an emergency, such as a fire emergency, occurs in an indoor environment, it is important both to monitor a change of the emergency situation and to know physical conditions of residents in the environment. In this scenario, service users (e.g., residents) wear physiological sensors and carry mobile phones. The service system analyzes a user's health conditions (e.g., heartbeat and posture) based on the sensed data. The mobile phone communicates with environmental sensors to monitor environmental conditions (e.g., air pollution level and temperature). If it detects the conditions are harmful for users, it notifies a rescue team of present user's situations.

3.2 Requirements

To realize the above service scenarios, we assume that a mobile sensor fusion platform is required to suffice for the following requirements.

Providing mobile services on user's cellular phone: Because user's everyday mobile phone is used for providing context-aware services, the platform is implemented on top of the mobile phones popularly used by ordinal people. It uses communication facilities of the phone to provide monitoring and notification services. It also uses a graphical user interface of the phone to shows analysis results, such as air pollution levels.

Wireless communication with surrounding sensors: The platform can collect and aggregate sensing data by using wireless communication. It communicates with wearable body sensors and surrounding sensor networks. It is required to speak common communication protocols to connect to various sensor devices in an ad-hoc manner.

Distributed Analysis of sensed data: The platform fuses collected sensor data and analyzes them to recognize users' contexts, and provides services based on the analytic results. Because complex analysis, such as motion recognition, consumes much computation resources which may not be available at a mobile phone, the complex analysis can be performed at a remote server on the Internet.

Management of sensed data: The platform manages the sensor data received from the sensor networks. Because some applications are required to analyze sensed data of the past hours/days, the service can store the sensed data on storage of the mobile phones, or on remote database systems.

3.3 Architecture

Considering mobile sensor fusion platform that suffices for the above requirements, we propose the following two types of architecture. We require both types of the architecture to realize our vision, and have been developing them.

Mobile sensing architecture: The architecture is shown in Fig. 1. This architecture uses a mobile phone carried by a user to communicate with surrounding environmental sensors. A mobile router attached to the mobile phone communicates with wireless sensors in ad-hoc manner. Although the router and phone are required to perform ad-hoc communication mechanisms, interaction styles of the sensors are intuitive for the user; the proximity based communication architecture is not required to manage user's locations. Under the vision of the architecture, we have been developing CONSORTS-S, a mobile sensing platform (Sashima et al., 2008). The CONSORTS-S platform is designed to confirm the validity of this architecture based on mobile phone popularly used in Japan and its network architecture (e.g., 3G network). Healthcare services for mobile users by accessing surrounding wireless sensors are implemented on the platform. The outline of the platform is described at section 4.

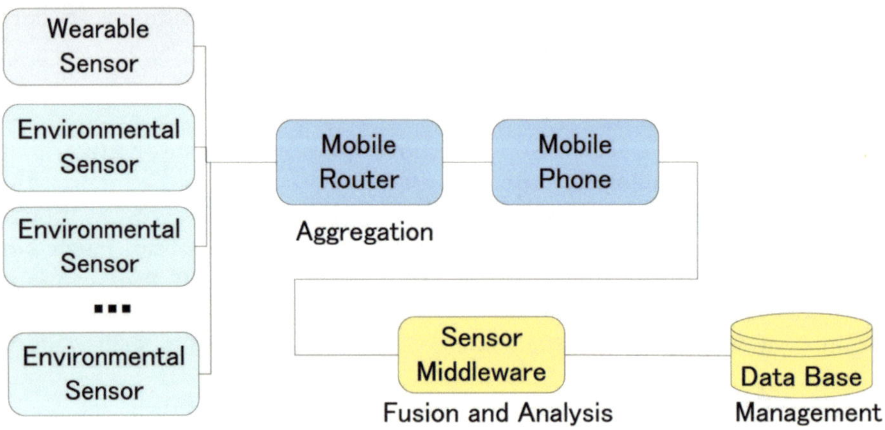

Fig. 1. Mobile sensing architecture: mobile phone communicates with environmental sensors in ad-hoc manner

Stable sensing architecture: The architecture is shown in Fig. 2. In this architecture, sensor middleware always communicates with predetermined environmental sensors, collects the sensed data, and stores them with locations where the data are sensed. To provide a service using the sensed data from user's surrounding sensors, sensor middleware must know user's location to retrieve the data. Hence, sensor middleware is required to manage user's location by using some location systems like GPS. Because the architecture does not use the ad-hoc connection to the wireless environmental sensors, communication mechanism can be simple. Under the vision of the architecture, sensor middleware, SENSORD (Sashima et al., 2008) has been developed to confirm the validity of this spatial sensor data management and analysis, namely spatial sensor fusion. An indoor temperature monitoring system has been implemented with the middleware (Sashima et al., 2008). Currently, sensing information of wearable sensors is not integrated into the system. Outline of the system is described at section 6.

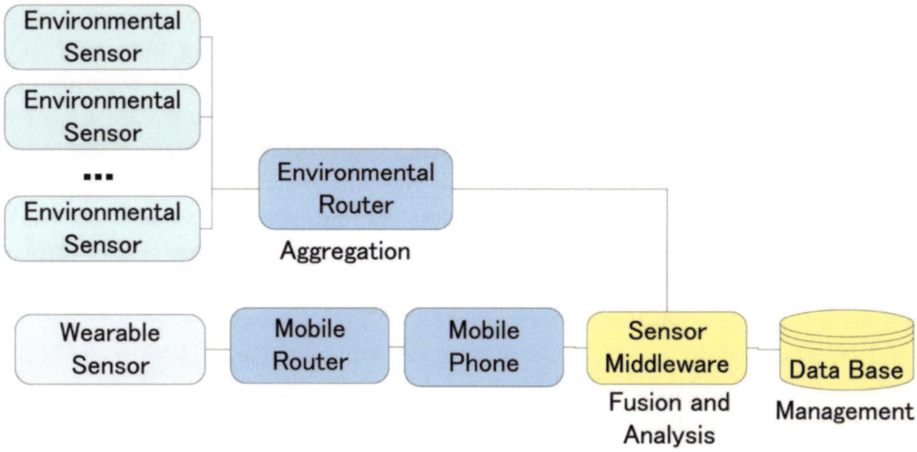

Fig. 2. Stable sensing architecture: sensor middleware communicates with predetermined environmental sensors

4. Mobile sensing platform: CONSORTS-S

The CONSORTS-S platform uses two additional components that work with mobile phones: *mobile sensor router* and *sensor middleware*. Fig. 3 shows the architecture of the platform. A mobile sensor router is attached to a mobile phone for the *communication*. Sensor middleware on a remote server performs *management* and *fusion and analysis of sensed data* coordinating with the software in the mobile phone.

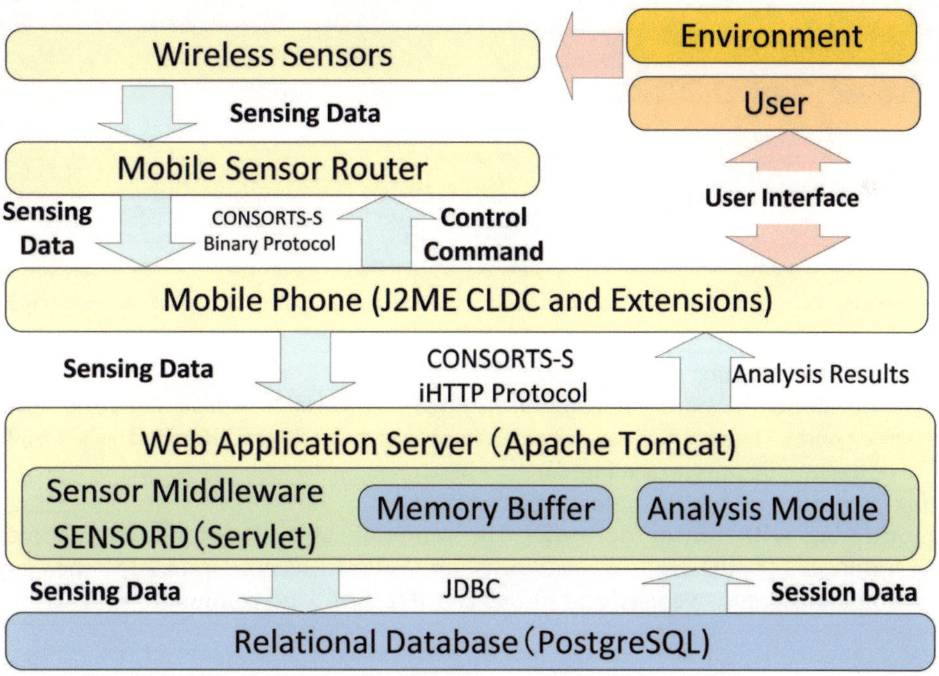

Fig. 3. Architecture of CONSORTS-S platform

4.1 Wireless sensors

We assume wireless sensor networks of two types communicating with CONSORTS-S: *embedded type sensors stayed in an environment* and *mobile type sensors worn or carried by a user*. The sensor networks are assumed to communicate with other nodes in a peer-to-peer manner. Sensors of several types are assumed: thermometers, hygrometers, vision systems, microphone array systems, and so on. Because the vision systems and microphone array systems might produce enormous raw sensor data continuously, we assume that the mobile phones receive not raw sensor data from the sensor systems but rather binary information, such as *exists/not-exists* and *passed/not-passed*, which is pre-processed at the sensor systems.

Wireless sensor units communicate with CONSORTS-S platform via an original 2.4 GHz ISM band communication. Currently, a wireless sensor unit[1] (see Fig. 4) is ready for such communication. The unit is a small wireless sensor unit that includes built-in sensors of three kinds: an electrocardiograph (potentiometer), thermometer, and 3-axis accelerometer. It is just a transmitter of sensed data; it has no function to receive communication signals. Maximum sensing rates of sensors are 204 Hz; the maximum wireless communication rate is about 1 Mbps. Its communication range is about 15 m.

The sensor unit is mainly designed for medical uses. However, it can be used as embedded type sensor (e.g., thermometer) stayed in an environment. We use the sensor for monitoring biological information and environmental information.

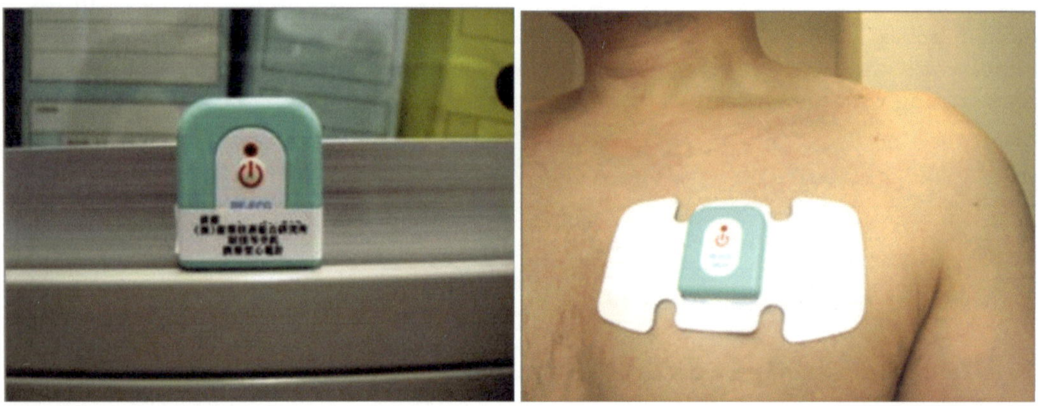

Fig. 4. Settings of wireless sensor: environmental sensor (left), physiological sensor (right)

4.2 Mobile sensor router

We have developed a board for communicating with wireless sensor networks, called a *mobile sensor router*. The router is a wireless communication board attached to a serial port (UART) of the mobile phone (see Fig. 5).

A mobile sensor router has the following functions:

Communicating with sensor networks The router must understand a communication protocol of the sensor networks to collect sensor data. In the current implementation, we used an original 2.4 GHz ISM-band communication.

[1] MESI RF-ECG http://www.mmdevice.co.jp/product_all.html#p1 (in Japanese)

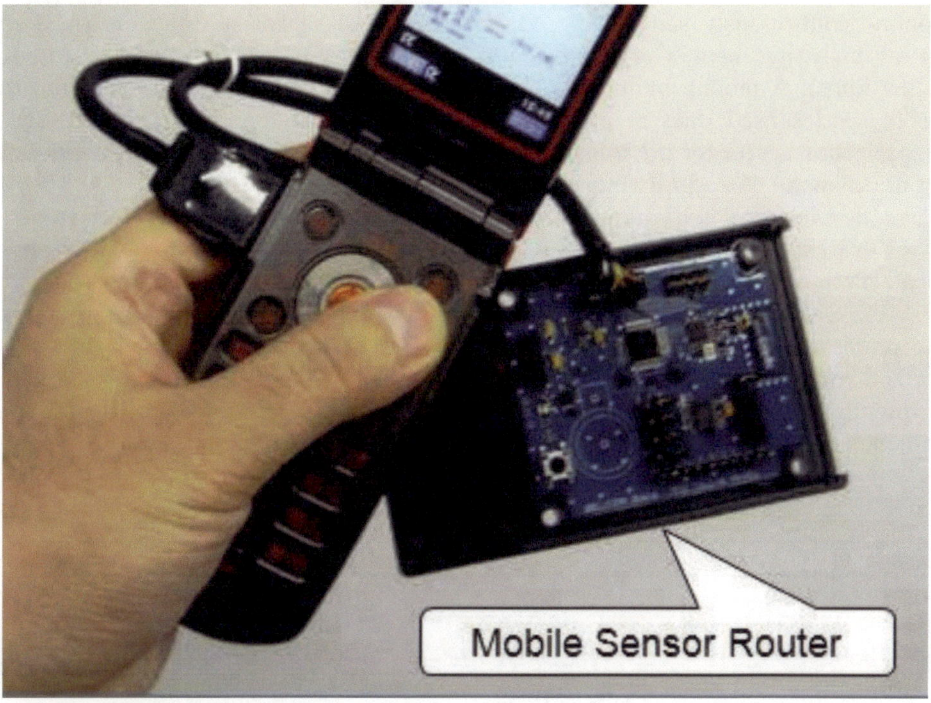

Fig. 5. Mobile sensor router.

Reducing the number of sensed data Although the router can receive full rates of the sensor data stream from the wireless biosensor described before, the mobile phone cannot receive such a data stream. Therefore, to compensate the limited computational ability of the mobile phone, the router sends not raw data received from the sensors but their reduced data at the router.

Communicating with a mobile phone The router is connected to a serial port of the mobile phone for communicated through the wire. The communication rate is 115000 bps. We have developed a content level communication protocol between them, called *CONSORTS-S-Binary Protocol*. It is a lightweight protocol for controlling the router function and obtaining sensed data.

4.3 Mobile phone

Mobile phones used popularly in Japan have a runtime environment in which a program downloaded from Web sites can be executed. We use a mobile phone[2] that can execute a Java program (J2ME CLDC edition with extensional APIs for accessing native functions). A CONSORTS-S program running at the runtime environment, and communicates to a mobile sensor router. It collects sensed data and sends the data to the remote web server. The program also provides a user interface of CONSORTS-S that controls its behaviors: starting (or stopping), setting up parameters, and so on. The interface shows contents received from the remote web server.

---

[2] NTT-docomo FOMA N903i http://www.nttdocomo.co.jp/support/utilization/product/n903i/index.html (in Japanese)

The phone continuously sends reduced sensor data to sensor middleware on a remote server for analyzing them. The phone sends data using W-CDMA wireless communication (Max 384 kpbs). A mobile phone of CONSORTS-S must make connections to the remote server to send sensed data to a sensor middleware on a remote server. We set up a web/application server for downloading the programs and providing proxy services of the sensor middleware. We adopt Tomcat 5.5[3] as the web/application server.

We have developed a communication protocol between mobile phone and web server, called *CONSORTS-S-iHTTP Protocol*. It is a lightweight protocol implemented on HTTP protocol. Because HTTP protocol is a connectionless protocol, each message of the CONSORTS-S-iHTTP protocol requires including some identification signals of users, their mobile phones, and sessions. In the CONSORTS-S-iHTTP protocol, a mobile phone is first authorized with login name, password, and subscriber ID, and receives a session cookie. Consequently, the mobile phone sends reduced sensor data with the subscriber ID and the session cookie to be identified by the server. Using this scheme, multiple mobile phones can access the same web server simultaneously. Table 1 summarizes communications of CONSORTS-S.

	Connections	Protocols	Data Rates
Sensor <=> Router	Wireless (2.4 GHz)	Original	1 M bps (Max.)
Router <=> Mobile Phone	Serial (UART)	CONSORTS-S Binary	115K bps (Max)
Mobile Phone <=> Web Server	W-CDMA + IP	CONSORTS-S iHTTP	7.2M bps (Max)

Table 1. Communications of CONSORTS-S

The phone shows analytic results of the sensed data and messages (e.g., recommendations) to users. The graphical user interface depends on implementation of the application and services; it does not depend on CONSORTS-S. Therefore, we describe details of the user interface with an example of mobile sensing services in section 5.

4.4 Sensor middleware: SENSORD

We adopt sensor event-driven service coordination middleware (SENSORD) (Sashima et al., 2006) as sensor middleware of the platform. A servlet program on the application server includes a SENSORD core module. It processes sensed data received on HTTP protocol. It analyses them by calling SENSORD API, such as FFT API. A SENSORD module stores sensed data into an in-memory data container to achieve fast and complex analysis (see Fig. 6). The analysis results of the module are sent back to the mobile phone as a HTTP response. The response is represented as a mobile-phone-friendly format, such as a HTML document. Because this transaction is a synchronous process, the HTTP communication process of the mobile phone waits to receive the results. The sensed data is stored in a relational database[4]. Sensor middleware of CONSORTS-S performs several signal processing and classification processes using machine learning techniques, such as Fast Fourier Transform (FFT), support vector machine (SVM), and nearest neighbor learning. Using such algorithms, the sensed data are analyzed statistically or classified into some qualitative categories. The analysis results are based on remote sensing data from users' surroundings.

[3] http://tomcat.apache.org/

[4] http://www.postgresql.org/

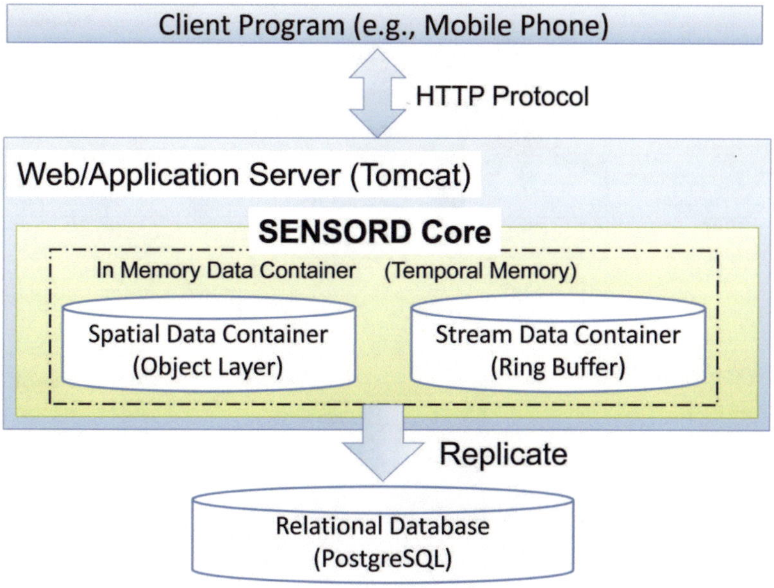

Fig. 6. SENSORD core module in web/application server

The module can store and retrieve spatial information (or geometric map), specifically locations of objects, humans, and sensor devices. Sensed data of CONSORTS-S is stored with spatial information: locations of the sensor devices. The locations are represented as using a widely used coordinate system, WGS84 latitude and longitude. The WGS84 coordinate system is used by GPS devices in mobile phones. Consequently, users' locations and their sensor data are managed easily on the CONSORTS-S platform.

5. Mobile healthcare services

In this study, we propose a services scenario to maintain and promote one's health condition by monitoring both environmental information (e.g. room temperature) and biological information (e.g., heartbeat, posture and skin temperature) from wireless sensors. We have implemented a prototype of the healthcare service considering the following scenarios (Sashima et al., 2008).

> Particularly, elderly people need preparation for unexpected health troubles. In this scenario, the service detects and prevents health troubles of older people, such as falling down and heart failure. Service users wear wearable biological sensors and carry mobile phones. The service system analyzes a user's health conditions (e.g., heartbeat, posture, and locomotion) based on the sensed data. Then it notifies the user. Doctors and family members can monitor the conditions remotely. In addition, the mobile phone communicates with environmental sensors to monitor whether environmental conditions (e.g., room temperature) are not harmful for users. The service supports a user's health based on both environmental information and biological information obtained from wireless sensors.

Fig. 7 depicts an outline of a prototype service that we have implemented to address the vision implied by the healthcare scenarios described above. It monitors a user's health

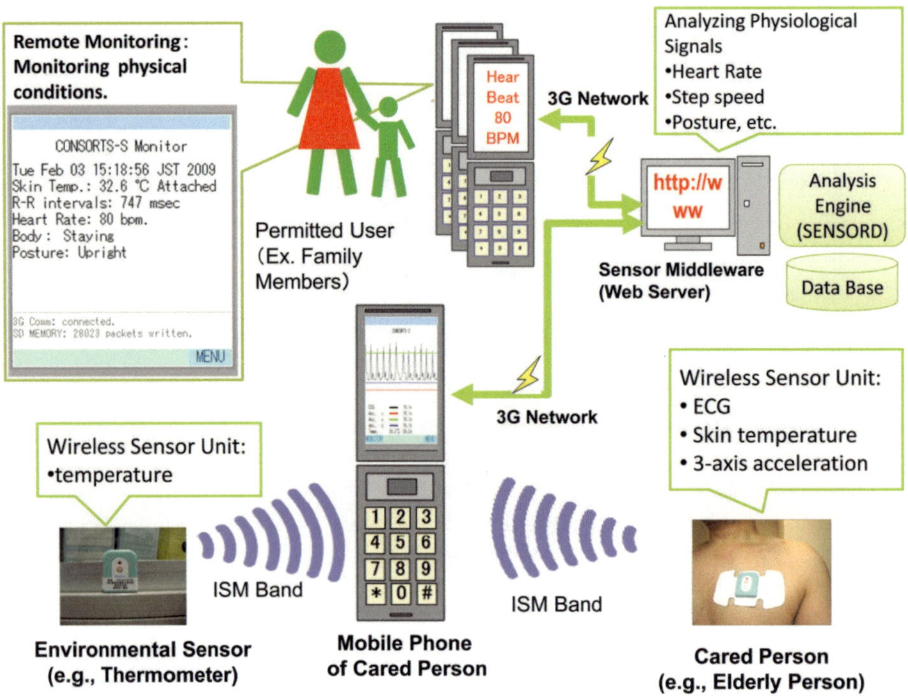

Fig. 7. Mobile healthcare services

conditions and room temperatures using popular 3G phones and wireless sensors. A sensor to monitor physiological signals must be attached to a user's chest by sticking electrodes of the sensor on tightly with a peel-off adhesive seal. Once it is attached to a user's chest, it can detect the inclination and movement of the upper half of a user's body using a 3-axis accelerometer. On the other hand, the sensor to monitor room temperature is set in a room. The temperature sensor is assumed to be set in each room where users will stay. The user can know the room temperature by communicating with the sensor.

The monitoring service has the following modes: *graph mode, multi sensor mode,* and *remote monitor mode*. Screen images of the modes are shown in Fig. 8.

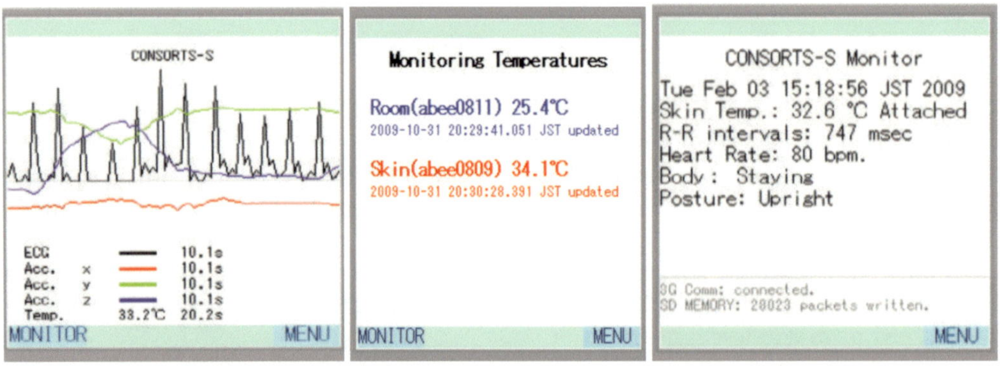

Fig. 8. Graphic user interface of the healthcare service: graph mode (left), multi sensor mode (middle), and remote monitor mode (right)

Sensed physiological signals are sent to the mobile phone through the mobile sensor router described in section 4.2. In *graph mode*, the mobile phone shows a graph of the physiological signals, such as electrocardiography (see the left image of Fig. 8).

In *multi sensor mode*, environmental information (e.g. room temperature) is shown (see the middle image of Fig. 8). The temperature information is obtained using the environmental sensors that can be communicated with the mobile phones. Locations and unique IDs of the sensors are also shown (e.g. room (abee0811)). Because the system communicates with one sensor at a time, it periodically switches from a communication channel for a sensor to other. In the current implementation, the system has a list of sensor devices (device id and location) that might be communicated with. This process interrupts data processing of the graph modes. Therefore, physiological signals are not shown when this mode is working.

In *remote monitor mode*, the monitoring software on a mobile phone of a remote user periodically accesses the sensor middleware and receives current analysis results of cared-person's physiological signals, such as the posture (see the right image of Fig. 8). In this mode, it analyzes sensing signals of electrocardiograph and calculates cared-person's heart rates as beat per minute (BPM). The heart-rates are calculated by Fast Fourier Transform (FFT) of finite length time series of sensed signals. In the current implementation, the length of the time series is about 16 seconds (128 samples).

Moreover, it shows user's the movement recognition, which classifies the signals into some qualitative statuses, for example, running, walking, standing-still, etc. In the movement recognition, the steps are recognized by calculating FFT of finite length time series of sensed data of the y-axis accelerometer. In the current implementation, the length of the time series is 8 seconds (64 samples). It also classifies user's statuses into three categories: *staying, walking, running* based on the results of FFT. When user's status is "walking" or "running," it also shows an average speed of user's movements as Steps Per Minute (SPM).

To detect cared-person's posture (e.g., standing-still, facing downward, and facing upward), it calculates the inclination of the upper half of user's body based on the sensed signals of the 3-axis accelerometer. The classification uses simple rule-based inference on the inclination.

In this section, we have described a prototype system of the mobile healthcare service by using mobile phones with surrounding wireless sensor networks. The demonstration has shown a first step of a mobile sensor fusion that enables mobile users to collect and publish their favorite sensing information anywhere and anytime. Although we have developed CONSORTS-S and confirmed a basic idea of mobile sensor fusion, fusion and analysis of sensed data have not been shown. In next section, we will show an example of such analysis by using SENSORD, a key component of CONSORTS-S. Although, the service does not use wireless sensors, analysis of collected sensor data is performed in an analogous fashion.

6. Indoor temperature monitoring system

An indoor temperature monitoring system has been developed under the vision of stable sensing architecture (Sashima et al., 2008). The experimental area of the floor is about 700 square meters. It analyzes sensed data of thermometers[5] placed in a floor of our laboratory building, and graphically shows distributions of temperature. Distributions of temperature are analyzed and monitored 24 hours a day.

[5] T&D TR72W: http://www.tandd.com/product/tr7w/index.html

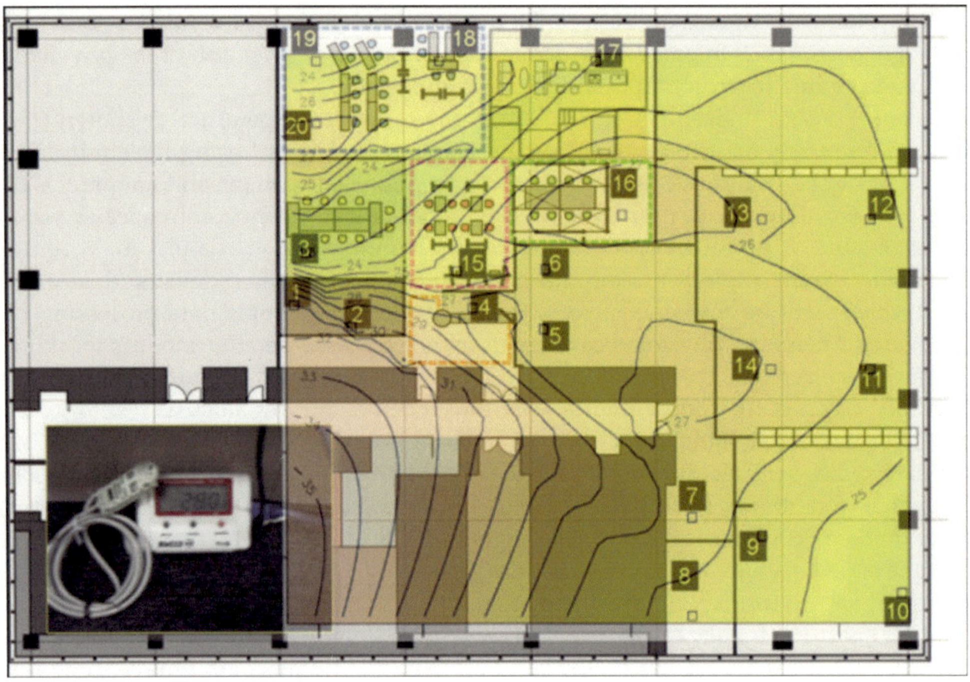

Fig. 9. A configuration of thermometers

Fig. 9 displays an overview of the configuration of 20 thermometers used for the system. The thermometer has a wired network interface (TCP/IP) to send sensed data to the middleware. A black box with a number shows a location of the sensor. A yellow area shows a monitoring area by analyzing sensor data.

Because the thermometers are irregularly placed on the floor, it is required to apply various types of interpolation functions in analyzing sensed data to achieve an appropriate 2-dimensional distribution of temperature. In addition, the interpolation algorithms use complex, numerical computing techniques so that the implementations are not easy. Thus, we have developed the system based on SENSORD/Stat (Sashima, Ikeda, Inoue & Kurumatani, 2008). SENSORD/Stat is an extension of SENSORD. In the SENSORD/Stat system, SENSORD cooperatively works with a statistical and numerical analysis environment, called R (Ihaka & Gentleman, 1996). Because the R environment provides various statistical analysis packages, users can try to apply them in the sensor data analyses. By using the SENSORD/Stat system, application developers can access to both statistical and numerical analyses of R and spatiotemporal sensor data management of SENSORD. Hence, spatial sensor fusion analysis can be performed on the system. Fig. 10 shows an outline of the analysis.

In the analyses, we have selected an interpolation function package, named *akima*[6]. It is a package for a linear or cubic spline interpolation for irregularly gridded data (Akima, 1996). Applying various add-on packages of R, we have easily developed the program that calculates appropriate 2-dimensional distributions of temperature. Fig. 11 shows an example of the distributions.

---

[6] http://cran.r-project.org/web/packages/akima/akima.pdf

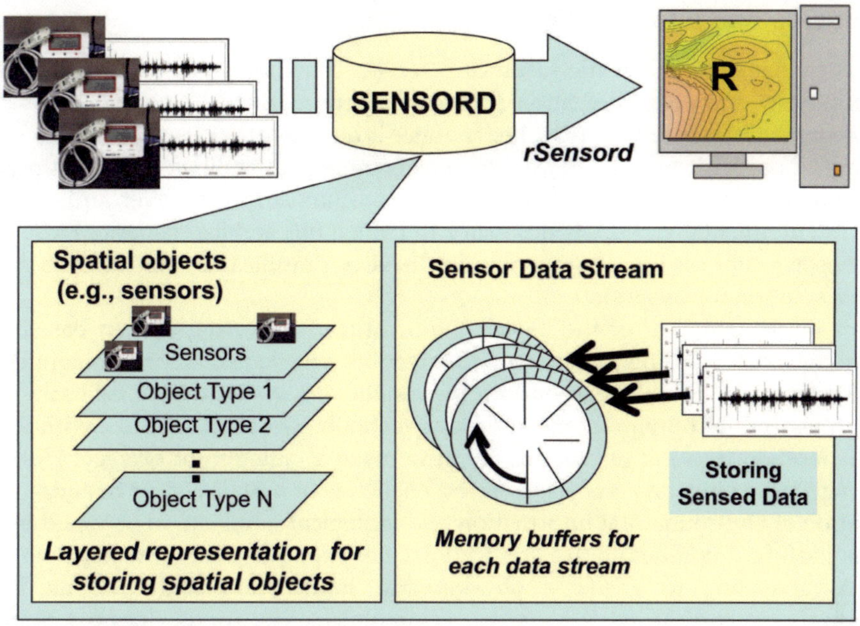

Fig. 10. Indoor temperature monitoring system

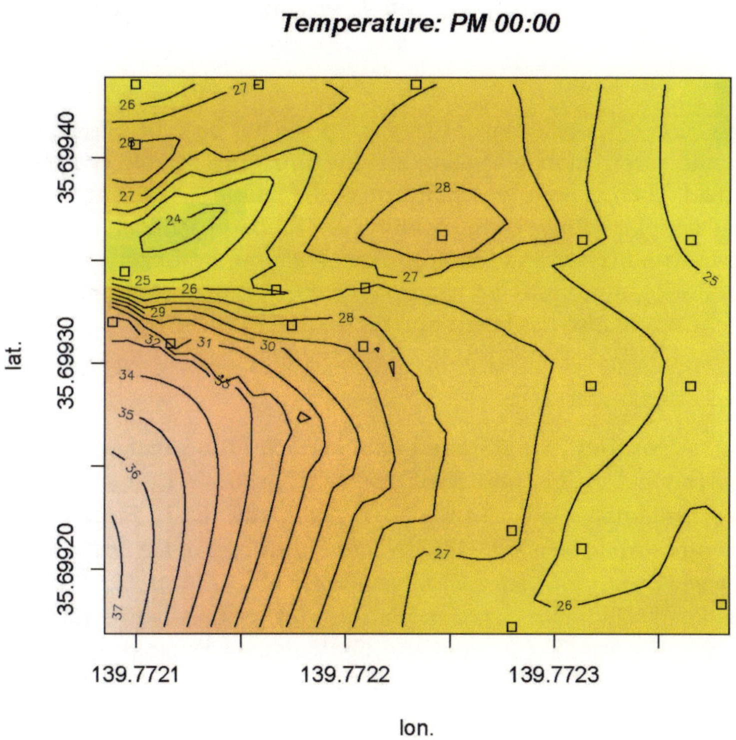

Fig. 11. 2-dimensional distribution of temperature

7. Discussion and future work

In current implementation of the healthcare service based on mobile sensing architecture, sensor discovery and communication protocols are predefined. How it can communicate with environmental sensors in an ad-hoc manner is an important issue. Users do not stay in their homes. They visit various places, such as commercial facilities. How can users access environmental sensors in such public spaces? A mechanism to discover and communicate with the environmental sensors is necessary to realize our service scenario. Developing the mobile sensor router on top of other standardized communication stacks, such as ZigBee[7], might be a solution for this issue.

In current implementation of the indoor temperature monitoring system based on stable sensing architecture, sensing information obtained by mobile users is not integrated into the system. To integrate the information into the monitoring system based on users' locations, we plan to use indoor human location tracking technologies, such as RFID, with the system. However, location tracking of humans is apt to make a violation of privacy. Hence, secure and privacy preserving data analysis is a next challenge of mobile sensor fusion.

Combination of environmental information and biological information obtained by wireless sensors is useful for non-healthcare applications. For example, energy management of home appliances according to a user's physiological information might be an interesting application. In the current implementation, the mobile sensor router does not communicate with multiple sensors simultaneously. Hence, the monitoring process of heartbeat can not work with the monitoring process of room temperatures. We plan to develop a new mobile sensor router that can communicate with multiple sensors to realize our scenario.

8. Conclusions

In this chapter, a vision of mobile sensor fusion platform has been proposed. First, two types of the fusion architecture: "mobile sensing architecture" and "stable sensing architecture" have been described. Then, a prototype platform of the mobile sensing architecture has been proposed. As an exemplar service of the prototype, a mobile healthcare service being aware of user's physical conditions and environmental status has been shown. An indoor temperature monitoring system as an example of the sensor fusion and analysis base on stable sensing architecture also has been shown.

9. References

Akima, H. (1996). Algorithm 761; scattered-data surface fitting that has the accuracy of a cubic polynomial, *ACM Trans. Math. Softw.* 22(3): 362–371.

Campbell, A. T., Eisenman, S. B., Lane, N. D., Miluzzo, E. & Peterson, R. A. (2006). Peoplecentric urban sensing, *WICON '06: Proceedings of the 2nd annual international workshop on Wireless internet*, ACM, New York, NY, USA, p. 18.

Chen, G. & Kotz, D. (2002). Solar: An open platform for context-aware mobile applications, *In Proceedings of the First International Conference on Pervasive Computing (Pervasive 2002*, pp. 41–47.

[7] http://www.zigbee.org/

Clarkson, B., Pentland, A. & Mase, K. (2000). Recognizing user context via wearable sensors, *Wearable Computers, IEEE International Symposium* 0: 69.

Garlan, D., Siewiorek, D., Smailagic, A. & Steenkiste, P. (2002). Project AURA: Toward distraction-free pervasive computing, *IEEE Pervasive computing* pp. 22–31.

Ihaka, R. & Gentleman, R. (1996). R: A language for data analysis and graphics, *Journal of Computational and Graphical Statistics* 5(3): 299–314. URL: *www.r-project.org*

Kawahara, Y., Kurasawa, H. & Morikawa, H. (2007). Recognizing user context using mobile handsets with acceleration sensors, *IEEE International Conference on Portable Information Devices. PORTABLE07*, pp. 1–5.

Krause, A., Horvitz, E., Kansal, A. & Zhao, F. (2008). Toward community sensing, *IPSN '08: Proceedings of the 7th international conference on Information processing in sensor networks*, IEEE Computer Society,Washington, DC, USA, pp. 481–492.

Leijdekkers, P. & Gay, V. (2006). Personal heart monitoring and rehabilitation system using smart phones, *ICMB '06: Proceedings of the International Conference on Mobile Business*, IEEE Computer Society,Washington, DC, USA, p. 29.

Lester, J., Choudhury, T. & Borriello, G. (2006). A practical approach to recognizing physical activities., *Proceedings of The Fourth International Conference on Pervasive Computing (PERVASIVE 2006)*, pp. 1–16.

Miluzzo, E., Lane, N. D., Fodor, K., Peterson, R., Lu, H., Musolesi, M., Eisenman, S. B., Zheng, X. & Campbell, A. T. (2008). Sensing meets mobile social networks: the design, implementation and evaluation of the cenceme application, *SenSys '08: Proceedings of the 6th ACM conference on Embedded network sensor systems*, ACM, New York, NY, USA, pp. 337–350.

Oliver, N. & Flores-Mangas, F. (2006). Healthgear: A real-time wearable system for monitoring and analyzing physiological signals, *Proceedings of the International Workshop on Wearable and Implantable Body Sensor Networks (BSN'06)*, IEEE Computer Society, Washington, DC, USA, pp. 61–64.

Roman, M., Hess, C., Ranganathan, A., Madhavarapu, P., Borthakur, B., Viswanathan, P., Cerquiera, R., Campbell, R. & Mickunas, M. D. (2001). GaiaOS: An infrastructure for active spaces, *Technical Report UIUCDCS-R-2001-2224 UILU-ENG-2001-1731*, University of Illinois at Urbana-Champaign.

Sashima, A., Ikeda, T., Inoue, Y. & Kurumatani, K. (2008). Sensord/stat: Combining sensor middleware with a statistical computing environment, *Proceedings of the 5th International Conference on Networked Sensing Systems (INSS 2008)*, pp. 123–126.

Sashima, A., Inoue, Y., Ikeda, T., Yamashita, T. & Kurumatani, K. (2008). CONSORTS-S: A mobile sensing platform for context-aware services, *4th International Conference on Intelligent Sensors, Sensor Networks and Information Processing (ISSNIP 2008)*, IEEE, Sydney, Australia, pp. 417–422.

Sashima, A., Inoue, Y. & Kurumatani, K. (2006). Spatio-temporal sensor data management for context-aware services: designing sensor-event driven service coordination middleware, *ADPUC '06: Proceedings of the 1st international workshop on Advanced data processing in ubiquitous computing (ADPUC 2006)*, ACM Press, New York, NY, USA, p. 4.

Van Laerhoven, K., Kilian, D. & Schiele, B. (2008). Using rhythm awareness in long-term activity recognition, *Proceedings of the eleventh International Symposium on Wearable Computers (ISWC 2008)*, IEEE Press.

4

SPR Imaging Label-Free Control of Biomineral Nucleation!?

Stancu Izabela-Cristina
Politehnica University of Bucharest, Faculty of Applied Chemistry and Materials Science
Romania

1. Introduction

Bone regeneration due to trauma and pathology, bone degeneration in aging population as well as osteporosis ellicit a societal need for new performant regenerative products. Although a wide range of biomaterials have been researched and applied for hard tissue repair and regeneration, there is still a high competition and challenge in improving their performances for *in vivo* applications.

To create high-quality orthopaedic implants, several approaches have been proposed; among them the self-biomineralizing scaffolds are intensively researched. Despite intensive studies and an impressive number of investigated structures, no optimum formulation has been yet set-up. This is why high-performing methods of controlling the biomineralization induction are still needed and researched. In this context, a deeper and broader understanding of the mineralization phenomenon induced on/inside different materials would be extremely useful.

The present chapter is aimed as the first attempt of investigation of biomaterials-induced biomineralization through the label-free Surface Plasmon Resonance Imaging (SPRi).

1.1 Biomineralization inductive materials

One of the most exciting and researched class of biomaterials for bone repair and regeneration is represented by polymer materials supporting or even better, enhancing mineral phase formation (Kamei et al., 1997; Shin et al., 2003; Stancu et al., 2004). The main advantage of these materials over classical bone fillers consists in their in situ transformation in polymer-hydroxyapatite composites, similar to natural bone. The advantages of the so-formed composites are evident when compared to synthetic composites prepared prior to implantation; the most important is that the hydroxyapatite is generated inside the bone tissue enhancing the further osteointegration of the implant. The mineralization of either natural or synthetic matrix is an extremely complex phenomenon. To date, there is no consensus over the nucleation processes responsible for materials' calcification (*calcification* is synonym with *biomineralization* when referring to bone mineral phase formation). All the hypotheses and the mechanisms researched have lead to a very important common conclusion: the sine-qua-non condition for biomineralization to occur is the presence of calcium and phosphate ions in the surrounding liquid environment. Calcium cations are provided by cells and physiological fluids while phosphate anions are generated through phosphoesters and phosphoproteins hydrolysis as well as from the body fluids (Whyte et al., 1995). Mineralization to occur needs nucleation to be induced by a perturbation like the ions' capturing by special molecules/species.

Based on the observation that natural phosphate-containing proteins are actively involved in naturally occurring mineralization and due to their calcium affinity, phosphate-containing polymers have been studied with respect to hydroxyapatite formation in physiological fluids (Stancu et al., 2004; Swart et al., 1976). The literature also presents the carboxylic functionalities from bone proteins (e.g. bone sialoprotein) and from some polymers as responsible for hydroxyapatite formation (Hunter et al., 2001; Filmon et al., 2002; Ganns et al., 1999).

To resume, negatively charged groups seem to elicit hydroxyapatite nucleation and growth through calcium capturing from body fluids (Vijayasekaran et al., 2000). Another important aspect deciding on the mineralization occurrence concerns the importance of the distribution and of the density of the negative groups inside/outside the support (Stancu et al., 2004).

Recently, starting from the idea that a defined chemical functionality could decide on the nucleation and on the mineral crystals' growth, dendrimers have been investigated as leading to mineral embedding the support materials, with predefined shape and properties (Donners et al., 2003). This hypothesis has opened a wide field of research and the present chapter subscribes this direction. Dendrimers are globular tridimensional macromolecules presenting a high number of branched structural units (dendrons) diverging from a central core. The branches end with superficial end groups which form the exterior functional shell of the dendrimer. This reactive shell may contain a diversity of functional groups: amines, carboxylic acids, alcohols, aldehydes, thiols, etc. The polyamidoamine dendrimers (PAMAM) have nano- dimensions and their immobilization on surfaces would lead to structural features within this dimensional range.

The present work represents an attempt of assessment of the biomineralization capacity of PAMAM dendrimers amino- and carboxylic-terminated immobilized on solid supports.

1.2 Importance of nano-dimension in bone regeneration

For a bone graft to be successful, it seems that a biomaterial with superficial nano-features and presenting a superior surface reactivity available for further growth factors and other biospecies to be immobilized could represent real advances. Nanomaterials domain covers a wide range of materials of different natures with dimensions under 100 nm or presenting structural features (particles, fibers) under this dimensional threshold. Considering the tissue regeneration behavior, nanomaterials have been studied with respect to the proteins and cells interactions. The success of these materials is based on the initially interaction with the proteins controlling the cellular functions. Several recent works report superior bone cells performances associated with nanoroughness and nanophase materials of various nature. Professor Dr. Webster T.J. could be considered as a real promoter of the positive effects of nanomaterials in tissue engineering and reconstruction, the research of his group in the last 7 years proving this affirmation. In this context, it has been constantly reported that these materials increase the recognition of the surfaces by the osteoblasts that are naturally accustomed with the nanostructured components of natural bone (HA crystals, fibrillar collagen etc.) (Price et al., 2003; Ward & Webster, 2006). To remember, bone is structured on three dimensional levels: 1) macroscopic (cortical, trabecullar), 2) microscopic (Haversian systems) and 3) nanometric (mineral crystals, noncollagenous proteins, collagen fibrils).

1.3 SPRi

SPR is a well known high-sensitive techniques specially used for the assessment of both ultrathin layers of biomolecules as well as for the analysis of biomolecular specific interactions. The principle of SPR is based on the detection of molecules' presence on a modified metallic surface through monitoring the change in the local reflectivity, without using molecular labels. In addition to the SPR spectrometer, the SPRi tool has an excellent efficiency and broader application since it allows for simultaneous and comparative investigation of the whole surface of the sensor in real time. The technique is still underexplored and its potential is far of being totally used. In this aim, the approach of mineralization monitoring through SPRi is perfectly justified and welcome. The technique provides high sensitivity, time-driven analysis of mineral phase formation, accuracy in mimicking the physiological conditions with respect to fluid environment providing and, nevertheless, simple operation.

The present work will try to go deeper in the description of biomineralization induced by PAMAM-coated substrates, as explored by SPRi.

2. Experiment design

2.1 Materials

Substrate. The biosensor substrate is based on commercially available SPR gold slides (sSens, Netherlands). These sensors (10 x 10 mm) are made out of borosilicate glass with a refractive index of 1.51 and 0.3 mm thick. They are compatible both with common commercial SPR instruments as well as with modular SPR set-up. The gold applied onto the sensor's surface is evaporated following an optimized procedure with respect to gold layer thickness and cristallinity; a thin titanium layer was applied in order to ensure a good adherence of the gold on the glass. Substrates' rinsing with piranha solution (prepared using 75% concentrated H_2SO_4 and 25% of H_2O_2 30%) should be performed for approximately 1 minute, followed by distilled water cleaning and drying under a nitrogen stream; this treatment should immediately precede the use. (Recommended time for rinsing with piranha is up to 5 minutes, in order to remove the contaminants and to avoid the increase of the superficial roughness (Ulman, 1991).

Thiols. Thiols are needed to chemically immobilize the dendrimer molecules onto the gold surface. Thiols with different chain lengths and presenting amino- or carboxyl- terminal functional groups may be utilized: Cysteamine, 3-Mercaptopropionic acid, 16-Mercaptohexadecanoic acid, 11-Mercaptoundecanoic amine etc. Thiols should be used without further purification and as freshly prepared ethanolic solutions (1 mM).

Activation mixture. The activation mixture was described elsewhere (Stancu et al., 2007). Briefly, the carboxylic groups can be activated with 20 mM solution of N,N-(3-dimethylaminopropyl)-N'-ethyl-carbodiimide hydrochloride (EDC) and 5 mM solution of N-hydroxysuccinimide (NHS) in phosphate buffer pH7.4.

Sensing phase. PAMAM dendrimers with amino- and carboxylic acid- external reactive shells are used as sensing phase. It should be remembered here that amino-terminal PAMAM is full generation and the acid-PAMAM is half generation according to their synthesis. The synthesis of these macromolecules starts from the ethylediamine (EDA) core, followed by Michael addition of methyl acrylate (MA) and amidation reactions of the resulting ester with large excess of EDA. Repetition of this sequence gives full generation g = 0,1,2,3,... (amino terminal groups), while the interruption of this sequence after the Michael addition leads to half generations g = 0.5, 1.5, 2.5,... (carboxyl-ended dendrimers) (Majoros et al., 2004). In this study two generations of PAMAM dendrimers both with amino- as well as with carboxyl- ending functionalities are used as sensing phase. Generations 1.5 and 3.5 are used for the dendrimers with -COOH functional end-groups (further referred as PAMAM-g1.5 and PAMAM-g3.5). Generations 2 and 4 are selected for the $-NH_2$ ending dendrimers (further referred as PAMAM-g2 and PAMAM-g4). All dendrimers are supplied from Sigma-Aldrich and used as received, as solutions in methanol. Generations 1.5 and 2 present 16 ending groups while generations 3.5 and 4 present 64 terminal groups.

Mother liquor inducing the mineralization. Two abiotic fluids of physiological pH (pH 7.4) are to be used as mother liquors from which the mineral is formed. Both are based on the natural mineral constituents and composition of human plasma (as shown in table 1) and are referred as Synthetic Body Fluid (SBF) and SBF 1.5x according to their composition: SBF has very similar composition as the human plasma while SBF 1.5x is 1.5 folds more concentrated; the latter is used in order to elicit an accelerated response only for the materials/surfaces proved to induce mineralization when exposed to SBF. Preparing SBF is based on the procedure set-up by Prof. Kokubo (Kokubo et al., 1990) and later used by our group (Stancu et al., 2004).

	Ionic concentration, mmol/dm^3		
Ions	SBF	SBF 1.5x	Human plasma
Na+	142.0	213.0	142.0
K+	5.0	7.5	5.0
Mg2+	1.5	2.25	1.5
Ca2+	2.5	3.75	2.5
Cl-	147.8	221.7	103.0
HCO3-	4.2	6.3	27.0
HPO42-	1.0	1.5	1.0
SO42-	0.5	0.75	0.5

Table 1. Ionic concentration of the mother liquors used in the study (Kokubo et al., 1990; Stancu et al., 2004); the composition of human plasma (Tsuru et al., 2001; Jaakkola et al., 2004) is indicated as control.

The pH of the prepared solutions is adjusted to 7.40, at 36.5^{o}C, using Tris (Tris(hydroxyamino)methane - $(CH_2OH)_3CNH_2)$) and HCl. Perfectly clean reservoirs are used to prepare SBF and SBF1.5x; they should be carefully cleaned with HCl solutions followed by rinsing with demineralized water prior to use. Table 2 indicates the amount of salts needed to prepare 1 L SBF; the salts should be dissolved successively in the Tris solution previously prepared in demineralized water. Dissolving is carried out under continuous stirring, at 36.5^{o}C. The pH's adjustement represent the last step of the procedure. The stability of the so-prepared solution ahould be checked prior its utilization. The presence of spontaneously formed precipitate corresponds to contaminated solution inappropriate to be used. Only freshly prepared solutions are recommended to be used.

Reagent	Amount needed
NaCl	7.996 g
$NaHCO_3$	0.350 g
KCl	0.224 g
$K_2HPO_4 \cdot 3H_2O$	0.228 g
$MgCl_2 \cdot 6H_2O$	0.305 g
1 kmol/m³ HCl	40 cm³
$CaCl_2$	0.278 g
Na_2SO_4	0.071 g
$(CH_2OH)_3CNH_2$	6.057 g
1 kmol/m³ HCl	To adjust the pH

Table 2. Receipe for 1L SBF.

2.2 Methods

2.2.1 PAMAM immobilization on the sensor's surface

PAMAM dendrimers with amino and carboxyl terminal functionalities bearing 16 and respectively 64 reactive end groups are immobilized on gold. The immobilization procedure depends on the ending functionality of the dendrimers. The exterior reactive shell of the selected dendrimers is chemically inactive with respect to gold. Thus, in order to create stable PAMAM coating on gold, self-assembled monolayers (SAMs) of amino- and carboxyl-ended thiols should be first created on gold.

Deposition of Thiol SAMs. This is realized through the direct exposure of neat gold surfaces to 1 mM freshly prepared thiol ethanolic solution (as schematically shown in Fig. 1); the spontaneous adsorption and self-organization of thiols is achieved after 24 hours, at room temperature. Further details on thiols SAMs preparation and characterisation on gold are presented elsewhere (Stancu et al., 2007). Thiol SAMs with acidic or amino terminal functions are realized.

Dendrimers immobilization. Following carboxyl-ended thiol SAMs formation, the immobilization of amino- PAMAM occurs through bioconjugation, after the intermediate activation of carboxylic groups with EDC/NHS mixture, for 30 minutes at room temperature and in the dark (schematically shown in Fig.1). One terminal primary amine from amino-PAMAM reacts with an activated carboxyl from the thiol SAMs creating a chemical linkage. Thus, the sensor surface is chemically coated with amino-PAMAM leading to homogeneous dendrimer layers of different morphology/topography and amino-density, according to the dendrimers generation. Rinsing with demineralised water is performed to remove unreacted species.

Carboxyl-ended dendrimers are first partially activated using EDC/NHS mixture, for 30 minutes at room temperature and in the dark; then, the amino-ending thiol SAMs are exposed to the activated COOH-bearing macromolecules to create COOH-PAMAM coatings on the sensor's surface (Fig. 2). Rinsing with demineralised water is performed to remove unreacted species.

The morphology and reactivity of the new formed surfaces depend on PAMAM's generation as well as shown in Fig.3.

The so created PAMAM surface-loaded sensors should be further characterised with respect to the surface nanoroughness, dendrimers density and distribution in order to provide the quantitative characteristics of the sensing phase, further useful to quantify the mineral nucleation occurrence/evolution. Atomic Force Microscopy and a wide range of chemico-physical methods for dendrimers' quantification are available with this respect but they are not the object of this work.

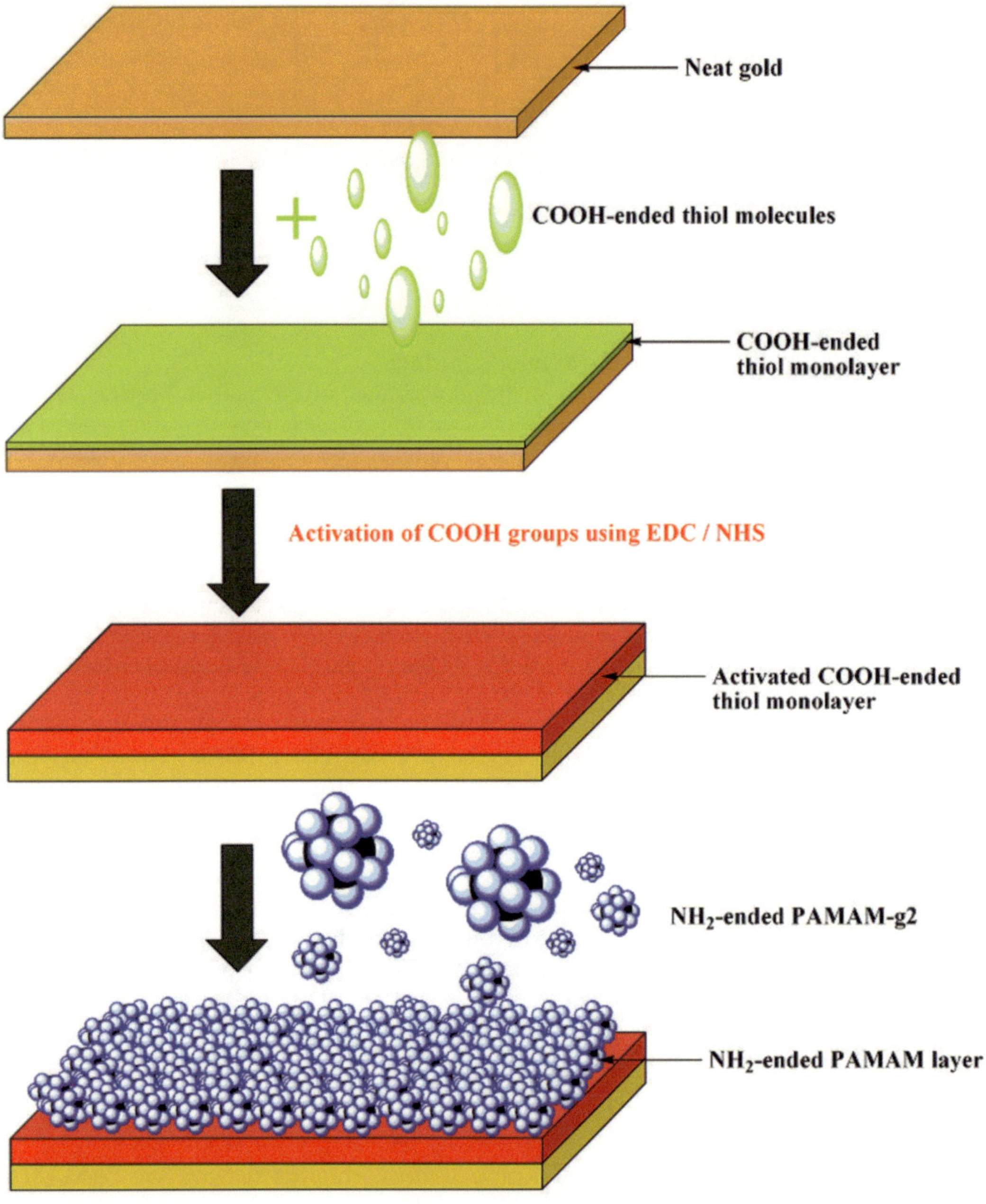

Fig. 1. Design of the NH_2-ended PAMAM sensors. Schematic view for PAMAM-g2

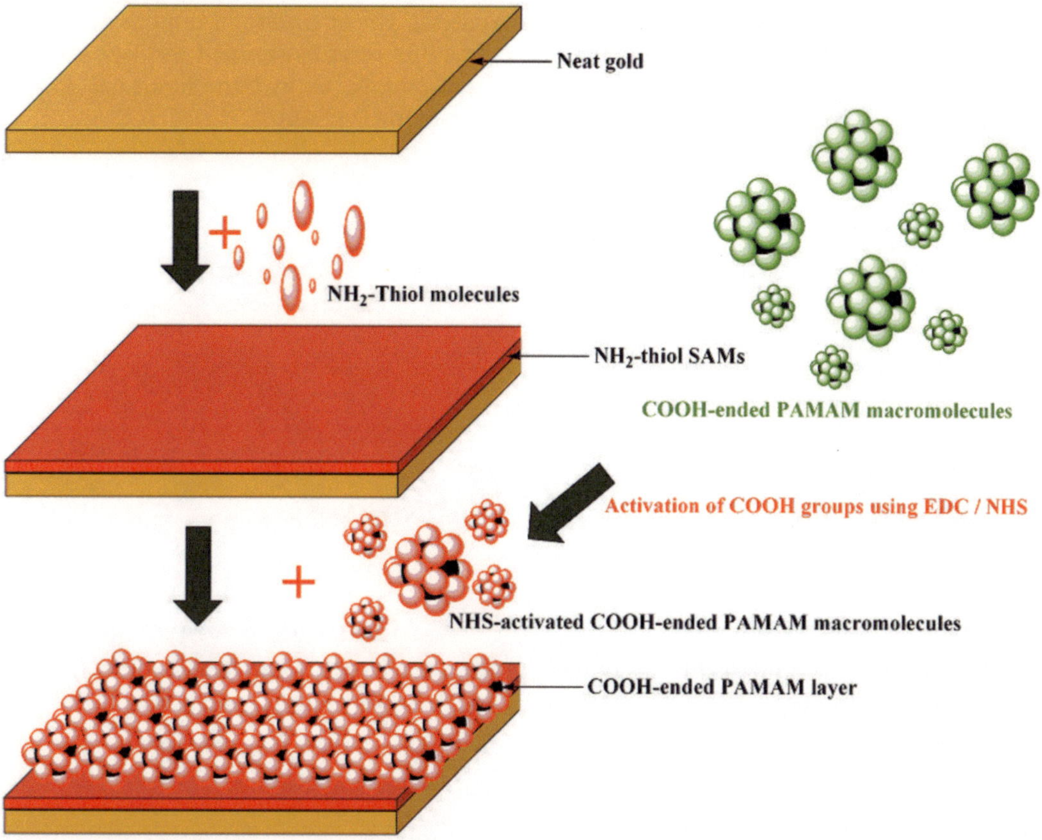

Fig. 2. Design of the COOH-ended PAMAM sensors. Schematic view for PAMAM-g1.5

2.2.2 SPRi principle and functioning

The SPRi principle is based on the label-free detection of the whole surface of the array, in a very sensitive manner, regardless the chemical nature of the immobilized molecules. Among commercially available devices one should mention the two GenOptics systems (InteractorTM and SPRiLAB TM) and the GWC SPRImager®II Array instrument. The researchers in the field of SPR imaging are usually building up their own modular instruments. The modular set-up used in this study was previously described in another work (Stancu et al., 2007); the set-up is presented in Fig. 4. Briefly, monochromatic light (wavelength 632,8 nm) is provided by a He-Ne laser LGK 7653-8 (LASOS GmbH, Ebersberg, Germany) (1 in Fig.4). The light beam is p-polyrised through the polaryser (2 in Fig. 3) and then expanded 10 times using the collimator (3 in Fig. 4).

Two tilting mirrors (4 in Fig.4) are guiding the light to the prism, under the convenient incident angle allowing for the SPR occurrence. The system contains a prism (5 in Fig.4) made of BK7 glass (n=1.51), 90°. The sensing system (7 in Fig.4) is fixed on the prism surface through a drop of oil (6 in Fig.4) with the same refractive index as the glass of the prism and of the sensor.

The reflected light is guided by another mirror (4 in Fig.4) on the CCD camera (Retiga 1300 Qimaging, Burnaby, British Columbia, Canada) (8 in Fig.4). The collected data are displayed in real time and they may be stored for further analysis. For operation in fluid as needed in this work, a flow cell (9 in Fig.4) is used. The circulating fluid is pumped through an inlet and evacuated through an outlet; the flow is 2 ml/minute, as in bone tissue, at 36.5°C. Operation under continuous flow or under stop-flow mode is possible.

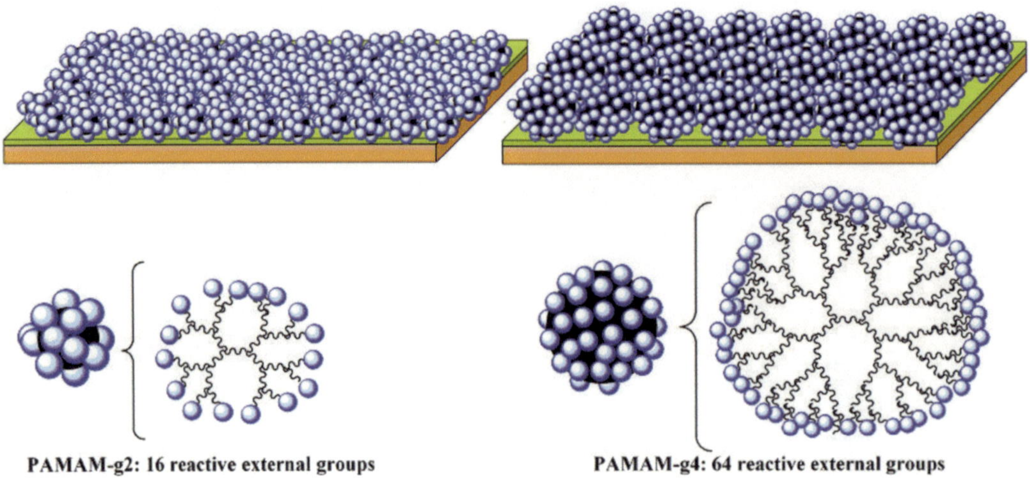

Fig. 3. Schematic view of the surfaces of the sensors coated with amino-terminal PAMAM; the morphology/topography of the sensor's surface depends on the generation of the dendrimer

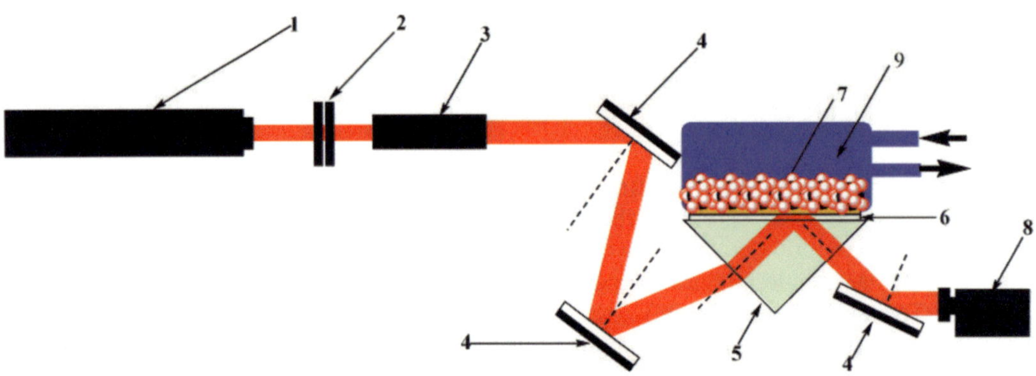

Fig. 4. SPRi modular set-up. Functioning principle - schematic view. 1 - He-Ne laser; 2 - polarysors; 3 - collimator; 4 - tilting mirrors; 6 - drop of oil; 7 - PAMAM-containing sensor; 8 - CCD camera; 9 - flow cell with inlet and outlet for analyte circulation

2.2.3 Mineralization occurrence

The PAMAM-containing sensors are fixed on the SPRi analysis platform as displayed in Fig.4 and then exposed to the experimental fluids, inside the thermostated flow cell. PAMAM macromolecules create nanorough surfaces with affinity towards calcium ions (through internal amide, and external amino and/or carboxyl groups). These macromolecules present an exterior reactive shell bearing $-NH_2$ or $-COOH$ and an intrinsic nanoporosity due to their hyperbranched tree-like structures divergent from a central core (see Fig. 3).

The architecture and the assembling of the molecules onto the gold surface are responsible for the creation of a porous layer expected to contain delineated cages in which mineral supersaturated solutions accumulates and determine the nucleation of the mineral phase.
The above mentioned functional groups (amide, amino and carboxyl) behave like ionic pumps capturing calcium ions from the test fluids; then calcium cations exert affinity towards phosphate anions and the repetition of that sequence generates calcium-phosphate mineral nuclei on the dendrimer surface; these inorganic structures develop themselves and continue to grow by ions capturing from the SBFs when the sensors are exposed to the mother liquors (left panels in Fig.5).

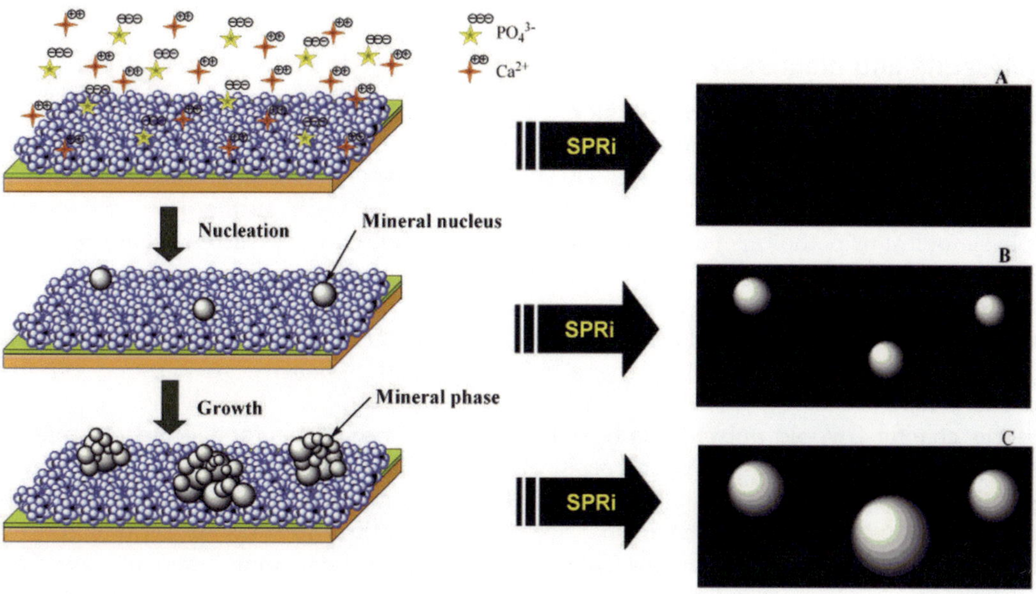

Fig. 5. Mineralization - occurrence and detection. Schematic view of: left - the evolution of the phenomenon with the formation of mineral clusters on the sensor's surface and right - the associated SPRi images as detected at PAMAM-coated gold SPR angle: A-minimum reflectivity at PAMAM-coated gold SPR angle; B – bright area due to nucleation; C – expanded bright spots due to mineral growth

2.2.4 Mineralization detection principle

The analysis tool SPRi is expected to be sensitive enough in order to provide important quantitative information on mineralization's occurrence and kinetics. The innovative SPRi detection of the mineralization is based on the specific mass change induced by the mineral nuclei formation and growth.
Of course, the technique is not adapted to distinguish between the origin/nature of the mass change, but only to sense the refraction index modification associated to that one. However, it should clearly be stated that, in that experiment, the only reason of mass change on the sensor's surface is the mineral precipitation due to nucleation and growth. These events are going to be detected and monitored as schematically presented in Fig.5.
The detection should be recorded at the SPR angle of the PAMAM-coated sensor (where the minimum reflectivity takes place leading to the darkest image of the whole sensor's surface)

as shown in panel A from Fig.5. Following nucleation in well distinct areas of the sensor a corresponding modification of the refractive index occurs and leads to the signals recorded on the image as displayed in panel B fig.5. Increasing the amount of mineral phase during the nucleation and growth leads to more intense signals schematically presented in panel C. The mineralization is not an instantaneous phenomenon. This is why, in a first attempt, the kinetics of the phenomenon should be explored in terms of induction time defined as the time, from the beginning of the experiment, needed to notice mineral nuclei formation (as the first detectable spots on the dark background). Since this might need long functioning time, it is recommended to operate the system at predetermined time intervals. Only then the experiment conditions may be optimized; data should be collected and then processed.

3. Results and discussion

3.1 Biomineralization – general considerations

Biomineralization represents the general phenomenon by which mineral formation occurs in living organisms. The process is extremely complex, it covers a multidisciplinary area and it presents specific features to each type of species involved; furthermore its nature (physiological or pathologic) and its localization in the body lead to distinct characteristics. Several researchers have tried a better understanding of the way this processes occurs. Without trying to explain here how and why biomineralization takes place, I would like to mention a reference book - *On biomineralization* written by Lowenstam and Weiner (Lowenstam & Weiner, 1989) giving a wide and comprehensive background on the phenomenon.

In this chapter I would only like to refer to the importance of macromolecules in mineral formation inside organisms. More specifically, mineral formation in bones occurs on a previously formed organic matrix consisting mainly in collagen and containing non-collagenic proteins as well. The main actors of the biomineralization are represented by cellular and acellular components functioning in an aqueous environment, but "no specialized cellular or macromolecular machinery" is known as set-up to induce mineralization (Lowenstam & Weiner, 1989); the phenomenon is generally induced even by minor perturbation of the liquid media. With respect to the acellular species involved in biomineralization, it is generally believed and demonstrated that naturally occurring polymers - mainly proteins from the hard tissue structure present special influences on the phenomenon. The functionality and the distribution of the reactive groups of these biopolymers play important roles in the induction of the nucleation and mineral growth. The use of PAMAM dendrimers offers the possibility to modify/modulate both the functionality and the distribution of the functional groups in the aim of enhancing the biomineralization response.

The here proposed experimental platform is based on homogeneous layers of PAMAM (different end-groups and different sizes/generations); more complex sensors may be designed, allowing the simultaneous investigation of several identical or different PAMAM. It is believed that PAMAM macromolecules will behave like ionic pumps with predefined shape and delineation cages, presenting affinity towards calcium and phosphate from the test fluid; the successive capturing of calcium and phosphate should lead the formation of hydroxyapatite(-like) mineral structures. The variation of parameters like the generation and the functionality should help the understanding of functional groups influence on biomineralization. It is expected that higher generation, corresponding of course to higher number of amide and amino or carboxylic ending groups, will lead to more intense calcification of the matrix. Differences between the effect of the different ending functionalities is also anticipated.

On the micro-patterned sensors containing both amino-PAMAM as well as carboxylic-PAMAM, the real time imaging of the local reflectivity should give details about who of the two chemical groups is more efficient in inducing and sustaining mineralization. Nucleation induction time should be recorded as well as the mineral growth kinetics depending of the number and type of functional shell of the tested dendrimers. Nevertheless, the best responsive PAMAM coating will be further available for implant coating.

3.2 Biomineralization – investigation tools – SPRi solution

Mineralization induction and control represent still a top-challenge in the field of hard tissue repair and regeneration. The interest on bone mineral phase formation has its start early in the biomedical field; Bronn and Buetchli cited by Lowenstam and Weiner (Lowenstam & Weiner, 1989) have performed an extraordinary work that marks the beginning of the biomineralization research, providing a solid background on mineralized structures despite their limited investigation tools: only light microscopy and chemical treatments. The modern biomineralization research started with the introduction of powerful tools such as X-ray diffraction and improved light microscopes combined with histological techniques that allow for improved access to tissue exploring. Other instruments and techniques have been added in time to the list of tools needed to help in morpho-functional biomineral and hard tissue evaluation: Scanning Electron Microscopy (SEM), Transmission Electron Microscopy (TEM), Micro-tomography. Energy dispersive X-ray spectrometer attached to electron microscopes (SEM or TEM) represents useful sensitive elemental analysis detector; however, it does not distinguish the mineral type. This latter task should be resolved with help from mineralogists. FT-IR spectroscopy and microscopy are nowadays also used to investigate the chemical structure of the biominerals.

In what concerns the induction of biomineral on different materials, sequential experiments have been presented in the literature. Basically the substrates believed to induce biomineral formation are immersed in one or several fluids with controlled composition, incubated under specific conditions (usually the physiological environment is mimicked) and at the end of the test the mineral formation is explored through the above mentioned techniques. Chemical analyses of the dissolved mineral are also an option, leading to information such as the molar ratios between different elements which in the case of calcium phosphates is very important (for instance a ration between Ca and P of 1.67 states for hydroxyapatite).

In order to obtain details on the biomineralization induction and kinetics, a high number of samples, important amounts of test materials and long experimental times are needed. To be more specific, an example will be presented. In a typical *in vitro* acellular biomineralization assay, in our group we use to explore at least 12 samples of each tested substrate; each sample is incubated in 50 ml SBF, under physiological temperature and pH, for at least 14 days (Stancu et al, 2004). Each 48 hours the incubation fluid is changed in order to provide enough ions available for the potential mineralization. At the end of the incubation time each sample is rinsed to remove non-bound mineral and debris and then the typical investigation of mineral formation is followed: SEM, TEM, EDS, FT-IR, chemical analyses, performed at least in triplicate (see details in Stancu et al, 2004).

Nevertheless, the analyses and the processing of the collected data at the end of the experiments are important.

With this respect, the present work introduces a totally new approach, based on the evaluation of one sensor at the time, using an important amount of SBF incubation fluid with constant composition, since the fluid is continuously renewed onto the sensor surface. The fluid is continuously pumped on the sensor's surface using a peristaltic pump with controlled flow of 2 ml/minute, like in natural bone tissue. Based on the investigator's expertise in what concerns the induction time (it is recommended to first explore the biomineralization induction time in order to start the detection just before its end), the sample can be monitored to record any mass change/refractive index change in real time. The samples are imaged and as soon as brighter spots appear on the dark background it can be concluded that the mineral nucleation took place. Then, increasing the intensity of the signals proves the mineral phase growth and spreading onto the tested material.
One major disadvantage of this method should be revealed here; it consists in the lack of specificity with regard to the chemical nature and complexity of the bound species. However, under controlled experimental conditions if the only source of mass change is represented by mineral formation, this disadvantage is minimized or even removed. Nevertheless, the sensor can be removed at the end of the experiment and its surface can be submitted to other specific investigation such as FT-IR or SEM to obtain complementary data on the deposited phase. A second problem associated to that method could be represented by too long operation times needed - this could be an important technical and economical problem when the light source consists in a He-Ne laser.
Now, that the most important disadvantages have been exposed, the advantages of the SPRi approach for the biomineralization investigation should be highlighted too. The high sensitivity of the SPRi tool, able to detect even few ppm of bound molecules, is an important parameter allowing to detect the presence of the early nucleation sites onto the surface of the sensor. This aspect is extremely useful since none of the previously presented techniques is able to identify that "at this moment is the real zero time and here is the zero point" of the mineral formation. Depending on the chemical nature and on the homogeneity of the analysed substrate one may explore the efficiency of a certain substrate against a different one, through micro-patterning of the sensor's surface followed by competitive monitoring of the places where the first nuclei appear (schematically displayed in Fig.6). The continuous flow of mother liquor needed to induce mineralization brings also a plus for the newly proposed method when compared with the classical ones. Typically, the old wide used methods based on the incubation of the samples in known amount of fluid (for instance 50 ml - (Stancu et al., 2004)) and the change of that one at regular time intervals (e.g. 48 hours) is not, of course, the best solution since the fluid may become poor in the needed ions and then the mineralization potential of the substrate may be misjudged. The new approach is using the continuous flow of fresh SBF and exposes the substrate to a considerable volume of 5768 ml of testing fluid in only 48 hours, which, of course, represent an advantage with respect to the accuracy of the estimation. Moreover, thin layers and respectively low amounts of sensing phase are needed in this experiment. PAMAM dendrimers that are used in this study as sensing phase are quite expensive and the evaluation of their mineralization potential when immobilized on different scaffolds would need an important budget if performed using the classical methods. If choosing the SPRi here proposed experiment, the same or even better results may be obtained with considerably lower amount of dendrimers. Nevertheless, their assembling onto the sensor may be performed on micro-domains leading to both reproducibility and competitive

results between different functionalities of the external shells in a simple experiment, on a 10 x 10 mm slide (see Fig.6).

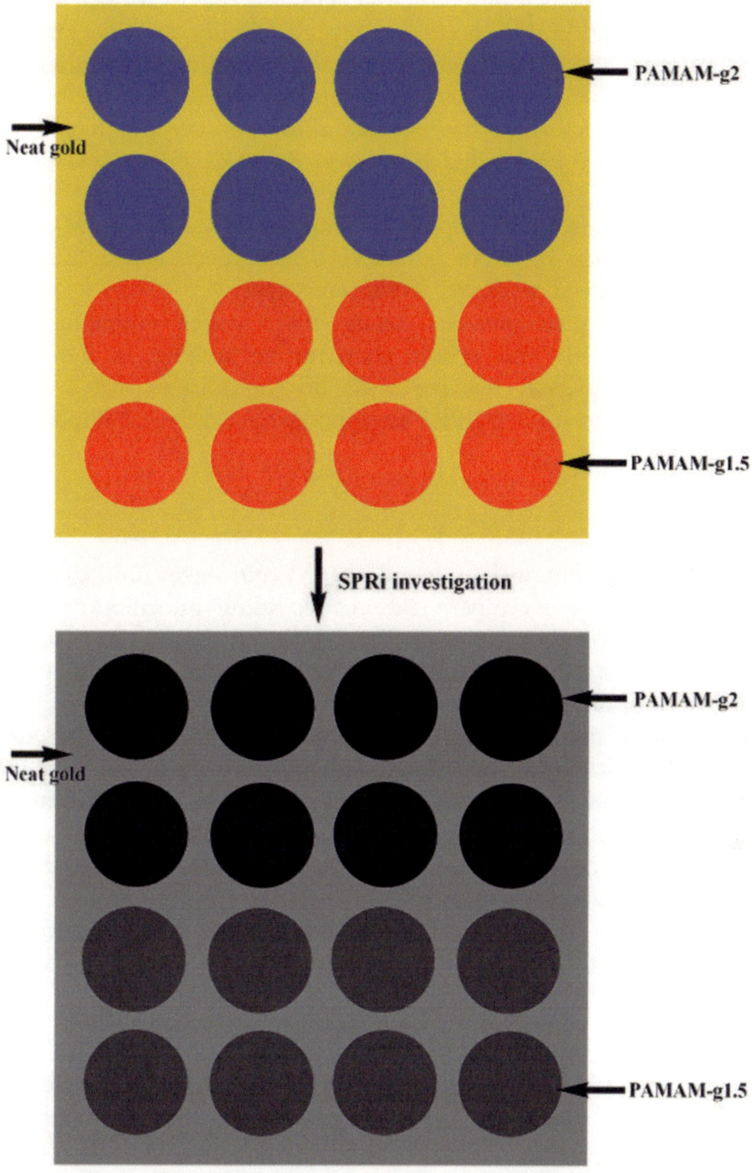

Fig. 6. Micro-patterned sensor bearing PAMAM-g2 and PAMAM-g1.5; up panel - sensor's schematic view; down - sensor imaged at SPR angle of the PAMAM-g2-coated substrate and under SBF before the nucleation occurs.

These practical aspects being mentioned, several design related features should be also emphasized. It is of maximum importance that the immobilization of the sensing phase takes place in a controlled manner, leading to ultrathin and homogeneous layers of dendrimers. Agglomeration of these macromolecules onto the sensor surface would lead to non-homogeneous signal that might make the observation of the mineralization impossible. Nevertheless, the important size of PAMAM molecules, increasing with the generation, limits the sensitivity of the sensor at too high generations due to surface's saturation. When micro-patterning is intended to check for reproducibility in the same experimental conditions, several spots of dendrimer should be created on the sensor; after exposure to the experimental fluid the results may be compared and the generated conclusion will be more precise. Moreover, the micro-paterning could allow for comparative studies between different immobilized species. In this latter case the start image will be similar to the schematic presented in Fig.6: darkest areas correspond to the PAMAM-g2-coated spots observed at their SPR angle under liquid; the images of the PAMAM-g1.5-coated spots appear brighter due to their different refractive index. When mineralization takes place, brighter signals will be noticed on the respective substrate.

The sensors may be designed/modified using different generation of dendrimers and different functionalities. This will enable comparative studies on the influence of the generation and of the external reactive shell on the mineralization occurrence. This information is extremely useful in further nano-patterning different implants with the best PAMAM coating.

4. Conclusion

The proposed SPRi assessment of the mineralization occurrence could be very useful in the better understanding of the biomineralization, providing information impossible to be revealed by the already existing techniques. The method is simple, clean, very sensitive and efficient, opening a new route to mineralization evaluation. Practical advantages are evident against some inherent disadvantages.

Versatility represents a major characteristic of this method since the set-up and the experimental conditions are easy to be changed depending on the investigator's choice. Nevertheless, the use of PAMAM nanostructured surfaces to induce biomineral formation has its novelty character too. Versatility is also the key attribute of the developed sensors since both the functionality and the generation of the dendrimers may be modified in order to get the best biomineralization answear.

To my knowledge, this is the first attempt of investigating mineralization through SPRi. Further development, improvements and experimental data will follow this approach.

5. Acknowledgements

The National Authority for Scientific Research from The Ministry of Education, Research and Youth of Romania is gratefully acknowledged for the financial support through the exploratory project "Polymeric Biomaterials for Bone Repair. Biomimetism through Nanostructured Surface", PN-II-ID-2008-2, number 729/19.01.2009

6. References

Donners J.J.J.M.; Nolte R.J.M.; Sommerdijk N.A.J.M. (2003). Control over calcium carbonate phase formation by dendrimer/surfactant templates. *Advanced Materials*, Vol.15, No. 4, 313-316, ISSN 0935-9648 (print) 1521-4095 (Online)

Filmon R.; Grizon F.; Basle M.F.; Chappard D. (2002). Effects of negatively charged groups (carboxymethyl) on the calcification of poly(2-hydroxyethyl methacrylate). *Biomaterials,* Vol. 23, No.14 (July 2002), 3053–3059

Ganss B.; Kim R.H.; Sodek J. (1999). Bone sialoprotein. *Critical Reviews in Oral Biology & Medecine,* Vol 10 (January 1999) 79 -98, ISSN 1544-1113 (online) 1045-4411 (print),

Hunter G.K.; Poitras M.S.; Underhill T.M.; Grynpas M.D.; Goldberg H.A. (2001). Induction of collagen mineralization by a bone sialoprotein- decorin chimeric protein. *Journal of Biomedical Materials Research,* Vol. 55, No.4 (June 2001) 496–502, ISSN 1552-4965 (online) 1549-3296 (print)

Jaakkola, T.; Rich, J.; Tirri, T.; Narhi, T.; Jokinen, M.; Seppala, J.; Yli-Urpo, A. (2004). In vitro Ca-P precipitation on biodegradable thermoplastic composite of poly(E-caprolactone-co-DL-lactide) and bioactive glass (S53P4). *Biomaterials.,* Vol. 25, No. 4 (February 2004) 575-581, ISSN 0142-9612

Kamei S.M; Tomita N.; Tamai S.; Kato K.; Ikada Y. (1997) Histologic and mechanical evaluation for bone bonding of polymer surfaces grafted with a phosphate-containing polymer. *Journal of Biomedical Materials Research,* Vol. 37, No.3 (December 1997) 384 -393, ISSN 1552-4965 (online) 1549-3296 (print)

Kokubo, T.; Ito, S.; Huang, Z. T.; Hayashi, T.; Sakka, S.; Kitsugi, T. and Yamamuro, T. (1990). Ca-P rich layer formed on high strength bioactive glass-ceramics. *Journal of Biomedical Materials Research.* Vol. 24, No.3 (March 1990) 331-343, ISSN 1552-4965 (online) 1549-3296 (print)

Lowenstam, H.A.; Weiner, S. (1989), *On biomineralization,* Oxford Academic Press, ISBN 0-19-504977-2 (U.S.), New York

Majoros, I.J.; Mehta, C.B.; Baker Jr., J. R. (2004). Mathematical Description of Dendrimer Structure. *Journal of Computational and Theoretical Nanoscience,* Vol. 1, No. 2 (September 2004), 193-198(6), ISSN 1546-1955, 1546-1963

Price, R.L.; Haberstroh, K.M. and Webster, T.J. (2003). Enhanced Functions of Osteoblasts on Nanostructured Surfaces of Carbon and Alumina. *Medical and Biological Engineering and Computing (Incorporating Cellular Engineering),* Vol. 41, No. 3 (May 2003) 372-375, ISSN 0140-0118 (Print) 1741-0444 (Online)

Shin H.; Jo S.; Mikos A.G. (2003). Biomimetic materials for tissue engineering. *Biomaterials* Vol. 24, No.13 (….2003) 4353- 4364, ISSN 0142-9612

Stancu, I. C.; Filmon, R.; Cincu, C.; Marculescu, B.; Zaharia, C.; Tourmen, Y.; Basle, M. F.; Chappard, D. (2004). Synthesis of methacryloyloxyethyl methacrylate phosphate copolymers and in vitro calcification capacity. *Biomaterials,* Vol. 25, No. 2 (January 2004) 205-213, ISSN 0142-9612

Stancu, I.C.; Fernandez-Gonzalez, A.; Salzer, R. (2007). SPR imaging antimucin-mucin bioaffinity biosensor as label-free tool for early cancer diagnosis. Design and detection principle. *Journal of Optoelectronics and Advanced Materials,* Vol. 9, No. 6 (June 2007) 1883-1889, ISSN 1454 - 4164, 1841 - 7132

Swart J.G.N.; Driessen A.A.; DeVisser A.C. (1976). Calcification and bone induction studies in heterogeneous pohosphorylated hydrogels. In: *Hydrogels for medical and related applications.* Andrade J.D. (Ed.), 151–161, ACS Symposium Series, No.31, Washington DC

Ulman, A. (1991), *An Introduction to Ultrathin Organic Films from Langmuir-Blodgett to Self-Assembly,* Academic Press, ISBN 0127082301, 9780127082301, 978-0127082301

Vijayasekaran S.; Chirila T.V.; Robertson T.A.; Lou X.; Fitton J.H.; Hicks C.R.; Constable I.J. (2000) Calcification of poly(2-hydroxyethyl methacrylate) hydrogel sponges implanted in the rabbit cornea: A 3-month study. *Journal of Biomaterials Science. Polymer Edition,* Vol. 11, No.6 (June 2000) 599–615, ISSN 0920-5063, 1568-5624 (Online)

Ward B.C.; Webster T.J. (2006). The effect of nanotopography on calcium and phosphorus deposition on metallic materials in vitro, *Biomaterials,* 27 (June 2006) 575-8, ISSN 0142-9612

Whyte M.P.; Landt M.; Ryan L.M.; Mulivor R.A.; Henthorn P.S.; Fedde K.N.; Mahuren J.D.; Coburn S.P. (1995). Alkaline phosphatase: Placental and tissue-nonspecific isoenzymes hydrolyze phosphoethanolamine, inorganic pyrophosphate, and pyridoxal 5-phosphate. Substrate accumulation in carriers of hypophosphatasia corrects during pregnancy. *Journal of Clinical Investigation,* vol. 95 (April 1995) 1440–1445, ISSN 0021-9738

5

Soft Computing Techniques in Modelling the Influence of pH and Temperature on Dopamine Biosensor

Vania Rangelova[1], Diana Tsankova[1] and Nina Dimcheva[2]

1Technical University – Sofia, branch Plovdiv

2University of Plovdiv

4000 Plovdiv

Bulgaria

1. Introduction

Biosensors represent very promising analytical tools that are capable of providing a continuous, fast and sensitive quantitative analysis in a straightforward and cost-effective way. According to the definition of IUPAC (International Union of Pure and Applied Chemistry) the biosensing analytical devices combine a biological element for molecular recognition with a signal-processing device (transducer). The transducer, which normally ensures the high sensitivity of the sensor, can be thermal, optical, magnetic field, piezo-electrical or electrochemical. On the other hand, the selectivity of detection is assured by the biological recognition element that might consists of either a bioligand (DNA, RNA, antibodies etc.) or a biocatalyst, such as some redox proteins, individual enzymes and enzymatic systems (cell membranes, whole microorganisms, tissues) (Castillo et al., 2004; Scheller et al. 2001). Electrochemical biosensors show two main advantages over the other types of biosensors: i) they are susceptible to miniaturization, and ii) the electrical response – current or potential, could be easily processed using not expensive and compact instrumentation.

Among the electrochemical biosensors, enzyme-based amperometric biosensors represents the most used group, which functions on the basis of monitoring the current variation at an polarised electrode, induced by the reaction/interaction of the biorecognition element with the analyte of interest. Then, amperometric enzyme-based biosensors on their part, can be classified into three categories (Castillo et al., 2004; Scheller et al., 2001), in accordance with the mode of action:

- *first generation biosensors*: the signal is generated upon the electrochemical reaction of an active reagent (monitoring the decrease of the current) or product (monitoring the increase of the current) that are involved in the biochemical transformation of the target compound- the enzyme substrate (Dimcheva et al., 2002 ; Dodevska et al., 2006; Horozova et al., 2009).
- *second generation biosensors*: the architecture of these biosensors includes a freely diffusing redox mediator (small molecular weight compounds, able to effectively shuttle electrons between the electrode surface and the enzyme active site) and in this

mode the concentration of the target analyte, that participate at the biochemical reaction, is proportional to the response resulted from the mediator oxidation/reduction at the electrode (Stoica et al., 2009).

- *third generation biosensors*: the biocomponent is capable of directly (mediatorsless) exchanging electrons between the active site of the enzyme and the transducer and as a result, the concentration of analyte is directly proportional to the redox current generated at the polarised electrode. The advantages of third generation biosensors are represented by the simplicity of construction, the exclusion of additional supportive substances (e.g. mediator), the increase of specificity for target analyte, the removal of interferences due to usually low polarization potential at the working electrode, etc. (Christensson et al., 2004; Stoica et al., 2005). Nevertheless, only limited number of enzymes (mostly heme - or copper - containing oxidoreductases) has been proven to work for the third generation biosensors and their common feature is that a metal-containing cofactor that functions either as a catalytic cofactor and/or as an intra-molecular electron transfer cofactor is embedded in the protein shell.

Despite the second and especially third generation biosensors ensure an exceptional selectivity of the analysis, first generation biosensors are the most widely spread, mainly because of the simplicity of their construction. A typical first generation biosensor can be easily constructed by assembling the biological recognition element onto a conventional electrode, which can be either an oxygen-sensitive probe to assay the consumption of oxygen, or a hydrogen peroxide – sensitive electrode to monitor the concentration of H_2O_2, produced upon the enzymatic conversion of the analyte. Assaying the biological oxygen demand (BOD) seems to be the most universal method for biosensing, since oxygen is the reagent consumed during biochemical transformations catalysed not only by individual oxidative enzymes or enzymatic systems, but also by whole aerobic microorganisms.

Modelling the processes taking place at the interfaces of the first generation amperometric biosensors as well as identifying the factors possessing strong impact on their response will facilitate to a great extent the optimisation of biosensors fabrication, which in turn will considerably shorten the period between R&D stage and their mass–market acceptance. The catalytic activity of the biological recognition element is known to depend strongly on pH and temperature, and therefore these factors are expected to affect the biosensor response as well. Similarly to the chemical reactions, the rate of enzyme-catalyzed reactions rises exponentially with increasing temperature, however this dependence passes through a maximum because at temperatures around 50 deg an irreversible thermal denaturation of the enzymes starts. The dependence of the biosensor response on pH represents a bell-shaped curve that reaches its maximum around the pH optimum of the bio-component. The peak might be broad or narrow, depending on the composition of the medium and temperature. Under the optimal conditions (pH and temperature) the biosensor response is stable and the sensitivity is high and hence, this environment shall be preferred for the measurements.

The modern intelligent devices typically possess the ability to compensate the influences of different kind such as temperature and pH as the later are among the most important factors for an optimal biosensor performance. Modelling the output current versus pH and temperature would provide the opportunity to improve their accuracy and usage while doing measurements under variable conditions.

In the present work a plant tissue biosensor for dopamine assay is considered as the model biosensor, based on a plant tissue immobilized onto an oxygen Clark probe (Rangelova et al., 2003). Such a biosensing system will be of high interest for the biomedical analysis because the dopamine levels in urine and blood plasma are indicative for diseases like ganglioneuroma, schizophrenia, manic-depressive psychosis, stress, and burn-out syndrome. The traditional analysis is made mainly by radioimmunoassay or chromatography, which are time and labour-consuming techniques, requiring tedious sample pre-treatment and costly equipment. Alternatively, an amperometric dopamine biosensor would provide a fast and straightforward assay of the analyte. Depending on the diffusion limitations the response time of such an amperometric biosensor can range from several seconds to 2-3 minutes.

The purpose of the present work is to model the influence of pH and temperature- separately and simultaneously, on the dopamine biosensor response by means of soft computing. The problem to solve is to find a way of increasing the accuracy (and the rapidity) of the modelling process, under a condition of insufficient experimental data. To this end, the following soft computing techniques were compared in MATLAB environment: (1) *Cerebellar Model Articulation Controller* (CMAC) neural network, (2) *neural network with backpropagation learning algorithm* (NNBP), (3) *fuzzy logic* (FL), and (4) *adaptive-network-based fuzzy inference system* (ANFIS). The relative errors over a few new experimental samples were calculated for validation of the proposed models.

2. The biosensor

2.1 Biosensor construction, the mechanism of enzyme action, experimental setup, measurement procedure, and factors affecting the biosensor performance

a) Biosensor preparation.

The detection principle of dopamine biosensing consists in measuring the oxygen consumption upon the oxidation of dopamine, catalysed by the enzyme polyphenol oxidase (PPO). The first-generation biosensor studied here, was constructed from a conventional oxygen probe (Clark type gold electrode, purity 99.95%, 1 mm diameter) used as transducer and a polyphenol oxidase (PPO) - containing membrane, fixed at the tip of the electrode. A thin banana (*musa acuminata*) slice was used as the source of PPO enzyme. The banana tissue was first homogenised, then immobilised onto a dederone mesh (thickness 70 μm), the mesh was placed over an oxygen-permeable Teflon membrane (10 μm thick) which was further assembled on the forehead of the oxygen electrode. To protect the biological material from leakage, the dederone mesh was covered by a 25 μm thick dialysis membrane and the so obtained triple-layer membrane was fixed with an O – ring onto the forehead of the working electrode.

b) Mechanism of enzyme action

The enzyme polyphenol oxidase (PPO) the physiological function of which is to convert phenolic compounds into *o*-quinones in the presence of molecular oxygen, consists of four subunits containing one atom of copper per subunit (Palmer, 1963), with a relative molecular weight of the tetramer of about 128 000 Daltons. It possesses two binding sites for aromatic compounds including phenolic substrates (Climent, 2001) and a distinct binding site for oxygen. The enzyme reaches its optimum activity at pH 7 when using it specific substrate dopamine - a phenolyc type neurotransmitter. The oxidation of dopamine with molecular oxygen, catalysed by the enzyme PPO is schematically represented by the following reaction (1):

$$\text{Dopamine} + 1/2\ O_2 \xrightarrow{\text{PPO}} \text{Dopamine-o-quinone} + H_2O \tag{1}$$

Or the corresponding general scheme of a bi-substrate enzyme –catalysed reaction:

$$\text{So} + \text{C} \xrightarrow{\text{E}} \text{P} \tag{2}$$

where So stands for the first substrate - dopamine, the dissolved oxygen gas (the co-substrate) is denoted with C, with E – the enzyme PPO; with P – the products: dopamine – o – quinine and the molecule of water released upon dopamine oxidation.

c) Experimental setup and apparatus.

The experimental setup is schematically depicted at Fig.1. (Rangelova et al., 2002). All the measurements were performed in a conventional dual-electrode electrochemical setup with the working bio-electrode and a reference Ag/AgCl electrode. Prior to use the biosensor was conditioned by dipping in a phosphate buffer (pH = 7) for one hour. Then the prepared biosensor was immersed in a single-compartment electrochemical cell (working volume 15 ml, filled with phosphate buffer) and polarised at a constant potential of - 800 ± 80 mV/ vs. Ag/AgCl. During the experiments the solution was permanently stirred at 600 rpm (*rpm-rotations per minute* stirring rate, with a magnetic stirrer). Transient currents were allowed to decay to a steady-state value within 2 - 3 min until a constant background current (the response in the buffer solution without substrate) of 104 nA ± 7.5 nA was established. The output current was measured by means of a microampermeter (Ф 195 accuracy ±1.5%, Russia, measuring range 50 nA - 100 μA). For monitoring the transient state a Y - t recorder (ENDIM 622.01, Germany) was used. The pH of the buffer solutions was adjusted with a

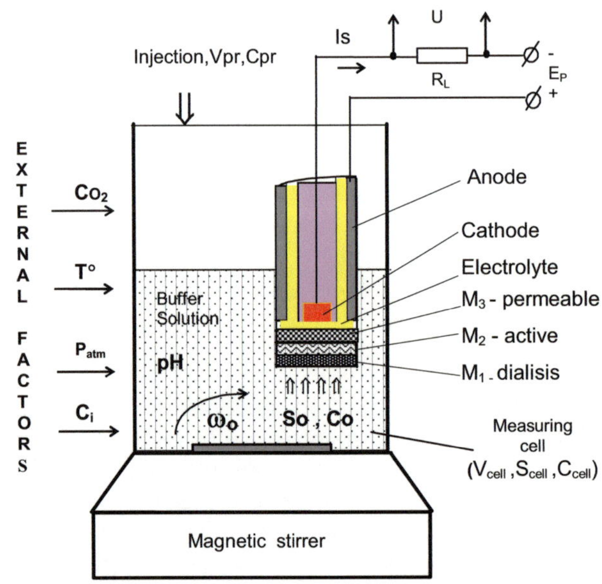

Fig. 1. Schematic representation of the dual-electrode experimental setup

pH-meter Piccolo (Hanna Instr., accuracy ± 0.1), while the temperature was monitored with a mercury thermometer (accuracy ± 0.05°C).
On Fig.1. the three membranes are indicated as follows: M_1 - dialysis, M_2 - the banana tissue-containing membrane and M_3 - the gas-permeable membrane. In the electrochemical cell the working electrode was negatively polarised and therefore functioned as the cathode, while the reference electrode was the anode. The potential difference between the electrodes was generated by applying an external voltage E_P. When the current Is passed through the loading resistance R_L an Ohmic drop U was generated.

d) Measurement procedure

In order to determine any unknown concentration of substrate in the cell ($S_{cell} = S_o$) a calibration graph was built by using the method of subsequent additions. For this purpose, the background current was first established at the chosen pH and temperature, then an aliquot of the substrate stock solution with a volume V_{pr} and concentration C_{pr} was added to the buffer in the cell (volume V_{cell}) and the current was allowed to decay to a steady-state value. Then new aliquots were injected in the cell and the corresponding biosensor responses were registered until the saturation of the enzyme layer with substrate was reached, i.e. until the electrode response stopped changing when a new injection was added. Upon injecting the substrate the transient current was registered with Y-t recorder until the steady state was reached and the readings of microampermeter were taken as electrode response. Usually, 12 additions with volume of 100 µl each, were made and the calibration graph was obtained by plotting the electrode response versus the substrate concentration at which it was registered. Single dopamine injection assures a final concentration of substrate in the cell of S_o=0.142 mM.
In order to provide the enzyme-catalysed reaction with a continuous flow of oxygen, which is the second substrate of PPO, the buffer solution was permanently stirred with a stirring rate ωo, ensuring also much faster mass-transfer of the substrate towards the enzyme layer (the membrane M_2). In this layer the measured substrate So is converted to the product P, a part of the dissolved oxygen is consumed during the dopamine enzymatic oxidation, while the rest of the oxygen passes through the gas-permeable membrane and is further depolarised on the cathode, resulting in an output current I_s. The measurements were performed in a steady-state regime.

e) The influencing factors

The main factors supposed to affect to a great extent the output current of the dopamine biosensor, are schematically depicted at Fig.2. (Rangelova et al., 2002). With block 1) is denoted the dissolution of the oxygen C_{O2} from the gas phase to the liquid phase Co. With block 2) is denoted the dilution of the sample concentration Ssm to the measured one So. With block 3) is denoted the conversion of the gas components C_G into the corresponding concentrations in the liquid phase Ci. In the active membrane from the membrane group 4) reaction catalyzed by the enzyme (E) takes place. With Pi is denoted the lateral product from the conversion of substrate S into the product P. They change the acidity of the medium to the value pH_R. In the active membrane, usually the optimal pH and temperature T are maintained. In the active membrane normally the optimal pH is given and for these reason it is changed with ΔpH. Because the system is co-substrate sensitive, through the membrane M_3 the residual concentration of oxygen Cx and only a part of obstructive substances $Ci^{(2)}$ is passing. The rest reagents with concentration $Ci^{(1)}$, product P and substrate S are returned

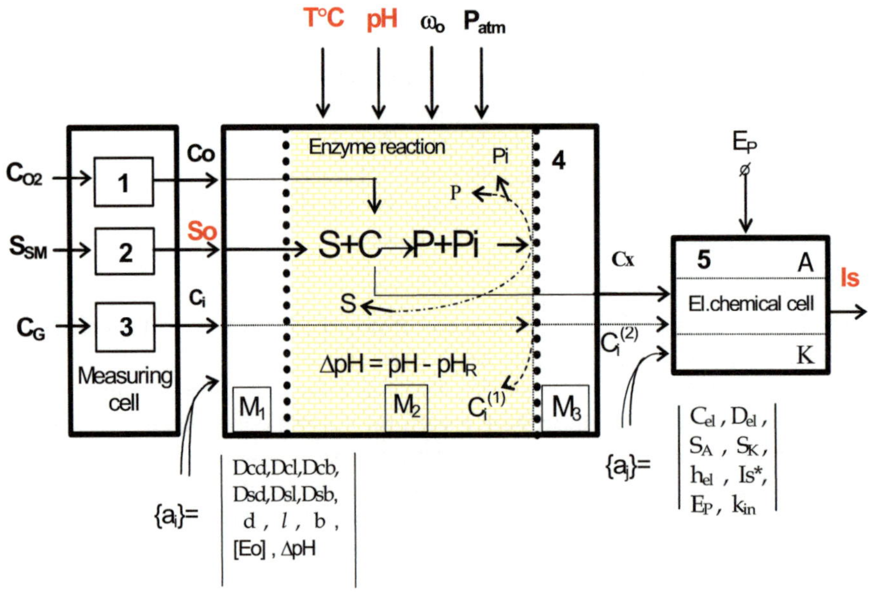

Fig. 2. Scheme of the factors influencing the biosensor responce.

to the active membrane. The electrochemical cell 5) is supplied by an external polarising voltage Ep. The output steady-state current is Is. **The main external factors possessing strong impact over the biosensor performance are: temperature t °C, pH, stirring rate ω_o and atmospheric pressure P_{atm}. They have significant effect over the processes into the measuring cell. For the practical measurements all these parameters are chosen very carefully and the measurements are done for some definite working conditions (depending on the task).** The constructive parameters can be divided into two groups. The *first one* $\{a_i\}$, includes all diffusions coefficients Dij, the thickness of membranes b, l, d, variation of ΔpH and concentration of enzyme [Eo]. The *second group* $\{a_j\}$ includes the parameters of the electrochemical cell: concentration of electrolyte Cel and the corresponding diffusion coefficients Del, the thickness of the electrolyte layer h_{el}, anode and cathode surface area- S_A and S_K, the initial value of the current I*, the value of the polarising voltage Ep and the rate constant of the electrochemical reaction Kin.

From the metrological point of view, the measurements with a biosensor can be presented with the model

$$y = F(x, \xi_{1,} ......\xi_m, T, a_1 ....a_n, \Delta F) \, , \tag{3}$$

where: x – is the measured value (concentration of substrate So);

$\xi_{1,} ......\xi_m$ - influencing factors (C_{O2} , C_G ,T, pH, ωo, P_{atm});

$a_1 ....a_n$ - constructive parameters ($\{a_i\}$, includes all diffusions coefficients Dij, the thickness of membranes b, l, d, variation of ΔpH, concentration of enzyme [Eo] and $\{a_j\}$ include the parameters of the electrochemical cell : concentration of electrolyte Cel and corresponding diffusion coefficients Del, the thickness of the electrolyte layer h_{el}, anode area S_A and cathode area S_K, the initial value of current Is*, the value of the polarising voltage Ep and the rate of the electrochemical reaction Kin.);

ΔF - error of the model.

For the given biosensor all constructive parameters are chosen after careful selection, depending on the task and usage, but the influencing factors depend on the circumstances and they may change during the measurement. Temperature and pH are the most important influencing factors. They have strong impact not only on the very enzymatic reactions (Ziyan & Pekyardimci, 2004; Shizuko et al., 2005; Burkert et al., 2006) but also on the diffusion parameters (Puida et al, 2009) and the oxygen concentration (Falck , 1997) and therefore the output current will be greatly dependent on them. Moreover, the temperature and pH significantly affect the biosensor response, causing *non-linearity* (maximum in our case) in the curve of the output current.

Thermostatic conditions can be achieved by either controlling the sample solution temperature or by regulating the temperature of the electrode itself so that the membrane and diffusion layers are at a constant temperature throughout an experiment (Falck , 1997). pH can be controlled too. But when the biosensor is used *in-situ* or *in-vivo* (in our case for measurement of neurotransmiter dopamine) the temperature and pH affect strongly the output reading. The body temperature may be higher or lower than the temperature at which the sensor is calibrated and the same is for the pH (depending on the person's acid-base status, the pH of urine may range from 4.5 to 8) thereby it can be invalidating the calibration curve (usually it has been done for constant pH and constant temperature). If thermostatic conditions are not feasible, temperature effects must be compensated. The most popular method is hardware method. Using a miniature thermistor probe, the temperature of the sensing system is measured simultaneously with the current of the biosensor and a normalised signal is calculated which does not depend on temperature (Skladal 1995, Patent Appl. No. 60/859,586, 2006). But those methods can not compensate the full process of measurement. First, pH can not be compensated during the in vivo measurement. Second, the measured current is very small - within the nA- range, where the drift of electronic devices will affect the precision of the whole system. If the biosensor is used for the biomedical purposes, where the accuracy of the device is of key importance, it is necessary to be sure that measured values are real and precise.

The soft computing methods propose a new type of modelling the influence factors over measurement quantity and that way the calibration surfaces for the certain range of them can be received. Those methods are intelligent and adaptive. Their advantages become more obvious when the data are complex.

2.2 Calibration graphs

The experimental data used in the work were derived under the following conditions: Calibration graphs were carried out in steady state regime, using the method of subsequent additions. Every addition was with volume 0.1 ml and corresponding to 0.142 mM dopamine concentration. Measurements were stopped when the saturation zone of the output current Is was reached, because the system became uninformative. *Five* calibration graphs were obtained for five different temperatures (15 24 26 35 and 50°C) at a constant pH=7 and 12 steps of substrate additions (Fig.3a). *Seven* calibration graphs were built up for seven different pH-values (4 4.8 5 5.4 5.8 7 7.5 and 8) at a constant temperature T=24°C and with the same steps of substrate additions (Fig.3b). Because the output current is a dropping function of substrate concentration it was centred to the zero of the scale. The vertical section of Fig.3a and Fig.3b for the given substrate concentration So=0.142 mM is shown in Fig.3c and Fig.3d, respectively.

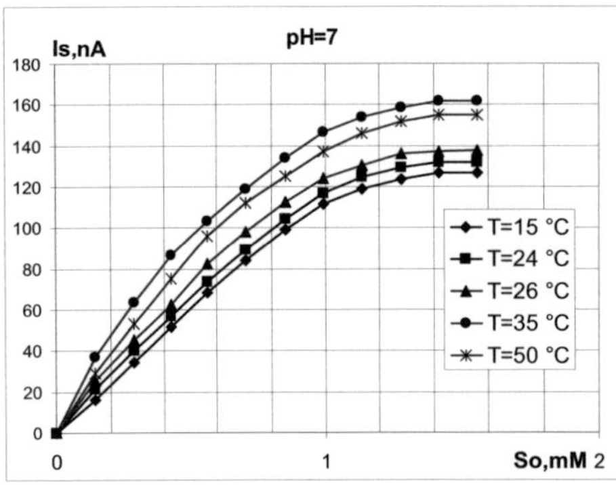

(a) Influence of temperature, pH =7

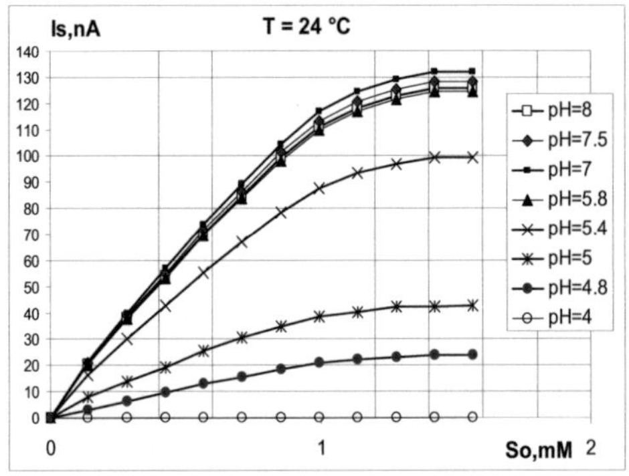

(b) Influence of pH, T = 24°C.

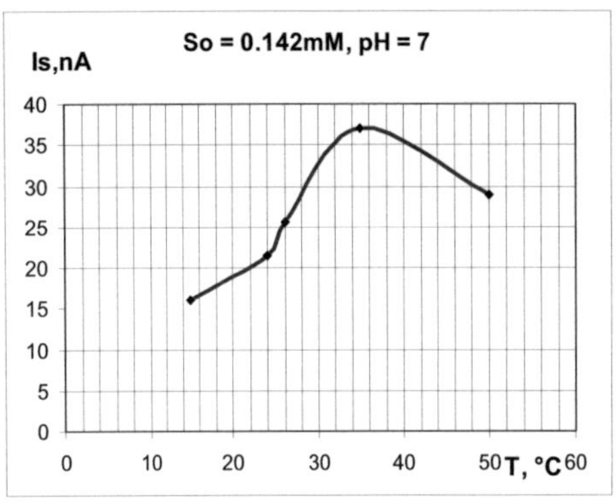

(c) Influence of temperature under constant So and pH

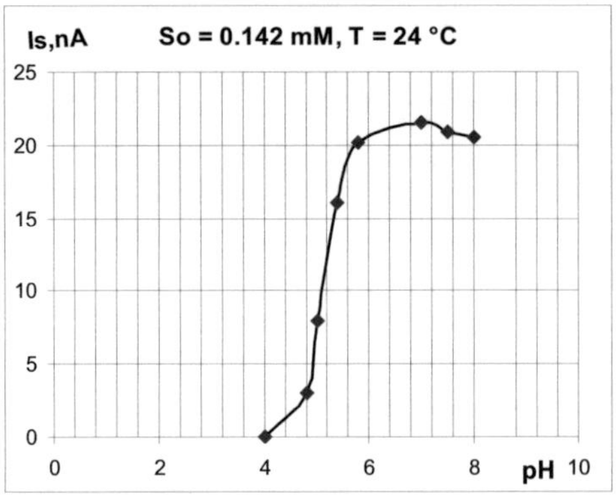

(d) Influence of pH under constant So and pH

Fig. 3. Experimental data: influences of temperature and pH on a dopamine biosensor

3. The task formulation and soft computing algorithms for its implementation

To some extent, the soft computing draws inspiration from natural phenomena. Its key areas include: neural networks, fuzzy systems, and evolutionary computation. The soft computing is usually robust under noisy input environments and has a high tolerance for imprecision in the data on which it operates. It is well known that neural networks are universal function approximators (Blum & Li, 1991). The approximation possibility of feedforward multilayered neural networks with backpropagation learning algorithm for modelling the biosensor's output voltage versus substrate concentration at different temperatures has been considered in (Ferreira et al., 2003). The same type of neural network has been used for pH estimation (Hitzman et al., 1997; Moatar et al.,1999) and control (Lamanna et al., 1996; Syu & Chen, 1998) with applications in ecology. Such neural networks have some drawbacks: (1) the proper number of hidden layers and the number of neurons in them are not known in advance, (2) the learning is a time consuming process, which often gets stuck in local minima, (3) the neural network could not generalize, if the training samples are insufficient. The CMAC-neural-network-based model of the biosensor input/output has overcome some of the drawbacks, however it needs sufficient number of experimental data for designing a large set of overlapping receptive fields. Additional samples obtained by linear interpolation have been applied for the CMAC training in (Rangelova & Tsankova 2007a). The use of interpolated data is justified under the lack of data, because of difficulties associated with their experimental acquisition, but it reduces the main advantage of a neural model - the high accuracy. Two fuzzy logic based models of a dopamine biosensor that take into account the influence of temperature (first model) and pH (the other) have been recently proposed in (Rangelova & Tsankova, 2007b) and (Rangelova & Tsankova, 2008), respectively. This technique has been found to perform well under imprecise and insufficient experimental data.

3.1 The task formulation

The overall goal of this scientific work is to propose an appropriate soft computing technique to model the influence of both the temperature and the pH on the input-output dependency of a biosensor for dopamine assay. Due to the difficulties associated with their experimental acquisition, only very limited number of experimental data are supposed to be available. Thus, in order to accomplish the target of the work the following directions were identified:

1. To investigate and model separately the influence of temperature and pH on the output current of the above described dopamine biosensor;
2. To explore four types of soft computing techniques - CMAC, NNBP, FL and ANFIS;
3. To determine the average relative error of a few new experimental data intended for a validation of the models;
4. To select the best performing under insufficient experimental data technique;
5. To apply the selected technique for modelling the influence of both the temperature and pH (simultaneously) on the dopamine biosensor.

Since in the literature have been proposed some intelligent models, considering the influence of the temperature and the pH on the same type of biosensor, some of the here made analyses have a confirmative character (Section 5) and give us a reason to expect, that under deprived information the fuzzy model performs better than the others. That is why the fuzzy logic has been chosen *a priori* as a means for modelling simultaneously the influence of the temperature and pH. A more precise design of this model (our particular contribution here) is given in Section 4. The next two Sections (3.2 and 3.3) treat in brief some neural and fuzzy algorithms used for the purposes of intelligent modelling.

3.2 Feedforward neural networks

In this Section two types of feedforward NNs are presented: (1) CMAC-based NN, and (2) NN trained by error backpropagation learning algorithm. They are used as universal function approximators.

CMAC functional block diagram for two-dimensional input space (Miller et al., 1990) is shown in Fig. 4. A large set of overlapping, multidimensional receptive fields with finite boundaries describes the operation of the Albus CMAC (Kraft et al., 1992). Any input vector falls within the range of some of the receptive fields and excites them. The response of the CMAC neural network to a given input is the average of responses only of receptive fields excited by that input. Neural network training for a given input vector affects the adjustable parameters of the excited receptive fields. The total collection of receptive fields is divided into C subsets (layers), which represent parallel N- dimensional hyperspaces for a network with N inputs. The receptive fields in each of the layers are organized so as to span the input space without overlapping. Any input vector excites one receptive field from each layer, which means C exited receptive fields per input. Each of the layers of receptive fields is offset relative to the others in the input hyperspace. The width of the receptive fields produces input generalization, while the offset of the adjacent layers of receptive fields produces input quantization (Miller & Glanz, 1994). The integer parameter C is determined as the *generalization parameter*. The ratio of the width of each receptive field (input generalization) to the offset between adjacent layers of receptive fields (input quantization) must be equal to C. Each receptive field is assumed to be a 'switch on/ switch off' type of content. If a receptive field is excited, its response is equal to the magnitude of a single adjustable weight assigned to that receptive field. If a receptive field is not excited, its response is zero. The CMAC output is the average of the adjustable weights of the excited receptive fields.

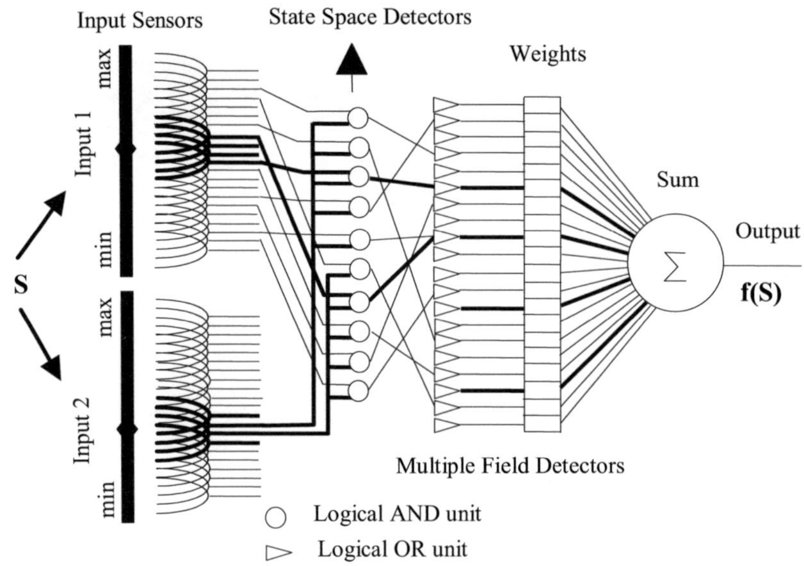

Fig. 4. CMAC functional block diagram (Kraft et al., 1992).

Consider Albus CMAC neural network with the following real valued input vector

$$\mathbf{S} = (s_1, s_2, ..., s_N)^{\mathrm{T}}, \tag{4}$$

where N is the dimension of input space. Let C be the generalization parameter (the number of simultaneously excited receptive fields for each input). The first step of the CMAC computing algorithm is to form a normalized integer input vector $\mathbf{S}'$ by dividing each component s of the input vector by an appropriate *quantization parameter* Δ_j:

$$\mathbf{S}' = (s'_1, s'_2, ..., s'_N) = (\mathrm{int}(s_1 / \Delta_1), \mathrm{int}(s_2 / \Delta_2), ..., \mathrm{int}(s_N / \Delta_N))^T. \tag{5}$$

The width of each receptive field along the jth axis is equal to $C \cdot \Delta_j$ in the original input space, and is equal to C along all axes in the normalized input space. The next step of the CMAC computing algorithm is to form the vector addresses $\mathbf{A}_i$ of the C receptive fields which contain the input point $\mathbf{S}'$:

$$\mathbf{A}_i = (s_1' - ((s_1' - i)\%C), s_2' - ((s_2' - i)\%C), ..., s_N' - ((s_N' - i)\%C))^T = (a_{i1}, a_{i2}, ..., a_{iN})^T, \quad i = 1,2,...,C, \tag{6}$$

where % represents the modulus operator, and the index i references the C parallel layers of receptive fields. $\mathbf{A}_i$ is the normalized N-dimensional address of one corner of the hypercubic region spanned by the single excited receptive field in layer i. Then the next step of the CMAC algorithm is forming the scalar physical addresses A_i' of the actual adjustable weights:

$$A_i' = h(a_{i1}, a_{i2}, ..., a_{iN}). \tag{7}$$

In this equation, $h(...)$ represents any pseudo-random hashing function which operates on the components a_{ij} of the virtual addresses of the receptive fields, producing uniformly distributed scalar addresses in the physical weight memory of size M. Finally, the CMAC scalar output $y(\mathbf{S})$ is calculated as:

$$y(\mathbf{S}) = \frac{1}{C}\sum_{i=1}^{C} W(A_i'). \tag{8}$$

Network training use the data pairs $\mathbf{S}$ and $y_d(\mathbf{S})$, where $y_d(\mathbf{S})$ is the desired network output in response to the input vector $\mathbf{S}$. The weights of memory are adjusted by ΔW, calculated as:

$$\Delta W = \beta(y_d(\mathbf{S}) - y(\mathbf{S})), \tag{9}$$

where the same value ΔW is added to the content $W(A')$ of each of the C memory cells, taking part in the computation of $y(\mathbf{S})$. β is a constant training gain (between 0 and 1).
NNBP is composed of one hidden layer, whose neurons have a hyperbolic tangent sigmoid transfer function, and one neuron with a linear transfer function in the output layer. The weights of the network connections and the biases of the neuron's transfer functions are trained by the classical error backpropagation learning algorithm. Because of the limited space and the popularity of the backpropagation learning algorithm, it will not be described here. A detailed description can be found in (Rumelhart et al., 1986; Krose & Smagt, 1996).

3.3 Fuzzy logic and ANFIS

A fuzzy system employing fuzzy if-then rules can model the qualitative aspects of human knowledge and reasoning without precise quantitative analyses. Consider a fuzzy system, which comprises of four principal components: fuzzifier, fuzzy rule base, fuzzy inference engine, and defuzzifier (Fig. 5). For the sake of simplicity of understanding the mechanism of fuzzy logic the system under consideration has two inputs and one output.

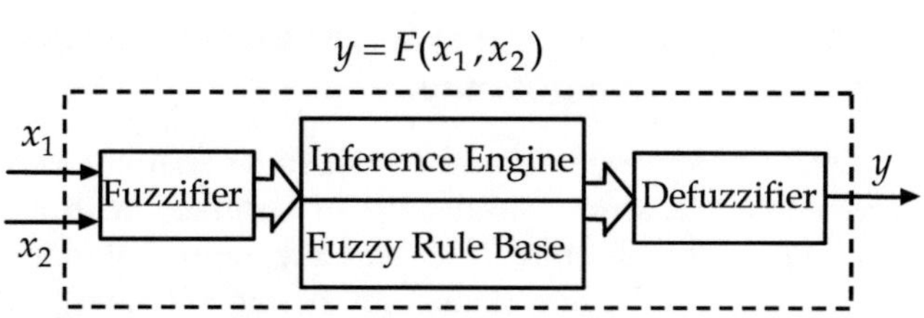

Fig. 5. Basic configuration of a fuzzy system.

Let $X_1, X_2, Y \subset R$ are universes of discourse of the variables x_1, x_2, and y, respectively. The fuzzifier performs a mapping from the observed crisp input spaces X_1 and X_2 to the fuzzy sets in these spaces. The fuzzy sets $X_1^i \in X_1$ ($i = 1,2,...,l$) and $X_2^j \in X_2$ ($j = 1,2,...,m$) are linguistic terms characterized by fuzzy membership functions $\mu_1^i(x_1)$ and $\mu_2^j(x_2)$, respectively. The two linguistic variables (for x_1 and x_2) with corresponding membership functions ($X_1^i, \mu_i(x_1)$, $X_1^{i+1}, \mu_{i+1}(x_1)$, $X_2^j, \mu_j(x_2)$, and $X_2^{j+1}, \mu_{j+1}(x_2)$) enter the fuzzy rule table. The fuzzy rule base consists of fuzzy if-then rules of Takagi and Sugeno's type (Takagi & Sugeno, 1983). The fuzzy rule set can be expressed in the following form:

$$\text{IF } x_1 \text{ } is \text{ } X_1^i \text{ } and \text{ } x_2 \text{ } is \text{ } X_2^j \text{ THEN } y = Y_{i,j}, \tag{10}$$

where $i = 1,2,...,l$ and $j = 1,2,...,m$. Four fuzzy sets of the output signal are obtained from the fuzzy rule table: $Y_{i,j}$, $\mu_{i,j}(y)$; $Y_{i,j+1}$, $\mu_{i,j+1}(y)$; $Y_{i+1,j}$, $\mu_{i+1,j}(y)$; and $Y_{i+1,j+1}$, $\mu_{i+1,j+1}(y)$. ($Y_{i,j}$ is assumed to be the variable in the cell arranged in i-th row and j-th column of the rule table).

The *fuzzy inference engine* is a decision making logic which employs fuzzy rules from the fuzzy rule base to determine a mapping from the fuzzy sets in the input spaces X_1 and X_2 to the fuzzy sets in the output space Y. The firing strength of p,q-th rule ($\mu_{p,q}(y)$) is obtained as the T-norm of the membership values on the premise part (by using a multiplication operator):

$$\mu_{p,q}(y) = \mu_p(x_1)\mu_q(x_2), \tag{11}$$

where $p = i,\ i+1$, and $q = j,\ j+1$.

The *defuzzifier* performs a back mapping of the output signal from the fuzzy sets to crisp points. So the overall output is computed as the weighted average of each rule's output:

$$y = \frac{\sum_{p,q} Y_{p,q}\mu_{p,q}(y)}{\sum_{p,q} \mu_{p,q}(y)}, \tag{12}$$

where $p = i,\ i+1$; $q = j,\ j+1$.

ANFIS has the same number of membership functions assigned to each of the two inputs as those of the fuzzy system. A supervisor gives the training input-output samples (experimental data). The ANFIS uses a combination of least-squares and backpropagation gradient descent methods for training membership function's parameters to model that set of training data. More detailed description of ANFIS can be found in (Jang, 1993).

4. Fuzzy logic based modelling the influence of both temperature and pH on the biosensor's input/output dependency.

According to (Kosko 1992) the representation theorem states that any continuous nonlinear function can be approximated to any desired level of accuracy with a finite set of fuzzy variables, values, and rules. This theorem describes the representational power of fuzzy modelling, but it does not answer the questions, how many rules are needed and how they can be found, which are of course essential to real-world problems and solutions (Driankov et al., 1993). In a conventional fuzzy system, the number of rules is decided by an expert who is familiar with the system to be modelled.

The experimental data needed for modelling the biosensor under consideration are given in Section 2.2 (Fig.3). The surface plot of the output current versus both pH and temperature for three different values of the substrate concentration, $S_0 = (0.142 \quad 0.426 \quad 0.710)\,\text{mM}$, is shown in Fig.6. The surfaces have the expected bell-shaped trend, forming maximum for pH=7 and temperature 35°C. Actually, only part of this experimental data, belonging to a region, that is important for the dopamine measurement, is used in the modelling process.

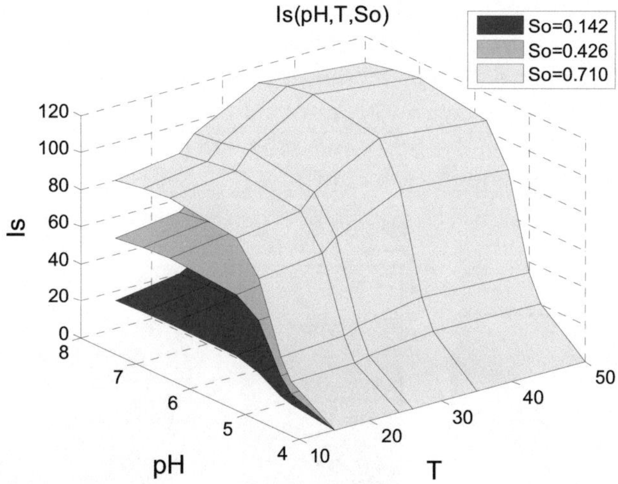

Fig. 6. Experimental data: Surface plots of the output current vs. both pH and temperature for three different values of the substrate concentration

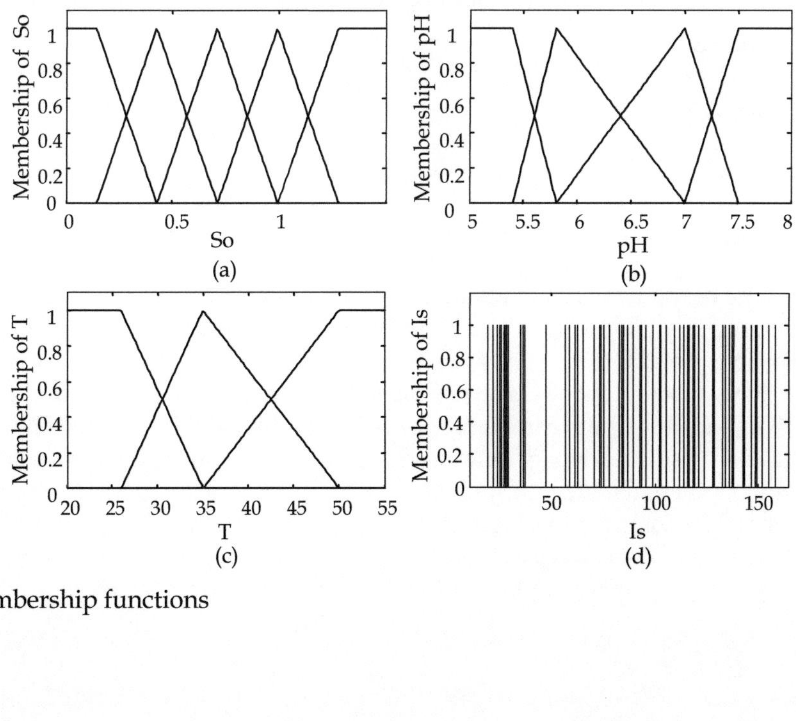

Fig. 7. Membership functions

The substrate concentration S_0, the pH and the temperature T are the three input variables of the fuzzy inference system, i.e. $x_1 \leftarrow S_0$, $x_2 \leftarrow pH$ and $x_3 \leftarrow T$. The fuzzy system described in Section 3.3 is used here, but adapted to three-dimensional input space. The number of membership functions assigned to each input variable is proposed to be equal to the number of corresponding measured values, i.e. $l = 5$ (S_0), $m = 4$ (pH) and $n = 3$ (T). In conformity with the results, reported in (Rangelova & Tsankova, 2007b; Rangelova & Tsankova, 2008) and confirmed in the next Section, the triangular shape of membership functions (Fig.7) and T-norm (using the multiplication operator) of the membership values on the premise part are chosen. The apexes of the triangles are exactly the measured values of substrate, pH and temperature. The fuzzy rule table can be filled in with all the experimental data for biosensor's output current ($y \leftarrow I_S$), which are $Y_{i,j,k} : l \times m \times n = 60$. The output current is presented by 60 different values. For the sake of convenience the values $Y_{i,j,k}$ in the fuzzy rule table are presented with 60-level gray scale squares (Fig. 8), corresponding to the values of $I_S = I_S(S_0, pH, T)$.

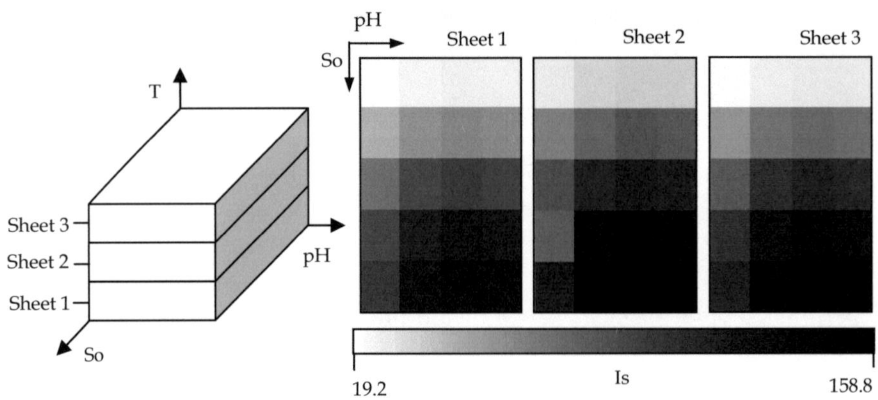

Fig. 8. Fuzzy rule table

5. Results and discussions

The next Sections 5.1 and 5.2 treat modelling the influence of the temperature and the pH separately on the biosensor's output current. The soft computing models investigated in those sections have been already proposed in the literature, and their presentation here has a confirmation character. On the basis of their comparative analysis, made in Section 5.3, the most proper type of model (sufficiently accurate under a small number of data) was chosen for the simultaneously modelling the influence of the temperature and pH on dopamine biosensor (Sections 4 and 5.4).

Fig. 9 shows the surface plots of the experimental data (Section 2.2) used in the modelling procedure of: (a) the temperature influence (pH=7), and (b) the pH influence (T=24°C).

All of the models using learning techniques need a large amount of data for training, otherwise they do not generalize incoming new data. A supervisor gives the training input-output samples. The basic samples are obtained experimentally (Fig.3, Fig9), but they are insufficient, because of difficulties associated with their experimentally deriving. This may result in a very coarse approximation or a lack of generalization. In the literature (Rangelova

& Tsankova, 2007a,b; Rangelova & Tsankova, 2008) additional samples obtained by linear interpolation have been used in training procedure.

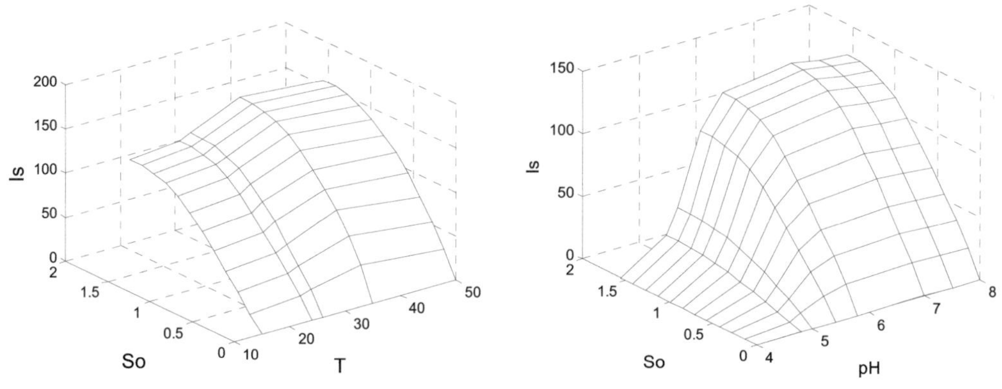

(a) (b)

Fig. 9. Surface plots of experimental data: (a) temperature influence (pH=7), and (b) *pH* influence (T=24°C)

The supervisors for both CMAC and NNBP, as well as ANFIS used the experimental data supplemented with additional samples obtained by linear interpolation with discrete parameters: (a) $0.071\,mM$ and 1^0C along substrate concentration S_0 and temperature T, respectively, in $I_S = I_S(S_0, T)$ models; and (b) $0.071\,mM$ and 0.1 along substrate concentration S_0 and pH, respectively, in $I_S = I_S(S_0, pH)$ models.
The validation of the considered aproximators is based on the average relative error over a few new experimental data (Section 5.3).

5.1 Neural networks based models of the influence of the temperature and the pH (separately) on the biosensor's output current

As it was mentioned above, in both models (the temperature influenced model and the pH influenced one), the supervisor for the CMAC neural network, as well as for the NNBP, used experimental data supplemented with additional samples.
The CMAC's generalization parameter and learning coefficient were chosen to be $C = 2$ and $\beta = 0.05$, respectively. The results obtained after 10000 learning epochs is shown in Fig.10a and Fig.10b, but after the first three thousands of iterations the accuracy of approximation was already satisfactory. The sum squared error (SSE) over the experimental data used in training (the interpolated samples are not included in the calculation of SSE) is $SSE_T^{CMAC} = 0.260$ for the temperature influenced model and $SSE_{pH}^{CMAC} = 0.423$ for the pH influenced one.
As it was mentioned in Section 3.2 the NNBP consists of one hidden layer, whose neurons posess hyperbolic tangent sigmoid transfer functions, and one output layer neuron with linear transfer function. The NNBP, modelling the temperatute influence, contained 500 neurons in its hidden layer, and the other NNBP, modelling the pH influence - 1000 neurons. After millions iterations the NNBPs were still not learned enough. The responces of the NNBP, modelling the temperatute influence and the other, modelling the pH influene (after prolonged training) are shown in Fig.10c and Fig.10d, respectively.

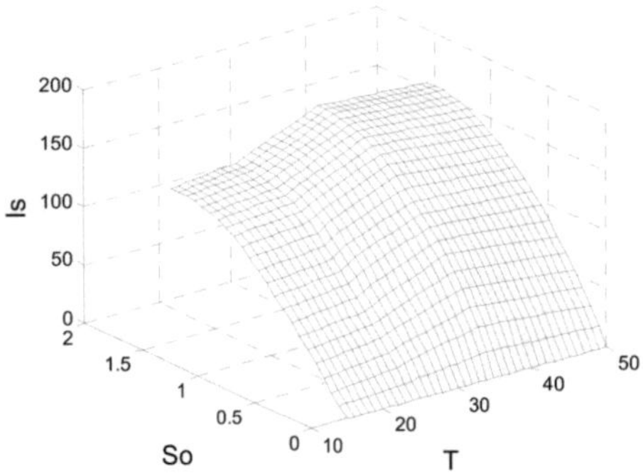

(a) CMAC model of T influence

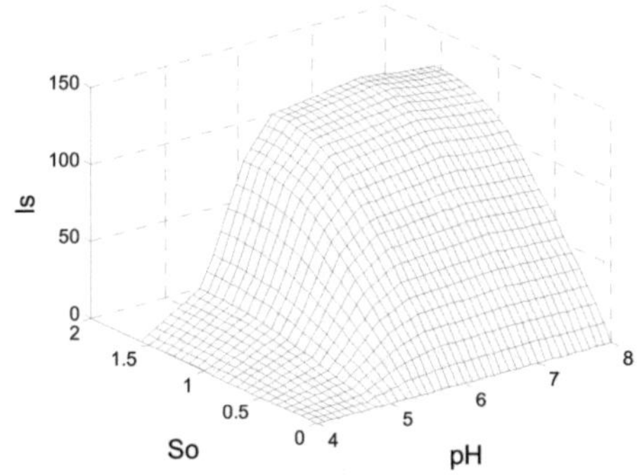

(b) CMAC model of pH influence

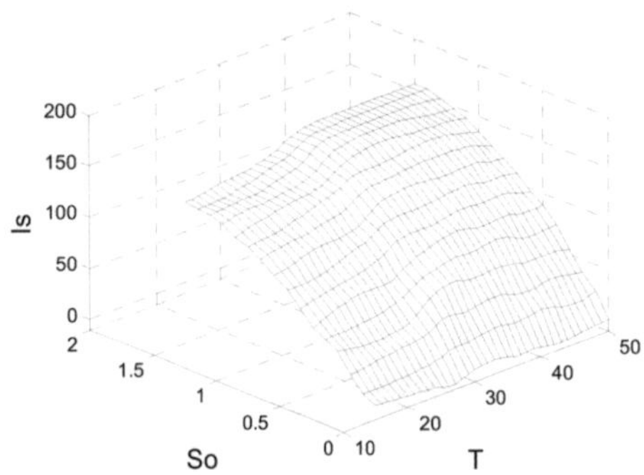

(c) NNBP model of T influence

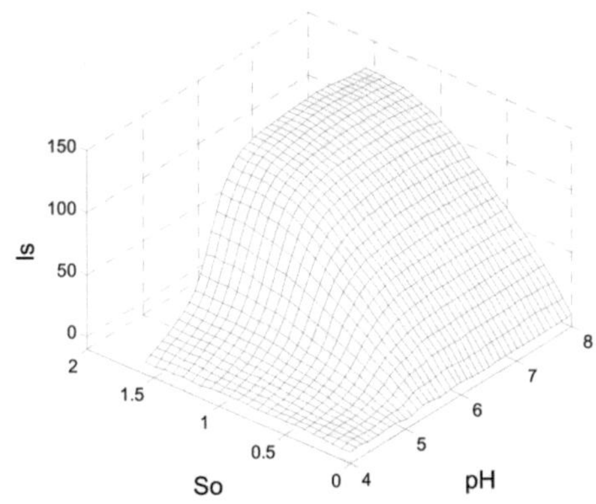

(d) NNBP model of pH influence

Fig. 10. NN-based approximation surfaces of the biosensor input/output dependency

5.2 Modelling the influence of the temperature and the pH (separately) on the biosensor's output current using fuzzy logic and ANFIS

Fuzzy logic based biosensor's model has two inputs: $x_1 \leftarrow S_0$ and $x_2 \leftarrow T \text{ or } pH$ - the substrate concentration and the temperature (for the first model) or the pH (for the second model), respectively, and one output – the biosensor's current $y \leftarrow I_S$. As it was described in Section 4 the number of membership functions assigned to each input variable is equal to the number of corresponding measured values, i.e., $l = 12$ and $m = 5 \text{ or } 8$ (for T or pH, respectively). The triangular form of membership functions and T-norm of the membership values on the premise part were chosen. The fuzzy rule table contained all the measurements of the biosensor's output current, which are $Y_{i,j} : l \times m = 60 \text{ or } 96$ (for T or pH, respectively).

The fuzzy approximations of the biosensor's input-output relation, taking into account the influence of the temperature and the pH (separately) are shown in Fig.11a and Fig.11b, respectively. For the sake of clarity of simulations and a good visualization, discrete steps 0.071 mM, 1^0C and 0.1 pH were used along the substrate concentration, the temperature, and the pH, respectively.

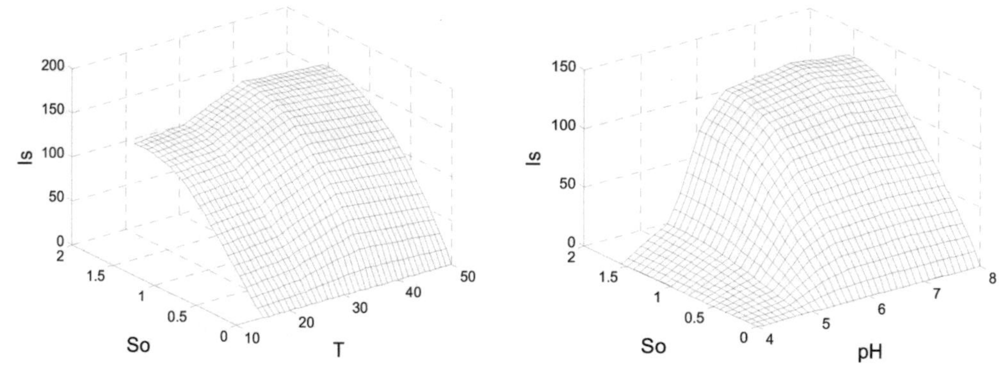

(a) (b)

Fig. 11. Fuzzy approximation surface of the influence of: (a) the temperature, and (b) the pH, on the biosensor's input-output dependency.

ANFIS had the same number of membership functions as the fuzzy approximator. Two types of membership function (MF), triangular and Gaussian curve membership functions, were heuristically chosen. The output membership function type was set up linear.

The performance of two variants of ANFIS-based approximators, one using triangular membership functions, and another - Gaussian curve based ones, is demonstrated in Fig.12a and Fig.12b, respectively. The former modelled the temperature influence on the biosensor's current, and the latter - the pH influence. In these two cases ANFIS *used only the experimental data*. Regardless of the shape of membership functions the ANFIS did not generalize under insufficient number of data. The modelling procedure was repeated with the same additional interpolated data as those used in the neural approximations. The resultant surfaces reffering to the temperatute influenced model and the pH affected one are shown in Fig.13a and Fig.13b. Both approximators shown in Fig.13 used triangular membership functions. All the ANFIS approximators were considered as trained after 20 epochs.

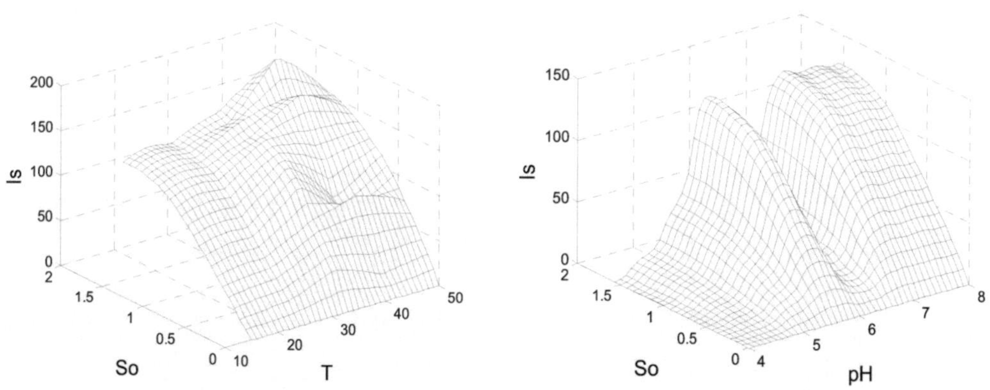

(a) ANFIS with triangular MF (model of T influence)

(b) ANFIS with Gaussian MF (model of pH influence)

Fig. 12. ANFIS-based approximation surfaces using only experimental data

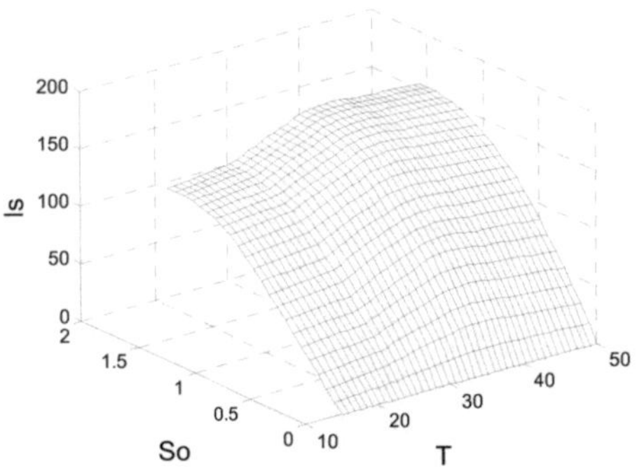

(a) ANFIS with triangular MF
(model of T influence)

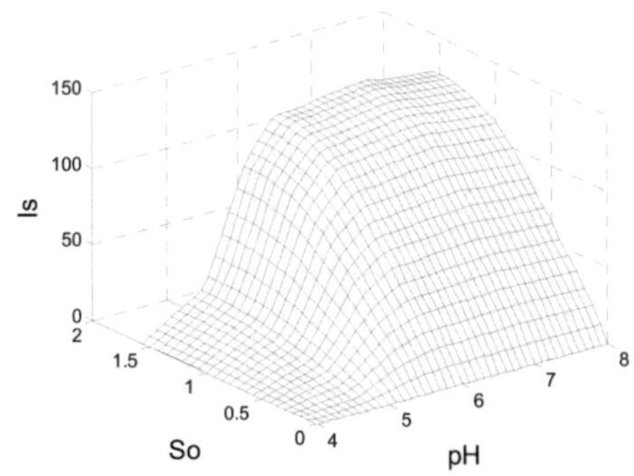

(b) ANFIS with triangular MF
(model of pH influence)

Fig. 13. ANFIS-based approximation surfaces using additional interpolated data

5.3 Comparative analysis of the investigated models

The generalization of the four soft computing techniques was verified on the one hand qualitatively, by a visual observation the shape of approximation surfaces, and on the other hand - quantitatively, by calculating the average relative error over three new experimental samples. The relative error of each of the new experiments is calculated as

$$\varepsilon = \frac{| I_S^{approx} - I_S^e |}{I_S^e} 100, \ \% \qquad (13)$$

where I_S^e and I_S^{approx} are the output current determined experimentally and by means of one of the four type of approximations. The validation results, represented by the relative error (13), are listed in Table 1 and Table 2, referring to the temperature influence model and the *pH* influence one, respectively.

No.	Test Data pH = 7			NN				Fuzzy Logic		ANFIS			
				BP		CMAC				Using additional interpolated data			
										Triangular		Gaussian	
	T	S_0	I_S	I_S^{NNBP}	ε^{NNBP}	I_S^{CMAC}	ε^{CMAC}	I_S^{FL}	ε^{FL}	I_S^{ANFIS}	ε^{ANFIS}	I_S^{ANFIS}	ε^{ANFIS}
	°C	mM	nA	nA	%	nA	%	nA	%	nA	%	nA	%
1	18	0.568	70.2	72.192	2.838	70.208	0.012	70.2	0	72.80	3.706	74.60	6.271
2	18	1.136	120.8	118.782	1.671	120.902	0.085	120.9	0.083	125.96	4.272	129.84	7.483
3	25	0.710	93.3	92.601	0.750	93.698	0.427	93.7	0.429	93.67	0.396	92.99	0.332
Average Relative Error [%]					1.75		0.18		0.17		2.79		4.69

Table 1. Results from validation test for **temperature** influence modelling.

No.	Test Data T = 24°C			NN				Fuzzy Logic		ANFIS Using additional interpolated data			
				BP		CMAC				Triangular		Gaussian	
	pH	S_0	I_S	I_S^{NNBP}	ε^{NNBP}	I_S^{CMAC}	ε^{CMAC}	I_S^{FL}	ε^{FL}	I_S^{ANFIS}	ε^{ANFIS}	I_S^{ANFIS}	ε^{ANFIS}
		mM	nA	nA	%	nA	%	nA	%	nA	%	nA	%
1	4.5	0.852	11.5	10.75	6.54	11.57	0.62	11.56	0.54	11.504	0.03	11.66	1.42
2	6.5	0.426	56.0	56.11	0.42	55.37	1.11	55.38	1.10	55.37	1.12	55.37	1.13
3	7.5	0.426	55.0	55.37	0.85	55.12	0.21	55.10	0.18	55.11	0.20	55.12	0.22
Average Relative Error [%]					2.60		0.65		0.61		0.45		0.92

Table 2. Results from validation test for ***pH*** influence modelling

It is evident from the two tables, that only the fuzzy approximator operates well under the small number of the experimental input/output samples. All the other approximators do not generalize under this circumstance. They need additional training data, which are obtained in this scientific work by linear interpolation of experimental data. The interpolated data predetermine the type of approximation surface and usually decrease the main advantage of neural models - the high accuracy. Using additional training data the models perform similarly to each other (with respect to accuracy), excepting the NNBP. Although the neural networks with backpropagation learning algorithm can approximate each function with sufficient high accuracy, practically, it is not so easy to determine the proper number of hidden layers and the number of neurons per each layer. Training is extremely time-consuming procedure, because it requires millions of iterations. Due to the gradient method there is a tendency the learning process to be trapped in local minima. The NNBP performs worse than the others, probably because of insufficient learning.

The fuzzy model performs better then the others: it is faster and easier to implement, works well under a small number of experimental data. These properties make it preferable for the particular purpose - to improve the accuracy of the dopamine measurement by taking into account both the temperature and the *pH* influences on the biosensor's output current.

5.4 Fuzzy modelling and validation of the simultaneous influence of temperature and pH on the biosensor's output current

The comparative analysis, made in the previous Section, shows that the most appropriate soft computing technique for our purpose (intelligent modelling the dependency $I_S = I_S(S_0, pH, T)$ using poor experimental data) is the fuzzy logic. Since this result was expected, having in mind the present publications, this model was developed and adapted to our purpose in advance in Section 4. So the membership functions of the three input variables (S_0, pH and T) and the output signal are presented in Fig.7a,b,c,d, respectively. The fuzzy rule table is shown in Fig.8. Only part of the experimental data, shown in Fig.3, is used in the fuzzy model. The samples, included in this part, correspond to the apexes of the membership functions of the input variables (Fig.7a,b,c), and more precisely written:

$$S_0 = (0.142 \quad 0.426 \quad 0.710 \quad 0.997 \quad 1.278)\ \text{mM}\,,\ pH = (5.4 \quad 5.8 \quad 7.0 \quad 7.5)\,,$$

$$\text{and}\ \ T = (26 \quad 35 \quad 50)\ {}^0\text{C}\,.$$

The fuzzy model was simulated in MATLAB environment using a number of assignment input samples and the result is shown in Fig. 14 (a qualitative validation test). For the sake of clarity two variants of a presentation (one using a gray scale, and another - colour scale) are proposed. The values of thus calculated output current I_S can be determined using the transformation bar (gray or colour bar), situated to the right of the pictures.

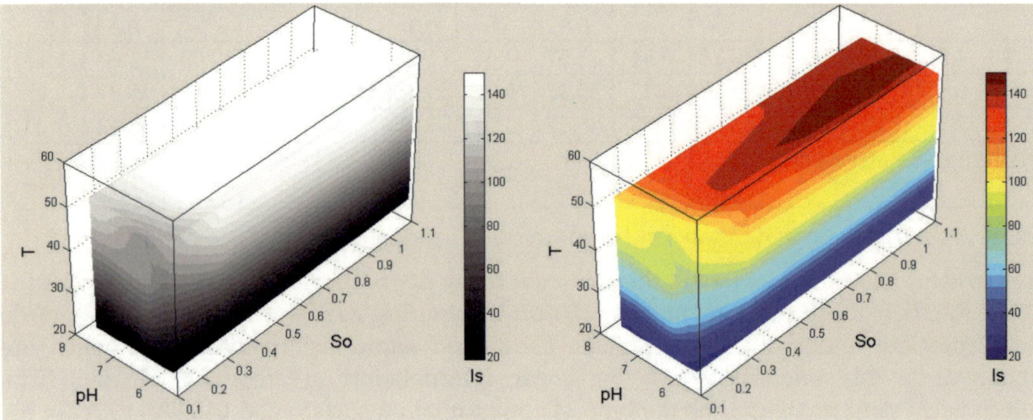

(a) (b)

Fig. 14. A plot of the biosensor's output current versus substrate concentration, temperature and pH: (a) in gray scale, and (b) in colour scale

The generalization of the fuzzy system was tested on three experimental data unused in the design process. The results are listed in Table 3 (a quantitative validation). The average relative error over the three test samples is $\bar{\varepsilon}_3^{FL} = 0.60\ \%$, and maximum relative error in this limited extract is $\varepsilon_{3,\max}^{FL} = 1.194\ \%$.

The proposed fuzzy model shows quite well results, having in mind the exceptional small extract of experimental data, needed for its design. The result inspires the idea for synthesizing a "quasi-inverse" fuzzy model in the form of $S_0 = S_0(I_S, pH, T)$, that could automate, facilitate and improve the accuracy of the dopamine measurement under variable temperature and pH.

No.	Test Data				Fuzzy Logic	
	T	pH	S_0	I_S	I_S^{FL}	ε^{FL}
	°C		mM	nA	nA	%
1	30	6.0	0.426	68.0	68.14	0.205
2	40	6.5	0.994	138.1	139.75	1.194
3	45	7.5	1.278	151.3	150.7	0.396
Average Relative Error ,%						0.60

Table 3. Results from a validation test for the simultaneous modelling the *pH* and *T* influences by means of fuzzy logic.

6. Conclusion

The presented work discusses the use of soft computing techniques for modelling the input-output dependency of a dopamine biosensor, which takes into account the simultaneous influence of pH and temperature over the output current. Under the conditions of insufficient experimental data the fuzzy approximator performs better than the others, regarding accuracy and rapidity. Besides, it does not need additional interpolated data. In order to generalize, all the other techniques, which undergo learning process, require more experimental (or interpolated) data. Moreover the learning of the NNBP is a very time consuming process and most probably could be trapped in local minima. The soft computing based modelling, as a whole, is able to improve the accuracy of a biosensor for measurement of dopamine by considering the simultaneous effect of pH and temperature on the output current. That way it provides the opportunity to have calibration surfaces for every value of the measured substrate. The algorithm can be easily programmed into a microcontroller and to be used for precise biomedical analyses. The future prospective of this work is foreseen in investigations on the simultaneous influence of the pH, temperature and dissolved oxygen concentration on the biosensor's response. The main benefit from these studies would be the possibility to expand and/or specifically adopt the resolved models over a large scale of sensing devices, sensitive to the dissolved oxygen concentration such as biosensors or microbial sensing platforms.

7. References

Blum, E. & Li, L. (1991). Approximation theory and feedforward networks, *Neural Networks*, Vol. 4, 511-515

Burket, J.; Kalil, S.; Maugeri Filho, F. & Rodrigues, M. (2006). Parameters optimization for enzymatic assays using experimental design, *Braz. J. Chem. Eng*, Vol.23, No.2, Sro Paulo Apr./June.

Castillo, J.;Gaspar, S.;Leth, S.; Niculescu, M.; Mortari, A.; Bontidean, I.; Soukharev, V.; Dorneanu, S.; Ryabov, A. & Csöregi, E. (2004). Biosensors for life quality. Design, development and applications, *Sensors and Actuators*, B 102, 179-194

Christensson, A.; Dimcheva, N.; Ferapontova, E.; Gorton, L.; Ruzgas, T.; Stoica, L.; Shleev, S.; Yaropolov, A.; Haltrich, D.; Thorneley, R. & Aust, S. (2004). Direct electron transfer between ligninolytic redox enzymes and electrodes, *Electroanalysis*, Vol.16, No.13-14, 1074-1092 (a review)

Climent, P.; Serralheiro, M. & Rebelo, M. (2001). Development of a new amperometric biosensor based on polyphenoloxidase and polyethersulphone membrane, *Pure Appl. Chem.*, Vol. 73, No. 12, 1993–1999

David, F.(1997). Amperometric Oxygen Electrodes, *Bioanalytical Systems, Inc.*, Vol. 16 No. 1

Dimcheva, N.; Horozova E. & Jordanova, Z. (2002). A Glucose Oxidase Immobilized Electrode Based on Modified Graphite. *Zeitschrift fur Naturforschung*, No. 57C, 705-711

Dodevska, T.; Horozova, E. & Dimcheva, N. (2006). Electrocatalytic reduction of hydrogen peroxide on modified graphite electrodes: application to the development of glucose biosensors. *Anal. Bioanal. Chem.*, Vol., 386, No.5, 1413-1418

Driankov, D.; Hellendoorn, H. & Reinfrank, M. (1993). *An Introduction to Fuzzy Control,* Springer-Verlag Berlin Heidelberg, USA

Ferreira, L.; Souza Jr, M.; Trierweiler, J.; Hitzmann, B & Folly, R.(2003). Analysis of experimental biosensor/FIA lactose measurements, *Brazilian Journal of Chemical Engineering,* Vol. 20, No. 1

Hitzmann, B. et al.(1997). Computational neural networks for the evaluation of biosensor FIA measurements, *Analytica Chimica Acta,* Vol.348, 135-141

Horozova, E.; Dodevska, T. & Dimcheva, N. (2009). Modified graphites: Application to the development of enzyme-based amperometric biosensors, *Bioelectrochemistry* , No.74 260 - 264

Jang, J.(1993). ANFIS: Adaptive-network-based fuzzy inference system, *IEEE Trans. on Systems, Man and Cybernetics,* Vol. 23, No. 3, pp. 665-685, May

Kosko, B. (1992). *Neural Networks and Fuzzy Systems. A Dynamical Systems Approach to Machine Intelligence,* Prentice-Hall Inc

Kraft, L, , Miller, W. & Dietz, D. (1992). *Development and application of CMAC neural network-based control,* Handbook of Intelligent Control. Neural, Fuzzy, and Adaptive Approaches. D.A. White, D.A. Sofge (Eds.), Multiscience Press, Inc., USA, 215-232

Krose, B. & Van der Smagt, P. (1996). *An Introduction to Neural Networks,* 8th ed., The University of Amsterdam, September 1996

Lamanna, R.; Uria, M.; Kelly, J. & Pinto, E.(1996). Neural network based control of pH in a laboratory-scale plant, International Workshop on Neural Networks for Identification, Control, *Robotics, and Signal/Image Processing (NICROSP '96),* pp.314-320

Moatar, F., Fessant, F. & Poirel, A. (1999) . pH modelling by neural networks. Application of control and validation data series in the Middle Loire river, *Ecological Modelling,* Vol. 120, No.2-3, 141-156

Miller, W., Glanz, F. & Kraft, L. (1990). CMAC an associative neural network alternative to backpropagation, *IEEE Proceedings* 78, 1561-1567

Miller, W. & Glanz, F.(1994). UNH_CMAC Version 2.1: The University of New Hampshire implementation of the Cerebellar model arithmetic computer - CMAC, http://www.ece.unh.edu/robots/ unh_cmac.ps

Palmer, J. Banana polyphenoloxidase. Preparation and Properties (1963) Preparation and properties, *Plant Physiology,* No.38, 508-513

Patent Application (2006) U.S. Provisional No. 60/859,586, filed Nov. 16, 2006, entitled "Temperature compensation for enzyme electrodes "

Puida, M.; Ivanauskas, F. & Laurinavicius, V. (2009), Mathematical modeling of the action of biosensor possessing variable parameters, *J Math Chem,* DOI 10.1007/s10910-009-9541-5, Springer Science+Business Media, LLC 2009

Rangelova, V., Kodjabashev,I. & Al. Neykov. (2002) Investigation of Repeatability and Error Instability Analysis of Tissue Biosensor, *Proceedings. of II Int. Symp. "Instrumentation Science and Technology- Isist2002",* 18-22 aug 2002, Jinan City, China, vol.3, pp.231-238

Rangelova, V. (2003). Investigation of influence of thickness of active membrane of constructed tissue biosensor. *Journal of TU-Plovdiv, Fundamental Sciences and Applications*, Vol.10, 23-28, Bulgaria

Rangelova, V. & Tsankova, D. (2007a). CMAC-based modelling the influence of temperature on tissue biosensor for measurement of dopamine, *Proc. of the 5th IASTED International Conference Biomedical Engineering (BioMED 2007)*, Innsbruck, Austria, pp.15-19.

Rangelova, V. & Tsankova, D. (2007b). Fuzzy-based modelling the influence of temperature on tissue biosensor for measurement of dopamine, *Proc. of the 15th Mediterranean Conference on Control and Automation - MED'07*, Athens, Greece, 27-29 June, 2007, Paper No. T12-008

Rangelova, V. & Tsankova, D. (2008). Soft computing techniques in modeling the influence of pH on dopamine biosensor, *Proc. of the 4th International IEEE Conference on Intelligent systems - IS'08*, Varna, Bulgaria, pp. 12-23

Rumelhart, D.E.; Hinton, G.E., & Williams, R.J. (1986). Learning internal representations by error propagation. In: *Parallel Data Processing*, Rumelhart, D.E. & McClelland, J., (Eds.), Vol.1, Ch. 8, pp. 318-362, Cambridge, MA: M.I.T. Press

Scheller, F.; Wollenberger, U.; Warsinke, A. & Lisdat, F. (2001). Research and development in biosensors, *Current Opinion in Biotechnology*, No 12, 35–40

Shizuko, H. et al., (2005). Biosensor Based on Xanthine Oxidase for Monitoring Hypoxanthine in Fish Meat, *American Journal of Biochemistry and Biotechnology*, Vol.1, No.2, 85-89

Syu, M.&Chen, B. (1998). Back-propagation neural network adaptive control of a continuous wastewater treatment process, *Ind. Eng. Chem. Res.*, Vol. 37, No. 9, pp. 3625 -3630

Skladal, P. (1995). Compensation of temperature variations disturbing performance of an amperometric biosensor for continuous monitoring. *Sensors and actuators. B, Chemical* , Vol. 28, No1, pp. 59-62

Stoica, L.; Dimcheva, N.; Haltrich, D.; Ruzgas, T. & Gorton, L.(2005). Electrochemical investigation of direct electron transfer between cellobiose dehydrogenase from new fungal sources on Au electrodes modified with different alkanethiols. *Biosensors and Bioelectronic,s* , No20, 2010–2018

Stoica, L., Dimcheva, N.; Ackermann, Y.; Karnicka, K.; Guschin, D.; Kulesza, P.; Rogalski, J.; Haltrich, D.; Ludwig, R.; Gorton, L. & Schuhmann, W. (2009). Membrane-less biofuel cell based on cellobiose dehydrogenase (anode)/laccase (cathode) wired via specific Os-redox polymers, *Fuel Cells* ,No.9, 53-62

Takagi, T. & Sugeno, M. (1983). Derivation of fuzzy control rules from human operator's control actions, *Proceedings. of the IFAC Symp. on Fuzzy Information, Knowledge Representation and Decision Analysis*, pp. 55–60, July

Ziyan, E. & Pekyardimci, S. (2004). Purifcation and Characterization of Pear Polyphenol Oxidase, *Turk J Chem*, No.28 , 547 - 557

Used denotations

ANFIS - Adaptive-network-based fuzzy inference system
BOD - Biological oxygen demand

CMAC - Cerebellar Model Articulation Controller
FL - Fuzzy logic
MF - Membership function
NNBP - Neural network with backpropagation learning algorithm
PPO - Polyphenol oxidase
SSE - Sum squared error

6

Non-invasive Electronic Biosensor Circuits and Systems

Gaetano Gargiulo [1,2], Paolo Bifulco[2], Rafael A. Calvo[1], Mario Cesarelli[2], Craig Jin[1], Alistair McEwan[1] and André van Schaik [1]
[1]*School of Electrical and Information Engineering, The University of Sydney, Sydney*
[2]*Dipartimento di Ingegneria Biomedica, Elettronica e delle Telecomunicazioni (D.I.B.E.T.)*
University of Naples, Naples,
[1]*(NSW) Australia*
[2]*Italy*

1. Introduction

An aging population has lead to increased demand for health-care and an interest in moving health care services from the hospital to the home to reduce the burden on society. One enabling technology is comfortable monitoring and sensing of bio-signals. Sensors can be embedded in objects that people interact with daily such as a computer, chair, bed, toilet, car, telephone or any portable personal electronic device. Moreover, the relatively recent and wide availability of microelectronics that provide the capabilities of embedded software, open access wireless protocols and long battery life has led many research groups to develop wearable, wireless bio-sensor systems that are worn on the body and integrated into clothing. These systems are capable of interaction with other devices that are nowadays commonly in our possession such as a mobile phone, laptop, PDA or smart multifunctional MP3 player. The development of systems for wireless bio-medical long term monitoring is leading to personal monitoring, not just for medical reasons, but also for enhancing personal awareness and monitoring self-performance, as with sports-monitoring for athletes. These developments also provide a foundation for the Brain Computer Interface (BCI) that aims to directly monitor brain signals in order to control or manipulate external objects. This provides a new communication channel to the brain that does not require activation of muscles and nerves. This innovative and exciting research field is in need of reliable and easy to use long term recording systems (EEG).
In particular we highlight the development and broad applications of our own circuits for wearable bio-potential sensor systems enabled by the use of an amplifier circuit with sufficiently high impedance to allow the use of passive dry electrodes which overcome the significant barrier of gel based contacts.

2. Advantages of biomedical signals long term monitoring

Monitoring of patients for long periods during their normal daily activities can be essential for the management of various pathologies. It can reduce hospitalization, improve patients'

quality of life, and help in diagnosis and identification of diseases. Long-term monitoring of activities can also be useful in the management of elderly people. Moreover, the combination of biomedical signals and motion signals allows estimation of energy expenditure (Gargiulo, Bifulco et al. 2008); (Strath, Brage et al. 2005). Hence, it could also enable the monitoring of human performance (e.g. athletes, scuba divers) in particular conditions and/or environments.
To accomplish these tasks the monitoring equipment will have to comply with some specific requirements such as: portability and/or wearability, low power, long lasting electrodes, data integrity and security, and compliance with medical devices regulation (e.g. electrical safety, electromagnetic compatibility) (Lin, Jan et al. 2004).

2.1 Long term of cardiac signals

Cardiology is one branch of medical science that could clearly benefit from long-term monitoring. It is well known that morphological changes or the presence of various arrhythmias in the long term electrocardiogram (ECG) have a strong correlation with heart and coronary artery diseases (Zheng, Croft et al. 2002). Also, the reoccurrence of atrial fibrillations after ablation is not uncommon and these can only be tracked using long term ECG monitoring (Hindricks, Piorkowsky et al. 2005).
Long term ECG monitoring in cardiology is not only useful for follow up of patients where their pathological status is already known, but also for the monitoring of athletes during exercise. The possibility that young, highly trained or even professional athletes may harbor potentially lethal heart disease or be susceptible to sudden death under a variety of circumstances seems counterintuitive. Nevertheless, such sudden cardiac catastrophes continue to occur, usually in the absence of prior symptoms, and they have a considerable emotional and social impact on the community (Basilico 1999). As a result of the ECG screening programs for athletes which are now compulsory in many countries, it is now known that many of these sudden deaths are due to a syndrome called "Athlete's heart". This syndrome may be associated with rhythm and conduction alterations, morphological changes of the QRS complex in the ECG, and re-polarization abnormalities resembling pathological ECG (Fagard 2003). However, it is broadly accepted that the standard 12 lead ambulatory ECG is not reliable enough during movement to clarify the origin of the ECG alteration, especially if this is triggered by the exercise(Kaiser & Findeis 1999). This makes a system that is able to record the ECG during exercise reliably and without interference desirable.
For standard ECG measurements electrodes are attached to the patient's skin after skin preparation, which includes cleaning, shaving, mechanical abrasion to remove dead skin, and moistening. A layer of electrically conductive gel is applied in between the skin and the electrodes to reduce the contact impedance (J. G. Webster 1998). However, in these so-called wet electrodes the electrolytic gel dehydrates over time which reduces the quality of the recorded signals. In addition, the gel might leak, particularly when an athlete is sweating, which could electrically short the recording sites. This is an even larger problem for monitoring athletes immersed in water. Securing the wet electrodes in place is also complicated, since the electrodes cannot directly be glued to the skin due to the presence of the gel. The use of dry or insulating electrodes may avoids or reduce these problems (Searle & Kirkup 2000).

2.3 Physical activity monitoring

There are many techniques to monitor human motion from self-reporting surveys, accelerometers, pedometers to constant video monitoring. Clinically it is interesting to measure gait, posture, rehabilitation from suffers of neurological conditions such as stroke(Uswatte, Foo et al. 2005), tremors associated with Parkinson's' disease and sleep(Mathie, Coster et al. 2004). However the most common aim for long term monitoring is to assess energy expenditure in physical activity due to its positive effects on health, decrease in mortality rates and aid with chronic diseases such as hypertension, diabetes and obesity(Murphy 2009). The gold standard measurement for energy expenditure is doubly labeled water which requires the ingestion of expensive water labeled with a non-radioactive isotope and the expensive and time consuming sampling of fluids such as blood, urine or saliva.

Accelerometry is becoming the widely accepted tool for assessment of human motion in clinical settings and free living environments as it has the following advantages: simple based on a mass spring system, low cost, small, light, unobtrusive, and reliable in the long term and for unsupervised measurements such as in the home. The most commonly used accelerometers for human movement are piezo-electric sensors that measure acceleration due to movement. They are also sensitive to gravitational acceleration which needs to be subtracted. They are normally manufactured using MEMs technology resulting in miniature, low cost and reliable devices. A tri-axial accelerometer can measure acceleration in three orthogonal dimensions and is able to describe movement in three directions. The use of solid state memories enables long term recording with commercial devices able to continuously record 1-minute epochs for longer than a year(Murphy 2009).

Home use is preferred to clinic studies to reflect normal functional ability of the subject. Activity monitoring with tri-axial accelerometers in a free living environment has been shown to correlate well with the gold standard(Hoos, Plasqui et al. 2003). Accelerometers also show little variation over time (drift) and can be easily recalibrated by tilting in gravitational field. They respond quickly to frequency and intensity of movement and are found to be better than pedometers which are attenuated by impact or tilt(Mathie, Coster et al. 2004).

Their main disadvantage is position dependence when whole body movement is desired. The common approach is to locate the sensor at centre of gravity (such as the waist or pelvis of a human subject) or for improved accuracy, locate many sensors in various positions over the body. Accelerometers are also sensitive to static position changes and movement. Most human movements are in the frequency band of 0.3 to 3.5Hz so most systems use a high pass filter with cut-off of 0.1 to 0.5 Hz to separate static orientation and body movement. As with any free-environment measurement, compliance is an issue as the data may not be used if the subject chooses or forgets to wear the sensor(Mathie, Coster et al. 2004). Some accelerometers measure the stationary tremor of the human body while others use skin conductance to detect when the sensor is being worn. It is also common to use signal processing to estimate compliance and remove non-compliant data segments (Murphy 2009).

To determine metabolic activity from accelerometer measurements various empirical models are have been proposed some of which rely on measurement of other variables such as mass, sex, age. However good correlations have been found with consumed oxygen in various populations with a model based solely on accelerometer counts (Pate, Almeida et al.

2006). Different activities such as running, walking, up-down stairs, cycling can be determined from accelerometer measurements but there is variability with accuracy ranging from 0.89 in house bound subjects to 0.59 for those in a free-living environment (Mathie, Coster et al. 2004). New technologies, including the combination of accelerometry with the measurement of physiological parameters, have great potential for the increased accuracy of physical-activity assessment (Corder, Brage et al. 2007).

2.2 Long term of brain signals

Long term monitoring of brain signals is used in neurology, cognitive science and psycho-physiological research. Its use in clinical EEG recordings improves diagnostic value by up to 90% (Logar, Walzl et al. 1994) One of its extended uses is in neuro-feedback or brain computer interfaces where the brain signals are interpreted as controls for a computer system (Gargiulo, Bifulco et al. 2008).

The clinical motivation to record brain signals long term has traditionally been to observe the Electroencephalogram (EEG) to aid in epilepsy or sleep studies. Epilepsy is an underlying tendency of the brain to produce sudden bursts of electrical activity that disrupt other brain function or a seizure. It is estimated that 10% will experience a seizure during their lifetime with 1% diagnosed with epilepsy. Seizures are variable in severity, frequency and the affected region of the brain and so difficult to diagnose (Waterhouse 2003).

Standard electrodes are small Ag/AgCl discs applied with conductive paste or gel to improve the conductivity of the contact. Collodium glue is often used in long term recording to ensure contact. The international 10-20 EEG electrode placement uses 30 electrodes arranged approximately in two concentric rings around the head and bio-potentials are recorded differentially using high gain, high input impedance FET input amplifiers usually arranged in an instrumentation amplifier circuit (J. G. Webster 1998). In modern systems the differential recording is converted using a high resolution analogue to digital converter so that difference voltages can be selected in computer software. This flexibility is important as clinicians tend to view the recordings as bipolar differences between sets of electrodes or differences from the reference or average of all electrodes. These are commonly referred to as montages(Waterhouse 2003).

EEG potentials recorded from electrodes placed on the scalp represent the collective summation of changes in the extracellular potentials of pyramidal cells. These are the most prevalent and largest cells in the cerebral cortex and are arranged in columns causing their activation currents to add. The resulting voltage is attenuated by about 10x by volume conduction through the tissues of the head: cerebrospinal fluid, skull, scalp and skin(J. G. Webster 1998).

The EEG signal normally ranges from 10 to 150uV and are commonly categorized in frequency bands which can indicate brain states and pathology depending on where they are recorded on the scalp: Delta 0.1-3.5 Hz, Theta 4-7.5 Hz, Alpha 8-13 Hz and Beta 14-22 Hz((Ed.) 2006). Exemplificative interpretations of such waveforms are: epilepsy seizure on-set (increased presence of 3 Hz spikes), the alpha wave replacement phenomenon, evoked potentials and the Mu-rhythm commonly used for BCI (Brain Computer Interface) applications.

Alpha wave replacement phenomenon is easy to elicit. As one of the most studied elicited mental states, it is also commonly used in clinical practice to ensure EEG setup validity.

It is well known that the closing of both eyelids in a relaxed subject is followed by alpha wave replacement in the EEG. In awake relaxed subjects the phenomenon presents a visible increase in the magnitude of alpha waves (8-13 Hz) that starts after the closing of both eyelids and stops with the opening of the eyes (J. G. Webster 1998).

The phenomenon is more apparent in the frequency domain as shown Figure 1. Observe the difference in the spectrum around 9 Hz between the eyes open (bold) and eyes closed cases (grey) as recorded by two electrodes placed on the scalp of a volunteer subject.

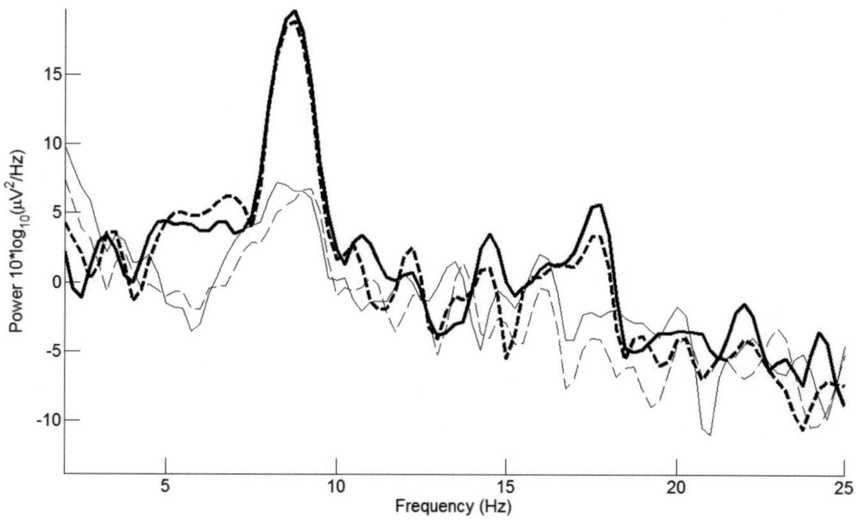

Fig. 1. Power spectral density showing alpha wave replacement.

Long term monitoring of EEG signals might also provide advantages for Brain Computer Interfaces (BCIs). An EEG based Brain-Computer Interface system seeks direct interaction between the human brain and machines, aiming to augment human capabilities by enabling people (especially those who are disabled) to communicate and control devices by merely "thinking" or expressing intent. Therefore, it is possible to say that the main aim of BCI researchers is to build a new communication pathway for the human brain that does not depends from its standard output channels such as nerves and muscles. (Millan, Renkens et al. 2004; Pfurtscheller, Brunner et al. 2006)

Such systems can be realized in two ways: in externally (stimulus)-paced mode (synchronous BCI) or in an internally paced mode (asynchronous BCI). Synchronous BCI requires that the subject achieves a specific mental state in response to an external event, within a predefined time window, whereas in asynchronous BCI is not required any time window constraint so the subject is free to intend a mental state or a specific thought. (Pfurtsheller & Neuper 2001) However, it is possible to say that both methodologies make use of classified EEG signals epochs,. Synchronous BCIs make use of oscillatory EEG activity (Pfurtscheller, Brunner et al. 2006) and slow cortical potential shifts (Hinterbergera, Küblera et al. 2003), while for asynchronous BCIs, various types of event-related potentials are used (Millán 2003).

Focusing on synchronous BCI, two types of oscillation seems to be the more usable: the Rolandic mu rhythm in the range 7–13 Hz and the central beta rhythm above 13 Hz, both originating in the sensorimotor cortex area, these phenomenon (known from the early '50 (Chatrian, Petersen et al. 1959)) are not only linked to the voluntary motor intentions, but as many recent studies confirm, they are linked to the mental imagination of movements. It has been shown that motor imagination involves similar brain regions/functions which are involved in programming and preparing such movement. (Jeannerod 1995)

Routine clinical EEG recordings are brief, typically a 20 minute recording, and unlikely to catch a sporadic seizure. They are also set in artificial environments such as a clinic. So ambulatory EEG: continuous recording over 72 hours has arisen with availability of solid state memories for easily storing data(Waterhouse 2003).

These allow long term brain signal recordings in a free- environment such as home use which is more convenient, less expensive, familiar environment. The extended recording time increases the chance to catch a seizure and recording time length correlates with number of seizures measured(Logar, Walzl et al. 1994). These have been found to be clinically useful in 75% of subjects with low false positives (0.7% in asymptomatic adults), they can detect normally up to 63% additional seizures over conventional recordings and can be used to validate therapy by showing a change from abnormal to normal EEG with treatment (Waterhouse 2003). They have been adopted for sleep monitoring and combined with EMG, ECG, respiration, oximetry to measure other sleep signals of interest.

3. Passive dry electrodes

As should be clear from what has been explained until now, it is urgent to find a solution to the number of issues raised by the use of conventional gel-based electrodes and skin preparations the so called 'wet electrodes' in biomedical signal recording. As mentioned a possible solution could be the use of the so called 'passive dry electrodes',(Gargiulo, Bifulco et al. 2008; Gargiulo, Bifulco et al. 2008; Bifulco, Fratini et al. 2009). These are distinct from active dry electrodes that require local active electronics, power supply over cables, additional manufacturing and hermetic enclosures. Passive dry electrodes have no local active electronics so it is possible to integrate them in garments or clothes resulting less obstruction in daily life activities.

A material with several particular attributes for dry electrodes is conductive rubber. Electrodes made from such material are durable, washable and re-usable, the carbon and silicon materials (commonly used in conductive rubber) are biocompatible, they provide a smoother and more uniform contact surface with the skin, they also can be thin, flexible and easily applied to a variety of substrates (Muhlsteff & Such 2004; Chang, Ryu et al. 2005). However, they also present much higher impedance with respect to conventional wet electrodes (Baba & Burke 2008).

Alternatively, textile electrodes, which can be embedded in clothes, can also be used as dry electrodes. These offer a high degree of patient autonomy and freedom of movement and are suitable for long term monitoring. Textile electrodes are typically made of synthetic materials which endure abrasion very well, do not irritate the skin, and are lightweight and washable. A major drawback is the high contact impedance of these electrodes, typically 1-5 $M\Omega/cm^2$, compared to a 10 $k\Omega/cm^2$ impedance for the disposable Ag/AgCl electrodes (Catrysse, Puers et al. 2003).

The high electrode impedance is a common issue with all types of dry electrodes. Therefore, to use these electrodes they must be connected to instrumentation amplifiers with extremely high input impedances (Prutchi & Norris 2005).

3.1 Active dry electrodes

Another possible solution to the entire above mentioned problem largely described in literature for many years is to buffer the electrode signal directly at the electrode to provide impedance conversion (Taheri, Knight et al. 1994; Harland, Clark et al. 2002; Valchinov & Pallikarakis 2004); this type of assembly is referred to as an active electrode. However, this approach exhibits a number of weaknesses. Firstly it is possible to observe that some rigid circuitry is fixed on the electrode, increasing the size of the electrode and resulting in an inflexible electrode that cannot be embedded in clothes e.g. Textile electrodes. Moreover, despite the various methodologies attempted to apply the electrode to the skin, particularly in EEG applications, dry electrodes signals are affected from large movement artifacts due to skin/electrodes stretch (Talhouet & Webster 1996) and electrode skidding that contributes to increases in the contact impedance imbalance. In "wet" electrodes this is mitigated by skin preparation and conductive paste interposition.

3.2 Physical activity monitoring

To monitor physical activity during daily life is not a trivial problem to solve. Current clinical assessments of physical activity monitoring and body energy expenditure are based on the evaluation of several parameters such as ECG, body temperature and oxygen consumptions. However, new perspective in physical monitoring are offered by novel M.E.M.S. (Micro Electro Machined Sensors) accelerometer sensors. Such kind of sensor is based on the changes in the value of a capacitor given geometrical variations. Often one plate of the capacitor is kept fixed whilst the other one is free to vary with the stimuli (in this case the acceleration). Nowadays such sensors are tiny, cheap, light weight and more important they are offered tri-axial and sensitive to the statically gravitational acceleration, so they are useful for orientation and position assessment in the gravitational field. Their use in daily life devices (such as gaming console or mobile phone and daily home-care (Freescale Semiconductor 2005)) is increasing and there are many examples in the available literature of their use as physical activity monitoring device.

Experimental evidence has shown that there are clear different pattern recordable by accelerometer sensors during different tasks and movements e.g. it is possible to distinguish between slow normal or fast walking simply looking at the signal magnitude end or its second derivate (Mühlsteff, Such et al. 2004). Moreover, rapid gradient changes and fast transients in the signal are useful for posture assessment and free fall recognition that are clearly useful in tele-medicine and home-care (Strath, Brage et al. 2005; Bifulco, Gargiulo et al. 2007; Giansanti 2007).

Measuring the acceleration, theoretically would be possible to calculate the velocity and then the position as function of the time, however, in order to calculate velocity and time two initial condition are needed. Furthermore, more than one sensor is needed to monitor anatomical segments such as arms and legs.

3.3 State of the art wearable biosensor systems

Many groups worldwide are developing wearable wireless biosensor systems for applications ranging from health care, athlete monitoring and vital signs in high risk environments. Most report on systems aimed at a particular application and these systems usually measure one or two physiological signals only (Pandian, Mohanavelu et al. 2008). Other groups are studying optimal network methods for body sensor networks (BSNs), body area networks or personal area networks (Hao & Foster 2008). The aims here are to develop a miniature, low power nodes, several of which are worn on the body and each capable of sampling, processing and communicating physiological or environmental measurements. In wireless BSNs the nodes wirelessly communicate to a central hub, removing the need for cables between sensors. While this improves long term monitoring from a comfort and practicality perspective, it does introduce challenging power and size requirements on the nodes.

A more immediate concern for long term monitoring of surface bio-potentials is the current need to use conductive gel. The "smart vest" introduced in (Pandian, Mohanavelu et al. 2008) is capable of monitoring a number of vital parameters in a single device, including ECG without the use of gel and cuff-less non-invasive blood pressure derived from the ECG and PPG. The vest is made of cotton or lycra with sensors embedded as to make good contact with the skin. The ECG sensor is custom made consisting of silicon rubber with pure silver filings and worn in the form of belts to acquire standard lead-II ECG. We would consider this design as a state of the art long term monitoring system, however it has not been combined with a physical activity monitor or accelerometer which is important in applications such as athlete monitoring.

4. A new wireless system based on passive dry electrodes

Our present research is focused on the use of passive dry electrodes mainly realized with conductive rubber. Hence, in order to successfully use such material to build electrodes we propose a bio-potential amplifier with an ultra-high input impedance. This high impedance allows our electrodes to overcome the barrier of the increased contact impedance and contact impedance imbalance that it is usually mitigated by the use of conductive gel or paste. The design, as reported later in this section, uses only commercial ICs and can thus be readily replicated by other researchers in the field. Laboratory and clinical tests demonstrate that the system is able to acquire the ECG and EEG of subjects as well as clinical ECG and EEG devices (0.95 correlation) and improved monitoring can be performed for at least 24 hours. The device (for ECG purposes), is shown to work even when the subject is fully immersed in water.

However, as mentioned, dry electrodes still suffer of many problems such as increased artifact sensitivity and high contact impedance value, which solutions are still the object of active international research.

4.1 The bio-amplifier hardware

We designed the biomedical front-end to provide a very high input impedance, and a selectable gain feature from ~1000 V/V for EKG/EMG up to ~70 kV/V for EEG applications. The bandwidth of the front-end is adjustable (from 0.05 or 0.5 Hz up to 40 Hz for EEG and EKG applications, or from 5 Hz up to 400 Hz for EMG applications). Bench testing shows that the front end current consumption is less than 1 mA when the circuit is powered by 4.5 V.

Figure 2 shows the implementation of a single analogue channel. The Burr-Brown INA-116 instrumentation amplifier is used for its extremely high input impedance. A virtual signal ground is derived from the battery (single power supply) using a voltage divider (R5/R6). The virtual ground is buffered to provide an optional driven ground connection for the right ear lobe (EEG) or for the right leg driver connection (EKG) via a calibrated coupling impedance Rcouple.

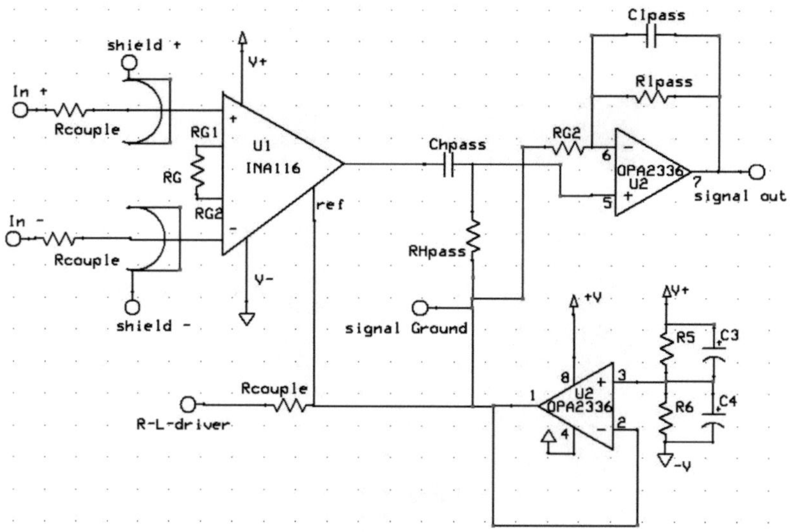

Fig. 2. Schematics of a single input channel

The INA116 is designed to work with a dual 9 V power supply, but because of the very low bandwidth requirement and the small amplitude of the biomedical signals, we were able to use it with a single voltage supply of only 2 V.

The cut-off frequency for the high pass filter is tuneable by changing the value of CHpass while RHpass is kept fixed at 390 kΩ. The second stage of amplification and filtering provides enough gain and high frequency suppression to directly feed the ADC. The cut-off frequency of the low pass filter is regulated by tuning CLpass while keeping RLpass fixed at 1 MΩ. The second stage amplification and the driven ground are implemented using the low-power, precision operational amplifier OPA2336 from Burr-Brown. The measured input referred noise for the proposed circuit (included electrodes) was less than 2 μVpp in the bandwidth up to 10 Hz. (Gargiulo, Bifulco et al. 2008; Gargiulo, Bifulco et al. 2008). A peculiarity of the amplifier is that it offers driven active guard shields (*shield+ and shield- in figure 2)* on each input to minimize capacitive signal leakage due to the PCB or cables. This ensures low input bias current and high input impedance which allow the recording of biopotentials from high contact impedance, dry electrodes connected by cables with driven shields. .

4.2 The passive dry electrode

Our electrodes are made with commercially available 1.5 mm thick silicone conductive rubber shaped in discs of 8 mm diameter. Figure 3 shows an illustrative diagram of the dry electrode. The active side of the electrode is capacitive coupled through a layer of insulating silicon rubber with a metal shield wired to the active guard shield. The impedance of the realized electrodes at 100 Hz is greater than 20 MΩ with a parasitic capacitance no greater than 2 pF. Laboratory tests demonstrate that even a tolerance of 20% for the electrode's impedance is acceptable and does not influence the quality of the measurement, even in a multi-channel montage. In order to avoid any accidental contact with the electrode's shield or with the optional grounded cable sleeve, a final layer of insulation rubber (not showed in Figure 3), is poured to cover them.(Gargiulo, Bifulco et al. 2008; Gargiulo, Bifulco et al. 2008)

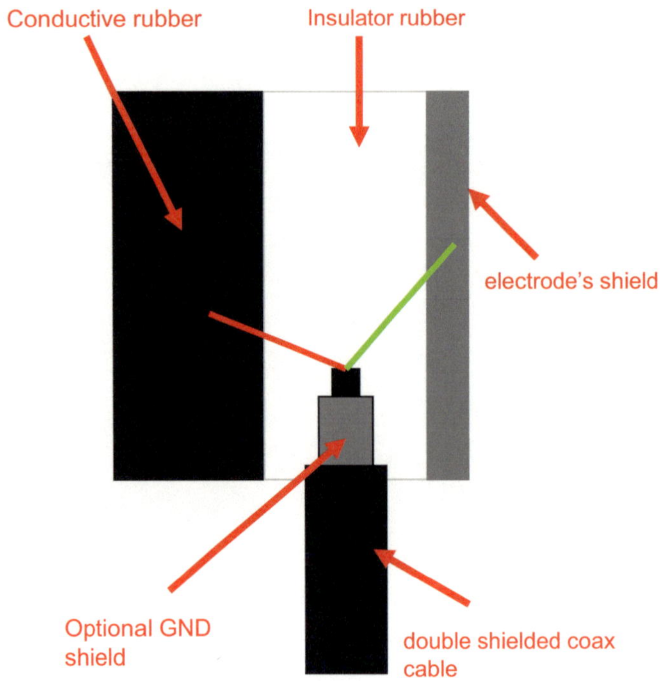

Fig. 3. Dry electrode illustrative diagram

The quality of the measurement it is not influenced by contact impedance imbalance between electrodes. It is possible to mix the electrodes - some dry and some wet - in our system.

4.3 Wearable personal monitor system

Wireless connectivity using a low-power ADC equipped with a Bluetooth module (currently approved for medical devices), was added in order to complete the system. The module is capable of acquiring up to eight analogue channels with a total sample rate of 4000 Hz transmitting data up to 25 m open field. The measured current consumption of the module operating in full mode (maximum sample rate available) is rated 35 mA when powered from a 4.5 V battery pack and 6.5 mA when operated in SNIFF mode. SNIFF mode is a standard Bluetooth low power modality that on the one hand reduces the power consumption, but also limits the data throughput of the device down to 500 Hz maximum sample rate. The general architecture of the realized device is depicted in Figure 4.
It is possible to observe data are acquired from a 3-axial accelerometer (for body or body parts motion sensing) and a number of bio-medical front ends in according with the application and the sample rate constraints.
In summary the prototype of our wearable personal monitor has the following specifications:

- Dimension: 43x60x15 [mm]
- Weight: 200 gr (battery excluded)
- Power consumptions: 40 mA @ 4.5 V reduced to 10 mA @ 5 V when SNIFF mode is used (M. Catrysse & H. van Egmondc 2004)

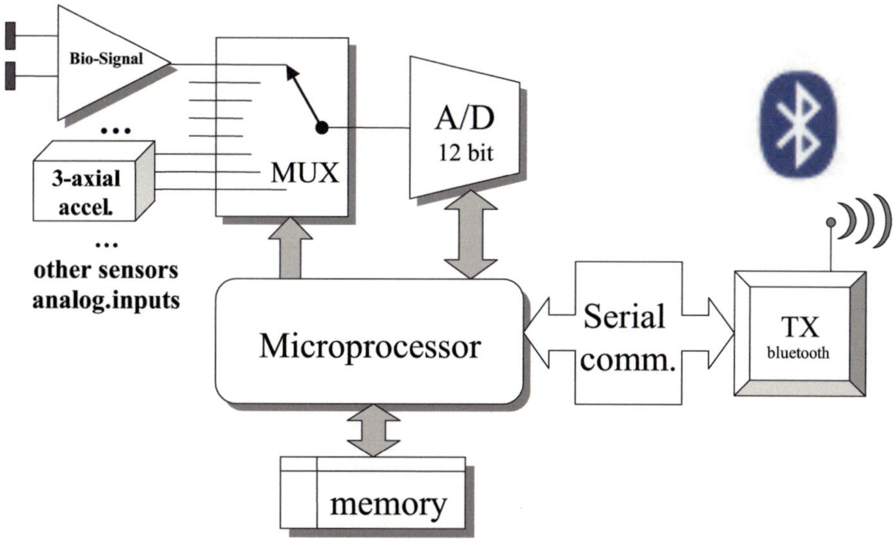

Fig. 4. System architecture

- AA batteries can provide up to 3000mAH, operation time is up to 300 hrs in SNIFF mode.
- Up to four configurable bio-front-ends
- Body motion detection with 3-axial MEMS accelerometer: 0.8 V per g (g=9.81 m/s^2)
- Customizable sample rate up to 4 KHz (500 Hz in SNIFF mode)
- Data security (Bluetooth 2001)
- Standard and wearable textile electrodes suitable.

4.3.1 ECG application

Acquiring data from a single Bio-medical front end configured as ECG (standard bandwidth of 0.5÷150 [Hz], sampling the data at 500 Hz or lower, it is possible to realize a very low power ECG monitor. Figure 5 shows an excerpt of data as they are recorded from a volunteer subject.

Then the qualitative performance of ECG system is assessed in parallel with standard commercially available ECG devices. In this comparative test, dry electrodes belonging to our system are placed on the chest of a volunteer subject as close as possible to standard wet electrode belonging to the control system. Skin preparation was used for wet electrodes but not performed for dry electrodes.

As shown in Figure 6, the signals were almost identical in freshly installed electrodes (fresh montage), with the correlation coefficient of the two signals scores 0.95. Correlation is calculated on the recorded workspace of ten minutes. Small differences in recorded signals come from the different filter orders and slightly different bandwidths (due to the variance of the components) and of course by the slight difference in electrode position. However, as shown in Figure 7, after 24 hours the differences between the two signals become evident. In particular it is possible to observe that the standard system (bottom panel) suffers from signal distortions from a loose contact between electrode and skin. Gel desiccation and adhesive problems do not affect our dry system since it does not rely on a full contact with the skin. (Gargiulo, Bifulco et al. 2008)

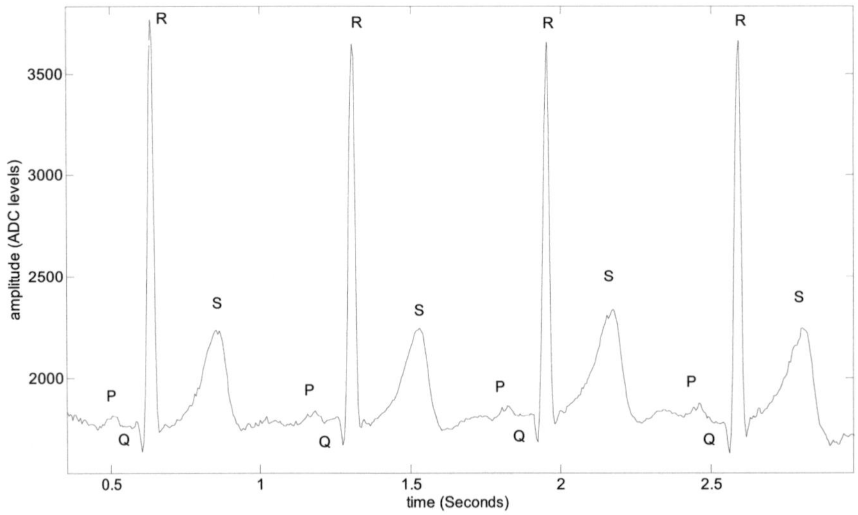

Fig. 5. ECG raw data acquired from a resting subject

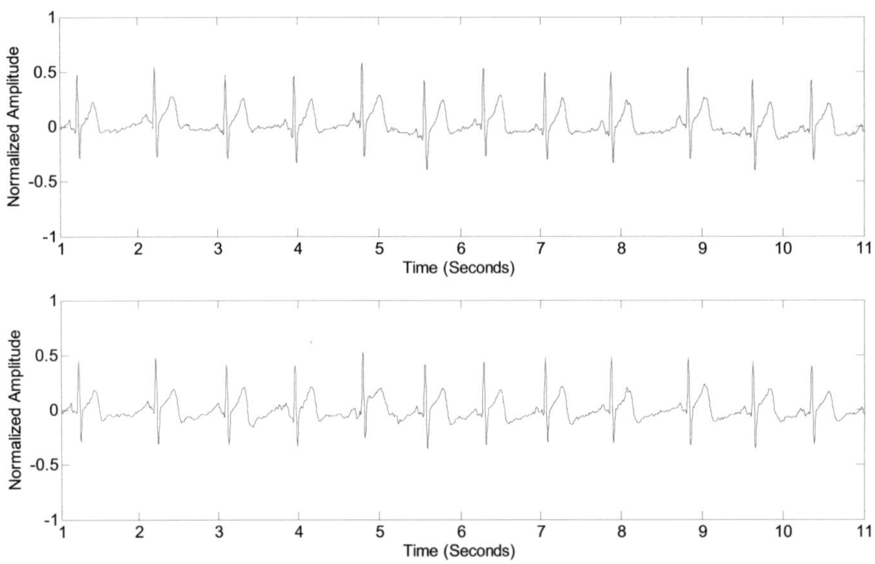

Fig. 6. Parallel ECG recording in fresh montage (Top panel: dry electrodes system)

4.3.2 EEG application

The realized system is been tested for EEG application during a BCI task; performance of the dry electrode system are assessed based on a parallel recording similar to the one performed for the ECG capabilities assessment. In this configuration, our system is able to acquire up to eight electrodes sampled at the maximum frequency of 128 Hz. Moreover, reference electrode circuitry was built without the use of additional circuitry, the shielding terminal of each electrode (referred as *shield+* and *shield-* in Figure 2) gives a replica of the sensed signal

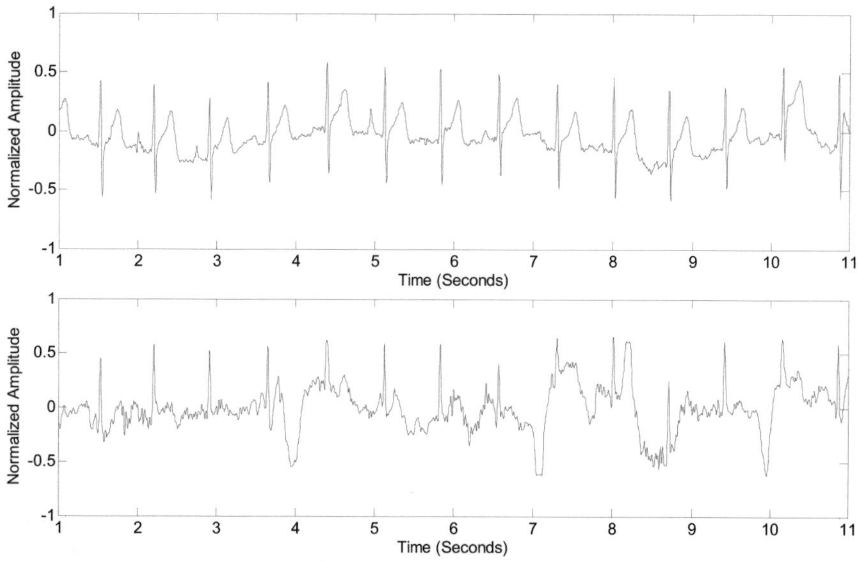

Fig. 7. Parallel ECG recording after 24 hours (Top panel: dry electrode system)

at the electrode (Horowitz & Hill 2002; Bifulco, Gargiulo et al. 2007; Gargiulo, Bifulco et al. 2008; Gargiulo, Bifulco et al. 2008), therefore, this terminal can be used to replicate the reference signal as depicted in Figure 8. To simplify the drawing, in Figure 8 is depicted only the pre-amplifier section of the first two channels.

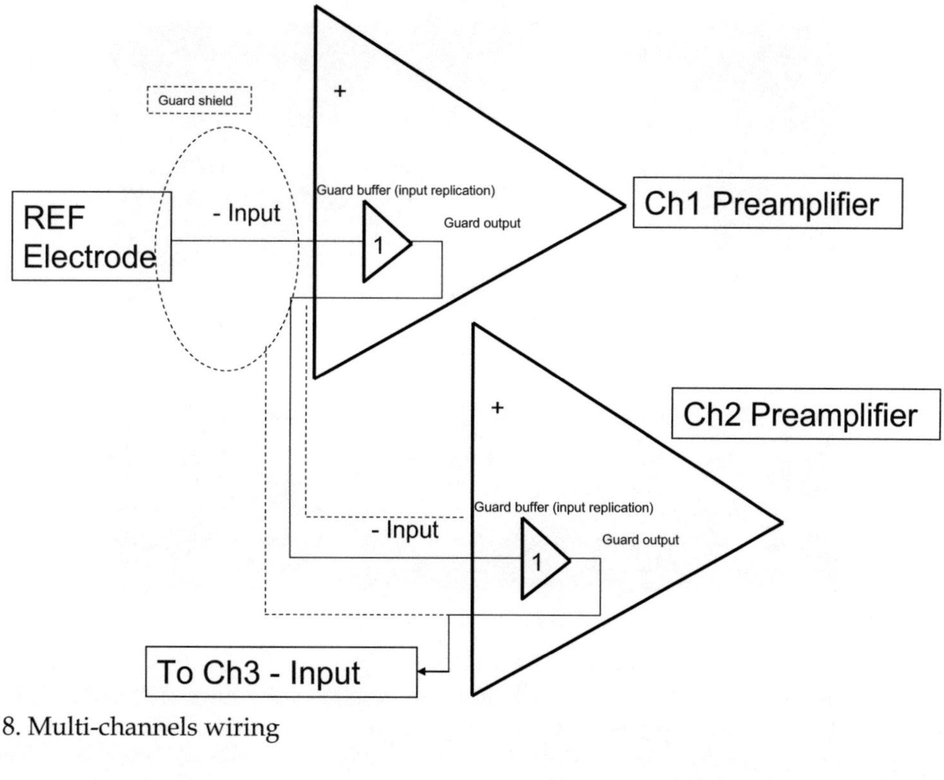

Fig. 8. Multi-channels wiring

A number of untrained subjects were asked to perform a BCI mono-dimensional cursor control task (left-right movement) with the following protocol consisting of three steps.
1) Familiarization trial (approximately 3 minutes): in this task the subjects were asked to manually depress a button with their right or left hand when a target appeared on the respective side;
2) Pre-BCI trial of 3-6 minutes, where the subjects were asked to imagine pressing the button when a target appeared on the respective side;
3) BCI L-R control tasks (until the subject got tired), where a cursor was moved based on the EEG signals recorded.

During the experiment EEG signals were recorded in parallel by both machines using the following montage: dry electrodes were placed at C3, C4, and Cz (also position used from the BCI classifier) and were surrounded by wet electrodes (belonging to the control machine) at Cp3, Cp4, Cpz, C1, C2, C5, C6, Fc3, Fc4 and Fcz.

Since we are interested in evaluating how the experimental burden is reduced using the new system, the time required to prepare the subjects was recorded, in particular, the preparation time per electrode was recorded separately for dry and wet electrodes. For the wet electrodes, full skin preparation, and contact impedance checking are required. The wet system required 2-3 minutes set-up time per electrode; wet electrode are kept in position using conductive adhesive paste and a bandage soaked in standard collodion. The dry system only required ten seconds per electrode, which was the time needed to dry the collodion applied directly to the surface of the electrode, Figure 9 shows the electrode montage, arrows indicate the dry electrodes.

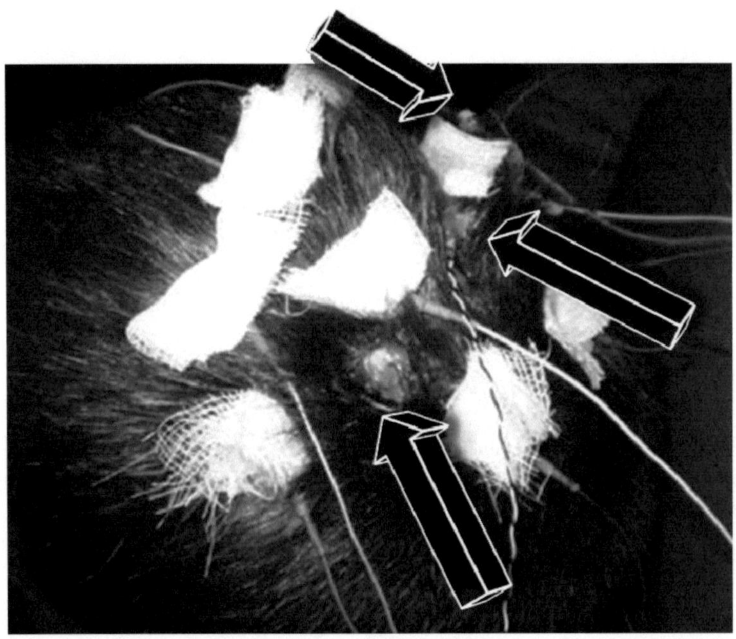

Fig. 9. Electrode montage, arrows indicate the dry electrode

In order to minimize the differences in the acquired signal due to hardware differences, the data were equalized in bandwidth to 0.5-35 Hz using a band pass filter (50th order FIR) and a 50 Hz IIR notch filter was applied to the recorded signals.

Time and frequency domain evaluation was performed on the data. In the time domain, in order to minimize the effect of clock misalignment and different ADC jitter in the two recording systems, an analysis based on the maximum of the correlation between signals recorded with the two systems was used. Using a one second long (256 samples) moving window, we calculate the correlation between electrode signals. We found that the maximum correlation of a 3 minute recording, i.e., when the two series are time aligned, was 0.90 when comparing electrodes from the same machine. The average of the maximum correlation between a dry electrode and the mean signal from its surrounding wet electrodes was 0.76.

We believe that the difference is mainly caused by the presence of artifacts that introduce high amplitude noise. Since each machine has slightly different recovery times and filter responses, these artifacts reduce overall correlation between the two systems. Figure 10 shows an excerpt of data where the subject was asked to strongly contract the jaw muscles, due to the absence of the gel able to mitigate the effect of the electrode bumping that follow the large artifacts, the response of the dry electrodes (represented in bold) is clearly different.

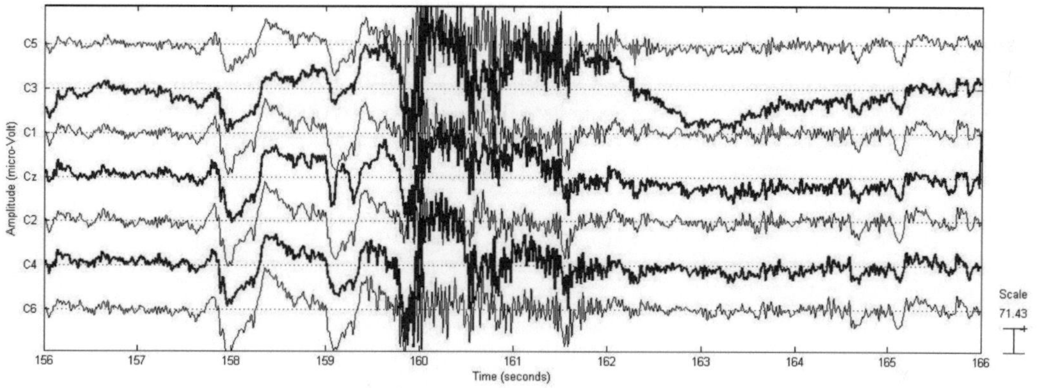

Fig. 10. Ten seconds EEG recording showing clear differences to artifacts between dry (bold line) and standard wet electrodes

Our hypothesis that the above artifacts account for the main differences between dry and wet recordings was tested in further analysis where the signals were visually inspected by a neurologist who was unaware which signals had been recorded by which system. They were asked to identify periods within the trials that contained artifacts and these were removed. Following the removal of artifacts, the average of the maximum correlation between a dry electrode and the mean signal from its surrounding wet electrodes increased from 0.76 to 0.94 (Gargiulo, Bifulco et al. 2008). Further tests show that the combined use of the amplifier and the passive dry electrode allows us to mix in the same montage dry and wet electrode. It is possible to record EEG using as reference a standard golden brass electrode applied as usual (conductive paste and collodion soaked bandage), while the active or exploring electrodes are dry passive ones. This montage superimposes a contact impedance imbalance of at least 100 kΩ (wet prepared electrodes usually offers a contact impedance smaller than 5 kΩ, while the passive dry electrodes contact impedance was always greater than 100 kΩ or even off the scale of the instruments).

4.2.3 Athlete monitoring

Configuring our system to acquire the tri-axial accelerometer and a single EMG channel at the sample rate of 500 Hz (that is the minimal sample rate for EMG applications (Ives & Wigglesworth 2003)), it is possible to realize a body part monitor. For example the accelerometer was installed on an athlete's wrist using an elastic band. Another band, containing two wearable electrodes for EMG recording, was installed on the biceps. The athlete executed several cycles of a standing biceps curl with supination. During these slow movements, the dominant acceleration is gravity, so that information of the orientation of the accelerometer can be extracted. A remote coach was able to gather information about the athlete performance from the acquired signals as follows:

- Rhythm and speed of the cycle's executions was determined by looking at the shape and time duration of the accelerometer's waveforms.
- As depicted in Figure 11 a single repetition cycle of the exercise can be divided into four sections. During section 1 (curling) the forearm is being raised and the acceleration on the red axis decreases, while the acceleration on the blue axis increases as the sensor is being tilted towards the horizontal. Next supination occurs when the lower arm turns, causing acceleration on the green axis to increase, while decreasing acceleration on the blue axis (section 2). This is followed by voluntary peak contraction (section 3) and relaxation that includes gradual pronation to return in the initial position (section 4).
- The presence of cheating, and the amount of cheating can be evaluated by abnormal acceleration just before a new curl is executed. This acceleration indicates that the arm is being swung prior to curling in order to increase the momentum to lift up the weight.

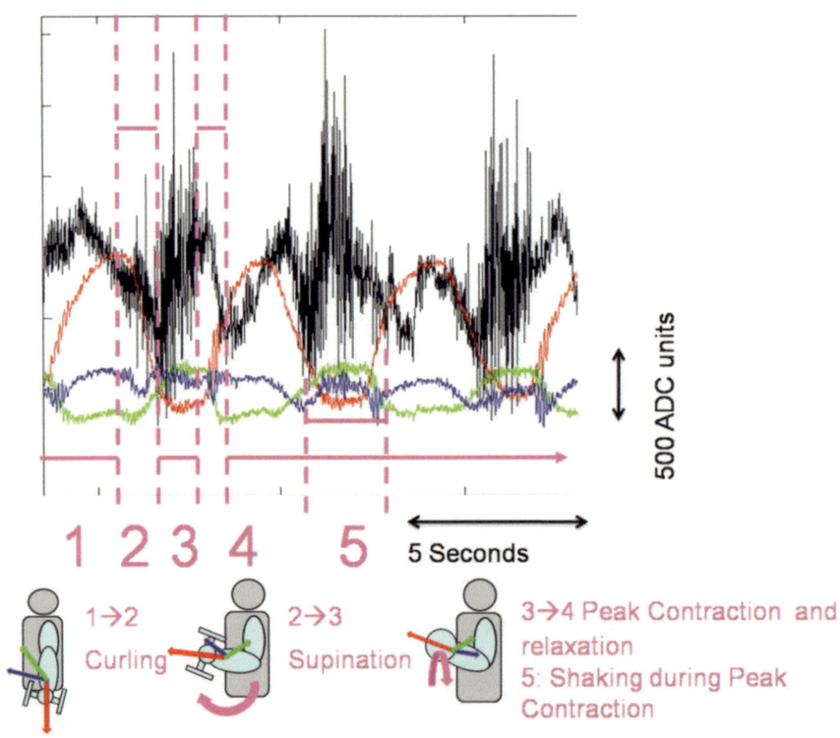

Fig. 11. Remote standing biceps curl assessment

- The voluntary peak contraction, denoted by the forearm shaking pattern (as it is evident in Figure 11, blue trace, section 5);
- The evaluation of the EMG signal (in particular its RMS value) will give information about muscular stress and fatigue across the cycles.

Configuring the hardware to acquire ECG and the tri-axial accelerometer, it is possible to obtain a full body exercises remote athlete management system or a general full body patient monitoring system.

A good example of athlete management is depicted in Figure 12, in this task the subject executes a squatting exercise. In this kind of exercise, the athlete usually carries a heavy weight on the shoulders and a loss of equilibrium over the horizontal axis (depicted in Figure 12 in turquoise) could be very dangerous. In addition, since during squatting the chest will bend forward, there is a high risk of overcharging the back muscles during return to the standing position. A remote coach can judge the quality of the exercise by evaluating several parameters such as:

- Recovery time between cycles from duration of the plateau on the vertical accelerometer axis (red trace).
- Lateral equilibrium loss denoted by the presence of peaks in the accelerometer's horizontal axis (turquoise trace)
- Recovery time in squatting position (length of simultaneous plateaus on the turquoise and green axes)
- Potentially dangerous charge of the back muscles during standing up. A hyperextension of the back will result in a negative deflection of the accelerometer's green axis.
- Additional information could also be gathered from the EKG such as heart rate and heart rate variability within cycles as well as the respiration rhythm.

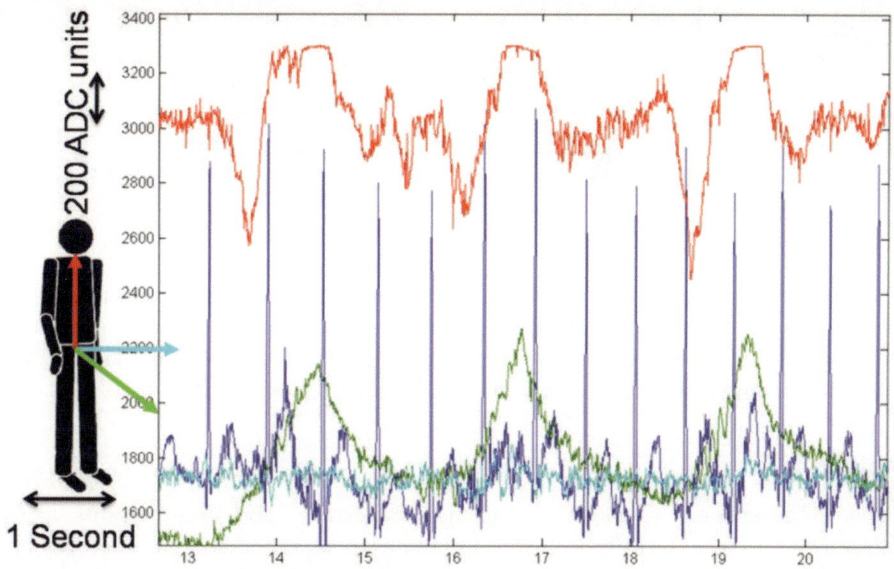

Fig. 12. Remote squatting exercise assessment

Even when the subject is not performing any particular task, since the accelerometer used is sensitive to gravity it is possible to transform the recorded acceleration along the three axes into tilt angles of each axis with respect to the direction of the gravity vector, for static positions, as well as during slow movements. This allows us to assess body posture in the gravitational field.

Figure 13 shows an example of posture assessment. In this trial, the signal recorded from the accelerometer positioned in the subject's belt and oriented as depicted, was translated in axis tilt with the gravity direction. Figure 13 shows the following body positions:

A: Standing up
B: Lying horizontally (face up)
C: Lying horizontally on the left side
D: Lying horizontally on the right side
E: Lying horizontally (face down)

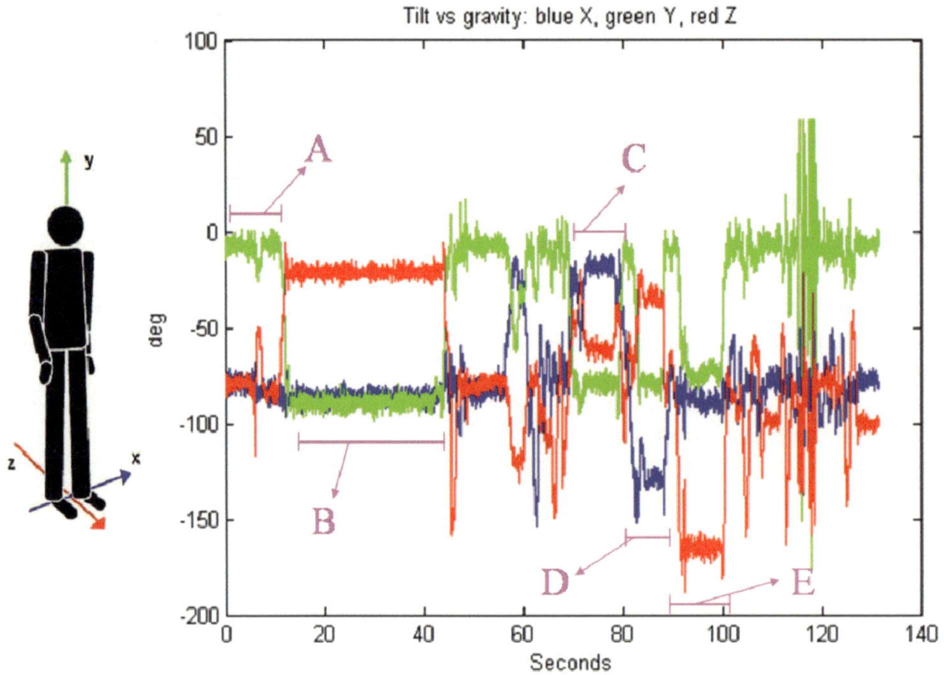

Fig. 13. Posture assessment

We found that that such a system is able to assess human performances and it may be useful in military and high risk zone operator monitoring and management. Moreover, it is possible to combine more than one system configured for different signals on the same subject to obtain more detailed information on the subject' performance.

5. Conclusion

Non-invasive biosensor systems are increasing in demand and many useful applications exist, particularly in long term monitoring One bottleneck is the current need for obtrusive 'wet electrodes' that fail to work in long term recordings. We have described a long term monitoring, wearable personal monitoring system that is wireless, low power and uses convenient dry electrodes. Its use for ECG and athlete monitoring has been demonstrated. This would be useful for those at risk of heart failure or health and activity monitoring in our increasingly sedentary and overweight society. We are currently assessing the system for EEG recordings, in particular for as a BCI device that would greatly assist the severely disabled and it may also be of use in epilepsy monitoring being able to track movement and record EEG in a comfortable environment.

6. Future researches

Currently our researches are focused on exploring all the possible uses of the proposed biomedical sensing system particularly in athlete and long term patient monitoring and BCIs.

6.1 Physical activity monitoring

Currently our research in physical activity monitoring is still focused on clinical assessment of human performance for long term monitoring particularly for full body assessment. It is well known that rapid changes in body orientation, such as during a free fall, may be identified from the information gathered by the accelerometer. Figure 14 shows an example using data recorded using our device. Moreover, being able to detect rapid changes in body orientation provides useful information for syncope detection, geriatric care and sport science.

In this evaluation the prototype was attached to the subject's chest using an elastic band with embedded dry electrodes. Our device was configured to acquire one EKG channel, a signal from the light reflected PPG (Photo PletysmoGraphic), unit, and skin temperature (not shown). The top section of Figure 14 shows the posture assessment gathered from the accelerometer during a passage from a lying down (face up) to a standing position. The lower section of Figure 11 shows the event related biological signals, i.e., ECG (1st lead, top trace) and PPG signals (bottom trace).

The passage from a lying position to a standing will cause a large blood pressure gradient inside the body (a vasovagal reaction) and this could be a cause for a syncope attack (Benditt, Ferguson et al. 1996).

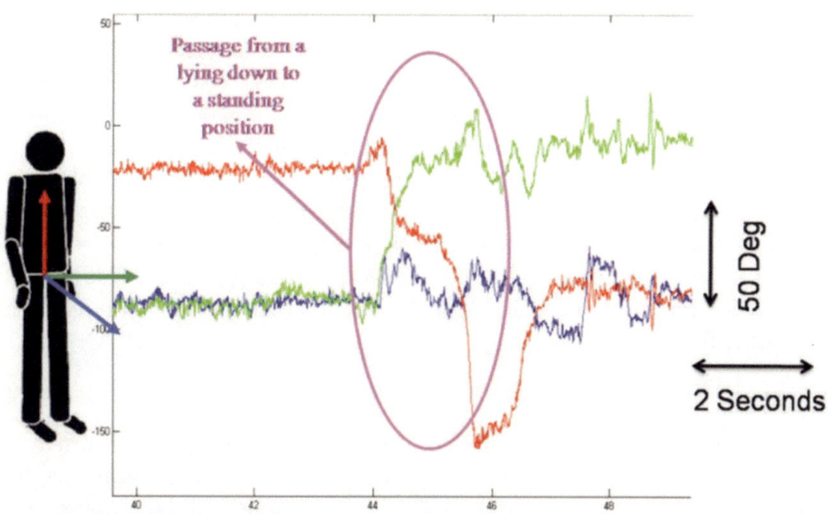

Fig. 14. Posture assessment, accelerometer signals

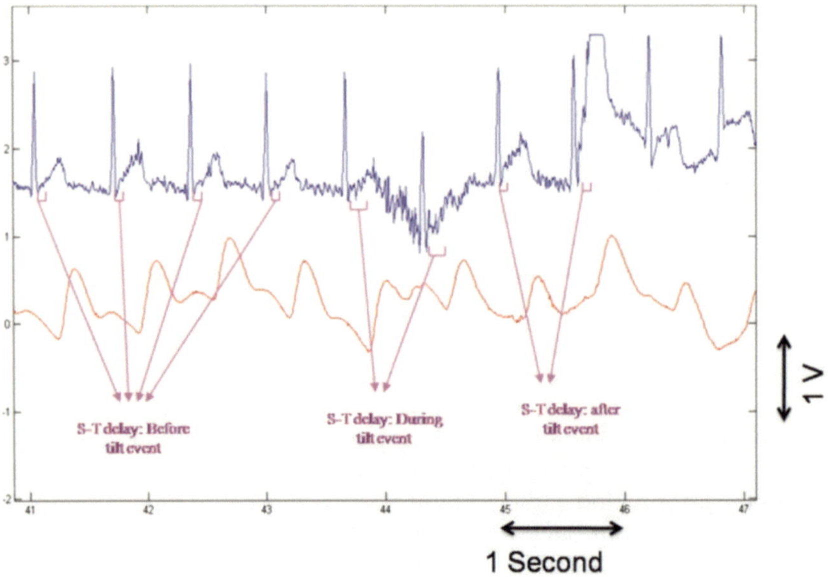

Fig. 15. Posture assessment, ECG and PPG signals

By wearing our device it will be possible to extract important information about the subject's health from the data recorded continuously each time that the subject changes from a resting position to an upright position. Evaluating the EKG signal (shape of a heart beat and delay between beats) during these events could improve therapies of at risk or elderly patients. Currently we are developing algorithms for the automated extraction of this information from long term monitoring periods (24hr or more). Recalling the well known Newton's formula that allows given the mass and the acceleration to calculate the force (F) as:

$$F = ma$$

Theoretically is possible to calculate the power (and then the calories expenditure) for a given exercise in a given time for a subject of known mass. It is worth to highlight that the calculation is not that trivial because it is obvious that the acceleration information that is possible to retrieve from the single posture sensor does not result enough to assess such estimation. However, further experiments using professional athlete in known tasks are scheduled to measure the error when comparing the calories expenditure calculated with the accelerometric sensors with the one calculated using standard equipments.

Moreover, an interesting link to the EEG, long term brain monitoring is the uses of accelerometers to detect seizure movements, as subjects usually have repeats of the same type of seizure the accelerometer could be placed on the known limb.. This might be able to serve as a proxy for the video used in clinical EEG, to correlate movements with spikes or the prediction of spikes.

6.2 ECG application

Our new focus in ECG application is the continuous monitoring of swimmers and divers. Usually this application requires water proofing of the electrodes because the water can short recording sites, moreover, water resistant glue must to be applied to keep the electrode in position.

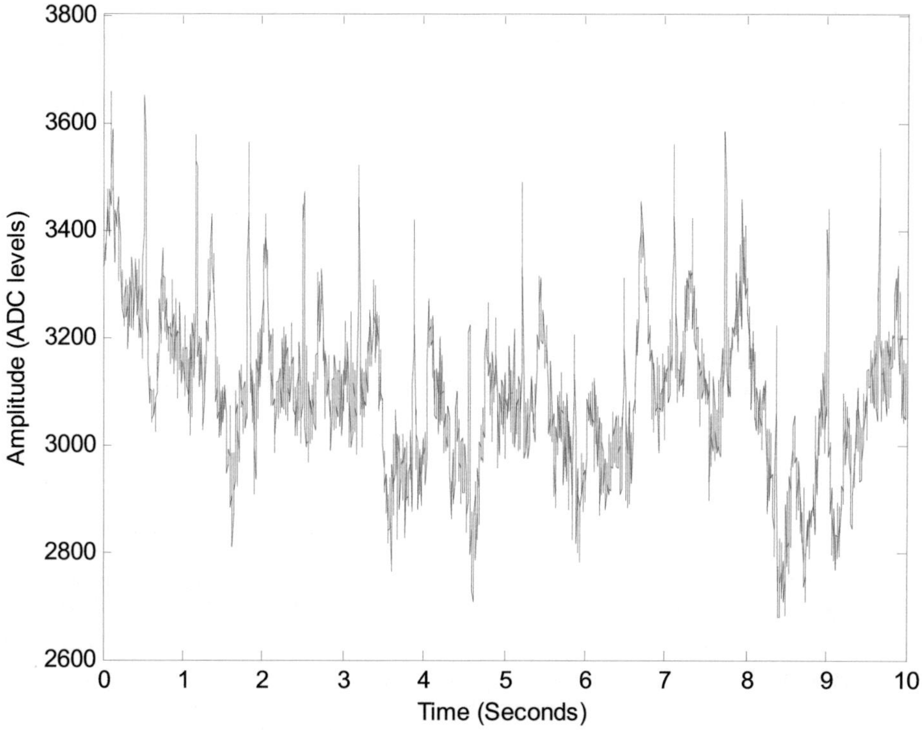

Fig. 16. Underwater ECG recording

The use of the proposed monitoring system opens a new monitoring scenario in this field as well. Even though our system is designed to operate in a dry environment, it can also be used in a wet environment it will even work when submerged in water. Figure 16 shows an excerpt of the data (raw) recorded from a subject totally submerged in fresh water, electrodes are placed on the chest. No special skin preparation was used and no waterproofing was performed at the electrode level. As it is possible to observe from the trace, the ECG signal is clearly recognizable, the baseline variation and the EMG artifacts clearly affecting the signal are due to the chest's muscles that the subject was using keep himself totally submerged (Gargiulo, Bifulco et al. 2008).

6.3 Long term of brain signals

Dry electrodes are obviously more convenient for long term EEG studies as gel melts as it heats up with body temperature, it smears shorting electrodes and is not convenient. Moreover EEG based BCI systems that ideally are to be worn as "plug and play" machine would have a great advantage from a system that result easy to install and remove, or even stable and reliable particularly when the subject is learning the BCI control. BCI training experiments can result tiredness and often the subject preparation takes longer that the experiment (in dense EEG montages). Therefore, beside the quest in finding a dry electrodes holding system able to work as good as the collodion glue (Gargiulo, Bifulco et al. 2008), without the mess caused from its repeated use, our current investigations are focused on the

role played from the feedback in BCI. Typically (but not always (Hinterberger, Neumann et al. 2004)) visual feedback is given to the user; however, it is broadly recognized that feedback plays an important role when subjects are learning to control their brain signals.
Moreover, it is worth highlighting that long term EEG monitoring could be part of a system that detects seizures and initiates automatic therapy (vagal nerve stimulator, deep brain stimulator or antiepileptic drugs) There is now even evidence that EEGs might predict seizures with inter-cranial electrodes (Waterhouse 2003).

7. References

(Ed.), J. G. W. (2006). ENCYCLOPEDIA OF MEDICAL DEVICES AND INSTRUMENTATION Vol 3, John Wiley & Sons, Inc., Publication.

Baba, A. and M. J. Burke (2008). "Measurement of the electrical properties of ungelled ECG electrodes." International Journal of Biology and Biomedical Engineering 2(3): 89-97.

Basilico, F. C. (1999). "Sudden Death in Young Athletes." THE AMERICAN JOURNAL OF SPORTS MEDICINE 27(1).

Benditt, D. G., D. W. Ferguson, et al. (1996). "Tilt Table Testing for Assessing Syncope." JACC 28(263).

Bifulco, P., A. Fratini, et al. (2009). A wearable long-term patient monitoring device for continuous recording of ECG by textile electrodes and body motion. 9th International Conference on Information Technology and Applications in Biomedicine (ITAB 2009). Larnaca, Cyprus, IEEE.

Bifulco, P., G. Gargiulo, et al. (2007). Bluetooth Portable Device for Continuous ECG and Patient Motion Monitoring During Daily Life. MEDICON, Ljubljana, Slovenia

Bluetooth, S. (2001) "Specification of the Bluetooth System - Core, version 1.1." Volume, DOI:

Catrysse, M., R. Puers, et al. (2003). Fabric sensors for measurement of physiological parameters. IEEE The 12th International Conference on Solid State Sensors, Actuators and Microsystems, Boston USA.

Chang, S., Y. Ryu, et al. (2005). Rubber electrode for wearable health monitoring. 2005 IEEE Engineering in Medicine and Biology 27th Annual Conference, Shanghai, China.

Chatrian, G. E., M. C. Petersen, et al. (1959). " The blocking of the rolandic wicket rhythm and some central changes related to movemnt." Electroencephalography and clinical Neurophysiology 11: 497-510.

Corder, K., S. Brage, et al. (2007). "Accelerometers and pedometers: methodology and clinical application." Curr Opin Clin Nutr Metab Care 10(5): 597-603.

Fagard, R. (2003). "Athlete's heart." Heart 89: 1455-1461.

Freescale Semiconductor, I. (2005) "MMA SERIES ACCELERATION SENSOR." Volume, DOI:

Gargiulo, G., P. Bifulco, et al. (2008). "Penso: equipment for a mobile BCI with dry electrodes." Submitted to IEEE Transactions on Neural Systems and Rehabilitation Engineering.

Gargiulo, G., P. Bifulco, et al. (2008). Mobile biomedical sensing with dry electrodes. ISSNIP, Sydney (NSW).

Gargiulo, G., P. Bifulco, et al. (2008). A mobile EEG system with dry electrodes. IEEE BIOCAS, Baltimore USA.

Giansanti, D. (2007). "Investigation of fall-risk using a wearable device with accelerometers and rate gyroscopes." PHYSIOLOGICAL MEASUREMENT 27: 1081–1090.

Hao, Y. and R. Foster (2008). "Wireless body sensor networks for health-monitoring applications." Physiological Measurement 29(11): R27-R56.

Harland, C. J., T. D. Clark, et al. (2002). "Electric potential probes—new directions in the remote sensing of the human body." Measurement science and technology journal. 13: 163-169.

Hindricks, G., C. Piorkowsky, et al. (2005). "Perception of atrial fibrillation before and after radiofrequency catheter ablation, relevance of asymptomatic arrythmia recurrence." Circulation 112: 307.

Hinterberger, T., N. Neumann, et al. (2004). "A multimodal brain-based feedback and communication system." Experimental Brain Research: 521-526.

Hinterbergera, T., A. Ku¨blera, et al. (2003). "A brain–computer interface (BCI) for the locked-in: comparison of different EEG classifications for the thought translation device." Clinical Neurophysiology 114: 10.

Hoos, M. B., G. Plasqui, et al. (2003). "Physical activity level measured by doubly labeled water and accelerometry in children." Eur J Appl Physiol 89(6): 624-6.

Horowitz, P. and W. Hill (2002). The Art Of Electronics, Cambridge.

Ives, J. C. and J. K. Wigglesworth (2003). "Sampling rate effects on surface EMG timing and amplitude measures." Clinical Biomechanics 18(6): 543-552.

J. G. Webster, (Editor) (1998). Medical Instrumentation application and design, John Willey.

Jeannerod, M. J. (1995). "Mental imagery in the motor context." Neuropsychologia 33(11).

Kaiser, W. and M. Findeis (1999). "Artifact processing during exercise testing." J Electrocardiol 32 Suppl: 212-9.

Lin, Y., I. Jan, et al. (2004). "A wireless PDA-based physiological monitoring system for patient transport." IEEE Trans Inf Technol Biomed. 8(4).

Logar, C., B. Walzl, et al. (1994). "Role of long-term EEG monitoring in diagnosis and treatment of epilepsy." Eur Neurol 34 Suppl 1: 29-32.

M. Catrysse, R. P., C. Hertleer, L. Van Langenhove, and a. D. M. H. van Egmondc (2004). "Towards the integration of textile sensors in a wireless monitoring suit." Sensors and Actuators 114: 302-314.

Mathie, M. J., A. C. Coster, et al. (2004). "Accelerometry: providing an integrated, practical method for long-term, ambulatory monitoring of human movement." Physiol Meas 25(2): R1-20.

Millán, J. d. R. (2003). Adaptive Brain Interfaces for Communication and Control. 10th International Conference on Human-Computer Interaction. Crete, Greece.

Millan, J. R., F. Renkens, et al. (2004). "Non invasive brain-actuated control of a mobile robot by human EEG." IEEE Transactions on Biomedical Engineering: 1026–1033.

Muhlsteff, J. and O. Such (2004). Dry electrodes for monitoring of vital signs in functional textiles. 26th Annual International Conference of the IEEE Engineering in Medicine and Biology Society (EMBC).

Mühlsteff, J., O. Such, et al. (2004). Wearable approach for continuous ECG and Activity Patient-Monitoring. 26th Annual International Conference of the IEEE EMBS San Francisco, CA, USA.

Murphy, S. L. (2009). "Review of physical activity measurement using accelerometers in older adults: considerations for research design and conduct." Prev Med 48(2): 108-14.

Pandian, P. S., K. Mohanavelu, et al. (2008). "Smart Vest: wearable multi-parameter remote physiological monitoring system." Med Eng Phys 30(4): 466-77.

Pate, R. R., M. J. Almeida, et al. (2006). "Validation and calibration of an accelerometer in preschool children." Obesity (Silver Spring) 14(11): 2000-6.

Pfurtscheller, G., C. Brunner, et al. (2006). "Mu rhythm (de)synchronization and EEG single-trial classification of different motor imagery tasks." NeuroImage 31: 153-159.

Pfurtsheller, G. and C. Neuper (2001). "Motor Imagery and Direct Brain–Computer Communication." PROCEEDINGS OF THE IEEE 89(7).

Prutchi, D. and M. Norris (2005). Design and development of medical electronic instrumentation, Wiley.

Searle, A. and L. Kirkup (2000). "A direct comparison of wet, dry and insulating bioelectric recording electrodes." Physiological Measurement 21: 271-283.

Strath, S. J., S. Brage, et al. (2005). "Integration of physiological and accelerometer data to improve physical activity assessment." Med Sci Sports Exerc. 37 (11 supp.): 563-571.

Taheri, B. A., R. T. Knight, et al. (1994). "A dry electrode for EEG recording." Electroencephalogrcphy and clinical Neuropltysiology 90: 376-383.

Talhouet, H. d. and J. G. Webster (1996). "The origin of skin-stretch-caused motion artifacts under electrodes." PHYSIOLOGICAL MEASUREMENT 17: 81-93.

Uswatte, G., W. L. Foo, et al. (2005). "Ambulatory monitoring of arm movement using accelerometry: an objective measure of upper-extremity rehabilitation in persons with chronic stroke." Arch Phys Med Rehabil 86(7): 1498-501.

Valchinov, E. S. and N. E. Pallikarakis (2004) "An active electrode for biopotential recording from small localized bio-sources." BioMedical Engineering OnLine Volume, DOI:

Waterhouse, E. (2003). "New Horizons in Ambulatory Electroencephalography." Engineering in Medicine and Biology Magazine, IEEE 22(3): 74-80.

Zheng, Z. J., J. B. Croft, et al. (2002). State specific mortality from sudden cardiac death Morbid Mortal Weekly Report: 51-123.

7

The Extraction of Symbolic Postures to Transfer Social Cues into Robot

P. Ravindra S. De Silva[1], Tohru Matsumoto[1], Stephen G. Lambacher[2], Ajith P. Madurapperuma[3], Susantha Herath[4] and Masatake Higashi[1]

[1]Toyota Technological Institute,
[2]Aoyama Gakuin University
[3]University of Moratuwa,
[4]St.cloud State University
[1,2]Japan
[3]Sri Lanka
[4]USA

1. Introduction

At present, the inclination of robotic researchers is to develop social robots for a variety of application domains. Socially intelligent robots are capable of having natural interaction with a human by engaging in complex social functions. The challengeable issue is to transfer these social functions into a robot. This requires the development of computation modalities with intelligent and autonomous capabilities for reacting to a human partner within different contexts. More importantly, a robot needs to interact with a human partner through human-trusted social cues which create the interface for natural communication. To execute the above goals, robotic researchers have proposed a variety of concepts that are biologically-inspired and based on other theoretical concepts related to psychology and cognitive science. Recent robotic research has been able to achieve the transference of social behaviors into a robot through imitation-based learning (Ito et al., 2007) (Takano & Nakamura, 2006), and the related learning algorithms have helped in acquiring a variety of natural social cues. The acquired social behaviors have emphasized equipping robots with natural and trusted human interactions, which can be used to develop a wide range of robotic applications (Tapus et al., 2007).

The transference of a variety of skills into a robot involves several diminutive and imperative processes: the need for efficient media for gathering human motion precisely, the elicitation of key characteristic of motion, a generic approach to generate robot motion through the key characteristics of motion, and the need for an approach to evaluate generated robot motions or skills. The use of media for amassing human motions has become a crucial factor that is very important for attaining an agent's motion within deficit noisy data. Current imitation research has explored ways of simulating accurate human motions for robot imitations through a motion capture system (Calinon & Billard, 2007(a)) or through image processing techniques (Riley et al., 2003). A motion capture system provides accurate data that is quieter than image processing techniques (Calinon & Billard, 2007(b)).

However, approaches using existing motion capture systems or image processing techniques have faced tedious problems. For example, when using a current motion capture system, markers must be placed on the subject's body, which sometimes causes discomfort for expressing natural motion. Also, image processing techniques utilize more than five cameras to detect human motions, which is a technically difficult task when processing information from five cameras simultaneously.

The earlier stage of imitation research (Hovel et al., 1996) (Ikeuchi et al., 1993) has focused on action recognition and detection of task sequences to teach a demonstrator's task to robots. They have mostly focused on developing perceptual algorithms for visual recognition and analysis of human action sequences. Perceptions were segmented into the actions for defining demonstrator tasks, and these sub-tasks (sequences) were repeated by the robot's arm. This work has dealt with a robot's arm for imitating a demonstrator's tasks, which has been convenient for generating a robot's arm motion in comparison to a robot's whole body motions. A human's body motions are complex when it performs tasks or behaviors, with the angle of their body parts dynamically changing (the kinematics of body motion), and each of the body angles have a relationship to each other. To transfer a demonstrator's motions into a robot, we must consider the above points, including the characteristics of motions.

In essence, an imitation approach must assort the characteristics of an agent's motion: the speed of the motion, the acceleration of motions, the distribution of motions, the changing point of motion directions, etc. Since recent robotic platforms have focused on developing the kosher mathematical model for extracting the characteristics of human motion, these extractions have evolved conveniently for transferring human motion into a robot (Aleotti & Caselli, 2005) (Dillmann, 2004). Kuniyoshi (Kuniyoshi et al., 1994) proposed a robot imitation framework that reproduces a performer's motion by observing the characteristics of motion patterns. A robot has reproduced a complex motion pattern through a recurrent neural network model.

Inamura (Inamura et al., 2004) proposed a robot learning framework by extracting motion segmentation. Motion segmentation has been employed by a Hidden Markov Model (HMM) for the acquisition of a proto symbol to represent body motion. These elicited motion segmentations with a proto symbol have been expended to generate a robot's motions. A problem with these contributions has been the patterns of motion have been assorted by observing the entire motion in each time interval. Instead of assorting the characteristics of motion via observation, it is important to design a mathematical model for selecting the characteristics of motion autonomously.

Another tendency of the proposed motion primitives is based on a framework for robot learning of complex human motions (Kajita et al., 2003) (Mataric, 2000). Recognizing primal motion primitives in each time interval is a decisive issue which is used for generating a whole robotic motion by combining the extracted motion primitives. In (Shiratori et al., 2004), the proposed robot learns dancing through motion primitives, and the forced assumption of an entire dance motion is a combination of determinate motion primitives. To disclose the motion primitives, the speed of the hands and legs during dancing and the rhythm of music are used. Most educed motion primitives are not meaningful and are difficult to replicate. The motion primitives-based techniques are able to cope with a variety of problems when motion primitives are extracted. Thus, there is a need to define diverse motion primitives and to yield to the whole motion through defined motion primitives. This procedure is able to procure different motion patterns that are dissimilar to the original agent's motions. Also, a motion primitive-based technique has to rely on a starting and end points of each motion primitive to generate a robot's motion accurately, which is contestable and arduous in this field.

Calinon & Billard (Calinon & Billard, 2007(c)) have proposed a robot imitation algorithm that projects motion data into a latent space, and the resulting data is employed by the Gaussian Mixture Model (GMM) in order to generate the robot's motion. In addition, a demonstrator is used to refine their motion while the robot reproduces the skills. Several statistical techniques, including a demonstrator motion and a motion-refined strategy were employed for generating the robot's motions. The proposed approach must process a demonstrator motion with recent motion-refined information simultaneously in order to successfully implement the imitation task. We believe their imitation task became too complicated, and another mathematical approach which combines the demonstrator's motion with a motion refine task (robot's motor information) for determining the robot's motions must be considered. The main emphasis of the robot imitation algorithm is that it relies on using less motion data (selecting symbolic postures), and it is necessary to conceive the robot limitation and environment using a simple mathematical framework for imitating human motion precisely.

In our approach, the robot does not use an agent's entire body motion to generate its motion. Instead, it selects preferable symbolic postures to re-generate the robot's motion through the dissimilarity values without any prior knowledge of social cues. Most existing imitation research attempts to transfer an agent's entire motion without considering a robot's limitations (e.g., motor information, body angles, and limitation of robot's motion). These methods are only applicable for predefined contexts, and are inconvenient to consider as a general framework for robot imitation in different contexts.

In contrast, our approach aims to extract symbolic postures, and through these elicited postures the robot generates the rest of the motions while its limitations are enumerated. Therefore, our proposed approach attempts to generate robot motion in different contexts without changing the general framework. Reinforcement Learning (RF) (Kaelbling et al., 1996) is utilized for finding optimal symbolic postures between two selected consecutive dissimilar postures.

2. Human motion tracking

Our approach needs to acquire human's motion information to transfer natural social cues into robot. To accomplish the above task, we have proposed the use of a single camera-based, image-processing technique to accurately obtain a agent's upper body motion. We attach a small color patch to a agent's head, right shoulder, right elbow right wrist, body/naval, left wrist, and left elbow (see Fig. 1). Through these markers, we estimate a agent's 12 upper body angles: hip front angle, shoulder font/rear angle (both left and right hand), shoulder twist angle (both left and right hand), elbow angle (both left and right hand), head front angle, neck twist angle, and neck tilt angle (see Fig. 1 for more details).

3. The extraction of symbolic postures

In this paper, we propose an approach capable of learning and eliciting the motions' segmentation points through postures dissimilarity values without any prior knowledge of

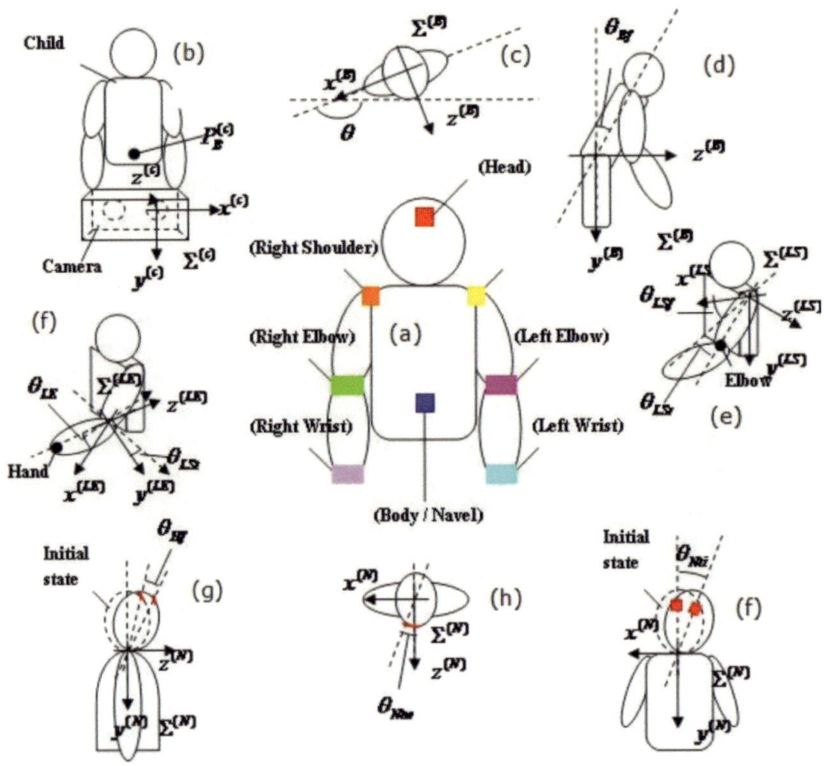

Fig. 1. (a): Attached color patch to the agent's upper body, (b): initial camera setup to detect each body position, (c): angle between camera and body, (d): hip front angle, (e): shoulder front/rear and right/left angle, (f): shoulder twist angle and elbow angle, (g): head front angle, (h): neck twist angle, (i): neck tilt angle.

the motions. Our approach assumes that the highest potential dissimilarity posture (points) can change the direction of the motion or the pattern of motion. Here we assumed that the characteristics of posture can be extracted through 12 upper body angles with the mean and variance of the postures in each frame. The postures' dissimilarity values can be computed according to the correlation of two consecutive postures. In this phase we explore the possible key-motion points which are capable of changing the motion pattern or motion directions.

First, we estimated the dissimilarity of two consecutive postures, and the highest dissimilarity values were directed to elicit dissimilarity postures from the entire motion. During this phase, we selected only higher dissimilarity postures which fulfill the $0.8 < \rho_{i\,i+1} \leq 1$ condition. Then, the earliest postures of consecutive postures were selected; for example, if posture number *i* and posture number *i+1* have the highest dissimilarity value ($max\ \rho_{i\,i+1}$), then only posture *i* was considered for further estimation. Here σ_i and σ_{i+1} represent the standard deviation of posture *i* and posture *i+1*, since β_{ij} is defined as the angle of postures *i* of joint angle *j*, $\bar{\beta}_i$ and represents the mean value of posture *i*. Similarly, β_{i+1j} is defined as the angle of posture *i+1* of joint angle *j* and $\bar{\beta}_{i+1}$ represents the mean value of posture *i+1* consorted with 12 upper body angles. The posture dissimilarity value (varying between $0 \leq \rho_{i\,i+1} \leq 1$) could be obtained through the following equation:

$$\rho_{i\,i+1} = \left| \left[(n-1)\, \sigma_i\, \sigma_{i+1} - \Sigma_{j=1..12} (\beta_{ij} - \bar{\beta}_i)(\beta_{i+1j} - \bar{\beta}_{i+1})\right] / (n-1)\, \sigma_i\, \sigma_{i+1} \right| \quad (1)$$

The significance of our approach was to estimate the possible key-motion points which are common for 12 upper body angles.

However, a study by (Calinon & Billard, 2007(d)) showed that it was necessary to consider each of the joint angles separately for extracting key-motion points. We believe that we have to consider the structure of the posture (combination of joint angles) to elicit key-motion points, since a posture provides information about how each of the joint angles are related in a particular frame. Accordingly, the selected key-motion points were considered as segmentation points of the demonstrator's motions.

4. Elicitation of optimal symbolic postures from reinforcement learning

In a study by (Calinon & Billard, 2007(d)) (Inamura et al., 2004) an HMM model was used for extracting dynamic features of a demonstrator's motions at states of the HMM to construct a robot's motions. Aude (Calinon & Billard, 2007(d)) used an HMM model with the Viterbi algorithm to elicit key-motion points from the entire motion. Here, the Viterbi algorithm searches the most significant state combinations from the inflexion point which are selected by local minimum or maximum points. As is generally known, a Viterbi algorithm searches an optimal state sequence to model motion or behavior. Moreover, the approach forces the Viterbi algorithm to select the best state sequence from inflexion points. But one problem is that the mechanism of the Viterbi algorithm does not consider eliciting the best state sequence, which includes the best key motion points to construct robot's motion. In that sense, there is a limitation in using an HMM for eliciting key motion points which can be considered as the best key motion points to generate a robot's motion - although HMM does provide the best sequence of states for modeling a human's motion or behaviors.

In our approach we used a Reinforcement Learning (Kaelbling et al., 1996) algorithm to learn and extract the most significant postures, which considered the individual difference of the postures. An RF mechanism is capable of directly considering the posture dissimilarity values to find the optimum postures (key motions) in order to construct the robot's motion for a given demonstrator's motion. This is the motivation for and advantage of using RF compared to a HMM, since RF learning extracts a few postures that have maximum individual differences of postures compared with entire postures. We estimated the postures dissimilarity values (p_{ii+1}) through equation 1. The estimated values are considred as the states in *Q-learning* ($p_{ii+1} \rightarrow s_i$), and the action is defined as the movemnet of state $s_i \rightarrow s_{i+1}$. We can define *Q-learning* function as:

$$Q\hat{}(s_i, a_i) \leftarrow (1-\alpha_i)\, r_i\, (s_i, a_i) + \alpha_i \left[R\,(s_i, a_i) + \gamma\, max^a\, Q(s_{i+1}, a_i)\right] \quad (2)$$

Where $R\,(s_i, a_i)$ is the reward matrix for each of the actions. The action a_i is defined as the movement of one state (posture) to another state (posture) and the element of the reward matrix is based on the value of the state transit (action) which is estimated using posture dissimilarity. In the *Q-learning* function, the action policy was defined as an essential part to find the optimal postures that have a maximum individual difference when compared with the other postures (motion points) or the optimal verdict to the *Q-learning* (see Fig.3). Accordingly, we defined two action policies: a state transit can move from one state s_i to another state s_k with $i<k$, and a state transit cannot be at a similar state (no link between s_i and s_i).

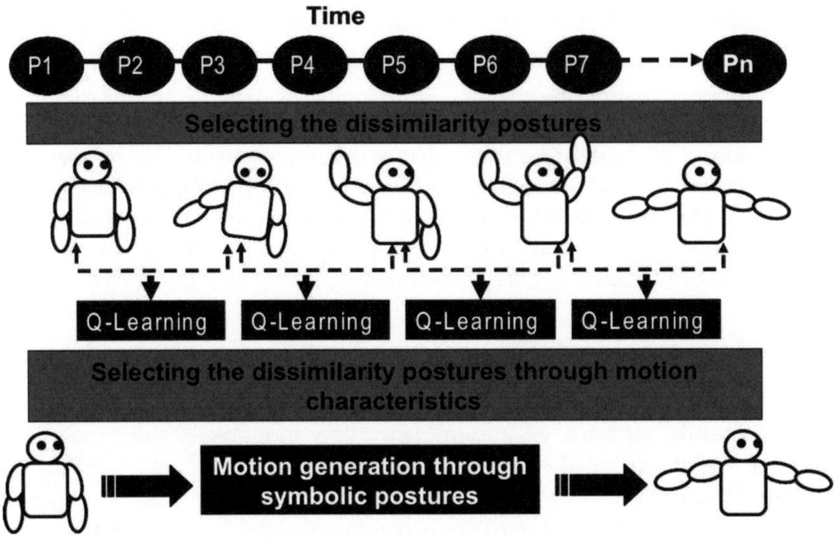

Fig. 2. An illustration of the proposed novel approach for generating the robot's social cues. First the symbolic postures are extracted through dissimilarity values and the *Q-learning* algorithm is utilized to find the optimal symbolic postures between selected postures in the previous step. In the final step, each angle is considered as a separately divisional cubic spline in order to generate robot motion through selected symbolic postures.

To process *Q-learning,* we must initialize the rewards matrix $R\ (s_i,\ a_i)$ whose estimatation is based on the individual difference of postures estimated by $\rho_{ik}= R(s_i \rightarrow s_k,\ a_i)$, where $i<k$. Consequently, if element of $R(s_i \rightarrow s_k,\ a_i)>0$, the initial reward matrix has a connection between s_i and s_k; otherwise, the reward matrix does not have a connection between s_i and s_k.

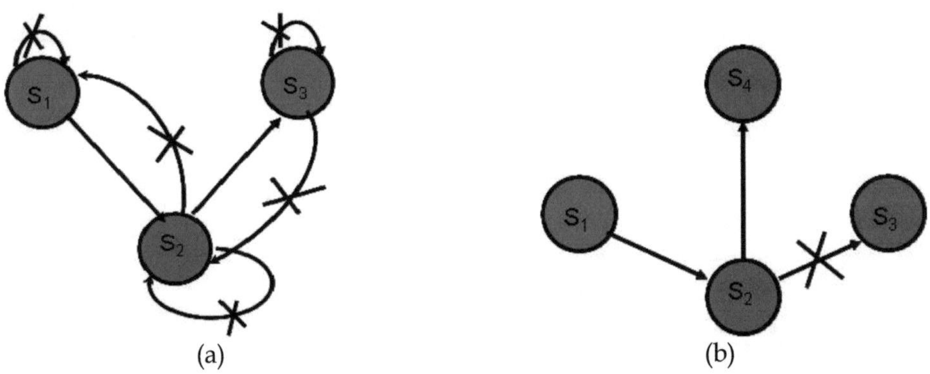

Fig. 3. (a) An illustration of the action policy of reinforcement learning to extract optimal symbolic postures. The action moves from one state to another $s_i \rightarrow s_k$ with $i<k$, and the action does not remain at the same state (no connection between s_i to s_i). For example, we do not have any connections from s_2 to s_1, and also from s_3 to s_2; and actions do not remain at the same states. (b) The initial reward matrix is defined according to: if $|s_i - s_k| >0$; the reward matrix then creates the connection between s_i and s_k. If $|s_i - s_k| = 0$, the reward matrix does not have a connection between those states. For example, if the above example satisfies $|s_1 - s_2| >0$ and $|s_2 - s_4| >0$, then the reward matrix has a connection for each state; but if $|s_2 - s_3| = 0$, then the reward matrix does not have a connection between them.

These policies are applied to the initial reward matrix. Here, we determine the learning rate α_t and the discount factor γ as 1. In the initial stage, we setup the *Q-matrix* $Q(s_t, a_t)$ as a zero matrix. Afterwards, we update $\hat{Q}(s_t, a_t)$ using the reward matrix. After updating the $\hat{Q}(s_t, a_t)$, we employed the epsilon greedy policy to find out the optimal state, and the corresponding key state was used as a guide to extract the optimal key-motion points (postures). RF is the concept of extracting postures that have the most individual difference values from motion sequences. In extracting these postures (key-motion), we assumed that the changing point of motion direction or motion pattern was also significant for constructing a robot's motion.

A similar mechanism is applied to the rest of the unlearned postures to extract optimal symbolic postures from the entire range of human motions. After extracting the optimal symbolic postures, our approach incorporates the divisional cubic spline interpolation for generating a robot's motion, considering each of angles as separate. Please refer to Fig.2 for further understanding of the proposed algorithm.

3. Generating robot motions

In this phase, we consider the trajectory of the angle (demonstrator) separately in the task space to construct each of the robot's angles, since we know the body scales of the robot and demonstrator are totally different. Indeed, both robot motion and demonstrator motion are proportional to each other when we capture motion through their joint angles because the body joint angles do not depend on the scale of the body. To construct the robot's motion, each of the angle trajectories are considered separately in task space, and selected key-motion points (common for every angle) are considered as reference points in the spline interpolation to construct the robot motions. We can define selected reference motion points as $(\beta_0, \beta_{1..}, \beta_n)$, where i= 0,1,..,n represents the selected key-motion points, and the corresponding time as $(t_1, t_2, .., t_n)$. The divisional cubic spline interpolation is defined as:

$$S_j = a_j(t-t_j)^3 + b_j(t-t_j)^2 + c_j(t-t_j) + d_j \tag{3}$$

where $t_j < t < t_{j+1}$, j= 0,1..., n-1 ; also a_j, b_j, c_j, and d_j are unknown parameters. Each cubic spline is generated by considering two consecutive points. To estimate a_j, b_j, c_j, and d_j, we need to define u_j, h_j, and v_j:

$$\begin{aligned} &S''(t_j) = u_j \\ &S''(t_0) = u_0 = S''(t_n) = u_n = 0 \\ &h_j = t_{j+1} - t_j,\ j = 0, 1, \ldots, n-1 \\ &v_j = 6\{[(\beta_{j+1} - \beta_j)/h_j] - [(\beta_j - \beta_{j-1})/h_{j-1}]\},\ j = 1,2,.., n-1 \end{aligned} \tag{4}$$

After estimating u_j, we compute a_j, b_j, and c_j in the following way;

$$\begin{aligned} &a_j = (u_{j+1} - u_j) / 6(t_{j+1} - t_j) \\ &b_j = u_j / 2 \\ &c_j = [(\beta_{j+1} - \beta j) / (t_{j+1} - t_j)] - (1/6)[(tj+1 - tj)(2uj + uj+1)] \\ &dj = \beta j \\ &\text{where } j = 0, 1, \ldots, n-1. \end{aligned} \tag{5}$$

Estimating the above parameters at time tj, where j= 0, 1,...,n we can generate an angle of robot's smooth motion. A similar approach is utilized for generating data of other angles for obtaining an entire robot's motion smoothly and precisely.

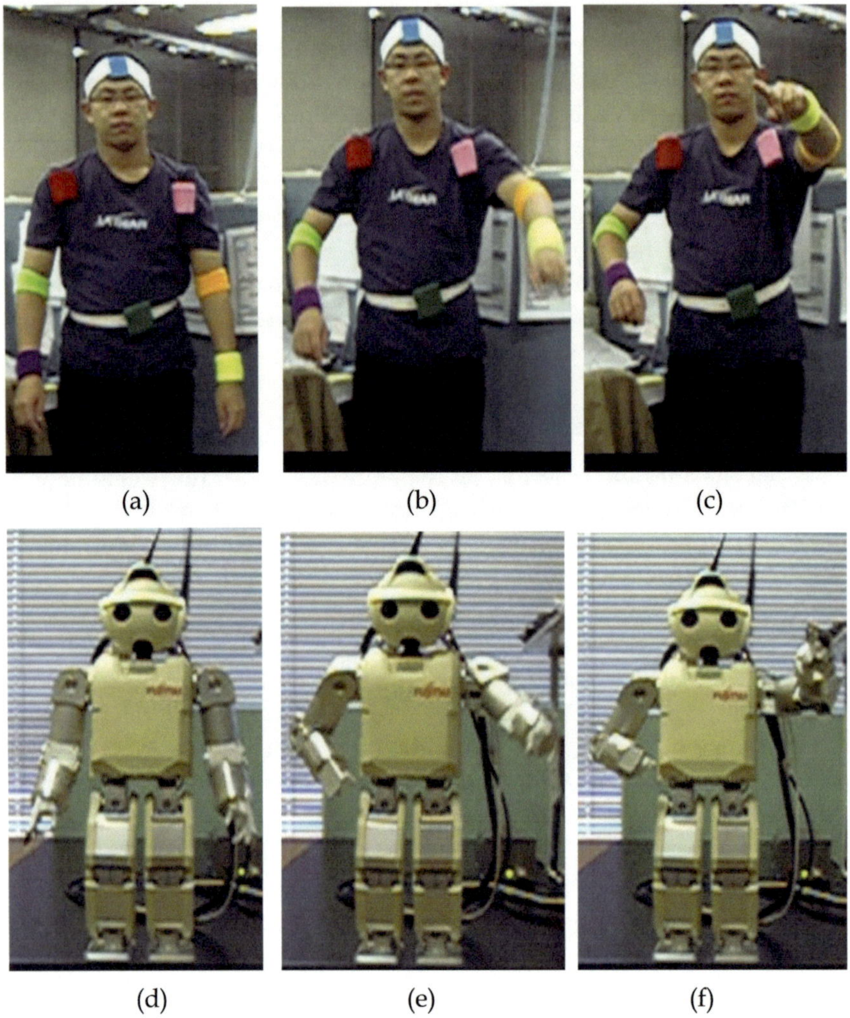

Fig. 4. The human agent expressing a "pointing gesture" in (a)(b)(c), and the robot successfully imitating the "pointing gesture" in (d)(e)(f).

5. Experimental protocol

The non-verbal communication channels help to transfer information interactively, and to provide more explicit elucidation to the meaning of verbal language. Since non-verbal communication is an essential channel in human communication for language understanding. Among these channels, a gesture-based channel plays a dominant role in human-human communication.

Recently, robotic research induced the development of a social cue-embodied robot to ameliorate the interface for natural human-robot interactions. A gesture-based channel can be used to more efficaciously and attractively create natural social cues embodied in a robot when in comparison with other communication channels, e.g., facial expressions. However, a gesture-based channel has played a major role in human-human communications, and we believe that a similar manner will work in human-robot interactions.

The experiment was conducted with a Fujitsu HOPE-3 robot with 28 degrees of freedom. The robot's leg DOF was set to a constant position. The human agent wore eight color patches and expressed three social cues in a natural way. Through an image processing technique, we estimated the position of the color patch within each frame. During the process, we first estimated the angle between the human body and camera position, which helped to estimate the 12 body angles.

Since, in our experiment, we attempt to transfer three social cues: a "pointing" gesture (see Fig. 4), "a gesture for explaining something attractively" (see Fig. 5) and a gesture for expressing "I don't know" (see Fig. 6), the human agent is used for transferring these selected social cues to the robot through the proposed imitation algorithm. The aforementioned gesture-based social cues are frequently used in human-human communication, and consequently for these social cues the robot would be used to create better natural human-robot interactions.

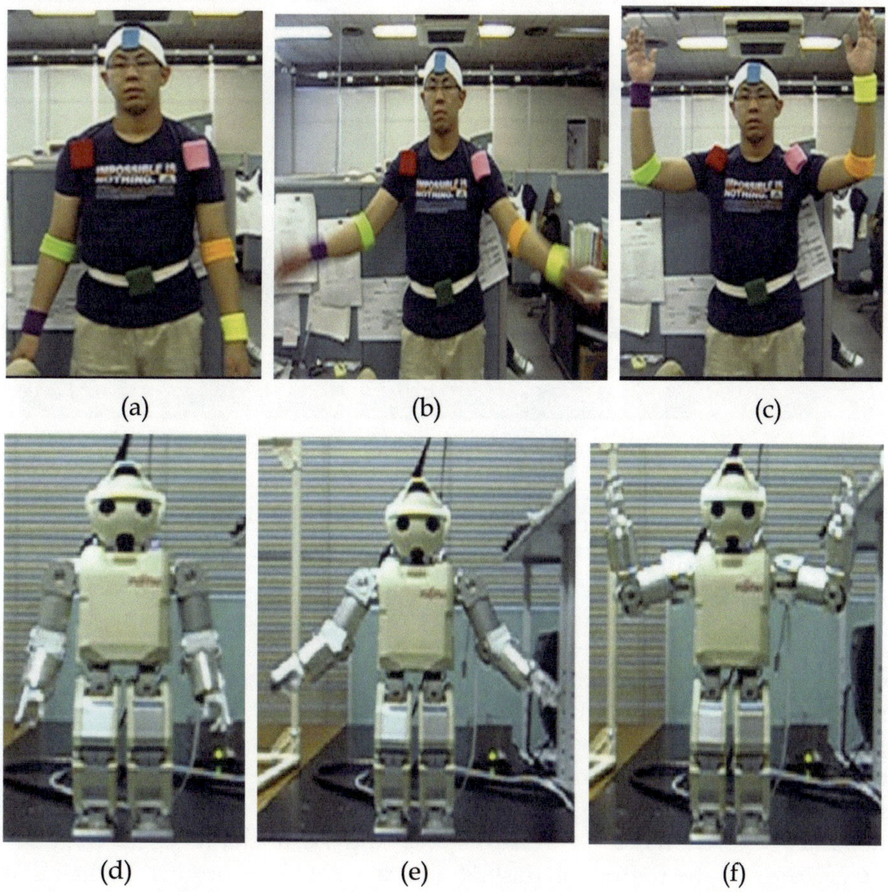

Fig. 5. The human expressing a "gesture for explaining something attractively," and the robot transferring the social cue precisely through the proposed imitation algorithm.

The dissimilarity values using the reinforcement learning method was applied to elicit symbolic key postures from the entire motions. Finally, we utilized the divisional cubic spline interpolation for generating robot motion considering each of the 12 angles separately. Fig. 4, Fig. 5, and Fig. 6 illustrate the expression of the agent's social cues and corresponding robot social generated by the proposed imitation algorithm. Our proposed algorithm precisely transferred the social cues into the robot. The robot obtained similar motion patterns of social cues when compared with the agent expressed motion.

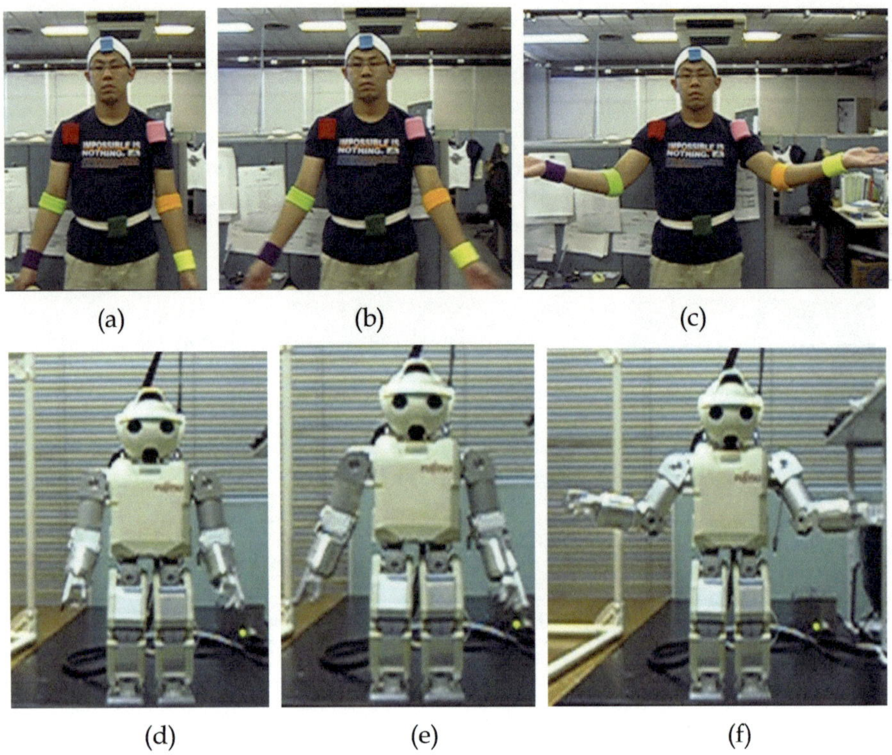

Fig. 6. The figure depicts the human expression of the social cue "I don't know" in (a)(b)(c), and the robot imitating the social cue precisely is shown in (d)(e)(f).

6. Experimental results

The novel part of the proposed method is its use of simple and accurate mathematical concepts with a few symbolic gestures for generating the whole robot motion. The robot required less computational complexity to precisely generate natural social cues. The generated robot social cues are commensurate to the patterns of the agent's social cues, and these can be validated by comparing the body angle data of the robot with the actual human body angle data (refer to Fig.7 – Fig.10 for a further description of the proposed algorithm).
Fig.7 illustrates the left hand front/rear angle, and right elbow angle (Fig. 8) for the "pointing gesture." In the figure, the dashed-line represents the original human angles and the solid-line represents the generated robot angles. In addition, the x-axis represents the time and the y-axis represents the radian values of angle. The pointing gesture has a quiet

simple motion when compared to the other social cues. However, the figures substantiated our claim that the robot-generated social cues had an almost similar pattern as that of the human-agent expressed social cues.

Also, according to the experimental results, some time intervals contained noisy data (see Fig. 7 at time 0.3 < t < 0.4). However, our proposed approach still did not consider these noisy data points in generating the robot's motion. The reason is that we compared the posture dissimilarity values extracted the key symbolic postures which consisted of all 12 body angles.

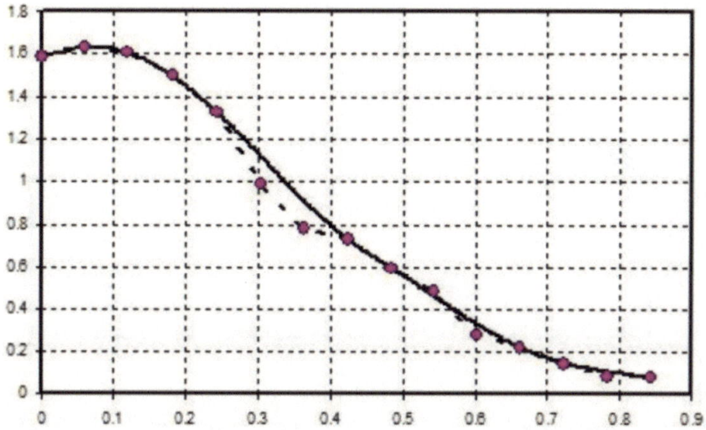

Fig. 7. An illustration of the motion of human social cue (constitute in dash-line) and generated robot motion (constitute in solid-line). The x-axis represents time and y-axis represents the radian value of angles. The angle of left hand front/rear angle data produced by the robot and the human for the "pointing gesture".

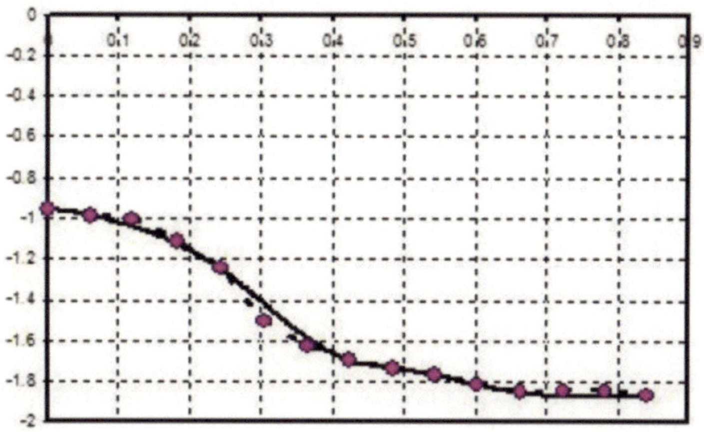

Fig. 8. The x-axis represents time and y-axis represents the radian value of angles. The motion data of the robot and human (right elbow angle) for expressing the "pointing gesture."

Also, a similar pattern was shown in Fig. 8 time range in 0.3 < t < 0.4 and 0.3 < t < 0.4. These results support our claim that the noisy data did not have a significant effect on generating accurate robot motion. In order to validate our proposed algorithm, the final social cues were transferred as the "I don't know" social cue. When carefully analyzing the angle of the right elbow (Fig. 9) and left front/rear (Fig. 10), the robot generated these motions more precisely than the other social cues.

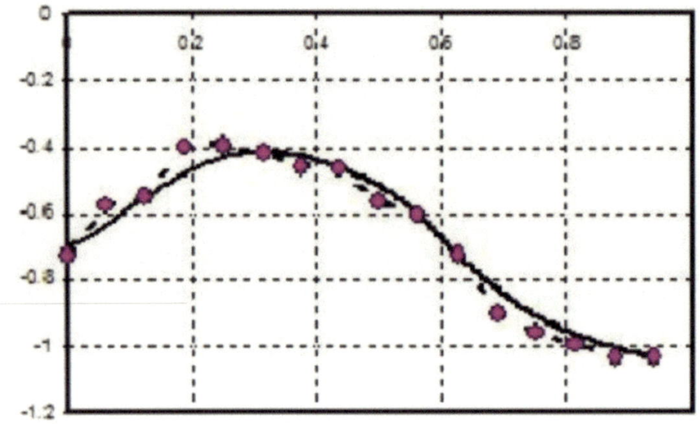

Fig. 9. An illustration of human and generated robot motions when the social cue of the "I don't know" gesture is expressed. The x-axis represents time and the y-axis represents the radian data of angles. Also, the solid line represents the robot generated motion and the dashed-line represents human motion for angle data of the right elbow.

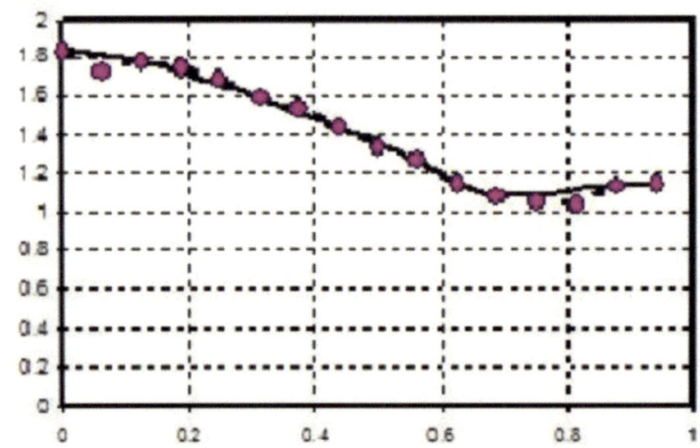

Fig. 10. The x-axis represents time and the y-axis represents the radian data of angles. Figure represent the angle data for the left hand front/rear angle is shown for social cue of ``I don't know" gesture is expressed.

The results of our experiment provide further evidence to validate that the noisy data did not have a significant effect on generating the robot motion precisely. This is demonstrated in Fig.11 and Fig.12, which represent the right hand elbow angle (Fig.11), and right hand shoulder twist angle (Fig.12). The data of the angles were obtained when the human demonstrator expressed the "gesture for explaining something attractively." Here, the "circle" symbol represents selected key motion points for the cubic spline in generating robot motions. Furthermore, Fig.12 shows certain noisy data that were not selected as key motion

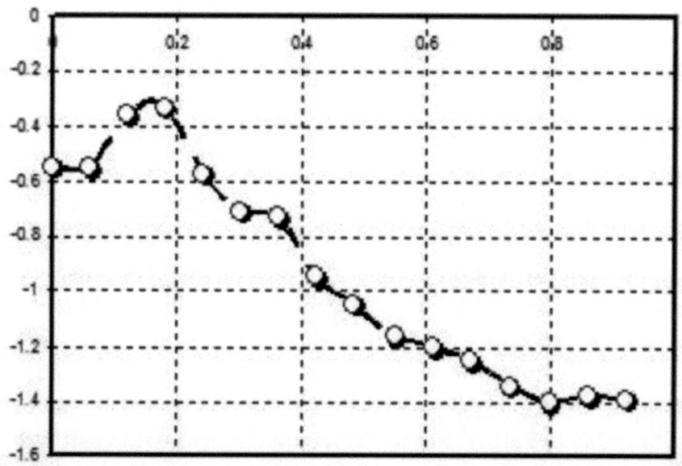

Fig. 11. Visualized data of selected body angles when the human expresses the gesture for "explaining something attractively". The "circle" symbol represents selected key motion points for generating robot motion through the cubic spline. The x-axis represents time and the y-axis represents the radian of angle data for right hand elbow angle

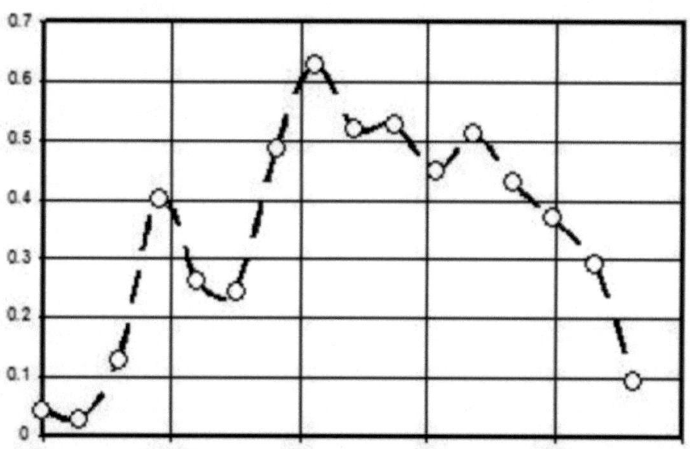

Fig. 12. An illustration of selected body angles when the human express "explaning something attractively". The "circle" symbol represents selected key motion points for generating robot motion through the cubic spline. The x-axis represents time and the y-axis represents the radian of angle data for right hand shoulder twist angle.

points. However, when considering the right hand twist angle (Fig.12) separately, that point still represents a point similar to the motion changing point. The concept of our proposed method includes considering and comparing all body angles to determine the key motion points (symbolic postures).

This manifests how our approach is capable of ignoring noised data efficiently. However, our mechanism did not select that point as a motion changing point. Overall, our results showed that the proposed imitation algorithm was able to generate the robot's social cues precisely, which corresponds to the agent's social cues, except during certain small time intervals.

7. Conclusion

In this paper, we presented a framework to transfer the natural gestural behaviors of a human agent to a robot through a robust imitation algorithm. The novelty of our proposed algorithm is the use of symbolic postures to generate the gestural behaviors of a robot ithout using any training data or trained model. The idea behind using symbolic postures is that a robot is flexibly able to generate its own motion.

The main challenge in robot imitation is identifying the changing points of motion direction at each time interval. In our approach, we estimated the changing points of motion direction through posture dissimilarity values and reinforcement learning at each time interval.

The image processing-based method obtained some noisy data that estimated the position of the colored patches. The noisy data did not have a significant effect on the accurate generation of the robot's motion, which was due to the fact that the imitation algorithm generated the robot's motion through only a small number of symbolic postures. Overall, the experimental results revealed that the proposed imitation algorithm imitated the human gestural behaviors quite accurately, except during only a few time intervals.

8. Acknowledgments

This research has been supported by both the Grant-in-Aid for Young Scientists (B)(19700477) from the Japan Society for the Promotion of science (JSPS) and the Grant-in-Aid for Sustainable Research Center of the Ministry of Education, Science, Sports and Culture of Japan.

9. References

Aleotti, J. & Caselli, S. (2005). Trajectory clustering and stochastic approximation for robot programming by demonstration, *Proceedings of IEEE-RAS international conference on intelligent robots and systems (IROS)*, pp. 1029-1034, August 2005, IEEE computer society

Calinon, S. & Billard, A. (2007)(a). Active teaching in robot programming by demonstration, *Proceedings of IEEE international symposium on robot and human interactive communication (RO-MAN)*, pp. 702-707, August 2007, IEEE computer society

Calinon, S. & Billard, A. (2007)(b). What is the teacher's role in robot programming by demonstration?- Toward benchmarks for improved learning, *Special issue on psychological benchmarks for improved learning, Interaction Studies,* Vol. 8, No. 3, pp. 441-464

Calinon, S. & Billard, A. (2007)(c). Incremental learning of gestures by imitation in a humanoid robot, *Proceedings of the ACM/IEEE international conference on human-robot interaction (HRI)*, pp. 255-262, 2007, ACM

Calinon, S. & Billard, A. (2004)(d). Stochastic gesture production and recognition model for a humanoid robot, *Proceedings of the international conference on intelligent robots and system*, pp. 2769-2774, 2004, IEEE computer society

Dillmann, R. (2004). Teaching and learning of robot tasks via observation of human performance, *Transaction on robotics and autonomous systems, IEEE, Vol.* 47, No. 3, pp. 109-116

Hovel, G. ; Sikka, P. & Mccarragher, B. (1996). Skill acquisition from human demonstration using a hidden markov model, *Proceedings of IEEE international conference on robotics and automation*, pp. 2706-2711, 1996, IEEE computer society

Ikeuchi, K. ; Kawade, M. & Suehiro, T. (1993). Assembly task recognition with planar, curved, and mechanical contacts, *Proceedings of IEEE international conference on robotics and automation*, pp. 688-694, 1993, IEEE computer society

Inamura, T.; Tanie, H. & Nakamura, Y. (2004). Embodied symbol emergence based on mimesis theory, *International journal of robotics research, SAGE, Vol.* 23, No. 5, pp. 363-377

Ito, M. ; Noda, K. ; Hoshino, Y. & Tani, J. (2007). Dynamic and interactive generation of object handling behaviours by a small humanoid robot using a dynamic neural network model, *Journal of Neural Networks, Elsevier Science,* Vol. 19, No. 3, pp. 323-337

Kaelbling, L. ; Littman, M. & Moore, A. (1996). Reinforcement learning: a survey, *Journal of artificial intelligence research, AAAI, Vol.* 4, No. 2, pp. 237-285

Kajita, S. ; Kanehiro, F. ; Kaneko, K. ; Fujiwara, K. ; Harada, K. ; Yokoi, K. & Hirukawa, H. (2003). Biped walking pattern generation by using preview control of zero-moment point, *Proceedings of IEEE international conference on robotics and automation*, pp. 1620-1626, 2003, IEEE computer society

Kuniyoshi, Y. ; Inaba, M. & Inoue, H. (1994). Learning by watching: extracting reusable task knowledge from visual observation of human performances, *Transaction on robotics and autonomous systems, IEEE, Vol.* 10, No. 6, pp. 799-822

Mataric, M. (2000). Getting humanoids to move and imitate, *IEEE intelligent systems, IEEE, Vol.* 15, No. 4, pp. 18-24

Riley, M. ; Ude, A. ; Wade, K. & Atkeson, C. (2003). Enabling real-time full-body imitation: a natural way of transferring human movements to humanoids, *Proceedings of IEEE international conference on robotics and automation*, pp. 2368-2374, May 2003, IEEE computer society

Shiratori, T.; Nakazawa, A. & Ikeuchi, K. (2004). Detecting dance motion structure through music analysis, *Proceedings of international conference on face and gesture recognition*, pp. 857-862, 2004, IEEE computer society

Takano, W. & Nakamura, Y. (2006). Humanoid robot's autonomous acquisition of proto-symbols through motion segmentation, *Proceedings of IEEE-RAS international conference on humanoid robots*, pp. 425-431, December 2006, IEEE computer society

Tapus, A.; Mataric, M. ; & Scassellati, B. (2007). *IEEE robotics and automation magazine, IEEE computer society Vol.* 14, No. 1, pp. 35-42

8

In-Vitro Magnetoresistive Biosensors for Single Molecular Based Disease Diagnostics: Optimization of Sensor Geometry and Structure

Seongtae Bae
Department of Electrical and Computer Engineering, Biomagnetics Laboratory (BML), National University of Singapore, 117576, Singapore
Singapore

1. Introduction

Detection of biological information using magnetoresistance (MR) sensors based on multilayered giant MR (GMR), or exchange biased GMR spin valves, operated by the magnetic field produced by magnetic nanoparticle sensor agents has been paid considerable attention in biomedical sensor technologies (Baselt et al., 1998; Tondra et al., 2000; Rife et al., 2003; Graham et al., 2004). The main reason for this interest is that MR based biosensors provide technical advantages such as high sensitivity, relatively fast and low-volume assay, and easy manipulation of the magnetic sensor agents under the externally applied magnetic field gradients (Graham et al., 2002; Lagae et al., 2002). These advantages lead to improved sensing performance, stimulating the development of functional *in-vitro* GMR based biosensors to obtain biological information and diagnose diseases more accurately in healthcare (Megen & Prins, 2005).

However, all the developed GMR biosensors so far were mostly focused on counting or indentifying multiple biomolecules such as a DNA counter and a bead array counter rather than single molecular detection (SMD) (Baselt et al., 1998; Miller et al., 2001; Graham et al., 2003; Li & Wang, 2003; Schepper et al., 2004; Wang et al., 2005; Shen et al., 2005). The main physical reason for this technical limitation is that the magnetic susceptibility of a single superparamagnetic nanoparticle sensor agent (SPNSA), which can be easily manipulated on the sensor surface without any serious agglomeration and easily retrieve magnetic stray field, is too small to generate a large enough field for acheiving a reasonably high SNR (Singal-to-Noise Ratio). Although superparamagentic microbeads have been attempted to obtain a larger stray field for higher SNR for SMD (Graham et al., 2002; Wirix-Speetiens et al., 2006), these agents were also revealed to have a technical drawback that they can not maintain one to one ratio between the microbead and the biomolecules due to a big mismatch in size. Hence, to develop more powerful in-vitro GMR bisoensor system for SMD, ferrimagentic nanoparticle (FN) sensor agents, which have a high remnant magentization expecting to producing a sufficient stray field for a higher SNR, and a high chemical stability as well as a high biocompatibility with living cells or biological entities, are currently considered as a feasible sensor agent to label the biomolecules. However, the applications of FN to a GMR biosensor agent has been limited for the past few years by a techical challenge relevant to a possible particle agglomeration while they are introducing into the microchannel. Fortunetely, as a new functional microfluidic channel with micromagnet, which can allow for effectively manipulating the FNs to flow into the channel one by one, has been recently developed (Lagae et al., 2002; Ramaden et al., 2006; Latham et al., 2007), the interests to apply a single FN sensor agent to an in-vitro GMR biosensor for SMD are dramtically increased in a molecular diagnostic biosensor system.

In this chapter, the physical characteristics of an in-vitro GMR biosensor with an immoblized single FNSA is mainly discussed to provide crucial information how to optimize its strucure for SMD. In chapter 2, the sensing performance of an in-vitro GMR biosensor with an immobilized FNSA or SPNSA is numerically analyzed based on the "Stoner-Wolfarth model" to evaluate which GMR biosensor system is more suitable for SMD. In chapter 3, the optimization of sensor geometry considering the spatial magentic field interaction between the FNSA and the FL as well as the physical correlation between the "effective sesning area" and SNR is introduced to successfully design an in-vitro GMR biosensor enabling to show maximized SNR for SMD. Finally, chapter 4 discusses the newly desgined sensoror structure of an in-vitro GMR biosensor with a specially designed magnetic shield layer (MSL) to explore its technical effectiveness for the diagnostic biosensor applications based on SMD.

2. An in-vitro GMR biosensor with an immobilized single FNSA or SPNSA for SMD

To confirm which sensor system is more promising for SMD, the sensing performance of an in-vitro GMR biosensor with an immobilized FNSA or SPNSA should be first clarified. Four physical sensing parameters: (1) the relative MR change (δR) relevant to the magnetization angle difference between the free layer (FL) (sensing layer) and the pinned layer in GMR spin-valves, (2) the interaction factor (IF) describing the magnetic spatial interaction between the FL and the nanoparticle sensor agent, (3) the distance between the single immobilized FNSA or SPNSA and the FL, and (4) the practically allowable sensor size considering the physical limit of current sensor fabrication technology, are mainly considered for the comparison of sensing performance. The numerical analysis is based on the "Stoner-Wolfarth model" describing that the magentizations of the FL in the GMR biosensors are coherently rotated under a globally applied magentic field with two-dimensional field components, which are homogeneous across the entire FL.

2.1 Physical model of spatial field distribution on an in-vitro GMR biosensor

The sensing mechanism of a GMR biosensor with an immobilized single FNSA or SPNA is illustrated in Fig. 1-(a). The sensor agents are captured on the FL surface of GMR biosensor through a bio-recognition process and the resistance of the GMR sensor is accordingly changed by the stray field produced from the magnetic nanoparticles. As shown in Fig. 1, the critical geometry parameters considered for the numerical calculation include the spacing between the SA and the sensor surface (h), and the geometry of FL, e.g. length (L), width (W), and thickness (t). Figure 1-(b) describes the magnetization configuration of FL in the GMR biosensor and the magnetic spatial interaction between the SA and the FL. The magnetization of pinned layer (PL) is exchange biased to the negative transverse direction (-y) and the easy axis (EA) of the FL is along the longitudinal direction (+x) due to shape anisotropy and crystalline anisotropy. To minimize the geometrically-induced magnetostatic coupling between the FL and the orthogonally coupled PL, the PL is considered as the "synthetic anti-ferromagnetic (AFM) layer", e.g. FM/non-magnetic/FM structure. The magnetization of FNSA is aligned in the positive transverse direction (+y) and the SPNSA is magnetized toward the positive transverse direction (+y) by the excitation field (+y) for comparison with the FNSA. In order to establish a physical model for the stray field induced by the magnetic nanoparticles, the single magnetic nanoparticle with spherical shape is assumed to be uniformly magnetized and has an effective dipole magnetic moment (m). The field intensity, H(H ≅ B in cgs unit) at a distance r can be expressed by equation (1) (Besse et al., 2002).

$$\overrightarrow{H(B)} = \frac{3\hat{r}(\hat{r} \times m) - m}{r} \tag{1}$$

The spatial distributions of the stray field induced by the magnetic nanoparticle on the FL of GMR biosensor are numerically calculated by considering the both longitudinal and transverse magnetic field components of an ideal dipole, as illustrated in Fig. 1-(b).

$$\begin{aligned} H_x(B_x) &= m \cdot \frac{2x^2 - y^2 - z^2}{(x^2 + y^2 + z^2)^{5/2}} \\ H_y(B_y) &= m \cdot \frac{3xy}{(x^2 + y^2 + z^2)^{5/2}} \\ H_z(B_z) &= m \cdot \frac{3xz}{(x^2 + y^2 + z^2)^{5/2}} \end{aligned} \tag{2}$$

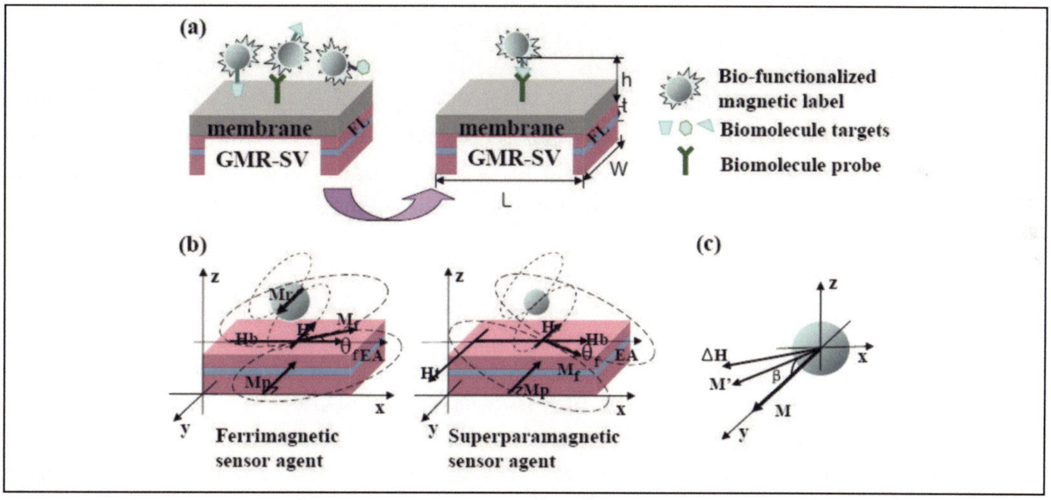

Fig. 1. A schematic diagram of an in-vitro GMR biosensor with a single nanoparticle sensor agent for SMD (a) the molecular recognition process on the GMR biosensor surface, (b) the magnetic spatial interaction between the magnetic nanoparticle agents and the FL of GMR biosensor. All the field components generated from the bias field, H_b, the excitation field, H_t and the magnetic nanoparticles are illustrated on the FL sensor surface, and (c) a schematic diagram of magnetization configuration of a single magnetic nanoparticle and its variation due to the magnetic dipole interaction caused by the x-component of FL magnetization to the FNSA or the SPNSA.

The total free energy in the FL is described by equation (3) based on the "Stoner- Wolfarth model" (Stoner & Wolfarth, 1948).

$$E = K_u \sin^2\theta + \frac{1}{2}(N_z - N_x)M_s \sin^2\theta - HM_s\cos(\psi-\theta) - H_t M_s \sin\theta - H_b M_s \cos\theta \qquad (3)$$

Where H is the stray field generated by the magnetic nanoparticles, which can be divided into H_x and H_y, respectively. The demagnetizing factors can be determined by equation (4) (William, 2001).

$$N_z = 8tw/l\sqrt{l^2+w^2}\ ,\ N_z = 8tw/w\sqrt{l^2+w^2} \qquad (4)$$

According to the "Stoner- Wolfarth model", the magnetization direction of the FL (FL is in a single domain state as the sensor size is in submicron range in this model) is determined by the minimization of the total free energy as shown in equation (3). Hence, the total free energy with respect to θ (Fig. 1-(c)) is minimized. Our method is to set up a discrete array of θ. The range of this array is from 0 to 2π and the step size is 0.00001. With such small step size, the range of θ can be considered as a continuous range. By substituting the array into equation (3), the minimized energy and the corresponding θ can be obtained using a simple algorithm. The next step is to use the following equation (5) to calculate the magnetoresistance (MR) ratio based on the magnetization (spin) configuration of GMR biosensor where the magnetization direction of PL is exchange biased to a fixed direction (-y).

$$\frac{\Delta R}{R} = \left(\frac{\Delta R}{R}\right)_0 \frac{1-\cos(\theta_f - \theta_P)}{2} \qquad (5)$$

Where θ_f and θ_p are the angles of the FL, and the PL with respect to EA, respectively; $(\Delta R/R)_0$ is the MR ratio of the GMR biosensor when the FL and PL is antiparallel with each other, which is also the maximum MR ratio for a GMR biosensor. To evaluate the sensing performance, the relative MR change, δR, is needed to be defined by equation (6).

$$\delta R = \left|\frac{(\Delta R/R)_{without} - (\Delta R/R)_{with}}{(\Delta R/R)_0}\right| \times 100(\%) = \frac{1}{2}\left|\sin\theta_{f,without} - \sin_{f,with}\right| \times 100(\%) \qquad (6)$$

Where $(\Delta R/R)_{with}$ indicates the MR ratio of GMR biosensors due to the nanoparticle sensor agents immobilized on the surface of FL, $(\Delta R/R)_{without}$ indicates the MR ratio without nanoparticle, especially SPNSA, on the surface of FL. Moreover, in equation (6), the $\theta_{f,without}$ is the angle between FL magnetization and EA when no sensor agent is on the sensor surface and the $\theta_{f,with}$ is the angle between FL magnetization and EA when the sensor agent is on the sensor surface. For FNSA, the $\theta_{f,without}$ is zero, thus δR can be written by $\delta R = 0.5\sin\theta_{f,with}$. For SPNSA, the $\theta_{f,without}$ is not zero due to the excitation field (see Fig. 1-(b)) and thus the δR can be rewritten by $0.5\cos\theta_f \cdot d\theta$, where, $d\theta$ is the angle difference before and after the SPNSA captured on the sensor surface ($d\theta = \theta_{f,without} - \theta_{f,with}$). The fringe field from the FL of GMR biosensors is also considered to affect the magnetic properties of nanoparticle sensor agent in both magnetization direction and magnetic moment due to the magnetic dipole interaction between the FL and the nanoparticles (see Fig. 1-(b)).

Accordingly, the effect of fringe field from the FL on the δR is included in this model to precisely interpret the sensing performance. To find out how many percentages the FL fringe field would influence on the magnetic moment of the magnetic nanoparticles, the interaction factor (IF) defined as $\alpha = (1 - m' \cos\beta / m) \cdot 100(\%)$ is employed, where m' is the magnetic moment considering the effect of the FL fringe field, m is the original magnetic moment and β is the angle difference between the original magnetization of sensor agent and the rotated magnetization due to the fringe field from FL as shown in Fig. 1-(c). In this model, the FNSA is considered as a $CoFe_2O_4$ nanoparticle. It has a remnant magnetization of 22 emu/g and a diameter of 26 nm (see Fig. 2-(a) and (b)). The magnetic moment of the $CoFe_2O_4$ nanoparticle is calculated using $\hat{m} = 4\pi M_r V$, where M_r is the remnant magnetization and V is the volume of the $CoFe_2O_4$ nanoparticle. Since the $CoFe_2O_4$ nanoparticle has a large remnant magnetization, the excitation field (H_t) is not required, thus the equation (3) can be simplified by equation (7),

$$E = K_u \sin^2\theta_f + \frac{1}{2}(N_z - N_x)M_f \sin^2\theta_f - H_x M_f \cos\theta_f - H_y M_f \sin\theta_f - H_b M_f \cos\theta_f \quad (7)$$

Due to the fringe field from the FL of GMR biosensor (ΔH), the induced magnetic moment of the $CoFe_2O_4$ nanoparticle becomes $\Delta m = \chi_f \cdot \Delta H$, where χ_f is considered as constant because the fringe field is relatively small. In addition, by considering the single domain state of $CoFe_2O_4$ nanoparticle agent, the magnetization direction of the $CoFe_2O_4$ nanoparticle can be calculated using the "Stoner- Wolfarth model" as below:

$$\begin{aligned} E &= \frac{1}{2}(H_u + H_d)m' \sin^2\beta - \Delta H_x m' \cos\beta - \Delta H_y m' \sin\beta - H_b m' \cos\beta \\ \Delta H_x &= \frac{M_f lwt \cos\theta_f}{(h + t/2 + D/2)^3}, \Delta H_y = \frac{M_f lwt \sin\theta_f}{(h + t/2 + D/2)^3} \end{aligned} \quad (8)$$

where $m' = m + \Delta m$, and ΔH_x, and ΔH_y are the longitudinal, and transverse component of the FL fringe field, respectively. As the saturation magnetization of the $CoFe_2O_4$ nanoparticle sensor agent is almost the same as the bulk $CoFe_2O_4$ ferrite, the anisotropy constant, K_1, of the sensor agent is assumed as bulk value of $CoFe_2O_4$ ferrite, which is a 2×10^6 erg/cm^3 and thus $H_u = 2K_1 / m'$. The demagnetizing factor is considered as $4\pi/3$ thus, $H_d = m' \cdot 4\pi/3$.

The SPN used in this model is also a single $CoFe_2O_4$ nanoparticle but the diameter is a 7 nm as shown in Fig. 2-(c) and (d). As can be seen in the inset of Fig. 2-(c), the magnetic susceptibility, χ, of the superparamagnetic $CoFe_2O_4$ nanoparticle is almost constant at a 0.041 independent of applied magnetic field. Using the experimentally obtained χ value, the magnetic moment of the superparamagnetic $CoFe_2O_4$ nanoparticle under the H_b and the H_t is determined at $\hat{m} = 4\pi r^3 \chi H_b \bar{x}/3 + 4\pi r^3 \chi H_t \bar{z}/3$ and the total free energy can be correspondingly re-written by equation (9).

$$\begin{aligned} E = {} & K_u \sin^2\theta_f + \frac{1}{2}(N_z - N_x)M_f \sin^2\theta_f - H_x M_f \cos\theta_f - H_y M_f \sin\theta_f - H_b M_f \cos\theta_f \\ & - H_t M_f \sin\theta_f \end{aligned} \quad (9)$$

As the χ value is constant and there is no magnetic anisotropy energy under no excitation field, the IF for the superparamagnetic $CoFe_2O_4$ nanoparticle sensor agent can be simplified as $\alpha_y = \Delta H_y / H_t$, where ΔH_y is the y component of the FL fringe field from GMR biosensor.

$$\alpha = \frac{M_s lwt \sin\theta_f}{(h + t/2 + D/2)^3 H_t} \times 100(\%) \tag{10}$$

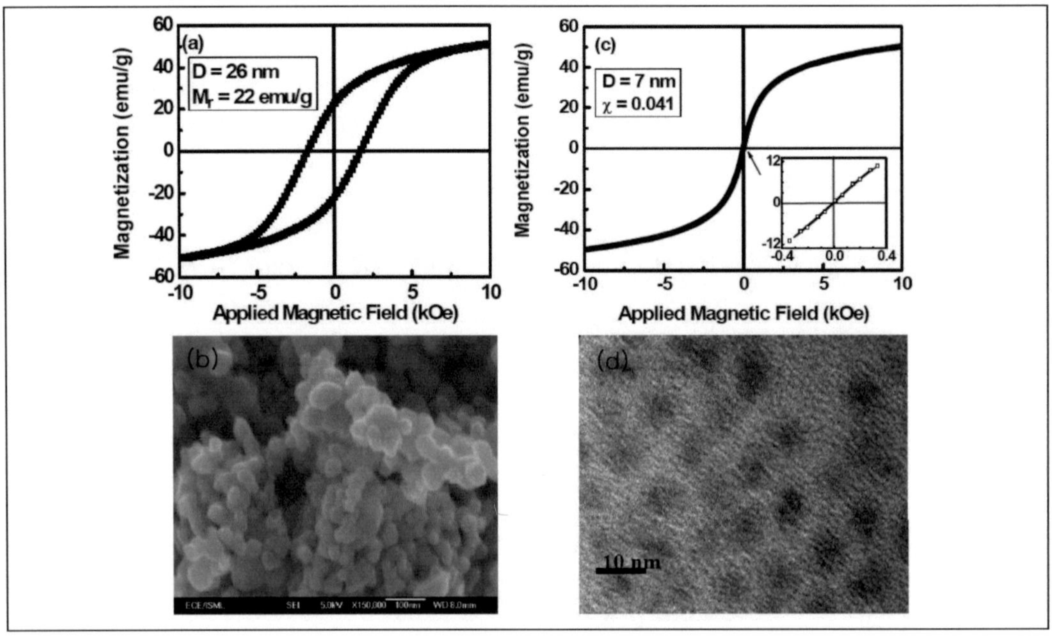

Fig. 2. (a) The hysteresis loop of $CoFe_2O_4$ FNSA with a 26 nm particle size, and (b) the SEM (Scanning Electron Microscopy) image of the $CoFe_2O_4$ FNSA, (c) the hysteresis loop of $CoFe_2O_4$ SPNSA with a 7 nm particle size. The inset shows the minor hysteresis loop measured at a ± 300 Oe, and (d) the TEM (Transmission Electron Microscopy) image of the $CoFe_2O_4$ SPNSA.

2.2 Comparison of sensing output performance

Based on the physical model developed in section 2.1, the sensing output performance of an in-vitro GMR biosensor with a single immobilized FNSA or SPNSA is calculated and compared. Figure 3 shows the dependence of sensor width at the fixed sensor geometry (sensor aspect ratio) on the δR and the IF of the in-vitro GMR biosensors. The sensor width, W, of the GMR biosensor is changed from 10 to 80 nm at the different aspect ratio (L : W) changed from 3 : 1 to 10 : 1. The purpose of changing the sensor aspect ratio is to explore the effects of vortex magnetization on the surface of FL due to the geometrically-induced demagnetizing factor (Girgis et al., 2000). The H_b, and the h are fixed at a 50 Oe, and a 30 nm, resepctively for precise comparison. The $CoFe_2O_4$ FNSA, and SPNSA has a mean particle size of 26 nm and 7 nm, resepctively. The δR and its variation due to the change of W is numerically analyzed by considering both the "effective sensing area", which is defined as the area formed on the FL surface whose magnetic spins can be coherently rotated by the stray magnetic field induced by the sensor agent, and the development of "inactive sensing area", which is not responded by the stray field, due to the increase of IF induced by the geometrically-increased magnetic anisotropy of FL.

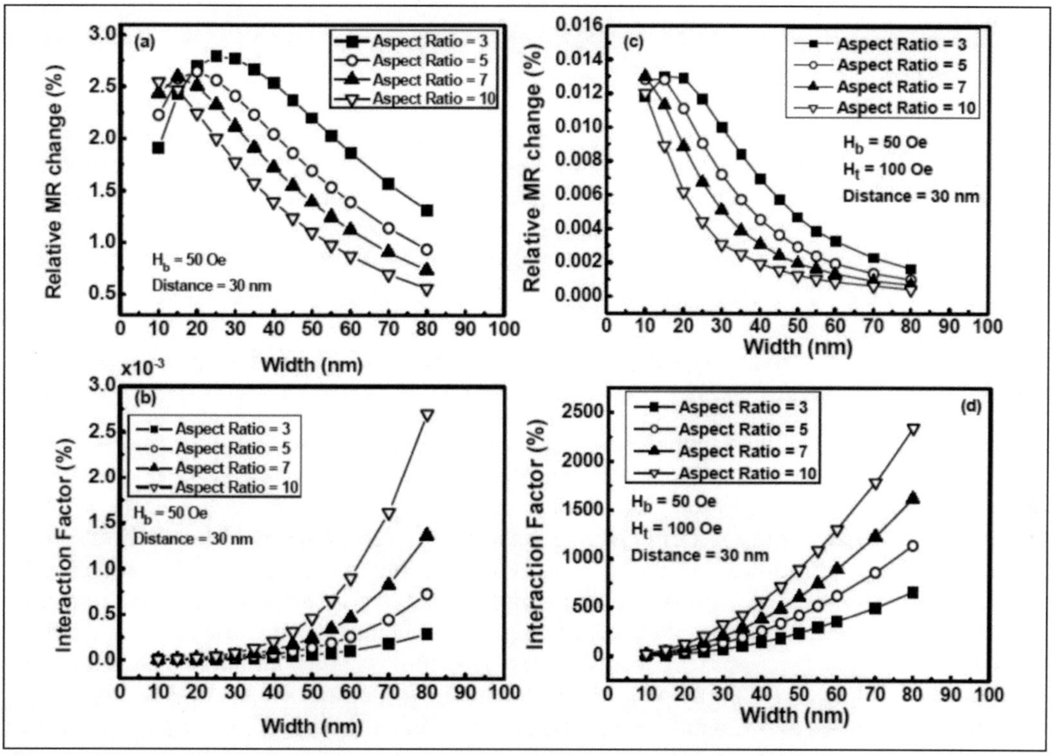

Fig. 3. The physical dependence of sensor width, W, on the relative MR, δR, and the interaction factor, IF, (a) δR, GMR biosensor with a FNSA, (b) IF, GMR biosensor with a FNSA, (c) δR, GMR biosensor with a SPNSA, and (d) IF, GMR biosensor with a SPNSA.

As shown in Fig. 3, the in-vitro GMR biosensors with an immobilized single FNSA or SPNSA exhibit the same physical characteristics that the δR is abruptly decreased above the maximized value obtained at the optimized sensor width, W_{op}, and that the IF is almost squarely increased, by increasing the W as well as the aspect ratio. This is supposed to be due to the increase of "inactive sensing area" and the magnetic anisotropy of FL induced by the increased sensor size proportional to the W. However, it is clearly noted that the absolute δR and IF values of the in-vitro GMR biosensor with a FNSA are much larger than those with a SPNSA. As can be clearly seen in Fig. 3-(a) and (c), the δR obtained from the in-vitro GMR biosensor with an aspect ratio of 3: 1 (75 nm (L) × 25 nm (W_{op})) and an immobilized FNSA is a 2.72 %, while the δR for the in-vitro GMR biosensor with a SPNSA, which has the same aspect ratio (45 nm (L) × 15 nm (W_{op})), is a 0.013 %. In addition, the variation of IF values depending on the W of the in-vitro GMR biosensor with a FNSA is negligibly small compared to those with a SPNSA as shown in Fig. 3-(b) and (d). The practically allowable sensor size based on the physical limit of current sensor fabrication technology, especially nanoelectronics technology, is another physical parameter to be considered in evaluating the sensing performance. Considering the patterning limit of EBL

(Electron Beam Lithography) technique (> 50 nm) and the geometrically-induced demagnetizing factor of FL directly relevant to the sensor aspect ratio and the IF, the minimum sensor size can be determined in the range between 150 nm (L) × 50 nm (W) and 250 (nm) × 50 nm (W). However, as verified in Fig. 3-(a) and (c), the δR values obtained from these sizes of in-vitro GMR biosensor with a SPNSA are too small to be considered for a real biosensor application.

According to the numerically analyzed sensing performance summarized in Fig. 3, it is clearly demonstrated that an in-vitro GMR biosensor with an immobilized single $CoFe_2O_4$ FNSA is more suitable for SMD due to its higher δR, less IF dependence, and practically allowable sensor size. The large remnant magnetization of single $CoFe_2O_4$ FNSA allowing to produce a sufficiently large stray field and to maintain extremly small variation of IF is the main physical reason for the technical promise of GMR biosensor with an immobilized single FNSA for SMD.

3. Optimizing the sensor geometry of an in-vitro GMR biosensor with an immobilized FNSA for SMD

In this chapter, the detailed spatial magnetic field interactions between the single $CoFe_2O_4$ FNSA and the FL of an in-vitro GMR biosensor is numerically analyzed to predict the optimized sensor geometry that maximizes the sensng perfromance for SMD prior to fabrication. In order to more accurately analyze the spatial magentic field interactions on the FL surface, the longitudinal and the transverse components of the stray field produced by the FNSA are considered. The optimized sensor geometry at a given remnant magentic moment of the FNSA is predicted by evaluating the "effective sensing area". The optimized sensor geometry is expressed in terms of the effective distance (δ), which includes the radius, *a*, of FNSA, the length of biological entities (especially, DNA including probe), membrane thickness, and the passivation layer, as well as the critical sensor length (l_c), and the critical sensor width (w_c). The experimentally demonstrated sensing performance of an in-vitro GMR biosensor with an immobilized $CoFe_2O_4$ FNSA is also compared to the numerically calculated sensing performance to confirm the effectiveness of the physical model introduced in this chapter.

3.1 Analytical model for optimizing sensor geometry and geometrical parameters

Figure 4 shows the schematic diagram of an in-vitro GMR biosensor with an immobilized single FNSA (a) and the typical MR curve (b) obtained from the $Si/Ta/Ni_{80}Fe_{20}/Ir_{22}Mn_{78}/Co_{84}Fe_{16}/Ru/Co_{84}Fe_{16}/Cu/Co_{84}Fe_{16}/Ni_{80}Fe_{20}/Ta$ exchange biased synthetic GMR spin-valve biosensor. For the numerical calculation, it is assumed that the $CoFe_2O_4$ FNSA has an a = 250 nm, and a mass density of 5.29 g/cm^3 (Lee et al., 2007). By considering only the logitudinal field compoent of the stray field produced by the immobilized single $CoFe_2O_4$ FNSA, B_x on the surface of FL along the x and y axis from equation (2) is simplified by equation (11) (Schepper et al., 2006).

$$B_{x,x-axis} = m \cdot \frac{2x^2 - z^2}{(x^2 + z^2)^{5/2}}$$
$$B_{x,y-axis} = m \cdot \frac{-y^2 - z^2}{(y^2 + z^2)^{5/2}} \tag{11}$$

The calculated magnetic field distribution and the two geometrically critical parameters, which are essential to determine the optimized sensor geometry, are also denoted in Fig. 4-(a). The geometrical parameters of the in-vitro GMR biosensor with an immobilized single FNSA are first determined by considering the longitudinal component of the stray field. The effective magnetization, β, is defined as the ratio of the total magnetization of the $CoFe_2O_4$ FNSA to the longitudinal field component of the stray field, $\beta = m/B_x$. The δ is defined as $\delta = h + a$. The geomtrical parameters, the l_c, and the w_c for achieving the optimized sensor geometry, which maximize the sensor output performance, are dependent on β and δ. These geometrical parameters, which determine the "effective sensing area", $l_c \times w_c$, are derived from equation (11) by considering x and y at the points where B_x is equal to the sensor switching field, B_{sw} (with $\beta_{sw} \equiv m/B_x$). The finally determined l_c, and w_c are given by,

$$l_c = |2x| = 2\sqrt{2}\delta\sqrt{\frac{\beta_{sw} - \delta^3}{4\beta_{sw} + 5\delta^3}}$$
$$w_c = |2y| = 2\sqrt{\beta_{sw}^{2/3} - \delta^2} \quad (12)$$

The insert in Fig. 4-(b) highlights the two characteristic parameters relevant to the operation of the in-vitro GMR biosensor; the B_{sw} and the detectable field limit (B_{DL}) directly associated with the exchange bias field of the in-vitro GMR biosensor, are defined in terms of the intensity of stray field produced by the single $CoFe_2O_4$ FNSA. The critical effective distance, δ_c, can be obtained by considering the operating conditions of the GMR biosensor including B_{sw}, B_{DL}, and the M_r of the single $CoFe_2O_4$ FNSA. If B_x is in the sensor operating range, $B_{sw}<B_x<B_{DL}$, δ can be expressed as a function of β. On the other hand, if B_x is smaller than B_{sw} ($B_{sw}>B_x$), then $l_c = w_c = 0$. Thus, the critical effective distance, δ_c, for the sensor

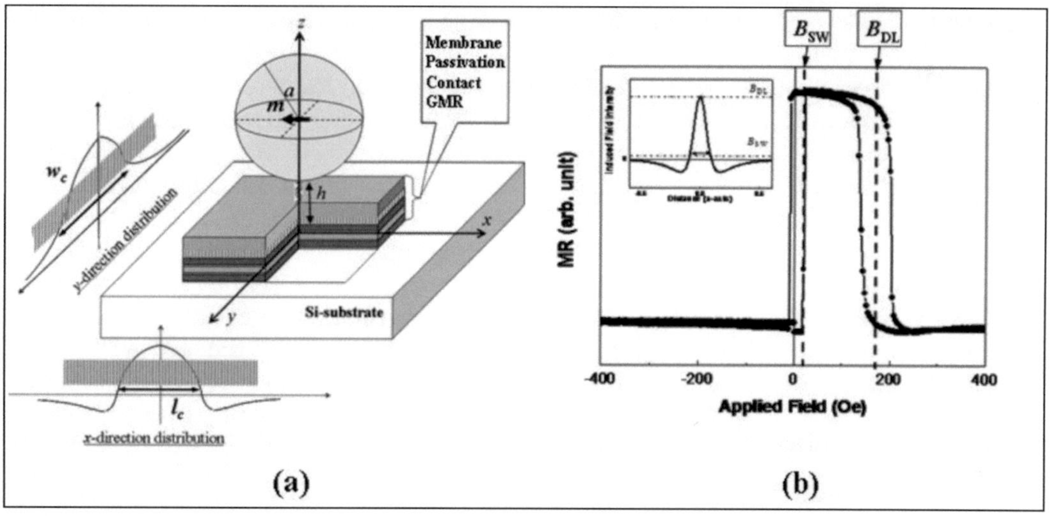

Fig. 4. (a) A schematic diagram of in-vitro GMR biosensor with an immobilized single FNSA, the field distribution , and the definition of geometrical parameters considering for optimizing sensor geometry, and (b) a typical MR curve of GMR biosensor and the definition of two sensing characteristics parameters.

operation based on the non-switching conditions: $B_{sw}>B_x$, and equation (12) can be determined at $\delta_c = \sqrt[3]{\beta}$. In addition, from equation (12), the aspect ratio, w_c / l_c for the optimized sensor geometry can be expressed by equation (13).

$$w_c / l_c = \frac{2\sqrt{\beta_{sw}^{2/3} - \delta^2}}{2\sqrt{2}\delta \cdot \sqrt{\dfrac{\beta_{sw} - \delta^3}{4\beta_{sw} + 5\delta^3}}} = \sqrt{\frac{(\beta_{sw}^{2/3} - \delta^2)\cdot(4\beta_{sw} + 5\delta^3)}{2\delta^2(\beta_{sw} - \delta^3)}} \qquad (13)$$

The numerically analyzed magnetic field distribution on the surface of the FL finally obtained by equation (13) clearly demonstrates that the optimized geometrical parameters, l_c, and w_c are directly relevant to δ and β_{sw}. In order to more accurately predict the optimized sensor geometry based on the "effective sensing area, $l_c \times w_c$", the numerical calculation is extended to two dimensional field component, both longitudinal and transverse field components, on the FL surface. The "Stoner- Wolfarth model" (or the "asteroid curve model") is employed for the detailed calculation (Hirota et al., 2002).

3.2 Optimizing the sensor geometry considering the one dimensional (longitudinal) field component

As described in the analytical model developed in section 3.1, the optimization of sensor geometry with an immobilized $CoFe_2O_4$ FNSA is based on the determination of l_c, and w_c by considering the longitudinal field component of B_x, and B_y, on the FL surface. Figure 5 shows the contour diagrams of the magnetic field intensity and its distributions, B_x, and B_y on the FL surface as a function of δ (for δ = 0.5, 1.0, and 2.0 μm). As can be seen in Figs. 5-(a), 5-(c), and 5-(e), the maximum B_x is rapidly decreased from 691.2 to 10.8 G by increasing δ from 0.5 to 2.0 μm. As shown in Fig. 4-(b), the in-vitro GMR biosensor considered in this model is operated at magnetic field intensity in the range from 12 G (B_{sw}) to 176 G (B_{DL}). Considering these the magnetic characteristics of GMR biosensor, the shaded region observed at δ = 0.5 μm due to the large field intensity (Fig. 5-(a)) and all the regions shown in Fig. 5-(e) do not contribute to the sensor operation. This indicates that the l_c and the w_c for the optimized sensor geometry based on equation (12) should be determined at δ_c < 0.79 μm, which corresponds to the sensor operating condition of $B_x \le B_{DL}$. Furthermore, by combining the calculated value of δ_c with the physical parameters of single $CoFe_2O_4$ FNSA and equation (12), the l_c, and the w_c are determined to be ~ 1.12 μm, and ~ 3.52 μm. Based on the numerical calculation, the aspect ratio (w_c / l_c) for the optimized sensor geometry of in-vitro GMR biosensor with an immobilized single $CoFe_2O_4$ FNSA (a = 250 nm) is determied at $w_c / l_c = 3.14$.

The calculation results shown in Fig. 5 clearly demonstrates that the geometrical and systematic design parameters (δ, l_c, and w_c) of the in-vitro GMR biosensor for producing a highly stable sensing performance can be precisely predicted prior to fabrication if the remnant magnetization of the single $CoFe_2O_4$ FNSA and the GMR characteristics of the sensor are known.

3.3 Optimizing the sensor geometry considering the longitudinal and transverse field components

Dependence of δ on the transverse component, B_y, is also estimated to confirm its physical contribution to the optimization of in-vitro GMR biosensor geometry. Figure 5-(b), 5-(d),

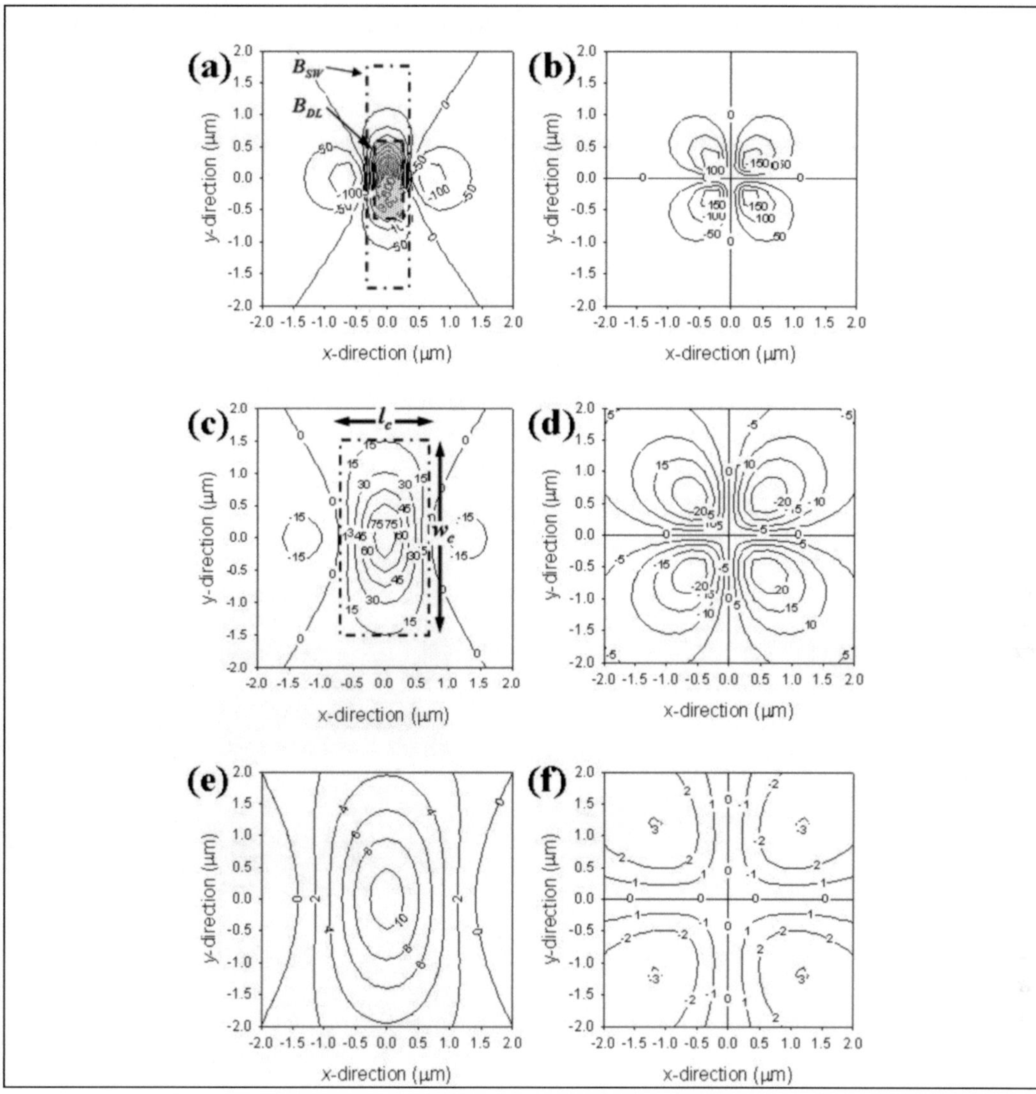

Fig. 5. Calculated contour diagrams of the longitudinal (left column) and transverse (right column) components of the magnetic field produced by an immobilized $CoFe_2O_4$ FNSA on the FL surface where δ is varied from 0.5 to 2.0 μm. The area defined by the dashed-dotted line and the shaded region show the optimized sensor geometry, and the undetectable region, respectively.

and 5-(f) show the contour diagrams of B_y as a function of δ changed from 0.5 to 2.0 μm. Similar to the calculation results shown in Figs. 5-(a), 5-(c), and 5-(e), the B_y has a strong dependence on δ. However, the distribution of B_y is completely different from B_x. The distribution of B_x on the FL surface shows an ellipsoidal shape with the major axis along the y-axis, while B_y exhibits a distribution that has a maximum and minimum field intensity of $B_{y,\max} \approx 1/3B_{x,\max}$ at the position of (±δ, ∓δ). The numerical comparison between B_x and B_y depending on δ suggests that both components of the stray field should be simultaneously considered for a more accurate prediction of the sensor geometry. Accordingly, the "Stoner-Wolfarth model": $H_k^{2/3} = H_x^{2/3} + H_y^{2/3}$, is employed to accurately analyze the spatial magnetic field distribution and intensity on the FL surface. Even though the "Stoner-Wolfarth model" assumes that the FL magnetizations are coherently rotated by the stray field and are homogneous across the entire FL surface, this model is considerably useful in interpreting the physical behavior of the in-vitro GMR biosensor under a highly localized magnetic dipole field from the immobilized single $CoFe_2O_4$ FNSA. Figure 6 shows the magentic field distribution and intesity considering both the logitudinal and transverse field components with different effective distances: δ = 0.5, 1.0, and 2.0 μm. Unlike the ellipsoidal shape of the "effective sensing area" shown in Fig. 5, the coherently rotated magnetization of the FL induced by two-dimensional magnetic field components shows a more complicated and extended "effective sensing area" due to the contribution of the transverse field component. Figure 7 shows the optimized sensor geometry (white line) and the "effective sensing area" (bright gray region) calculated by considering the one-dimensional

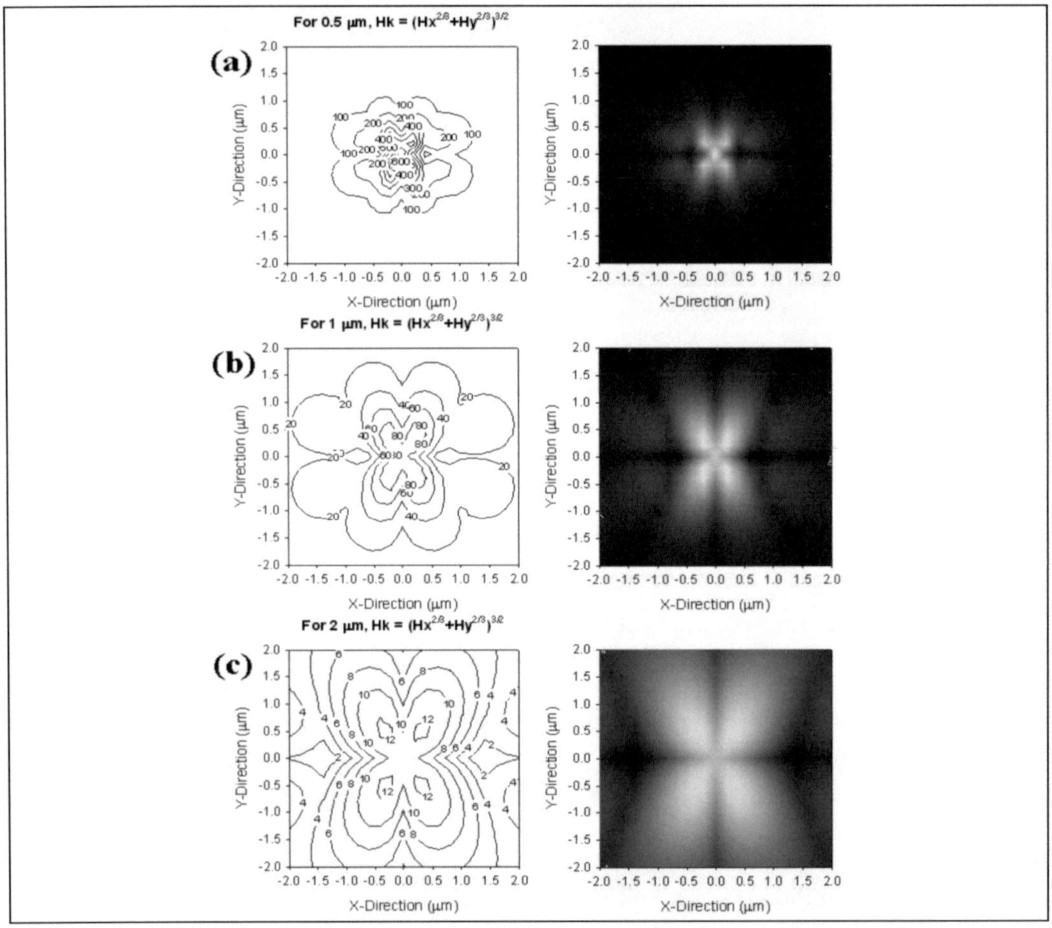

Fig. 6. The magnetic field distribution and intensity on the FL surface calculated by considering the longitudinal and transverse field components at the different effective distance of δ. (a) 0.5, (b) 1.0, and (c) 2.0 μm

(Fig. 7-(a)) and the two-dimensional components (Fig. 7-(b)) based on the "Stoner- Wolfarth model". Although the numerical values of optimized geometrical parameters determined at the effective distance of δ = 0.79 μm are the same as l_c = 1.12 μm, and w_c = 3.52 μm, the "effective sensing area" directly relevant to the sensing output performance is completely different. As can be seen in Fig. 7-(b), the "effective sensing area" is extended due to the transverse field component. This correspondingly results in enhancing the output signal of the in-vitro GMR biosensor. However, as can be also seen in Fig. 7-(b), an undetectable area in the vicinity of center of the optimized sensing area is developed due to the spatial magnetic field interaction. Making a GMR biosensor with a larger exchange bias field and introducing a specially designed sensor structure with a high permeability magnetic shield layer are suggested as an effective solution for the undesirable technical problem.

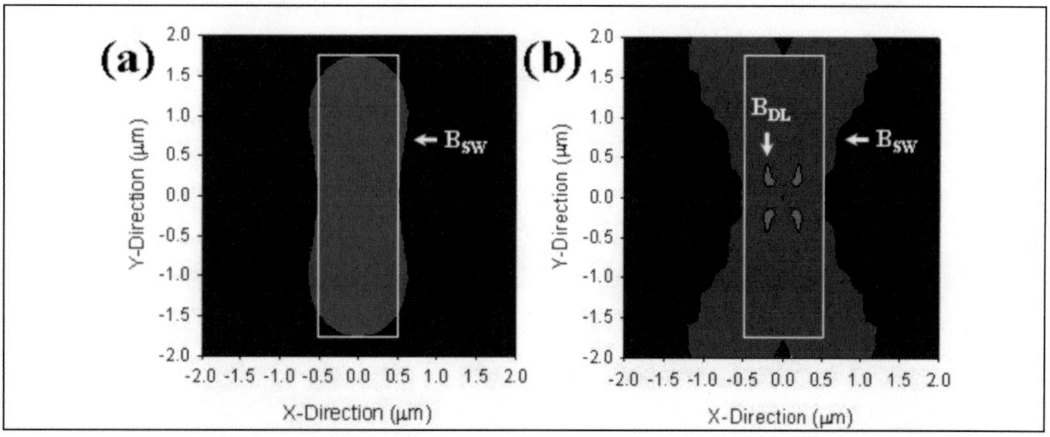

Fig. 7. Comparison of the optimized sensor geometry (square region) and the "effective sensing area" calculated by considering the (a) one-dimensional filed component, and (b) two-dimensional field component on the FL surface.

3.4 Demonstration of sensing performance of the in-vitro GMR biosensors with optimized sensor geometry

The sensing performance of an in-vitro GMR biosensor with an immobilized $CoFe_2O_4$ ferrimagentic nanobead SA geomtrically optimized by the analytical model developed in chapter 3.1 is demontrated to confirm its practical effectiveness. The $CoFe_2O_4$ nanobead with a mean raius, a, of 925 nm synthesized by using a modified sol-gel mehtod is considered as a ferrimagentic nanobead SA. The optimized sensor geomtry of the in-vitro GMR biosesnor based on the equations (11) ~ (13) as well as considering a 925 nm of mean nanobead size is calcuated to determine the "effective sensing area, $l_c \times w_c$ ". The sensing output performance of the optimized GMR biosensors is evaluated as a function of sensor length, l, at the fixed w_c by controlling the size of $CoFe_2O_4$ nanobead SA, which is systematically varied in the range of a = 925 nm ± 20.5 % as shown in Fig. 8-(a).

The controlled nanobead size leads to changing the l at the fixed w_c due to the variation of stray field intensity caused by the change of effective distance. The GMR biosensor used for this demosntration has a strucutre of Si/Ta(5)/$Ni_{80}Fe_{20}$(2)/$Ir_{22}Mn_{78}$(20)/$Co_{84}Fe_{16}$(2)/ Ru(0.75)/$Co_{84}Fe_{16}$(2)/Cu(2.3)/$Co_{84}Fe_{16}$(0.5)/Ni_{80} Fe_{20}(2.5)/Ta(3 nm) and is patterned by using an electron beam lithography (EBL) and a typical photolithography. The patterned

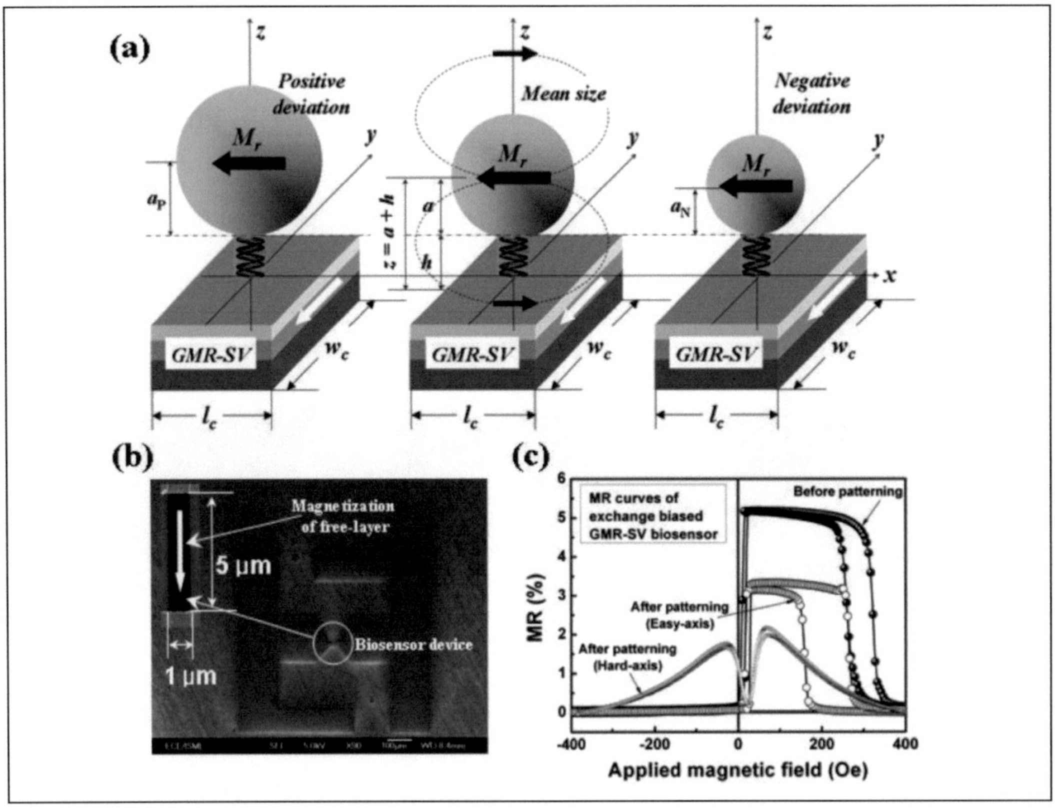

Fig. 8. (a) Schematic diagram of in-vitro GMR biosensors with an immobilized $CoFe_2O_4$ ferrimagentic nanobead SA with different bead sizes controlled in the range of a = 925 nm ± 20.5 %, (2) the patterned GMR biosensor with the geomtry of l = 1 μm, and w_c = 5 μm, and (c) GMR behaviour.

GMR biosensor structure and its GMR behaviour for the before and after patterning, and for the hard axis response are shown in Figs. 8(b), and (c), respectively. As can be seen in Fig. 8-(a), the magnetization of FL is orthogonally coupled to the pinned layer, and the stray field produced by the single $CoFe_2O_4$ nanobead SA is applied to the hard axis of FL magnetization for the detection of output sensing signal.

On the basis of the numerical analysis, the intensity of stray field produced by the $CoFe_2O_4$ nanobead SA with a radius of 750 (-20.5 %, negative standard deviation), 925 (mean nano bead size), and 1150 nm (+20.5 %, positive standard deviation) is calculated by considering the experimentally obtained M_r values to determine the l_c. The calculated maximum field intensity is a 67.8, 116.5, and 177.1 Oe (G), respectively and the l_c is revealed to be a 0.85, 1.08, and 1.31 μm, respectively at the fixed w_c = 5 μm. Figure 9 shows the detected output signal obtained from the in-vitro GMR biosensor shown in Fig. 8-(b). The detected signal is captured by using an oscilloscope. As can be clearly seen in Fig. 9-(a), when a DC magnet with a constant field of 103 Oe (G) is brought proximity to the GMR biosensor, an output signal of V_{out} = 6.13 mV (V_{output} = 613 mV after 100 times amplication using a 741 OP-AMP) is successfully achieved. This is attributed to the MR change of the GMR biosensor, $\Delta R/R_0$ = 2.2 %, which is exactly equal to the maximum MR ratio obtained along the hard-axis of the patternd GMR biosensor shown in Fig. 8-(c). At a 103 Oe (G) of field intensity, the "effective sensing area", $l_c \times w_c$ induced by the DC magnetic field intensity is larger than the patterned sensor geomtry of l = 1 μm, and w = 5 μm. This indicates that all the FL magnetizations are fully rotated by the applied DC magnetic field resulting in exhibiting the maximum MR ratio of 2.2 %. In contrast, the output signals obtained from the in-vitro GMR biosensors activated by the $CoFe_2O_4$ nanobead SAs show a strong dependence on the size of nanobead SA. As can be seen in Figs. 9-(b), (c), and (d), the output voltage and the $\Delta V_{out}/V$ of the GMR biosensor activated by the $CoFe_2O_4$ nanobead SA with a size of 750, 925, and 1150 nm are V_{out} = 6.07 mV ($\Delta V_{out}/V$ = 1.2 %), V_{out} = 6.12 mV ($\Delta V_{out}/V$ = 2.0 %), and V_{out} = 6.10 mV ($\Delta V_{out}/V$ = 1.7 %), respectively. Even though the non-uniformity and the position dependent stray field intensity produced by the nanobead SA can be considered to be partially influenced on the variation of output sensing signal, the observed sensing signal depending on the size of nanobead SA is primarily interpreted in terms of two physical parameters: (a) the change of stray field intensity relevant to the switching field, and (b) the "inactive sensing area" as well as the development of "undetectable sensing area". As can be

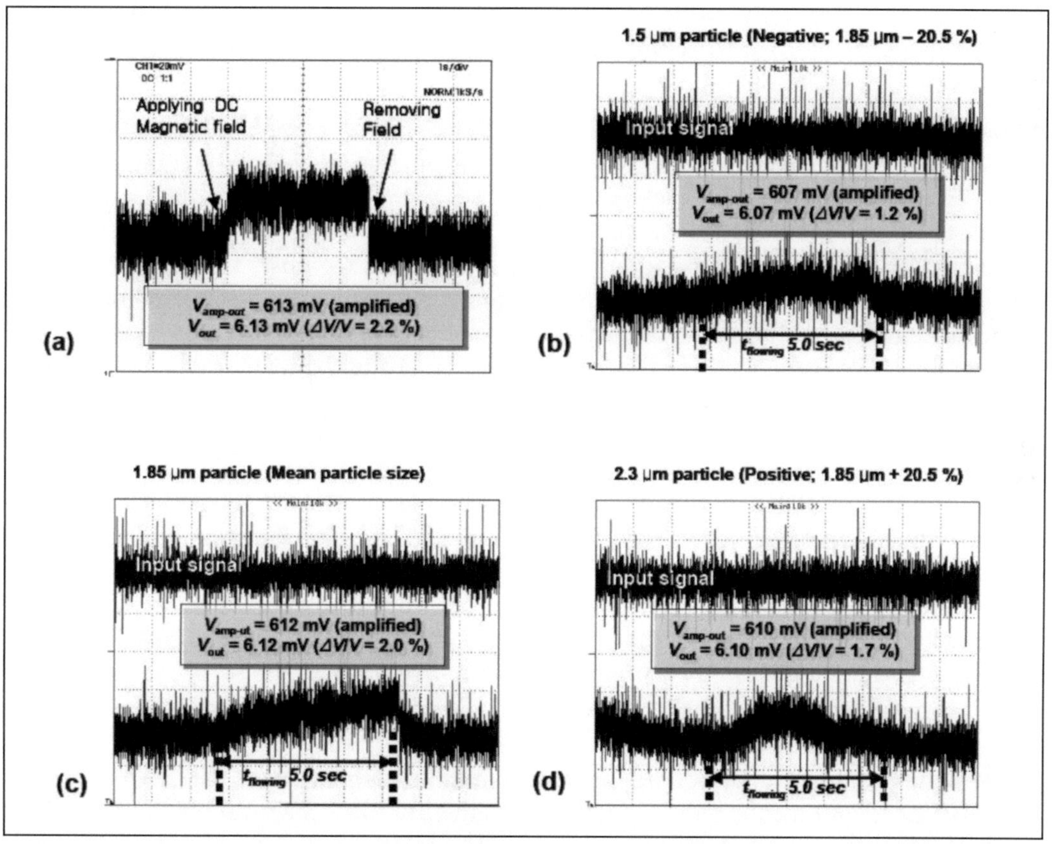

Fig. 9. Output sensing signal captured from the in-vitro GMR biosensor with geometry of l = 1 μm and w = 5 μm. (a) activated by DC magnet, (b) activated by 750 nm size $CoFe_2O_4$ nanobead SA, (c) activated by 925 nm size $CoFe_2O_4$ nanobead SA, and (d) activated by 1150 nm size $CoFe_2O_4$ nanobead SA.

confirmed from the calcualtion results, the 0.85 μm of l_c determined by the 750 nm size of nanobead SA at the fixed w_c = 5 μm is smaller than the geometry of patterned GMR biosensor, l = 1 μm and w = 5 μm, that results in the reduction of MR ratio due to the "inactive sensing area". In addition, the reduced stray field intensity due to the decrease of nanobead size leads to the reduction of switching field that results in a lower output sensing signal as shown in Fig. 8-(c). The slight decrease of output sensing signal obtained from the GMR biosensor with an 1150 nm size nanobead SA is thought to be due to the development of "undetectable sensing area" as shown in Fig. 7-(b). The large stray field intensity, around 177.1 Oe (G), obtained from the large size of nanobead SA is comparable to the exchange bias field of the patterned GMR biosensor. This induces the partial magnetic reversal of pinned layer resulting in a slight MR degradation. Furthermore, the spatial magnetic field interaction due to the large stray field intensity causes to form an undesirable "undetectable sensing area" at the central region of FL surface of the patterned GMR biosensor that leads to the reduction of MR ratio as well as the output sensing signal.

4. Effects of a specially designed magnetic shield layer (MSL) on the sensing performance of an in-vitro GMR biosensor with an immobilized single FNSA for SMD

As previously discussed, the in-vitro GMR biosensor with an immobilized single $CoFe_2O_4$ FNSA is suitable for SMD. However, accoridng to the numerical analysis on the spatial field interaction of the stray field, which is produced by a single FNSA, on the FL surface, the field distribution is found to be so complicated and non-uniform that it can not be easily interpreted. In particular, the creation of "undershoot field regions", which are formed at both edges of the maximum field intensity regions as well as the central regions of FL surface resulted from the spatial magnetic field interaction, is revealed as the most severe problem to induce the reduction of output sensing signal and the sensing stability of the in-vitro GMR biosensor. Thus, a new sensor structure, which can solve this technical challenge, is urgently required in a molecular based diagnostic GMR biosensor system for achieving more stable SMD.

In this chapter, a new structure of in-vitro GMR biosensor with a specially designed magnetic shield layer (MSL) is introduced and discussed based on the numerically analyzed calculation results to explore its effectiveness for the improvement of sensing performance as well as the sensing stability. The effects of MSL thickness including magnetic permeability of MSL, and gap width of MSL on the change of "undershoot field" as well as the "stray field intensity" are primarily discussed to demonstrate the physical contribution of MSL to the sensing performance of the in-vitro GMR biosensor considering for SMD.

4.1 Designing of in-vitro GMR biosensor with magnetic shield layer (MSL)

Figure 10-(a) shows a schematic diagram of an in-vitro GMR biosensor with a specially designed MSL. As shown in Fig. 10-(a), the in-vitro GMR biosensor has a single $CoFe_2O_4$ FNSA immobilized on the FL surface with a distanace of h μm, which is defined as the distacne between the FNSA and the FL surface of the GMR bionsensor. Accoridng to the physical model nuemrically developed in chapter 3.1 (Schepper et al., 2006), the h can be expressed as equation (14),

$$h = (4\pi \times m \frac{1}{B_{DL}})^{1/3} - a$$
$$m = \frac{4\pi}{3} a^3 M_r \tag{14}$$

In this numerical calculation, an IrMn based exchange biased GMR spin-valve device is considered as a sensing element. Thus, to achieve a stable sensing performance, the maximum field intensity produced by the single FNSA should be adjusted to be lower than the exchange bias field of the GMR biosensor. Considering this sensor operating condition, B_{DL} is determined based on the experimentally obtained exchange bias field from the patterned GMR biosensor.

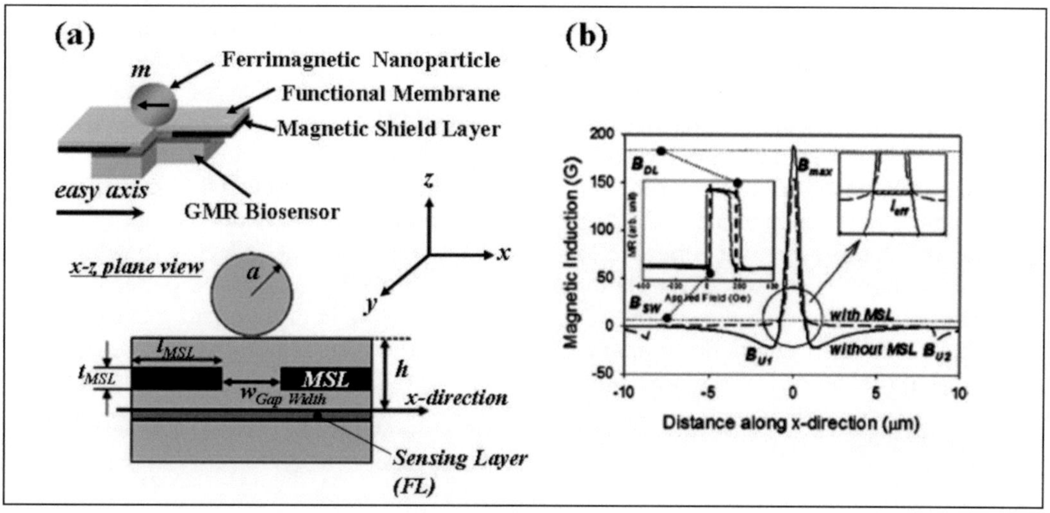

Fig. 10. (a) A schematic diagram of an in-vitro GMR biosensor with a specially designed MSL, and (b) the distribution of x-component of stray field produced by an immobilized single $CoFe_2O_4$ FNSA, with (solid line) and without (dashed line) MSL

For the numerical calculation based on equation (14), a radius of 250 nm size $CoFe_2O_4$ FNSA, an 176 G of exchange bias field, and a 0.48 μm of *h* are considered. As can be seen in Fig. 10-(a), the calcualted *h* value includes FL/passivation layer (40 nm)/MSL (0 ~ 300 nm)/Al_2O_3 functional membrane (140 nm; including a length of biological entities such as ten sequence of DNA: 34 nm). The Al_2O_3 functional membrane layer in this sensor structure is used for both maintaing the *h* depending on the variation of MSL thickness and immobilizing the FNSA using a membrane probe. The high magnetic permeability of materials such as supermalloy and permally are considered as a MSL in this structure. Figure 10-(b) shows a longitudinal field component (x direction) of stray field intesity on the FL surface without (solid line) and with (dashed line) MSL. The distribution of magentic field intensity shown in Fig. 10-(b) is calcualted as a function of distance from the center point of FNSA to the edge of GMR biosensor along the x direction. In addition, B_{max}, B_{U1}, B_{U2}, and l_{eff} are denoted as a maximum magentic field intensity, an undershoot field, an outer undershoot field, and an effective detectable length, which is the region enabled to be reversed by the stray field, respectively.

4.2 Effects of magnetic shield layer (MSL) on the sensing performance of in-vitro GMR biosensor for SMD

The MSL has a basic geometry of 300 nm thickness, a permeability of supermalloy (5.2×10^5), 1.2 μm gap width, and 8 μm length. To explore the effects of MSL on the sensing performance, the physical parameters of the MSL including its thickness, its gap width, and its permeability are changed from the basic structure. Figure 11 shows the dependence of MSL thickness on the sensing performance compared in terms of the physical sensing parameters such as B_{U1}, B_{max}, l_{eff}, and B_{U2}. As can be seen in Fig. 11-(a), the undesirable "undershoot field region", B_{U1}, is dramatically reduced when the MSL has a 1 nm of thickness. By further increasing its thickness, B_{U1} is sharply decreased and then it is completely removed above t_{MSL} = 100 nm. This indicates that the MSL needs to have a critical thickness to build up a close magnetic flux between the FNSA and the MSLs allowing for a distinct magnetic shielding effect. Figure 11-(b) shows the dependence of MSL thickness on the change of B_{max}. When the MSL has a 10 nm of thickness and above, the B_{max} is decreased down to 158 G and then it saturates at 153 G by further increasing the MSL thickness above 100 nm. This numerical result along with the increase of l_{eff} shown in Fig. 11-(c) indicates that the effects of MSL on the improvement of sensing performance of the in-vitro GMR biosensor are quite prominent. The reduction of B_{max} from 188 G (above B_{DL}) to 155 G (below the exchange bias field degradation point) and the increase of l_c of the sensing area due to the MSL shielding effects allow the dramatic increase of "effective sensing area" on the FL surface that leads to the increase of sensing output signal of the patterned GMR biosensor. However, as can be seen in Fig. 11-(d), the magnetic dipole field induced in the MSL due to its high magnetic moment generates another undesirable small "undershoot field", B_{U2} at the vicinity of the MSL edges. Even though its numerical value is small below

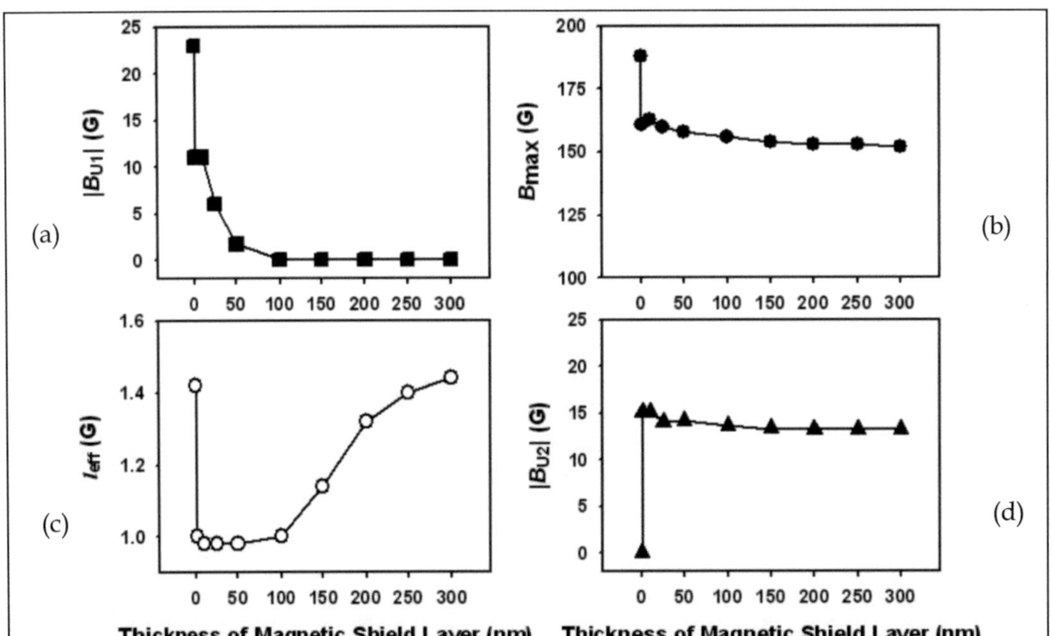

Fig. 11. Effects of MSL thickness on the sensing performance of an in-vitro GMR biosensor with an immobilized 250 nm size $CoFe_2O_4$ FNSA. (a) B_{U1}, (b) B_{max}, (c) l_{eff}, and (d) B_{U2}

12 G, it should be carefully controlled when the MSL is used for especially multi-array sensor architecture. The effects of MSL permeability on the sensing performance is not discussed in details in this chapter as all the physical sensing parameters have the same dependence on the permeability of MSL. However, the numerical calculation results obtained from the GMR biosensor with geometry of a 300 nm MSL thickness, a 1.2 μm of gap width, and a 8 μm of MSL length demonstrates that the MSL with magnetic permeability of at least 100 shows obvious shielding effects. Figure 12 shows the dependence of MSL gap width, which is changed from 0.2 to 2.0 μm, on the sensing performance of an in-vitro GMR biosensor with an immobilized $CoFe_2O_4$ FNSA. As shown in Fig. 12-(a), the B_{max} is dramatically increased from 150 G to 260 G, which is beyond the sensing limit, B_{DL}, by decreasing the gap width from 0.8 to 0.2 μm. The dramatic increase of magnetic field intensity at the gap width below 0.8 μm is mainly thought to be attributed to the increase of fringe field produced from the gap between two MSLs (This is quite similar to the "fringe field" produced by the head gap from the writer in magnetic recording technology) (Bertram, 1994). The high permeability of two MSLs, which are closely faced each others with small gap, can produce a strong "deep gap bubble field" due to a high magnetic flux density. This leads to increasing the "fringe field" on the surface of MSL gap that would be diverged into the FL surface resulting in the increase of magnetic field intensity on the FL (sensing layer) surface.

As shown in Figs. 12-(b) and 12-(c), the B_{U1} and the l_{eff} are also strongly influenced by the MSL gap width. The B_{U1} is obviously re-developed when the MSL gap width is increased above 1.4 μm. Moreover, l_{eff} is sharply decreased when the MSL gap width is increased above 1.2 μm. The serious degradation of sensing performance relevant to the dramatic

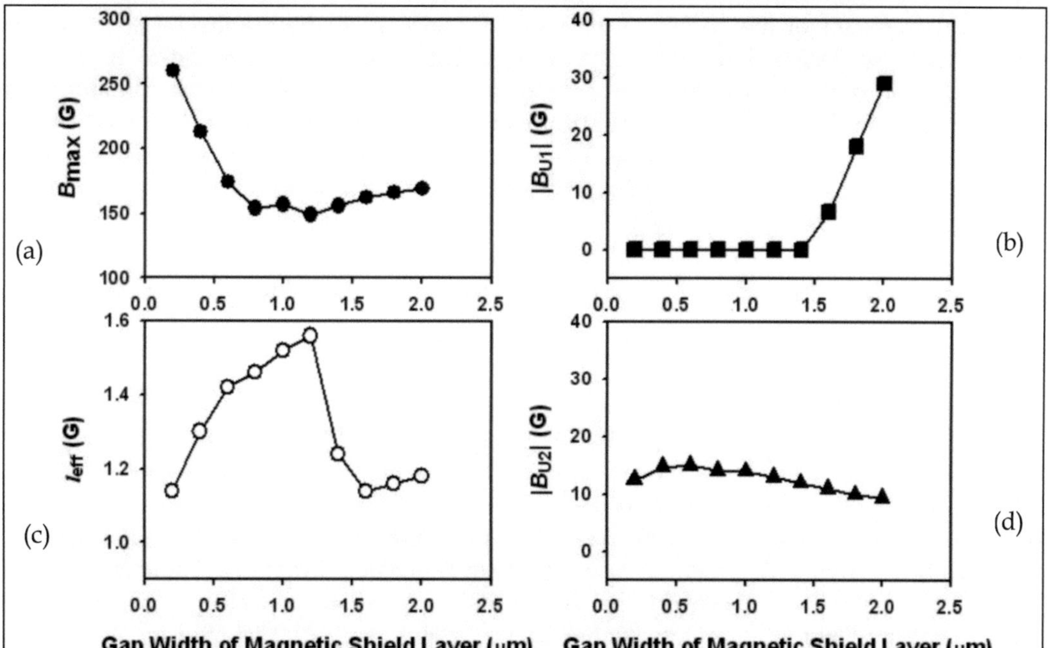

Fig. 12. Effects of MSL gap width on the sensing performance of an in-vitro GMR biosensor with an immobilized 250 nm size $CoFe_2O_4$ FNSA. (a) B_{U1}, (b) B_{max}, (c) l_{eff}, and (d) B_{U2}

reduction of "effective sensing area" on the sensor surface due to both the re-development of "undershoot field region" and the reduction of critical length, l_c, are mainly attributed to the reduction of shield gap flux density, which is inversely proportional to the MSL gap width. However, considering that the l_c (~1.56 μm), which is numerically determined based on the same geometry and configuration of in-vitro GMR biosensor system, is found to be much larger than that without MSL (~1.12 μm), it can be readily understood that shielding effects of MSL on the improvement of sensing performance is quite significant.
In summary, it is numerically demonstrated that the MSL is effective to improve the output sensing performance of an in-vitro GMR biosensor with an immobilized FNSA, because it can successfully remove an undesirable "undershoot field region" and enhance the "effective sensing area" due to the increase of l_c. This indicates that an in-vitro GMR biosensor with a specially designed MSL structure can be considered as a promising sensor structure for SMD due to its achievable high sensing signal and stability.

5. Conclusion

The physical sensing characteristics of an in-vitro GMR biosensor with an immobilized single FNSA have been introduced and discussed to explore its feasibility to a single molecular based disease diagnostic biosensor system. According to the theoretically and experimentally analyzed results, the in-vitro GMR biosensor with a FNSA was revealed to be more suitable for SMD than that with a SPNSA due to its higher relative MR, less interaction factor dependence, and practically allowable sensor size. In addition, the analytical models developed in this chapter allowed to readily predicting the optimized sensor geometry of an in-vitro GMR biosensor with a FNSA prior to fabrication if the physical parameters of the FNSA are provided. In particular, the in-vitro GMR biosensor with a specially designed magnetic shield layer (MSL) was demonstrated to be able to effectively control the undesirable "undershoot sensing region" as well as the "undetectable sensing area" on the FL surface. These promising sensing characteristics improved by the newly designed sensor structure allow for achieving both maximized output sensing signal and higher sensor stability that lead to accelerating the more practical applications to the SMD based diagnostic biosensor system.

6. References

Baselt D. R.; Lee G. U.; Natesan M.; Metzger S. W.; Sheehan P. E. & Colton R. J., (1998). A biosensor based on magnetoresistive technology. *Biosensors and Bioelectronics*, Vol. 13, pp. 731-739, ISSN 0956-5663

Besse P.; Boero G.; Demierre M.; Pott V. & Popovic R., (2002). Detection of a single magnetic microbead using a miniaturized silicon Hall sensor. *Applied Physics Letters*, Vol. 80, No. 22, pp. 4199-4201, ISSN 0003-6951

Bertram, N. (1994). *Theory of magnetic recording*, Cambridge, ISBN 0-521-44512-4, New York

Girgis E.; Schelten J.; Shi J., Tehrani S. & Goronicin H., (2000). Switching characteristics and magnetization vortices of thin-film cobalt in nanometer-scale patterned arrays. *Applied Physics Letters*, Vol. 76, No. 25, pp. 3780-3782, ISSN 0003-6951

Graham D. L.; Ferreira H.; Bernardo J.; Freitas P. P. & Cabral J. M. S., (2000). Single magnetic microsphere placement and detection on-chip using current line designs with integrated spin valve sensors: Biotechnological applications. *Journal of Applied Physics*, Vol. 91, No. 10, pp. 7786-7788, ISSN 0021-8979

Graham D. L.; Ferreira H. A.; Freitas P.P. & Cabral J. M. S., (2003). High sensitivity detection of molecular recognition using magnetically labeled biomolecules and magnetoresistive sensors. *Biosensors and Bioelectronics*, Vol. 18, pp. 483-488, ISSN 0956-5663

Graham D. L.; Ferreira H. A. & Freitas P.P., (2004). Magnetoresistive-based biosensors and biochips. *TRENDS in biotechnology*, Vol. 22, No. 9, pp. 455-462, ISSN 0167-7799

Hirota E.; Sakakima H. & Inomata K., (2002). *Giant Magnetoresistance Device*, Springer, ISBN 3-540-41819-9, Berlin

Lagae L.; Wirix-Speethens R.; Das J.; Graham D. L.; Ferreira H.; Freitas P. P.; Borghs G. & Boeck J. De., (2002). On-chip manipulation and magnetization assessment of magnetic bead ensembles by integrated spin-valve sensors. *Journal of Applied Physics*, Vol. 91, No. 10, pp. 7445-7447, ISSN 0021-8979

Latham A. H.; Tarpara A. N. & Williams M. E., (2007). Magnetic field switching of nanoparticles between orthpgonal microfluidic channels, *Analytical Chemistry*, Vol. 79, pp. 5746-5752, ISSN 10.1021

Lee S.; Bae S.; Takemura Y.; Shim I. B.; Kim T. M.; Kim J.; Lee H. J.; Zurn S. & Kim C., (2007). Self-heating characteristics of cobalt ferrite nanoparticles for hypertheria application. *Journal of Magnetism and Magnetic Materials*, Vol. 310, pp. 2868-2870, ISSN 0304-8853

Li G. & Wang S. X., (2003). Analytical and micromagnetic modeling for detection og a single magnetic microbead or nanobead by spin valve sensors. *IEEE Transaction on Magnetics*, Vol. 39, No. 5, pp. 3313-3315, ISSN 10.1109

Megens M. & Prins M., (2005). Magnetic biochips: a new option for sensitive diagnostics. *Journal of Magnetism and Magnetic Materials*, Vol. 293, pp. 702-708, ISSN 0304-8853

Miller M. M.; Sheehan P. E.; Edelstein R. L.; Tamanha C. R.; Zhong L.; Bounnak S.; Whiteman L. J. & Colton R. J., (2001). A DNA array sensor utilizing microbeads and magnetoelectronic detection. *Journal of Magnetism and Magnetic Materials*, Vol. 225, pp. 138-144, ISSN 0304-8853

Ramadan Q.; Samper V.; Poenar D. & Yu C., (2006). Magnetic-based microfluidic platform for biomolecular separation, Biomedical Microdevices, Vol. 8, No. 4, pp. 151-158, ISSN 10.1007

Rife J. C.; Miller M. M.; Sheehan P. E.; Tamanaha C. R.; Tondra M. & Whitman L. J., (2003). Design and performance of GMR sensors for the detection of magnetic microbeads in biosensors. *Sensors and Actuators A*, Vol. 107, pp. 209-218, ISSN 0924-4247

Schepper W.; Schotter J.; Bruckl H. & Reiss G., (2004). Analyzing a magnetic molecule detection system - computer simulation. *Journal of Biotechnology*, Vol. 112, pp. 35-46, ISSN 0168-1656

Schepper W.; Schotter J.; Bruckl H. & Reiss G., (2006). A magnetic molecule detection system—A comparison of different setups by computer simulation. *Physica B*, Vol. 372, pp. 337-340, ISSN 0921-4526

Shen W.; Liu X.; Mazumdar D. & Xiao G., (2005). In-situ detection of singl micron-sized magnetic beads using magnetic tunnel junction sensors. *Applied Physics Letters*, Vol. 86, pp. 253901-253903, 0003-6951

Stoner E. C. & Wöhlfarth, (1948). A mechanism of magnetic hysteresis in heterogeneous alloys. *Philosophical Transactions of the Royal Society A*, Vol. 240, pp. 599-642, ISSN 1471-2961

Tondra M.; Porter M. & Lipert R. J., (2000). Model for detection of immobilized superparamagnetic nanosphere assay labels using giant magnetoresistive sensors. *Journal of Vacuum Science and Technology A*, Vol. 18, No. 4, pp. 1125-1129, ISSN 0734-2101

Wang S. X.; Bae S. Y.; Li G.; Sun S.; White R. L., Kemp J. T. & Webb C. D., (2005). Towards a magnetic microarray for sensitive diagnostics. *Journal of Magnetism and Magnetic Materials*, Vol. 293, pp. 731-736, ISSN 0304-8853

William E. M., (2001). *Design and analysis of magnetoresistive recording heads*, John Wiley & Sons, ISBN 0-471-36358-8, New York

Wirix-Speetjens R.; Fyen W.; Boeck J. D. & Borghs G., (2006). Single magentic particle detection: Experimental verification of simulated behavior. *Journal of Applied Physics*, Vol. 99, No. 103903, pp. 1-4, ISSN 0021-8979

Mercaptobenzothiazole-on-Gold Organic Phase Biosensor Systems: 3. Thick-Film Biosensors for Organophosphate and Carbamate Pesticide Determination

V. Somerset[1], P. Baker[2] and E. Iwuoha[2]
[1]*Natural Resources and the Environment (NRE), Council for Scientific and Industrial Research (CSIR), Stellenbosch, 7600,*
[2]*SensorLab, Department of Chemistry, University of the Western Cape, Bellville, 7535, South Africa.*

1. Introduction

The last few decades has seen an increase in the use of pesticides in order to increase crop yields. This has resulted in the increased use of organophosphorous (OP) and carbamate (CM) pesticide compounds since they result in much lower bioaccumulation and higher biodegradability, therefore they have replaced organochlorine as the most popular pesticides. However, as with the overuse of many pesticides, the OP and CM compounds leave residues in the soil, crops and surface water, which in turn exert a great threat to the environment and human health. The OP and CM compounds enter organisms and then inhibit the activity of acetyl cholinesterase (AChE) by irreversibly binding to the active site of this enzyme, which is important for the transmission of nerve impulses (Wu et al., 2009; Somerset et al., 2009; García de Llasera et al., 2009; Mavrikou et al., 2008; Liu et al., 2008; Boon et al., 2008; Pinheiro & De Andrade, 2009).

A broad range of adverse effects can result from AChE inhibition and it includes abdominal pain and cramps, glandular secretions, skeletal muscle twitching, flaccid paralysis, tiredness, nausea, blurred vision, drowsiness, eye pain, convulsions, respiratory failure and untimely death. Furthermore, OP and CM compounds are now also known to have mutagenic, carcinogenic and teratogenic effects and have been included in the list of known endocrine disruptor compounds (Luo & Zhang, 2009; Wu et al., 2009; Liu et al., 2008; Fu et al., 2009; Caetano & Machado, 2008).

Due to the increasing toxicity and adverse effects of pesticides, many countries are now monitoring environmental and food samples for pesticides and have established maximum residue levels (MRLs) for various pesticides in food products (Hildebrandt *et al.*, 2008). Some of the conventional methods used for chemical analysis of pesticides include spectrophotometry, infrared spectrometry, flow-injection chemiluminescence, fluorimetry, fluorescence spectrometry, mass spectrometry, but mainly chromatographic techniques, such as gas chromatography-mass spectrometry (GC–MS) and high-performance liquid

chromatography (HPLC) (Wu et al., 2009; García de Llasera et al., 2009; Mavrikou et al., 2008; Liu et al., 2008; Caetano & Machado, 2008).
There is no doubt that these methods are highly efficient and allow discrimination among different types of OP and CM compounds, but they require tedious sample pre-treatments, highly qualified technicians and sophisticated instruments. Furthermore, these methods are also known to be time consuming and not suitable for field analysis of multiple samples (Liu et al., 2008; Hildebrandt et al., 2008).
For this reason several rapid, relatively inexpensive, sensitive screening analytical techniques that need little sample pre-treatment are constantly being developed for the identification and quantification of OP and CM compounds (Liu *et al.*, 2008). Biosensors have filled the gap in this regard and these analytical devices are based on the intimate contact between a bio-recognition element that interacts with the analyte of interest and a transducer element that converts the bio-recognition event into a measurable signal. Among the different types of biosensors, the electrochemical sensors are of special interest due to the high sensitivity inherent to the electrochemical detection and the possibility to miniaturise the required instrumentation, thereby making the construction of compact and portable analysis devices possible (Campàs et al., 2009; Mavrikou et al., 2008).
In this paper, we describe the application of a mercaptobenzothiazole-on-gold biosensor system for the analysis of OP and CM pesticide compounds. The aim of this work was to improve the detection limit of these insecticides with an AChE biosensor, applied to various water miscible organic solvents. The activity of the AChE immobilized in the biosensor construction was measured by amperometry based on the detection of thiocholine produced in the enzymatic hydrolysis of acetylthiocholine as substrate. The biosensor study was carried out in aqueous organic media to ascertain the role of organic phase on the reactivity of the enzyme and the performance of the biosensor for detecting both OP and CM pesticide compounds.

2. Materials and methods

2.1 Reagents and materials

The reagents aniline (99%), potassium dihydrogen phosphate (99+%), disodium hydrogen phosphate (98+%) and diethyl ether (99.9%) were obtained from Aldrich, Germany. The acetylthiocholine chloride (99%) was obtained from Sigma, Germany. The mercaptobenzothiazole (MBT), acetylcholinesterase (AChE, from Electrophorus electricus, EC 3.1.1.7; ~ 850 U/mg), acetylcholine chloride (99%) and acetone (>99.8%, pestanal) were obtained from Fluka, Germany. The hydrogen peroxide (30%) and the organic solvents ethanol (99.9%, absolute grade), acetonitrile (99.9%, pestanal grade) were purchased from Riedel-de Haën, Germany. The potassium chloride, sulphuric acid (95%), and hydrochloric acid (32%) were obtained from Merck, South Africa. Organophosphorous pesticides used in this study include chlorpyrifos, malathion and parathion-methyl. Carbamate pesticides include carbaryl, carbofuran and methomyl. These pesticide standards were purchased from Riedel-de Haën, Germany. Platinum (Pt) wires as counter electrodes were obtained from Sigma-Aldrich, South Africa. Alumina micropolish and polishing pads that were used for the polishing of the working electrode were obtained from Buehler, IL, USA (Somerset et al., 2007; Somerset et al., 2009).

2.2 Instrumentation

All electrochemical protocols were performed and recorded with a computer interfaced to a BAS-50/W electrochemical analyser with BAS-50/W software (Bioanalytical Systems, Lafayette, IN, USA), using either cyclic voltammetry (CV), Oysteryoung square wave voltammetry (OSWV), differential pulse voltammetry (DPV) or time-based amperometric modes. A conventional three electrode system was employed. The working electrode was a gold disc electrode (diameter: 1.6 mm; area: 2.01 x 10^{-2} cm^2; Bioanalytical Systems, Lafayette, IN, USA). Silver/silver chloride (Ag/AgCl - 3 M NaCl type) was used as the reference electrode and a platinum wire was used as auxiliary electrode (Morrin et al., 2004 ; Somerset et al., 2006).

2.3 Electrode surface preparation

Prior to use, gold electrodes were first polished on aqueous slurries of 1 μm, 0.3 μm and 0.05 μm alumina powder. After thorough rinsing in deionised water followed by acetone, the electrodes were etched for about 5 minutes in a hot 'Piranha' solution {1:3 (v/v) 30 % H_2O_2 and concentrated H_2SO_4} and rinsed again with copious amounts of deionised water. The polished electrodes were then cleaned electrochemically by cycling the potential scan between - 200 and + 1500 mV (vs. Ag/AgCl) in 0.05 M H_2SO_4 at the scan rate of 40 mV.s^{-1} for 10 min or until the CV characteristics for a clean Au electrode were obtained. The platinum (Pt) counter electrode was regularly cleaned before and after synthesis and in between synthesis and analysis. This involved flaming the Pt electrode in a Bunsen burner until it was white hot, followed by rinsing with copious quantities of deionised water (Michira et al., 2007; Somerset et al., 2007).

2.4 Preparation of mercaptobenzothiazole self-assembled monolayer on gold electrode

A self-assembled monolayer (SAM) of mercaptobenzothiazole (MBT) was formed by immersing the cleaned Au electrode into an ethanol solution containing 10 mM of MBT for 2 hours. After deposition the SAM electrode was rinsed extensively with ethanol and water and kept in 0.1 M phosphate buffer (pH 7.2) for later use. This electrode was then referred to as Au/MBT (Mazur et al. 2003; Somerset et al., 2007).

2.5 Electropolymerisation of polyaniline (PANI) films onto an Au/MBT electrode

A three electrode arrangement was set up in a sealed 10 ml electrochemical cell. Polyaniline (PANI) films were prepared by electropolymerisation from a 0.2 M aniline solution dissolved in 1 M hydrochloric acid (HCl) onto the previously prepared Au/MBT-modified electrode. The aniline/HCl solution was first degassed by passing argon (Ar) through the solution for approximately ten minutes and keeping the Ar blanket during electropolymerisation. Initial optimisation of the potential window for electropolymerisation was performed. During electropolymerisation the potential was scanned from an initial potential (E_i) of – 200 mV to a switch potential (E_λ) of +1200 mV, at a scan rate of 40 mV/s vs. Ag/AgCl as a reference. The polymerisation process was stopped after 10 voltammetric cycles, to ensure a smooth and relatively thin polymer film surface was obtained. The Au/MBT-polyaniline modified electrode was then rinsed with deionised water and used as the working electrode in subsequent studies. The electrode will be referred to as Au/MBT/PANI for the gold-MBT-PANI modified electrode (Somerset et al., 2007; Somerset et al., 2009).

2.6 Preparation of Au/MBT/PANI modified enzyme electrode

Following the electropolymerisation of a fresh PANI polymer film on an Au/MBT electrode, the Au/MBT/PANI electrode was transferred to a batch cell, containing 1 ml argon degassed 0.1 M phosphate buffer (pH 7.2) solution. The PANI polymer film was then reduced at a potential of - 500 mV (vs. Ag/AgCl) until a steady current was achieved, which took approximately thirty minutes. Electrochemical incorporation of the enzyme acetylcholinesterase (AChE) onto the PANI film was carried out next. This involved the addition of 60 µL of AChE to the 0.1 M phosphate buffer (pH 7.2) solution. After the enzyme solution was argon degassed, enzyme immobilisation was achieved by oxidation of the PANI film in the presence of AChE at a potential of + 400 mV (vs. Ag/AgCl) until a steady current was achieved, which took approximately fourty minutes.

During the oxidation step, the enzyme AChE was electrostatically attached to the polymer film via an ion-exchange process. The biosensor was then rinsed with deionised water to remove any unbound enzyme and stored in the working 0.1 M phosphate buffer (pH 7.2) solution at 4 °C. The resulting biosensor will be referred to as Au/MBT/PANI/AChE biosensor.For the Au/MBT/PANI/AChE bioelectrode, after enzyme incorporation the bioelectrode was arranged vertically and then coated with a 2 μL drop of poly(vinyl acetate) (PVAc) solution (0.3 M) prepared in acetone and left to dry for 1 min. The resulting biosensor will be referred to as Au/MBT/PANI/AChE/PVAc biosensor (Somerset et al., 2006; Somerset et al., 2009).

2.7 Electrochemical measurements using AChE-based biosensors in the presence of acetylthiocholine as substrate

The electrochemical cell used for the electrocatalytic oxidation of acetylthiocholine (ATCh) consisted of Au/MBT/PANI/AChE/PVAc bioelectrode, platinum wire and Ag/AgCl as the working, counter and reference electrode, respectively. A 1 ml test solution containing 0.1 M phosphate (0.1M KCl, pH 7.2) solution was degassed with argon before any substrate was added and after each addition of small aliquots of 0.01 M acetylthiocholine (ATCh). Cyclic, square wave and differential pulse voltammetry were used to measure the responses of the AChE-based biosensor towards ATCh as substrate Cyclic voltammetry (CV) was performed at a slow scan rate of 10 $mV.s^{-1}$ to study the catalytic oxidation of ATCh by applying a linear potential scan between - 400 mV and + 1800 mV (vs. Ag/AgCl). The cyclic voltammogram was first obtained in the absence of the substrate ATCh, followed by analysis in the presence of ATCh as substrate. Sequential 20 ml aliquots of 0.01 M acetylthiocholine (ATCh) were then added to the 1 ml of 0.1 M phosphate buffer (0.1 M KCl, pH 7.2) solution, degassed with argon and a blanket of gas was kept for the duration of the experiment. The phosphate buffer solution was stirred after each addition of ATCh. This was done to ensure homogeneity of the solution before measurements were taken.

Osteryoung-type square wave voltammetry (OSWV) was performed immediately after cyclic voltammetric analysis with the AChE-based biosensor in 1 ml of 0.1 M phosphate buffer (0.1 M KCl, pH 7.2) solution, containing different concentrations of ATCh as the substrate under anaerobic conditions (system kept under an argon blanket). The anodic difference square wave voltammogram (SWV) was collected in an oxidation direction only by applying a linear potential scan between - 400 mV and + 1800 mV (vs. Ag/AgCl), at a step potential of 4 mV, a frequency of 5 Hz, and a square wave amplitude of 50 mV. The SWV was first obtained in the absence of the substrate ATCh, followed by analysis in the presence of ATCh as substrate.

Differential pulse voltammetry (DPV) immediately followed SWV analysis with the AChE-based biosensor in 1 ml of 0.1 M phosphate buffer (0.1 M KCl, pH 7.2) solution, containing different concentrations of ATCh as the substrate under anaerobic conditions (system kept under an argon blanket). The anodic difference differential pulse voltammogram (DPV) was collected in an oxidation direction only by applying a linear potential scan between - 400 mV and + 1800 mV (vs. Ag/AgCl), at a scan rate of 10 mV.s^{-1} and a pulse amplitude of 50 mV. The sample width, pulse width and pulse period were 17 ms, 50 ms and 200 ms, respectively. The DPV was first obtained in the absence of the substrate ATCh, followed by analysis in the presence of ATCh as substrate (Pritchard et al. 2004; Joshi et al. 2005; Sotiropoulou et al. 2005; Somerset et al., 2007; Somerset et al., 2009).

2.8 Inhibitory studies of AChE-based biosensors in the presence of pesticide inhibitors

A new Au/MBT/PANI/AChE/PVAc biosensor was prepared each time a new organophosphorous or carbamate pesticide was studied. A new biosensor was also prepared for each of the six concentrations of the OP and CM pesticides studied. The electrochemical cell consisted of Au/MBT/PANI/AChE/PVAc bioelectrode, platinum wire and Ag/AgCl as the working, counter and reference electrode, respectively. A 1 ml test solution containing 0.1 M phosphate (0.1 M KCl, pH 7.2) solution was degassed with argon before any substrate was added and after each addition of small aliquots of 0.01 M acetylthiocholine (ATCh).

Inhibition plots for each of the OP and CM pesticides detected were obtained using the percentage inhibition method. The following procedure was used. The biosensor was first placed in a stirred 1 ml of 0.1 M phosphate (0.1 M KCl, pH 7.2) solution (anaerobic conditions) and multiple additions of a standard acetylthiocholine (ATCh) substrate solution was added until a stable current and a maximum concentration of 2.4 mM were obtained. This steady state current is related to the activity of the enzyme in the biosensor when no inhibitor was present. This was followed by incubating the biosensor in anaerobic conditions for 20 min with a standard pesticide phosphate buffer-organic solvent mixture. This was followed by multiple additions of a standard ATCh substrate solution (anaerobic conditions), to a fresh 1ml of 0.1 M phosphate (0.1 M KCl, pH 7.2) solution (anaerobic conditions) and multiple additions of a standard acetylthiocholine (ATCh) substrate solution was again added, until a stable current was obtained. The maximum concentration of acetylthiocholine (ATCh) was again 2.4 mM. The percentage inhibition was then calculated using the formula (Albareda-Sirvent et al., 2001; Sotiropoulou and Chaniotakis 2005; Wilkins et al., 2000; Somerset et al., 2009):

$$I\% = \frac{(I_1 - I_2)}{I_1} \; X\,100 \tag{1}$$

where I% is the degree of inhibition, I_1 is the steady-state current obtained in buffer solution, I_2 is the steady-state current obtained after the biosensor was incubated for 20 min in phosphate buffer-organic solvent mixture.

Cyclic, square wave and differential pulse voltammetric measurements were performed after each addition of ATCh up to a maximum concentration of 2.4 mM. Cyclic voltammetry (CV) was performed at a scan rate of 10 mV.s^{-1} by applying a linear potential scan between – 400 mV and + 1800 mV (vs. Ag/AgCl). For some experimental runs the anodic difference

square wave voltammogram (SWV) was collected in an oxidation direction only by applying a linear potential scan between – 400 mV and + 1800 mV (vs. Ag/AgCl), at a step potential of 4 mV, a frequency of 5 Hz, and a square amplitude of 50 mV.
The anodic difference differential pulse voltammogram (ADPV) was collected in an oxidation direction only by applying a linear potential scan between – 400 mV and + 1800 mV (vs. Ag/AgCl), at a scan rate of 10 $mV.s^{-1}$ and a pulse amplitude of 50 mV. The sample width, pulse width and pulse period were 17 ms, 50 ms and 200 ms, respectively (Somerset et al., 2007; Somerset et al., 2009).

2.9 Optimisation of acetylcholinesterase (AChE) enzyme loading

The operation of the Au/MBT/PANI/AChE/PVAc biosensor was evaluated at different amounts of AChE enzyme incorporated into the biosensor. To achieve this, 0.1 M phosphate buffer, 0.1 M KCl (pH 7.2) solutions were prepared and used. Following the electropolymerisation of a fresh PANI polymer film on an Au/MBT electrode, the Au/MBT/PANI electrode was transferred to a batch cell, containing 1 ml argon degassed 0.1 M phosphate buffer (pH 7.2) solution. The PANI polymer film was then reduced at a potential of – 500 mV (vs. Ag/AgCl) until a steady current was achieved, which took approximately thirty minutes. Electrochemical incorporation of the enzyme acetylcholinesterase (AChE) onto the PANI film was carried out next. This involved the addition of 40 µL of AChE to the 0.1 M phosphate buffer (pH 7.2) solution. After the enzyme solution was argon degassed, enzyme immobilisation was achieved by oxidation of the PANI film in the presence of AChE at a potential of + 400 mV (vs. Ag/AgCl) until a steady current was achieved, which took approximately fourty minutes. The Au/MBT/PANI bioelectrode was arranged vertically and then coated with a 2 μL drop of poly(vinyl acetate) (PVAc) solution (0.3 M) prepared in acetone and left to dry for 1 min.. The same procedure was followed to incorporate 60 and 80 µL of AChE enzyme into the PANI polymer surface.
Voltammetric characterisation was performed at a slow scan rate of 10 $mV.s^{-1}$ to study the catalytic oxidation of ATCh by applying a linear potential scan between – 400 mV and + 1800 mV (vs. Ag/AgCl). The voltammograms were first obtained in the absence of the substrate ATCh, followed by analysis in the presence of ATCh as substrate. Sequential 20 ml aliquots of 0.01 M acetylthiocholine (ATCh) were then added to the 1 ml of 0.1 M phosphate buffer (0.1 M KCl, pH 7.2) solution, degassed with argon and a blanket of gas was kept for the duration of the experiment. The phosphate buffer solution was stirred after each addition of ATCh. This was done to ensure homogeneity of the solution before measurements were taken (Nunes et al. 1999; Somerset et al., 2007; Somerset et al., 2009).

2.10 pH Optimisation for acetylcholinesterase (AChE) immobilised in Au/MBT/PANI/AChE biosensor

The operation of the Au/MBT/PANI/AChE/PVAc biosensor was evaluated at different pH values. To achieve this, 0.1 M phosphate buffer, 0.1 M KCl solutions were prepared at different pH values of 6.0; 6.5; 7.2; 7.5 and 8.0. A 1 ml test solution containing 0.1 M phosphate buffer, 0.1 M KCl solution was degassed with argon before any substrate was added. The Au/MBT/PANI/AChE/PVAc biosensor was then evaluated in the 1 ml test solution with small aliquots of the substrate consisting of 0.01 M acetylthiocholine (ATCh) being added to the test solution, followed by degassing. The maximum current response of the biosensor was then obtained at the different pH values after 2 mM of the ATCh substrate was added to the Au/MBT/PANI/AChE/PVAc biosensor (Albareda-Sirvent et al., 2001; Pritchard et al., 2004; Bucur et al., 2005; Somerset et al., 2009).

2.11 Long-term stability investigation of Au/MBT/PANI/AChE biosensor

The operation of the Au/MBT/PANI/AChE/PVAc biosensor was evaluated at different time intervals of 7 day periods for a total of 30 days, using one specific biosensor. A 1 ml test solution containing 0.1 M phosphate buffer, 0.1 M KCl solution was degassed with argon before any substrate was added. The Au/MBT/PANI/AChE/PVAc biosensor was then evaluated in the 1 ml test solution with small aliquots of the substrate consisting of 0.01 M acetylthiocholine (ATCh) being added to the test solution, followed by degassing. The maximum current response of the biosensor was then obtained after 2 mM of the ATCh substrate was added to the Au/MBT/PANI/AChE/PVAc biosensor. This procedure was performed on 0, 7, 14, 21 and 28 days using one specific Au/MBT/PANI/AChE/PVAc biosensor (Albareda-Sirvent et al., 2001; Somerset et al., 2009).

2.12 Temperature stability investigation of Au/MBT/PANI/AChE biosensor

The temperature stability of the Au/MBT/PANI/AChE/PVAc biosensor was evaluated at different temperature values. To achieve this, the optimum temperature for AChE activity in the constructed biosensor was determined by assaying the biosensor at various temperatures of 10, 15, 20, 25, 30, and 35 °C. A 1 ml test solution containing 0.1 M phosphate buffer, 0.1 M KCl solution was degassed with argon before any substrate was added, and incubated in a small water bath for approximately 10 minutes at a specific temperature. The Au/MBT/PANI/AChE/PVAc biosensor was then evaluated in the 1 ml test solution with small aliquots of the substrate consisting of 0.01 M acetylthiocholine (ATCh) being added to the test solution, followed by degassing. The maximum current response of the biosensor was then obtained after 2 mM of the ATCh substrate was added to the Au/MBT/PANI/AChE/PVAc biosensor. This procedure was performed at 10, 15, 20, 25, 30, and 35 °C using different Au/MBT/PANI/AChE/PVAc biosensors (Ricci et al., 2003; Kuralay et al., 2005; Somerset et al., 2009).

2.13 Determination of the Limit of Detection (LOD)

A 1 ml test solution containing 0.1 M phosphate buffer, 0.1 M KCl solution was degassed with argon before any substrate was added. The AChE-biosensor was then evaluated in the 1 ml test solution by performing 10 replicate measurements on the 0.1 M phosphate buffer, 0.1 M KCl solution, or on any one of the analyte (standard pesticide) solutions at the lowest working concentration. A calibration graph of current (A) versus saline phosphate buffer or analyte concentration was then constructed for which the slope and the linear range was then determined. The limit of detection (LOD) was then calculated with the following equation:

$$LOD = \frac{3 \cdot \sigma_{n-1}}{m} = \frac{3 \cdot s}{m} \tag{2}$$

where s is the standard deviation of the 10 replicate measurements on the 0.1 M phosphate buffer, 0.1 M KCl solution, or on any one of the analyte (standard pesticide) solutions at the lowest working concentration. The variable m represents the slope of the calibration graph in the linear range that is also equal to the sensitivity of the measurements performed (Somerset et al., 2007; Somerset et al., 2009).

3. Results and discussion

3.1 Biosensor design for pesticide detection

Different technologies have been developed over the years for the manufacturing of thick-film biosensors for pesticide detection. The major technologies can be divided into three categories of (i) multiple-layer deposition with biological deposition by hand or electrochemically, (ii) using screen-printing techniques of composite inks or pastes in two or more steps with biological deposition done by screen-printing, (iii) using a one-step deposition layer also called the biocomposite strategy. This work has seen the development of an electrode that can be exposed to organic solutions containing potential inhibitors without having the polymer layer separating from the electrode surface after use. Therefore the use of poly(vinyl acetate) as the binder was employed to circumvent this problem. Cellulose acetate is known to be used as a synthetic resin in screen-printing inks to improve printing qualities or as a selective membrane over platinum anodes to reduce interferences (Hart et al. 1999; Albareda-Sirvent et al. 2000; Albareda-Sirvent et al. 2001; Joshi et al. 2005; McGovern et al. 2005).

The detection of pesticides in non-aqueous environments has been reported but few publications refer to the use of immobilised AChE biosensors in non-aqueous media. Organophosphorous and carbamate pesticides are characterised by a low solubility in water and a higher solubility in organic solvents. It is for this fact that the extraction and concentration of pesticides from fruits, vegetables, etc. are carried out in organic solvents. It is known that some enzymes, e.g. glucose oxidase, work well in both water and organic solvents, while other enzymes require a minimum amount of water to retain catalytic activity. To circumvent the problem of hydrophilic solvents stripping the enzymes of essential water of hydration necessary for enzymatic activity, it is recommended that 1 - 10% water be added to the organic solvent for sufficient hydration of the active site of the enzyme (Somerset et al., 2007; Somerset et al., 2009).

In the amperometric sensor design, we have used polyaniline (PANI) as a mediator in the biosensor construction to harvest its dual role as immobilisation matrix for AChE and use its electrocatalytic activity towards thiocholine (TCh) for amperometric sensing. The biosensor mechanism for the Au/MBT/PANI/AChE/PVAc biosensor is shown in Figure 1.

Figure 1 displays the schematic representation for the Au/MBT/PANI/AChE/PVAc biosensor mechanism. It further shows that as acetylthiocholine (ATCh) is catalysed by acetylcholinesterase (AChE), it forms thiocholine (TCh) and acetic acid. Thiocholine is electroactive and is oxidised in the reaction. In return the conducting PANI polymer reacts with thiocholine and also accepts an electron from mercaptobenzothiazole as it is oxidised through interaction with the gold electrode (Somerset et al., 2007; Somerset et al., 2009).

3.2 Successive substrate addition to Au/MBT/PANI/AChE/PVAc biosensor

The functioning of the biosensor was established with the successive addition of acetylthiocholine (ATCh) aliquots as substrate to the Au/MBT/PANI/AChE/PVAc biosensor. Cyclic voltammetric (CVs) results were collected by applying sequential linear potential scan between - 400 to + 1800 mV (vs. Ag/AgCl), at a scan rate of 10 mV.s^{-1}. The CVs were performed at this scan rate to ensure that the fast enzyme kinetics could be monitored. The three CVs for successive 0.01 M ATCh substrate additions to Au/MBT/PANI/AChE/PVAc biosensor in 1 ml of 0.1 M phosphate buffer, KCl (pH 7.2) solution are shown in Figure 2 (Somerset et al., 2007; Somerset et al., 2009).

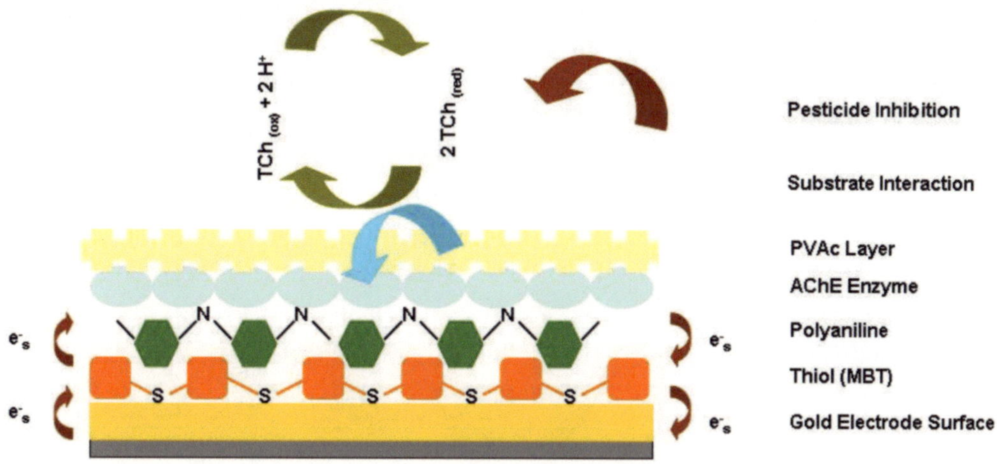

Fig. 1. The schematic representation of the Au/MBT/PANI/AChE/PVAc biosensor reaction occurring at the gold SAM modified electrode.

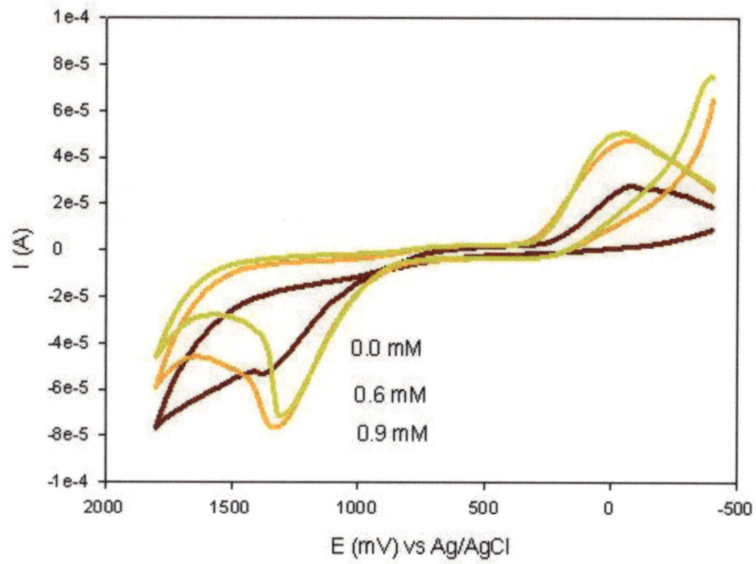

Fig. 2. CV response of successive ATCh substrate addition to Au/MBT/PANI/AChE/PVAc biosensor in 0.1 M phosphate buffer, KCl (pH 7.2) solution at a scan rate of 10 mV.s^{-1}.

A clear shift in peak current (I_p) was observed as the concentration of the substrate, ATCh, was increased indicating the electrocatalytic functioning of the biosensor. The results in Figure 2 further illustrate that in increase in the reductive current is also observed, but the magnitude is smaller when compared to the increases in oxidative current. This clearly illustrates that the oxidative response of the biosensor to ATCh addition is preferred (Somerset et al., 2007; Somerset et al., 2009).

The cyclic voltammetric (CV) results of the Au/MBT/PANI/AChE/PVAc biosensor were substantiated with the collection of differential pulse voltammetric (DPV) results. The DPV results obtained for the biosensor in a 1 ml of 0.1 M phosphate buffer, KCl (pH 7.2) solution are shown in Figure 3.

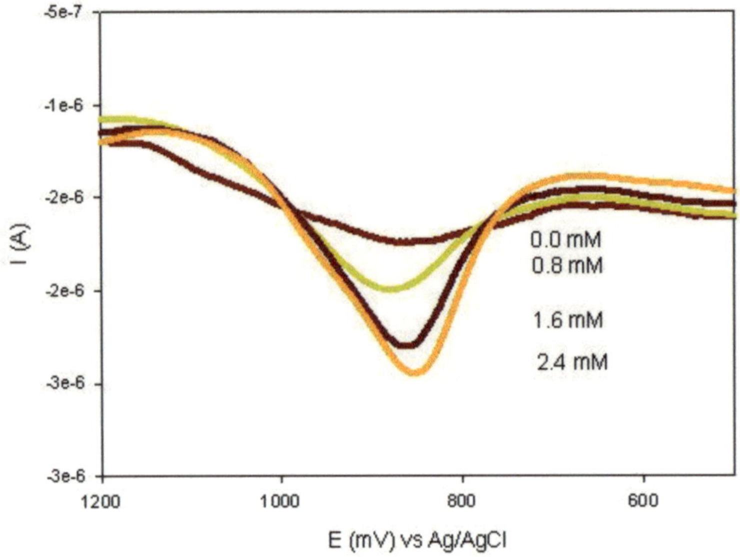

Fig. 3.DPV response of successive ATCh substrate addition to Au/MBT/PANI/AChE/PVAc biosensor in 0.1 M phosphate buffer, KCl (pH 7.2) solution at a scan rate of 10 $mV.s^{-1}$, and in a potential window of + 500 to + 1200 mV.

The DPV results in Figure 3 were collected in a shorter potential window to highlight the observed increase in anodic peak current. The results show the voltammetric responses for the electrocatalytic oxidation of acetylthiocholine at the Au/MBT/PANI/AChE/PVAc biosensor. The DPV responses shows an increase in peak current heights upon the successive additions of ATCh as substrate, with the results more pronounced around a specific potentials as compared with those observed in the CV responses in Figure 2 (Somerset et al., 2007; Somerset et al., 2009).

3.3 Optimum enzyme loading investigation

One of the variables optimised for the constructed biosensor, was the amount of enzyme incorporated during the biosensor development. The results obtained for 3 of the different amounts of the enzyme AChE incorporated into the biosensor are shown in Figure 4.

The results in Figure 4 show that the biggest increase in current for the successive addition of ATCh substrate, was experienced when the biosensor had 60 μL of AChE dissolved in 1 ml of 0.1 M phosphate buffer (pH 7.2) solution. The results obtained when 80 μL of AChE was used, does not show a very big difference in the current response when compared to the use of 60 μL of AChE. In both these cases it is observed that the biosensor response to ATCh substrate addition starts to level off after 1.0 mM of the substrate has been added. When the results for the use of 60 and 80 μL of AChE is compared to that of the 40 μL of

AChE, a big difference in the amperometric response was observed. It was then decided to use 60 μL of AChE in the biosensor construction (Somerset et al., 2007; Somerset et al., 2009).

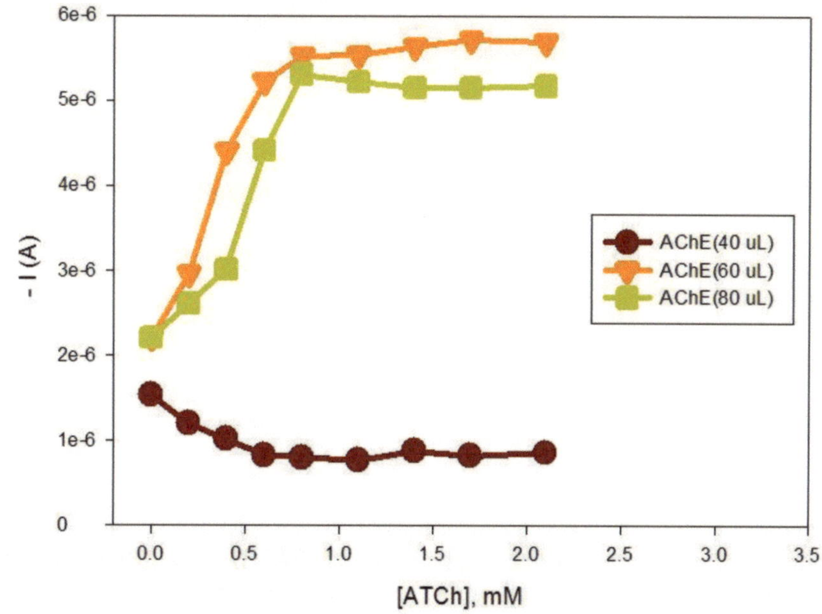

Fig. 4. The amperometric response of the AChE biosensor to different amounts of enzyme incorporated into the biosensor. These responses were measured in a 0.1 M phosphate buffer, KCl (pH 7.2) solution at 25 °C.

3.4 Optimisation of various biosensor parameters

The pH value of the working solution is usually regarded as the most important factor in determining the performance of a biosensor and its sensitivity towards inhibitors (Yang et al. 2005).

For this reason the operation of the biosensor was evaluated at different pH values. In Figure 5 the results for the investigation into the effect of different pH values on the working of the Au/MBT/PANI/AChE/PVAc biosensor can be seen.

The results in Figure 5 indicate that the highest anodic current was obtained at pH = 7.2, while the result for pH = 7.5 show a small difference. The response profile thus indicate that an optimum pH can be obtained between 7.0 and 7.5, which falls within the range reported in literature for the optimum pH of the free enzyme activity in solution (Arkhypova et al. 2003; Sen et al. 2004; Somerset et al., 2007; Somerset et al., 2009).

The parameters for long-term stability and increasing temperature on the functioning of the biosensor were also investigated. To determine the long-term stability of the biosensor, it was stored at 4 °C for a length of approximately 30 days and the biosensor was tested every 7 days by adding the substrate ATCh to a 1 ml of 0.1 M phosphate buffer, KCl (pH 7.2) solution, containing the biosensor, and measuring the current at every addition. This was followed by investigating the response of the Au/MBT/PANI/AChE/PVAc biosensor to successive additions of the substrate ATCh in a 1 ml of 0.1 M phosphate buffer, KCl (pH 7.2) solution, at different temperatures varying from 10 to 35 °C (Somerset et al., 2007; Somerset et al., 2009).

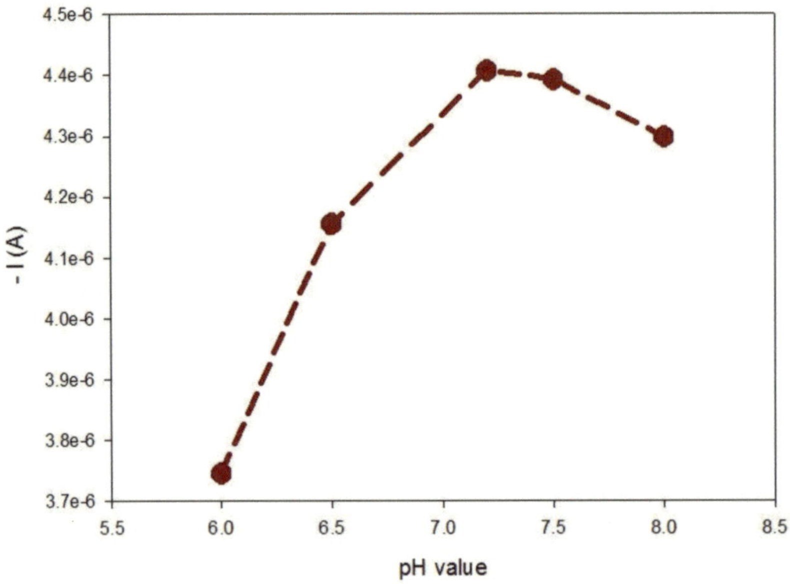

Fig. 5. Graph displaying the effect of pH on the Au/MBT/PANI/AChE/PVAc biosensor in 0.1 M phosphate buffer, KCl (pH 7.2) solution with 2 mM of ATCh added.

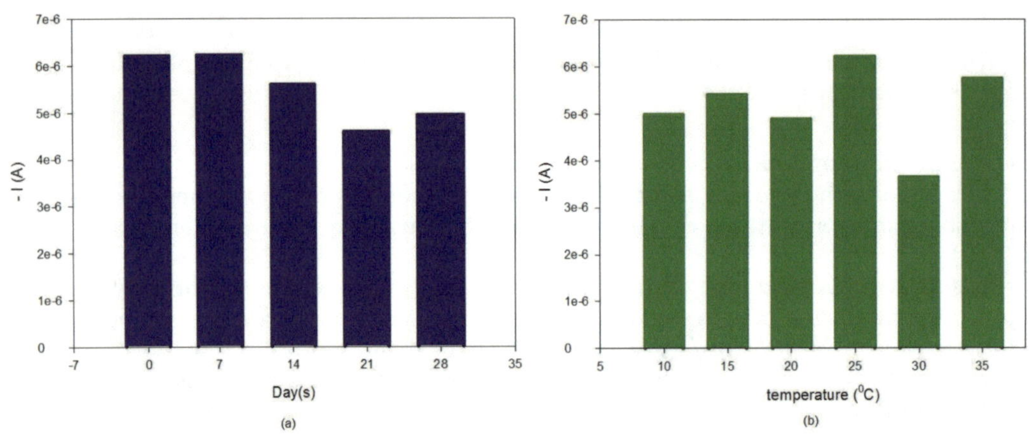

Fig. 6. Graph displaying the results for the long-term (a) and temperature (b) stability of the Au/MBT/PANI/AChE/PVAc biosensor in a 0.1 M phosphate buffer, KCl (pH 7.2) solution for successive additions of the ATCh substrate.

The results in Figure 6 (a) have shown that the biosensor responses reach a maximum current (I_{max}) within 0.6 mM of substrate added to the 0.1 M phosphate buffer, KCl (pH 7.2) solution. Not shown here is the fact that after 0.6 mM of substrate added, the biosensor response reaches a plateau and minimum changes in the current was observed. The results further indicate that at a substrate concentration of 0.6 mM, the maximum current (I_{max}) response show relatively minimum changes with one order magnitude difference between the initial current response, compared to the results obtained after 28 days.

The results for the temperature stability investigation in Figure 6 (b) have shown that for the six temperatures investigated, maximum current (I_{max}) was also reached within 0.6 mM of ATCh substrate added. These results indicate that the enzyme AChE responded favourably to most temperatures evaluated, ranging from 10 to 35 °C (Somerset et al., 2007; Somerset et al., 2009).

3.5 Biosensor behaviour in organic solvents

The influence of organic solvents on the activity of the enzyme AChE in the constructed Au/MBT/PANI/AChE/PVAc biosensor has been studied in the presence of polar organic solvents containing a 0 - 10% aqueous water solution. The polar organic solvents investigated in this study include acetonitrile, acetone and ethanol. The response of the Au/MBT/PANI/AChE/PVAc biosensor was first measured in a 0.1 M phosphate buffer, KCl (pH 7.2) solution, in the presence of a fixed concentration of ATCh. The biosensor was

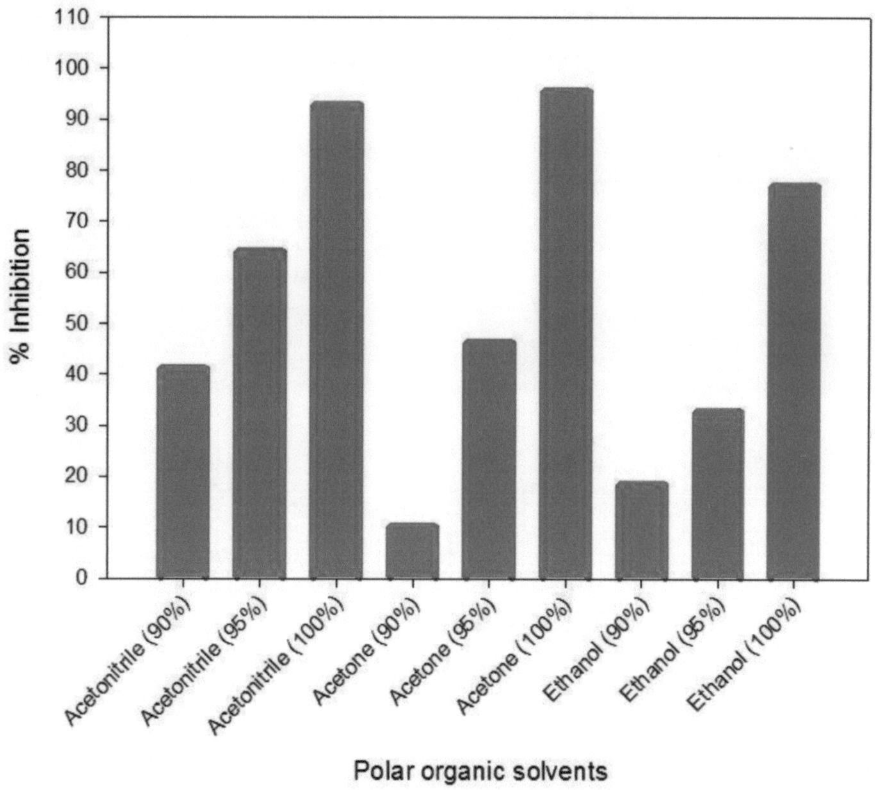

Fig. 7. Results obtained for the inhibition of AChE in the Au/MBT/PANI/AChE/PVAc biosensor after 20 minutes of incubation in (a) 10% water-organic solvent mixture, (b) 5% water-organic solvent mixture, and pure organic solvent. The ATCh concentration was 2.0 mM.

thereafter incubated for 20 minutes in an aqueous-solvent mixture or the pure organic solvent. The response of the Au/MBT/PANI/AChE/PVAc biosensor was then again measured in a 0.1 M phosphate buffer, KCl (pH 7.2) solution, in the presence of a fixed concentration of ATCh. The results of the two respective measurements were then used to calculate the percentage inhibition using the formula in equation (1) (Somerset et al., 2007; Somerset et al., 2009).
The results obtained in Figure 7 shows that for the three different 10% water-organic solvent mixtures investigated, the lowest decrease in catalytic activity of the enzyme AChE was observed in acetone, compared to acetonitrile and ethanol. For the 5% water-organic solvent mixtures, ethanol had the lowest decrease in the catalytic activity of AChE, while in the pure polar organic solvent it was again observed that ethanol had the lowest decrease in the catalytic activity of AChE (Somerset et al., 2007; Somerset et al., 2009).

3.6 Inhibition studies of standard organophosphorous pesticide samples

Inhibition plots for each of the three organophosphorous pesticides investigated were constructed using the percentage inhibition method. The method for the inhibition studies is described in section 2.8. Graphs of percentage inhibition vs. – log [pesticide] concentration were constructed and the results are shown in Figure 8.

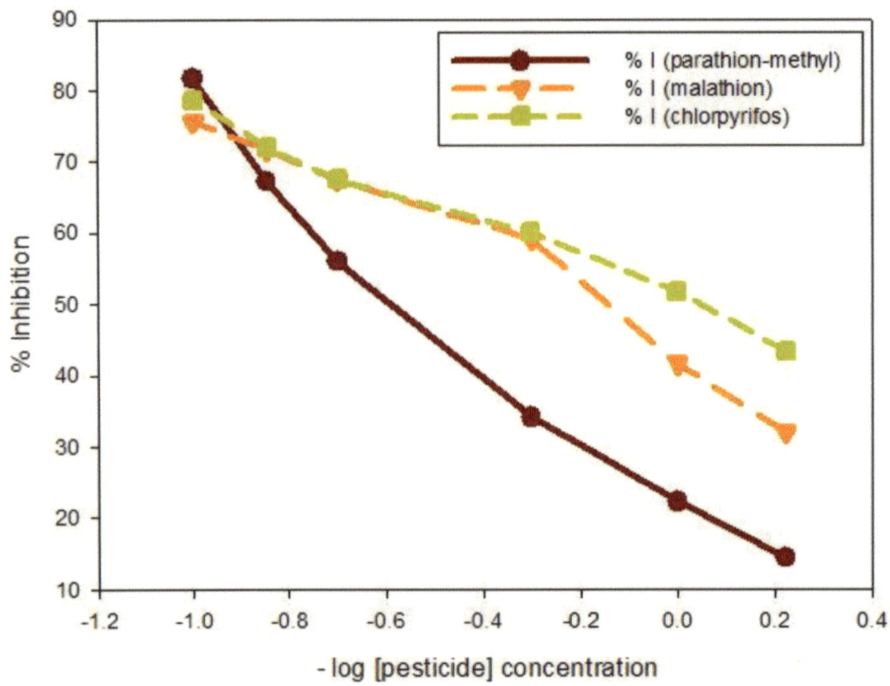

Fig. 8. Graph of percentage inhibition vs. – log [pesticide] concentration for three different organophosphorous pesticides investigated with the Au/MBT/PANI/AChE/PVAc biosensor.

The results shown in Figure 8 are that for the combined plot of the percentage inhibition vs. - log [pesticide] concentration results for the three different organophosphorous standard pesticide solutions investigated. The inhibition results for the pesticides called malathion and chlorpyrifos on the AChE biosensor response are relatively similar, for 4 of the concentrations investigated. It was also observed that the percentage inhibition results for malathion and chlorpyrifos, are higher compared to that obtained for parathion-methyl for most of the concentrations investigated. Further analyses of the inhibition plots and pesticide data were done and the results for the sensitivity, detection limits and regression coefficients are shown in Table 1 (Somerset et al., 2007; Somerset et al., 2009).

Organophosphorous pesticides			
Pesticide	Sensitivity (%I/decade)	Detection limit (nM)	Regression coefficient
parathion-methyl	-53.66	1.332	0.9766
Malathion	-35.24	0.189	0.9679
Chlorpyrifos	-26.68	0.018	0.9875

Table 1. Results for the different parameters calculated from the inhibition plots of the Au/MBT/PANI/AChE/PVAc biosensor detection of standard organophosphorous pesticide solutions (n = 2).

The results in Table 1 shows the parameters for the sensitivity and detection limit estimated from the inhibition plots in Figure 8. The highest sensitivity was obtained for chlorpyrifos as pesticide, while the lowest sensitivity was obtained for parathion-methyl as pesticide. Chlorpyrifos represents a more powerful organophosphate than the rest of the three pesticides studied (due to the three chlorine atoms substituted in its pyridine ring structure) and with the constructed Au/MBT/PANI/AChE/PVAc biosensor, a very good sensitivity was obtained. The best detection limit of 0.018 nM was also obtained for chlorpyrifos as pesticide (Somerset et al., 2007; Somerset et al., 2009).

3.7 Inhibition studies of standard carbamate pesticide samples

Similarly, inhibition plots for each of the three carbamate pesticides detected were obtained using the percentage inhibition method. Graphs of percentage inhibition vs. - log [pesticide] concentration were constructed and the results are shown in Figure 9.

The results for the combined plot of the percentage inhibition vs. - log [pesticide] concentration for the three different carbamate standard pesticide solutions investigated are shown in Figure 9. Analysis of the results shows that carbaryl had the lowest inhibition results for most of the concentrations investigated, while carbofuran had the best inhibition responses. Further analyses of the inhibition plots and pesticide data were done and the results for the sensitivity, detection limits and regression coefficients are shown in Table 2 (Somerset et al., 2007; Somerset et al., 2009).

Table 2 shows the results for the sensitivity and detection limit estimated from the inhibition plots shown in Figure 9. The highest sensitivity results were obtained for methomyl and carbaryl, while the results for carbofuran are the lowest. The difference between the sensitivity results for methomyl and carbaryl, showed also relatively small differences. The best detection limit of 0.111 nM was also obtained for methomyl as pesticide (Somerset et al., 2007; Somerset et al., 2009).

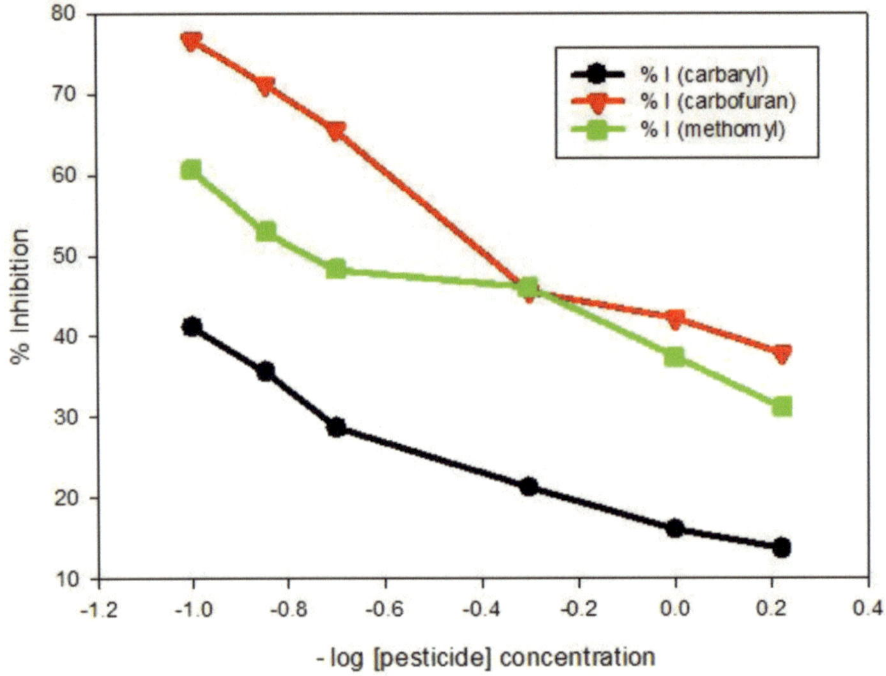

Fig. 9. Graph of percentage inhibition vs. – log [pesticide] concentration for three different carbamate pesticides investigated with the Au/MBT/PANI/AChE/PVAc biosensor.

Carbamate pesticides			
Pesticide	Sensitivity (%I/decade)	Detection limit (nM)	Regression coefficient
carbaryl	-21.92	0.880	0.9581
carbofuran	-33.20	0.249	0.9590
methomyl	-21.04	0.111	0.94552

Table 2. Results for the different parameters calculated from the inhibition plots of the Au/MBT/PANI/AChE/PVAc biosensor detection of standard carbamate pesticide solutions (n = 2).

4. Conclusion

The results described in this paper have successfully demonstrated the construction and use of an Au/MBT/PANI/AChE/PVAc thick-film biosensor for the detection of organophosphorous and carbamate pesticides in polar organic solvents. This study has also shown that self-assembled monolayers can be applied in thick film biosensor construction and that the poly(vinyl acetate) film does not interfere with the PANI-AChE electrocatalytic activity towards thiocholine. Furthermore, very good detection limits for the standard OP and CM pesticide standard samples were obtained with the Au/MBT/PANI/AChE/PVAc biosensor. The results for the detection limit values for the individual organophosphate pesticides were 1.332 nM (parathion-methyl), 0.189 nM (malathion), 0.018 nM (chlorpyrifos). The detection limit values for the individual carbamate pesticides were 0.880 nM (carbaryl), 0.249 nM (carbofuran) and 0.111 nM (methomyl).

5. Acknowledgements

The authors wish to express their gratitude to the National Research Foundation (NRF), South Africa for financial and student support to perform this study. The assistance of the researchers in the SensorLab, Chemistry Department and staff in the Chemistry Department, University of the Western Cape are also greatly acknowledged.

6. References

Li, B.; Xu, Y. & Choi, J. (1996). Title of conference paper, *Proceedings of xxx xxx*, pp. 14-17, ISBN, conference location, month and year, Publisher, City

Siegwart, R. (2001). Name of paper. *Name of Journal in Italics*, Vol., No., (month and year of the edition) page numbers (first-last), ISSN

Arai, T. & Kragic, D. (1999). Name of paper, In: *Name of Book in Italics*, Name(s) of Editor(s), (Ed.), page numbers (first-last), Publisher, ISBN, Place of publication

Wu, H-Z.; Lee, Y-C.; Lin, T-K.; Shih, H-C.; Chang, F-L. & Lin, H-P. (2009). Development of an amperometric micro-biodetector for pesticide monitoring and detection. *Journal of the Taiwan Institute of Chemical Engineers*, 40, 113–122

Somerset, V.; Baker, P. & Iwuoha E. (2009). Mercaptobenzothiazole-on-gold organic phase biosensor systems: 1. Enhanced organosphosphate pesticide determination. *Journal of Environmental Science and Health Part B*, 44, 164–178

García de Llasera, M.P. & Reyes-Reyes, M.L. (2009). Analytical Methods. A validated matrix solid-phase dispersion method for the extraction of organophosphorus pesticides from bovine samples. *Food Chemistry*, 114, 1510–1516

Mavrikou, S.; Flampouri, K.; Moschopoulou, G.; Mangana, O.; Michaelides, A. & Kintzios, S. (2008). Assessment of Organophosphate and Carbamate Pesticide Residues in Cigarette Tobacco with a Novel Cell Biosensor. *Sensors*, 8, 2818-2832

Liu, S.; Yuan, L.; Yue, X.; Zheng, Z. & Tang, Z. (2008). Review paper. Recent Advances in Nanosensors for Organophosphate Pesticide Detection. *Advanced Powder Technology*, 19, 419–441

Boon, P.E.; Van der Voet, H.; Van Raaij, M.T.M. & Van Klaveren, J.D. (2008). Cumulative risk assessment of the exposure to organophosphorus and carbamate insecticides in the Dutch diet. *Food and Chemical Toxicology*, 46, 3090–3098

Pinheiro, A.D. & De Andrade, J.B. (2009). Development, validation and application of a SDME/GC-FID methodology for the multiresidue determination of organophosphate and pyrethroid pesticides in water. *Talanta*, 79, 1354–1359

Luo, Y. & Zhang, M. (2009). Multimedia transport and risk assessment of organophosphate pesticides and a case study in the northern San Joaquin Valley of California. *Chemosphere*, 75, 969–978

Fu, L.; Liu, X.; Hu, J.; Zhao, X.; Wang, H. & Wang, X. (2009). Application of dispersive liquid-liquid microextraction for the analysis of triazophos and carbaryl pesticides in water and fruit juice samples. *Analytica Chimica Acta*, 632, 289–295

Caetano, J. & Machado, S.A.S. (2008). Determination of carbaryl in tomato "in natura" using an amperometric biosensor based on the inhibition of acetylcholinesterase activity. *Sensors and Actuators B*, 129, 40–46

Hildebrandt, A.; Bragos, R.; Lacorte, S. & Marty, J.L. (2008). Performance of a portable biosensor for the analysis of organophosphorus and carbamate insecticides in water and food. *Sensors and Actuators B*, 133, 195–201

Campàs, M.; Prieto-Simón, B. & Marty, J-L. (2009). A review of the use of genetically engineered enzymes in electrochemical biosensors. *Seminars in Cell & Developmental Biology*, 20, 3–9

Somerset, V.S.; Klink, M.J.; Baker, P.G.L.; Iwuoha, E.I. (2007). Acetylcholinesterase-polyaniline biosensor investigation of organophosphate pesticides in selected organic solvents. *Journal of Environmental Science & Health B*, 42, 297–304.

Somerset, V.S.; Klink, M.J.; Sekota, M.M.C.; Baker, P.G.L. & Iwuoha, E.I. (2006). Polyaniline-Mercaptobenzothiazole Biosensor for Organophosphate and Carbamate Pesticides. *Analytical Letters*, 39, 1683–1698

Morrin, A.; Moutloali, R.M.; Killard, A.J.; Smyth, M.R.; Darkwa, J. & Iwuoha, E.I. (2004). Electrocatalytic sensor devices: (I) cyclopentadienylnickel(II) thiolato Schiff base monolayer self-assembled on gold. *Talanta*, 64, 30–38

Michira, I.; Akinyeye, R.; Somerset, V.; Klink, M.J.; Sekota, M.; Al-Ahmed, A.; Baker, P.G.L. & Iwuoha, E. (2007). Synthesis, Characterisation ofnNovel Polyaniline Nanomaterials andApplication in AmperometricnBiosensors. *Macromolecular Symposia*, 255, 57–69

Mazur, M.; Tagowska, M.; Pays, B. & Jackowska, K. (2003). Template synthesis of polyaniline and poly(2-methoxyaniline) nanotubes: comparison of the formation mechanisms. *Electrochemistry Communications*, 5, 403–407

Pritchard, J.; Law, K.; Vakurov, A.; Millner, P. & Higson, S.P.J. (2004). Sonochemically fabricated enzyme microelectrode arrays for the environmental monitoring of pesticides. *Biosensors & Bioelectronics*, 20, 765–772

Joshi, K.A.; Tang, J.; Haddon, R.; Wang, J.; Chen, W. & Mulchandania, A. (2005). ADisposable Biosensor forOrganophosphorus Nerve Agents Based on Carbon Nanotubes Modified Thick Film Strip Electrode. *Electroanalysis*, 17, 54–58

Sotiropoulou, S.; Fournier, D. & Chaniotakisa, N.A. (2005). Genetically engineered acetylcholinesterase-based biosensor for attomolar detection of dichlorvos. Short Communication. *Biosensors & Bioelectronics*, 20, 2347–2352

Albareda-Sirvent, M.; Merkoci, A. & Alegret, S. (2001). Pesticide determination in tap water and juice samples using disposable amperometric biosensors made using thick-film technology. *Analytica Chimica Acta*, 442, 35–44

Sotiropoulou, S. & Chaniotakis, N.A. (2000). Lowering the detection limit of the acetylcholinesterase biosensor using a nanoporous carbon matrix. *Analytica Chimica Acta*, 530, 199–204

Wilkins, E.; Carter, M.; Voss, J. & Ivnitski, (2000). D. A quantitative determination of organophosphate pesticides in organic solvents. *Electrochemistry Communications*, 2, 786–790

Nunes, G.S.; Barcel ´ o, D.; Grabaric, B.S.; Diaz-Cruz, J.M. & Ribeiro, M.L. (1999). Evaluation of a highly sensitive amperometric biosensor with low cholinesterase charge immobilized on a chemically modified carbon paste electrode for trace determination of carbamates in fruit, vegetable and water samples. *Analytica Chimica Acta*, 399, 37–49

Pritchard, J.; Law, K.; Vakurov, A.; Millner, P. & Higson, S.P.J. (2004). Sonochemically fabricated enzyme microelectrode arrays for the environmental monitoring of pesticides. *Biosensors & Bioelectronics*, 20, 765–772

Bucur, B.; Danet, A.F. & Marty, J-L. (2005). Cholinesterase immobilisation on the surface of screen-printed electrodes based on concanavalin A affinity. *Analytica Chimica Acta*, 530, 1–6

Ricci, F.; Amine, A.; Palleschi, G. & Moscone,D. (2003). Prussian Blue based screen printed biosensors with improved characteristics of longterm lifetime and pH stability. *Biosensors & Bioelectronics*, 18, 165–174

Kuralay, F.; Ozyoruk, H. & Yildiz, A. (2005). Potentiometric enzyme electrode for urea determination using immobilized urease in poly(vinylferrocenium) film. *Sensors & Actuators B*, 109, 194–199

Albareda-Sirvent, M.; Merkoci, A. & Alegret, S. (2000). Configurations used in the design of screen-printed enzymatic biosensors.Areview. *Sensors & Actuators B*, 69, 153–163

McGovern, S.T.; Spinks, G.M. & Wallace, G.G. (2005). Micro-humidity sensors based on a processable polyaniline blend. *Sensors & Actuators B*, 107, 657–665

Hart, A.L.; Matthews, C. & Collier, W.A. (1999). Estimation of lactate in meat extracts by screen-printed sensors. *Analytica Chimica Acta, 386*, 7–12

Yang, M.; Yang, Y.; Yang, Y.; Shen, G. & Yu, R. (2005). Microbiosensor for acetylcholine and choline based on electropolymerization/sol–gel derived composite membrane. *Analytica Chimica Acta*, 530, 205–211

Arkhypova, V.N.; Dzyadevych, S.V.; Soldatkin, A.P.; Elukaya, A.V.; Martelet, C. & Jaffrezic-Renault, N. (2003). Development and optimisation of biosensors based on pH-sensitive field effect transistors and cholinesterases for sensitive detection of solanaceous glycoalkaloids. *Biosensors & Bioelectronics*, 18, 1047–1053

Sen, S.; Gulce, A. & Gulce, H. (2004). Polyvinylferrocenium modified Pt electrode for the design of amperometric choline and acetylcholine enzyme electrodes. *Biosensors & Bioelectronics*, 19, 1261–1268

10

Analysis of Pesticide Mixtures using Intelligent Biosensors

Montserrat Cortina-Puig, Georges Istamboulie, Thierry Noguer and Jean-Louis Marty
Université de Perpignan Via Domitia, IMAGES EA4218
France

1. Introduction

Pesticides are widely used in agricultural crops, forests and wetlands as insecticides, fungicides, herbicides and nematocides. Many of them are considered to be particularly hazardous compounds and toxic because they inhibit fundamental metabolic pathways.

Due to their high acute toxicity and risk towards the population, some directives have been established to limit the presence of pesticides in water and food resources. Concerning the quality of water for human consumption, the European Council directive 98/83/CE (Drinking Water Directive) has set a maximum admissible concentration of 0.1 $\mu g\ L^{-1}$ per pesticide and 0.5 $\mu g\ L^{-1}$ for the total amount of pesticides.

Organophosphates (OPs) are a class of synthetic pesticides developed from the Second World War, which are used as insecticides and nerve agents (Bajgar et al., 2004; Raushel, 2002). Since the removal of organochlorine insecticides from use, OPs have become the most widely used insecticides. They are normally used for agricultural, industrial, household and medical purposes. OPs poison insects and mammals by phosphorylation of the acetylcholinesterase (AChE) enzyme at nerve endings (Dubois, 1971; Ecobichon, 2001). Inactivation of this enzyme results in an accumulation of acetylcholine leading to an overstimulation of the effector organ (Aldridge, 1950; Reigart et al., 1999).

The hazardous nature of OPs and their wide usage has led to concerted efforts for developing highly sensitive detection techniques as well as efficient destruction methods for these compounds (Gill et al., 2000). Detection techniques are fundamental in order to accurately determine the level of contamination of waters by pesticides. They are classically based on extraction, cleanup and analysis using gas chromatography (GC) or liquid chromatography (LC) coupled to sensitive and specific detectors (Ballesteros et al., 2004; Geerdink et al., 2002; Kuster et al., 2006; Lacorte et al., 1993). Although they are very sensitive, these techniques are expensive and time consuming (involve extensive preparation steps), they are not adapted for in situ and real time detection and often require highly trained personnel. In addition, these methods are not able to provide any information concerning the toxicity of the sample.

AChE biosensors appear as a rapid and simple alternative method for the detection of OPs insecticides. A successful AChE biosensor for toxicity monitoring should offer comparable or even better analytical performances than the traditional chromatographic systems. Ideally, such sensors should be small, cheap, simple to handle and able to provide reliable information in real-time without or with a minimum sample preparation.

2. Acetylcholinesterase-based biosensors

An alternative to elaborated chromatographic methods is the use of enzymatic determination based on AChE inhibition. Detection kits have been successfully designed based on this principle (Andreescu et al., 2006; No et al., 2007). The most advanced systems described so far are based on the biosensor technology. Numerous sensors have been described for OPs determination based on the inhibition of cholinesterases (ChEs) (Andreescu et al., 2006); some of them involving recombinant AChEs specially tailored to enhance their sensitivity to specific inhibitors (Istamboulie et al., 2007). The mechanism of inhibition of AChE by OP and carbamate compounds is well-known (Aldridge, 1950). The inhibitor phosphorylates or carbamoylates the active site serine and the inhibition can be considered as irreversible in the first 30 min (Boublik et al., 2002).

$$E + PX \overset{K_d}{\leftrightarrow} E^*PX \overset{k_2}{\rightarrow} EP + X$$

where E = enzyme, PX = carbamate or OP and X = leaving group.
This scheme can be simplified using the bimolecular constant $k_i = k_2/K_d$:

$$E + PX \overset{k_i}{\rightarrow} EP + X$$

Two types of ChEs are known and have been used for designing biosensors: AChE and butyrylcholinesterase (BuChE). BuChE has a similar molecular structure to that of AChE but is characterized by different substrate specificity: AChE preferentially hydrolyses acetyl esters such as acetylcholine, while BuChE hydrolyses butyrylcholine. Another aspect that distinguishes AChE from BuChE is the AChE inhibition by excess of substrate. This property is related to substrate binding and the catalytic mechanism. Apart from the natural substrates, ChEs also hydrolyse esters of thiocholine such as acetylthiocholine, butyrylthiocholine, propionylthiocholine, acetyl-β-methylthiocholine as well as o-nitrophenylacetate, indophenylacetate and α-naphtyl acetate. Many of these substrates have been used in different ChE biosensor configurations. AChE enzymes extracted from the *Drosophila melanogaster* and electric eel are commercially available and are the most widely used for biosensor fabrication. ChEs have been extensively used in biosensor configurations based on amperometric detection. Basically, the first devices described were coupling a ChE with a choline oxidase, the detection being based on either the oxidation of H_2O_2 or the reduction of oxygen. This complicated system was further simplified using a synthetic substrate of AChE, acetylthiocholine, which produces under hydrolysis an easily oxidisable compound, thiocholine, according to the following reactions:

$$\text{Acetylthiocholine} \rightarrow \text{Thiocholine} + CH_3COOH$$

$$2\ \text{Thiocholine} + \text{Med (ox)} \rightarrow \text{Dithiobis(choline)} + 2\ H^+ + \text{Med (red)}$$

with Med = electronic mediator,

$$\text{Med (red)} \rightarrow \text{Med (ox)} + 2\,e^-$$

The use of an appropriate mediator, like tetracyanoquinodiemethane (TCNQ) or cobalt phatalocyanine (CoPC) allows decreasing the detection potential to values lower than 100 mV vs. Ag/AgCl. The mediator can be used in solution but it is generally incorporated in the working electrode material. The most versatile method for manufacturing the electrode is probably the screen-printing method. This technology allows the production of screen-printed three-electrode system with a low cost and a high reproducibility.
The detection principle of AChE-based biosensors leads on the blocking of thiocholine production by OP insecticides. Typically, amperometric measurements are performed in stirred PBS solution at pH values comprised between 7 and 8. After applying the appropriate potential for mediator oxidation, the current intensity is recorded in the presence of a saturating concentration of substrate acetylthiocholine. The time necessary to reach the plateau is 2–3 min. The measured signal corresponds to the difference of current intensity between the baseline and the plateau. The cell is washed with distilled water between measurements. The pesticide detection is made in a three step procedure: first, the initial response of the electrode to acetylthiocholine (1 mM) is recorded two times, then the electrode is incubated in a solution containing a known concentration of insecticide, and finally the residual response of the electrode is recorded again. The percentage of the inhibition is then correlated with the insecticide concentration.
Based on this method, highly sensitive biosensors have been developed in our group using recombinant enzymes and appropriate immobilization methods. We have mainly focused our attention on two insecticides of interest: chlorpyrifos (CPO) and chlorfenvinfos (CFV), which are included in a list of priority substances in the field of water policy (decision 2455/2001/EC) (Istamboulie et al., 2007). The developed sensors allowed the detection of pesticides concentrations as low as $1.3\ 10^{-11}$ M (Istamboulie et al., 2009b).

3. Artificial neural networks

One shortcoming in present stage of biosensors development using inhibition of AChE is the fact that various OP and carbamate pesticides inhibit this enzyme to a different extent, rendering calibration for an unknown mixture virtually impossible. To overcome this problem, we have recently described a biosensor associating a highly sensitive genetically-modified *Drosophila melanogaster* AChE (B394) with a phosphotriesterase (PTE) (Istamboulie et al., 2009b). This enzyme allows hydrolysing OP compounds with various affinities. The developed device has been shown to allow the discriminative detection of CPO and CFV in a wide range of concentrations. However, the determination of mixtures of pesticides was shown to be impossible without further analysis (Istamboulie et al., 2009b). A detection system capable of discriminating and quantifying several inhibitors in a mixture should provide a more reliable and robust biosensor analysis. In this sense, the use of a sensor array coupled with a chemometric tool, such as an Artificial Neural Network (ANN) employed for data treatment, could substantially improve biosensor selectivity and allow exact identification of the inhibitor present in a sample (Bachmann et al., 2000; Bachmann et al., 1999).

An ANN is a systematic procedure of data processing inspired by the nervous system function in animals. It tries to reproduce the brain logical operation using a collection of neuron-like entities to perform processing of input data (Cartwright, 1993).
The basic processing unit of an ANN is called perceptron (Svozil et al., 1997), which is a crude approximation to the biological neuron, the cell in the nervous system. It is a decision-making unit with several input connections and a single output, as shown in Figure 1. A signal p_i which is delivered from an input i is multiplied on arrival by a connection weight w_i, so that each signal appears at the perceptron as the weighted value $w_i\, p_i$. The perceptron sums the incoming signals and adds a bias b to give a total signal n. To this sum, a transfer function, usually a step-function, is applied to produce the output a. Inspired on its physiology, if the sum of inputs reaches the threshold level, the neuron is turned "on" and a message is sent out. If the sum is below the threshold value, the neuron is quiescent and remains "off". This process is summarized in Equation 1.

$$a = f\left(b + \sum_{j=1}^{i} w_i p_i\right) \quad (1)$$

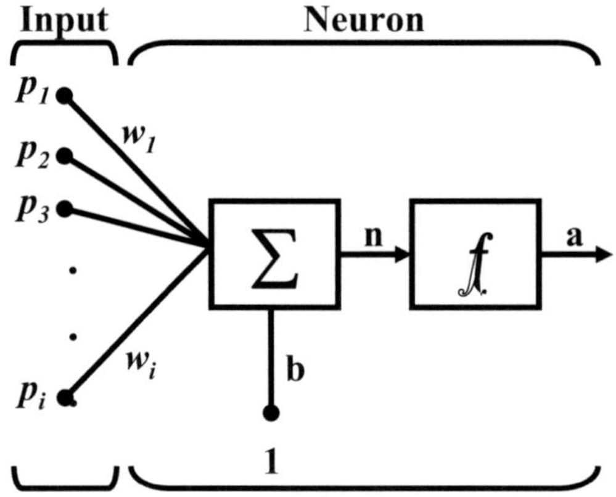

Fig. 1. Schematic representation of the perceptron

A unique condition must be fulfilled: the problem has to be linearly separable. However, most significant scientific problems are not. The failure of the perceptron to solve real-world scientific problems highlights the rather resemblance between it and the brain. The rich network of neurons that makes the brain suggested that a promising step would be to add more perceptrons. This can be done in two different ways: first giving the perceptrons neighbours to form a layer of units which share inputs from the environment; and secondly by introducing further layers, each taking as their input, the output from the previous layer. In this way, the most common ANN used for numerical models is known as the multilayer feedforward network, and is shown in Figure 2.
The path of the departure information begins entering an input layer, whose purpose is just to distribute incoming signals to the next layer; it does not perform any thresholding, thus the units are not perceptrons in its right sense. The perceptrons in the second layer constitute a hidden layer since they communicate with the environment only by sending or

receiving messages to units in the layers to which they are connected. The output layer provides a link between the artificial network and the outside world, submitting the processed information. Every perceptron is connected to all units in the adjoining layers, but there are no connections between units in the same layer. For this reason it is called a fully-connected layered feedforward.

As can be seen in Figure 2, all units have at least one input and one output. Their output may consist of the sum of their inputs but usually a transfer function is applied to this sum. Actually, the non-linear modelling capabilities arise because of these transfer functions. In the hidden layer, sigmoid functions are often used, whereas in the output layers, linear functions are used in quantification problems. Some of the transfer functions that can be used are shown in Figure 3.

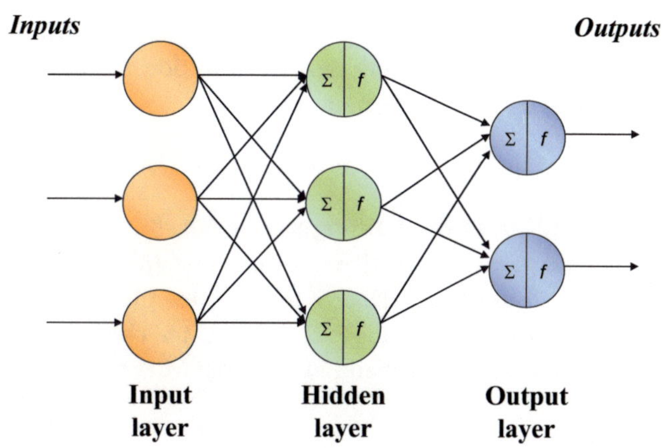

Fig. 2. Schematic structure of an ANN

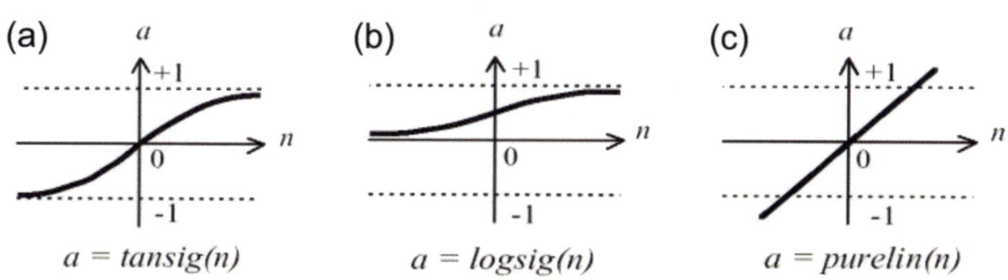

Fig. 3. Representation of three commonly used transfer functions: tan-sigmoid (a), log-sigmoid (b) and linear (c)

The output of a unit is sent with an attenuation factor (weight) to a unit in the next layer. These weights are randomly initialized before training. The model is built by repeatedly showing training instances (samples) to the network and adapting the weights so that the difference between the output units and the target values is minimized. Usually, the complete training set should be offered many times before a reasonable model is obtained. One pass of the randomly ordered instances in the training set is called an epoch. A vast number of different training algorithms exist (Rumelhart et al., 1986). The most well-known is called the back-propagation learning rule, whose objective is to adjust connection weights in a fashion which reduces the error function E_p (Equation 2):

$$E_p = \frac{1}{2}\sum(t_{pj} - o_{pj})^2 \tag{2}$$

where o_{pj} is the certain instant output and t_{pj} is the target output, for each neuron j and each set training member p.
A way to accomplish this is by using the gradient-descent algorithm, an iterative optimisation procedure in which the connection weights are adjusted in a fashion which reduces the error most rapidly, by moving the system downwards in the direction of maximum gradient (Bishop, 1995). The weight of a connection at stage (t + 1) of the training is related to its weight at stage (t) by the Equation 3:

$$w_{ij}(t+1) = w_{ij}(t) + \alpha \cdot \delta_{pj} o_{pj} \tag{3}$$

where α is a gain term, known as the training rate factor, δ is the size of change and the product $\delta_{pj} \cdot o_{pj}$ represents the gradient contribution. The training rate factor varies between 0 and 1 and accelerates or slows down the descent towards the global minimum of the system. It is possible to derive expressions prescribing the size of the changes that must be made at the connection weights to reduce the error signal (Rumelhart et al., 1986).
For the output layer:

$$\delta_{pj} = ko_{pj}(1 - o_{pj})(t_{pj} - o_{pj}) \tag{4}$$

For the hidden layer:

$$\delta_{pj} = ko_{pj}(1 - o_{pj})\sum_k \delta_{pk} w_{jk} \tag{5}$$

These expressions, which are known as the generalized delta rule, show that the extent of the adjustment of connection weights to hidden layers depends upon errors in the subsequent layers, so modifications are made first to the output layer weights, and then the error is then propagated successively back through the hidden layers – this is referred to as backpropagation (of error). Each unit receives an amount of the error signal which is in proportion to its contribution to the output signal, and the connection weights are adjusted by an amount proportional to this error.
Backpropagation by gradient descent is generally a reliable procedure; nevertheless, it has its limitations: it is not a fast training method and it can be trapped in local minima. To avoid the latter, a variant of the above algorithm called gradient-descent with momentum (GDM) introduces a third term, β:

$$w_{ij}(t+1) = w_{ij}(t) + \alpha \cdot \delta_{pj} o_{pj} + \beta \Delta w_{ij}(t) \tag{6}$$

The term β, referred to as the momentum, takes a fixed value between 0 and 1 and serves to reduce to the probability of the system being trapped in a local minimum.

A more efficient minimization algorithms is the Levenberg-Marquardt (LM) (Demuth et al., 1992; Rao, 1984), which is between 10 and 100 times faster than gradient-descent, since it employs a second-derivative approach, while GDM employs only first-derivative terms. As the calculation of the Hessian matrix (matrix of the second derivatives of the error in respect of the weights) is a very cumbersome task, LM algorithm employs an approximation starting with a Jacobian matrix (matrix of the first derivatives of the error in respect of the weights), since it is much easier to calculate the Jacobian than the Hessian matrix (Levenberg, 1944; Marquardt, 1963). Therefore, the weights can be calculated as:

$$w_{ij}(t+1) = w_{ij}(t) - \left[J^T J + \mu I\right]^{-1} J^T e \qquad (7)$$

where J stands for the Jacobian matrix, μ for an adjustment factor, I for the identity matrix and e for a vector of network errors. When μ is large, this becomes gradient descent with a small step size. Thus, the aim is to keep μ as small as possible. This way, if μ is decreased after every epoch, this becomes a very effective algorithm (Demuth et al., 1992).

One of the problems that may occur during neural network training is called overfitting (Freeman et al., 1991; Svozil et al., 1997). This situation occurs when the error on the training set is driven to a very small value, but when new data is presented to the network the error is large. Two different methods can be used to avoid overfitting:

1. Bayesian Regularization (BR): This technique searches for the simplest network which adjusts itself to the function to be approximated, but which also is able to predict most efficiently the points that did not participate in the training (Mackay, 1995). In contrast to gradient descent, in this case not only the global error of the ANN is taken into consideration, but also the value of every single weight of the network. Therefore, the values of the weights are minimized, and the network's complexity is reduced, the responses are smoothened and overfitting is avoided. Furthermore, certain neurons are pruned if all its weights are equal to zero.
2. Early stopping: This technique employs additional data to avoid the undesired overfitting. In this case the available data is divided into three subsets. The first subset is the training set, which is used for computing the gradient and updating the network weights and biases, viz. to accomplish learning of the ANN. The second subset is the validation set, which is used during the training process to check the trend presented by this error from data not used for training. The validation error will normally decrease during the initial phase of training, as does the training set error. However, when the network begins to overfit the data, the error on the validation set will typically begin to rise. When the validation error increases for a specified number of iterations, the training is stopped, and the weights and biases at the minimum of the validation error are returned. The test set error is a third subset, not used at all during the training process or its internal monitoring, but it is used to compare performance of different models. If the error in this external test set reaches a minimum at a significantly different iteration number than the validation set error, this may indicate a poor division of the data set.

4. Multicomponent determination of pesticides based on enzymatic inhibition

Several intelligent biosensors for the resolution of mixtures of pesticides have been developed based on the principle of the AChE inhibition and chemometric data analysis using ANNs.

Bachmann et Schmid (Bachmann et al., 1999) developed a sensitive screen-printed amperometric multielectrode biosensor for the rapid discrimination of the insecticides paraoxon and carbofuran in mixtures. For this purpose, four types of native or recombinant AChEs (Electric eel, bovine erythrocytes, rat brain and *Drosophila melanogaster*) were immobilized by screen printing on four-electrode thick film sensors in sets containing each AChE. The sensors registered a detection range for both analytes of 0.2–20 μg L^{-1} with an overall assay time of less than 60 min. The individual inhibition pattern of each AChE–analyte combination enabled the discrimination of both analytes by the use of ANNs. Thus, paraoxon and carbofuran in mixtures displaying a concentration range of 0–20 μg L^{-1} for each analyte could be analysed with prediction errors of 0.9 μg L^{-1} for paraoxon and 1.4 L^{-1} for carbofuran.

The same group improved the multianalyte detection by selecting different AChE mutants (Bachmann et al., 2000). They developed two different multisensors: the first one included the wild-type Drosophila AChE and mutants Y408F, F368L and F368H; in the second one, the use of the mutant F368W instead of the F368H increased the sensor's capacity even further. Both multisensors were used for inhibition analysis of binary paraoxon and carbofuran mixtures in a concentration range 0–5 μg L^{-1}, followed by data analysis using feedforward ANNs. The two analytes were determined with prediction errors of 0.4 μg L^{-1} for paraoxon and 0.5 μg L^{-1} for carbofuran. A complete biosensor assay and subsequent ANN evaluation was completed within 40 min. In addition, the second multisensor was also investigated for analyte discrimination in real water samples. Finally, the properties of the multisensors were confirmed by simultaneous detection of binary OP mixtures. Malaoxon and paraoxon in composite solutions of 0–5 μg L^{-1} were discriminated with predication errors of 0.9 and 1.6 μg L^{-1}, respectively.

Our group has developed different amperometric systems to resolve pesticide mixtures (Cortina et al., 2008; Istamboulie et al., 2009a; Valdés-Ramírez et al., 2009). These systems have been termed as electronic tongues, since they combine a sensor array to generate multidimensional data and their proper processing to obtain more detailed information (Holmberg et al., 2004). The combined response of these electrodes was always modelled by means of ANNs.

Firstly, an electronic tongue to quantify dichlorvos and carbofuran pesticide mixtures was developed (Cortina et al., 2008). In that case, the signal was generated from a three biosensor array that used different AChE enzymes: the wild type from Electric eel and two different genetically modified enzymes (B1 and B394). Mean values of concentration of evaluated pesticides were 0.79 nM for dichlorvos and 4.1 nM for carbofuran. The developed electronic tongue was also applied to the determination of dichlorvos and carbofuran in real water samples. Both pesticides could be determined with low errors from a direct measurement step.

Secondly, a bioelectronic tongue was developed to resolve pesticide mixtures of two OP pesticides: dichlorvos and methylparaoxon (Valdés-Ramírez et al., 2009). The biosensor array also used three different AChE enzymes: the wild type from Electric eel and two different genetically modified enzymes, B1 and B394 mutants, from *Drosophila melanogaster*. In this case, the biosensor array was used in a flow injection system, permitting to perform automatically the inhibition assay of the pesticide mixture. The inhibition response triplet was trained with mixture solutions that contained dichlorvos from 10^{-4} to 0.1 μM and methylparaoxon from 0.001 to 2.5 μM. When applied to real samples, the two pesticides could be determined with low errors using an extremely simple procedure.

Finally, an amperometric AChE biosensor array was developed to resolve mixtures of two OP insecticides: CPO and CFV (Istamboulie et al., 2009a). Three different biosensors were built using the wild type from Electric eel, the genetically modified *Drosophila melanogaster* AChE B394 and B394 co-immobilized with a PTE. Specifically two different ANNs were constructed. The first one was used to model the combined response of B394 + PTE and Electric eel biosensors and was applied when the concentration of CPO was high and the other, modelling the combined response of B394 + PTE and B394 biosensors, was applied with low concentrations of CPO. In both cases, good prediction ability was obtained. The developed system was also applied to the determination of CPO and CFV pesticides in real water samples. Both pesticides could be quantified with low errors from a direct measurement step.

5. Conclusions

Acetyl- and butyl-cholinesterases have been described for many years as sensitive tools for the detection of many neurotoxic compounds such as insecticides (OPs and carbamates), chemical weapons and toxins (anatoxin-a(s)). They have been extensively used in biosensor configurations based on amperometric detection. Basically, the first devices described were coupling a cholinesterase with a choline oxidase, the detection being based on either the oxidation of H_2O_2 or the reduction of oxygen. This complicated system was further simplified using a synthetic substrate of AChE, acetylthiocholine, which produces under hydrolysis an easily oxidisable compound, thiocholine. Since then, the sensitivity of AChE-based sensors has been greatly improved, mainly due to the use of genetically modified AChEs, which were specifically modified for their sensitivity to special classes of inhibitors. However, the described devices often lack of selectivity and specificity, mainly due to the fact that AChE enzymes are globally sensitive to a class of inhibitors. The selectivity of AChE-based sensors can be tuned by the use of PTE, an enzyme hydrolysing specifically some OP compounds. This enzyme has been successfully coupled to AChE for designing sensors selective to two OP compounds of great environmental concern: CPO and CFV. Despite this progress, the main problem still remained the analysis of pesticide mixtures, which can be solved in some cases by the use of a sensor array coupled with a chemometric tool. In this sense ANNs have been found to be powerful tools, particularly suited for various tasks in information processing. ANNs are non-parametric calibration methods specially created to process non-linear information. It has been demonstrated that by combining native and recombinant variant of AChE with ANNs data processing, a sensitive multianalyte detection is possible.

6. References

Aldridge, W.N. (1950). Some properties of specific cholinesterase with particular reference to the mechanism of inhibition by diethyl p-nitrophenyl thiophosphate (E 605) and analogues. *Biochemical Journal,* 46, 451-60

Andreescu, S. & Marty, J.-L. (2006). Twenty years research in cholinesterase biosensors: From basic research to practical applications. *Biomolecular Engineering,* 23, 1-15

Bachmann, T.T., Leca, B., Vilatte, F., Marty, J.-L., Fournier, D. & Schmid, R.D. (2000). Improved multianalyte detection of organophosphates and carbamates with disposable multielectrode biosensors using recombinant mutants of Drosophila acetylcholinesterase and artificial neural networks. *Biosensors and Bioelectronics,* 15, 193-201

Bachmann, T.T. & Schmid, R.D. (1999). A disposable multielectrode biosensor for rapid simultaneous detection of the insecticides paraoxon and carbofuran at high resolution. *Analytica Chimica Acta,* 401, 95-103

Bajgar, J. & Gregory, S.M. (2004). Organophosphates/nerve agent poisoning: Mechanism of action, diagnosis, prophylaxis, and treatment. *Advances in Clinical Chemistry,* Volume 38, 151-216

Ballesteros, E. & Parrado, M.J. (2004). Continuous solid-phase extraction and gas chromatographic determination of organophosphorus pesticides in natural and drinking waters. *Journal of Chromatography A,* 1029, 267-73

Bishop, C.M. (1995). *Neural Networks for Pattern Recognition,* Oxford University Press, 0-19-853864-2, Oxford

Boublik, Y., Saint-Aguet, P., Lougarre, A., Arnaud, M., Villatte, F., Estrada-Mondaca, S. & Fournier, D. (2002). Acetylcholinesterase engineering for detection of insecticide residues. *Protein Engineering,* 15, 43-50

Cartwright, H.M. (1993). *Applications of artificial intelligence in chemistry,* Oxford University Press, 0-19-855736-1, New York

Cortina, M., Del Valle, M. & Marty, J.-L. (2008). Electronic Tongue Using an Enzyme Inhibition Biosensor Array for the Resolution of Pesticide Mixtures. *Electroanalysis,* 20, 54-60

Demuth, H. & Beale, M. (1992). *Neural Network Toolbox, for Use with MATLAB,* Mathworks Inc, Natick, MA, USA

Dubois, K.P. (1971). The toxicity of organophosphorous compounds to mammals. *Bulletin of the World Health Organization,* 44, 233-40

Ecobichon, D.J. (2001). Toxic effects of pesticides. In: *Casarett & Doull's Toxicology: The Basic Science of Poisons,* Klaassen, C. (Ed.), 763-810, Mc Graw-Hill, New York

Freeman, J.A. & Skapura, D.M. (1991). *Neural Networks: Algorithms, Applications and Programming Techniques,* Addison-Wesley, 0-20-151376-5, Reading, MA, USA

Geerdink, R.B., Niessen, W.M.A. & Brinkman, U.A.T. (2002). Trace-level determination of pesticides in water by means of liquid and gas chromatography. *Journal of Chromatography A,* 970, 65-93

Gill, I. & Ballesteros, A. (2000). Degradation of organophosphorous nerve agents by enzyme-polymer nanocomposites: Efficient biocatalytic materials for personal protection and large-scale detoxification. *Biotechnology and Bioengineering,* 70, 400-10

Holmberg, M., Eriksson, M., Krantz-Rulcker, C., Artursson, T., Winquist, F., Lloyd-Spetz, A. & Lundstrom, I. (2004). 2nd Workshop of the Second Network on Artificial Olfactory Sensing (NOSE II). *Sensors and Actuators B: Chemical,* 101, 213-23

Istamboulie, G., Andreescu, S., Marty, J.-L. & Noguer, T. (2007). Highly sensitive detection of organophosphorus insecticides using magnetic microbeads and genetically engineered acetylcholinesterase. *Biosensors and Bioelectronics,* 23, 506-12

Istamboulie, G., Cortina-Puig, M., Marty, J.L. & Noguer, T. (2009a). The use of Artificial Neural Networks for the selective detection of two organophosphate insecticides: Chlorpyrifos and chlorfenvinfos. *Talanta,* 79, 507-11

Istamboulie, G., Fournier, D., Marty, J.-L. & Noguer, T. (2009b). Phosphotriesterase: A complementary tool for the selective detection of two organophosphate insecticides: Chlorpyrifos and chlorfenvinfos. *Talanta,* 77, 1627-31

Kuster, M., López De Alda, M. & Barceló, D. (2006). Analysis of pesticides in water by liquid chromatography-tandem mass spectrometric techniques. *Mass Spectrometry Reviews,* 25, 900-16

Lacorte, S., Molina, C. & Barceló, D. (1993). Screening of organophosphorus pesticides in environmental matrices by various gas chromatographic techniques. *Analytica Chimica Acta,* 281, 71-84

Levenberg, K. (1944). Method for the Solution of Certain Problems in Least Squares. *Quarterly of Applied Mathematics,* 2, 164-68

Mackay, J.C. (1995). Probable networks and plausible predictions: a review of practical Bayesian methods for supervised neural networks. *Network: Computation in Neural Systems,* 6, 469-505

Marquardt, D. (1963). An algorithm for least-squares estimation of nonlinear parameters. *SIAM Journal on Applied Mathematics,* 11, 431-41

No, H.-Y., Kim, Y.A., Lee, Y.T. & Lee, H.-S. (2007). Cholinesterase-based dipstick assay for the detection of organophosphate and carbamate pesticides. *Analytica Chimica Acta,* 594, 37-43

Rao, S.S. (1984). *Optimization: Theory and applications,* Halsted Press, 0-47-027483-2, New York

Raushel, F.M. (2002). Bacterial detoxification of organophosphate nerve agents. *Current Opinion in Microbiology,* 5, 288-95

Reigart, R. & Roberts, J. (Eds.) (1999). *Recognition and Management of Pesticide Poisonings,* U.S. Environmental Protection Agency, USA

Rumelhart, D.E., Hinton, G.E. & Williams, R.J. (1986). Parallel Distributed Processing: Explorations in the Microstructure of Cognition (Vol 1: Foundations). In: *Learning internal representations by error propagation,* Rumelhart, D.E. & Mcclelland, J.L. (Eds.), MIT Press, 0-262-68053-X, London

Svozil, D., Kvasnick, V. & Pospichal, J. (1997). Introduction to multi-layer feed-forward neural networks. *Chemometrics and Intelligent Laboratory Systems,* 39, 43-62

Valdés-Ramírez, G., Gutiérrez, M., Del Valle, M., Ramírez-Silva, M.T., Fournier, D. & Marty, J.L. (2009). Automated resolution of dichlorvos and methylparaoxon pesticide mixtures employing a Flow Injection system with an inhibition electronic tongue. *Biosensors and Bioelectronics*, 24, 1103-08

11

Enzyme vs. Bacterial Electrochemical Sensors for Organophosphorus Pesticides Quantification

Margarita Stoytcheva
Universidad Autónoma de Baja California, Instituto de Ingeniería
México

1. Introduction

The worldwide increasing use of organophosphorus (OP) pesticides which are powerful neurotoxins and the resulting environmental and public concerns (CDC, 2005) created a demand for the development of reliable, fast, sensitive, simple and low-costing methods for their quantification, appropriate for on-line and on-site measurements. The conventional chromatographic, spectroscopic and immunoassay techniques for OP compounds determination, despite of their accuracy and sensitivity, are not well suited to these tasks. In contrast, the electrochemical biosensors based methods fulfill all the mentioned requirements.

The biosensors are relatively new analytical devices developed taking advantage of the progress in the biotechnology and the material science, in particular, in association with the modern principles of transduction of the chemical information. They represent a variety of chemical sensors, transforming the concentration of the quantified substance into an analytically useful signal (Thévenot et al., 1999).

The electrochemical biosensors provide selective quantitative or semi-quantitative analytical information using a biological recognition element (enzymes, whole cells, organelles or particles, tissues, etc.), in direct spatial contact with an electrochemical transducer, converting the signal produced by the interaction between the bioreceptor and the analyte, into electrical one (Thévenot et al., 1999).

A great variety of electrochemical biosensors quantifying the organophosphorus pesticides have been designed over the last decades. This review gives a survey on the state of the art of organophosphorus compounds detection using enzyme- and bacterial-based electrochemical sensors.

The survey includes the presentation of the OP pesticides structure and biochemical action, as well as the sources of pollution and the regulatory norms.

The current chromatographic and immunoassay methods for OP analysis are briefly discussed. The emerging during the last decades electrochemical biosensors based techniques are presented as their alternative.

The analytical performances of the two main types of enzyme-based electrochemical sensors for OP determination (the organophosphorus hydrolase and the acylcholinesterases ones), involving respectively the direct enzyme transformation of the analyte, and the inhibition of the enzyme activity, are summarized.

The recent trends in the development and in the increasing application of bacterial sensor systems for OP analysis are revised.
The advantages and the limitations of the enzyme-based vs. the bacterial electrochemical sensors are discussed.

2. The organophosphorus pesticides

The chemical compounds including stable functional groups that contain the carbon-phosphorus bond or that are organic derivatives of inorganic phosphorus acids are known as organophosphorus (Quin, 2000). Most of them, with the following general structure (Corbett et al., 1984; Eto, 1974; Hassall, 1982):

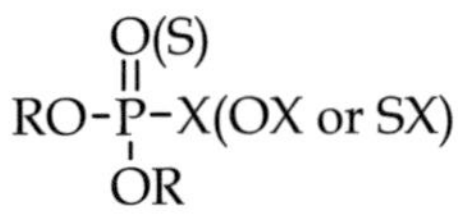

are highly toxic and are used as chemical warfare agents and pesticides (insecticides, herbicides, fungicides, rodenticides, moluscocides, nematocides, and regulators of vegetal growth, among other).
According to their chemical constitution, the organophosphorus pesticides could be classified into several types (Gupta, 2006). Some representative structures are shown in Fig. 1.

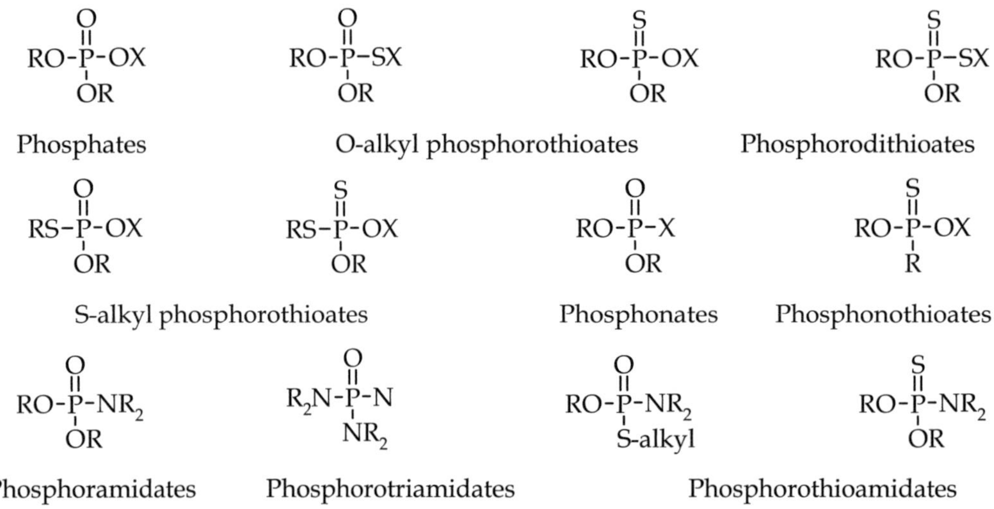

Fig. 1. Main types of organophosphorus pesticides (R is usually methyl or ethyl group and the leaving group X is aliphatic, homocyclic or heterocyclic one).

The OPs structural variety is reflected in their physicochemical and biological properties (Corbett et al., 1984; Hassall, 1982; WHO, 1986). Data on individual OPs could be found in Dictionary of organophosphorus compounds (Edmundson, 1988), Handbook of pesticide toxicology (Hayes, 1991), The Pesticide manual: A world compendium (Worthing & Hance, 1991), at http://www.pesticideinfo.org/, etc.
The biochemical mode of action of the organophosphorus pesticides primarily involves the inhibition of the acetylcholinesterase occurring throughout the central and peripheral

nervous system of vertebrates, through phosphorylation of the serine hydroxyl moiety of the enzyme active site, thus preventing the hydrolysis of the neurotransmitter acetylcholine, performed in an analogous manner (Corbett et al., 1984; Fukuto, 1990; Gupta, 2006; Matsumura, 1980), as shown in Fig. 2. The resulting acetylcholine accumulation at the nerve synapses disrupts the nerve impulses propagation.

Slow recovery of the acetylcholinesterase activity could be observed, because of the spontaneous hydrolysis of the phosphorylated enzyme (Fig. 2B). The nucleophilic attack of the phosphorylacetylcholinesterase by some reagents (hydroxylamine, oximes) leads to quicker enzyme reactivation. "Aging" consisting in loss of an alkyl group from an alkoxy group on a phosphoryl residue attached to the active-site serine causes irreversible enzyme inhibition (Fig. 2C).

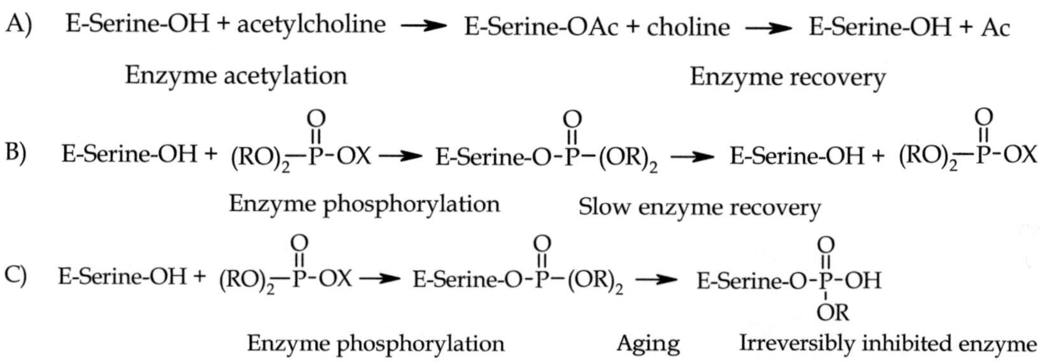

Fig. 2. A) Acetylcholine enzymatic hydrolysis; B) Acetylcholinesterase inhibition by OP and its reactivation; C) Acetylcholinesterase inhibition by OP and aging. (E-Serine-OH represents the enzyme acetylcholinesterase)

OPs are among the most acutely toxic pesticides. They belong to the toxicity class I (highly toxic) or toxicity class II (moderately toxic), according to the EPA classification. Although less persistent than the organochlorine pesticides, their widespread usage poses risk to man and his environment. Pesticides pollution results from agricultural practices, from industrial waste or discharge, from seepage of buried toxic wastes, and from run-off during spraying (Larson et al., 1997; Majewski & Capel, 1995; Vighi & Funari, 1995). Pesticides production, distribution, use, exposure, environmental levels, and maximum permissible levels in drinking water and food are subject of regulations in accordance with the national and international legislations. The primary involved organizations are the US Environmental Protection Agency (EPA), the EU Commission, the World Health Organization (WHO), the Food and Agricultural Organization of the United Nations (FAO), and the Codex Alimentarius Commission.

The high acute toxicity of the OPs, rapid absorption by the organism, and fast degradation in the environment call for the development of adequate analytical tools for their "*in situ*" determination. The commonly used methods for OPs quantification include various chromatographic techniques, such as gas-chromatography, gas chromatography with mass spectrometry detection, thin-layer chromatography, and high performance liquid chromatography (Jeannot & Dagnac, 2006; Schlecht & O'Connor, 1994), requiring time-consuming extraction, preconcentration, and clean-up procedures, skilled personnel and expensive laboratory equipment. Immunoassays (Van Emon, 2006) applied for OPs quantification involve numerous washing steps and long analysis time (one to two hours). Thus, these methods are not suitable for in field determinations and continuous monitoring. Nowadays, the devices of choice for organophosphorus pesticides "*in situ*" analysis, because of the inexpensive instrumentation, the simple operation procedure and the high sensitivity, are the emerged during the last decades electrochemical biosensors, applicable as well as for real-time and on-line determinations.

3. The electrochemical biosensors for OPs quantification

The electrochemical biosensors for OP pesticides analysis could be classed into two great groups according to the nature of the biological recognition element – enzymes or bacteria.

3.1 Enzyme electrochemical sensors

The function of the acylcholinesterases (acetylcholinesterase or butyrylcholinesterase) and phosphatases (acid or alkaline) electrochemical sensors is based on the ability of the OP compounds to inhibit these enzymes. The quantification is realized measuring the variation of the enzyme activity as a function of the organophosphorus pesticide concentration, applying electrochemical techniques. Thus, according to the transduction mode, the reported biosensors are mainly potentiometric or amperometric.
The potentiometric acylcholinesterase sensors involve the following reaction:

$$\text{R}'\text{-choline} + H_2O \xrightarrow{\text{ChE}} \text{choline} + \text{R}'\text{-COOH} \qquad (1)$$

where R′ is an acetyl or butyryl moiety and ChE is the acylcholinesterase.
The pH change of the solution, resulting from the acid release during the enzyme catalyzed hydrolysis of the choline esters is recorded as a sensor response, the latter depending on the cholinesterase activity.
Another potentiometric system is that developed by Ghindilis (Ghindilis et al., 1996), based on mediatorless bioelectrocatalysis:

$$\text{R}'\text{-choline} + H_2O \xrightarrow{\text{ChE}} \text{choline} + \text{R}'\text{-COOH} \qquad (2)$$

$$\text{choline} + 2O_2 + H_2O \xrightarrow{\text{ChO}} \text{betaine} + 2H_2O_2 \qquad (3)$$

$$H_2O_2 + 2H^+ + 2e^- \xrightarrow{\text{HRP}} 2H_2O \qquad (4)$$

(ChO is the enzyme choline oxidase and HRP is the enzyme peroxidase)
The H_2O_2 electrocatalytical reduction causes a shift in the electrode potential. This tri-enzyme sensor allowed detecting $2\text{x}10^{-13}$ mol L^{-1} trichlorfon.
The amperometric acylcholinesterase sensors, providing in general faster response, as well as higher sensitivity and accuracy than the potentiometric do, are developed in two directions:

a. First generation ChE amperometric sensors

They exploit the bienzymatic processes described by Eq. 2 and Eq. 3. The current of H_2O_2 oxidation or O_2 reduction, depending on the substrate concentration and the enzyme activity, is recorded as a sensor response. However, since the H_2O_2 oxidation is carried out at a potential of +0.60 V/SCE, many substances contained in biological liquids and submitted to an oxidation at the same potential (glutathione, ascorbates, urates, etc.) interfere, corrupting the determination. The output signal is influenced by the fluctuations in the oxygen concentration, too.

b. Second generation ChE amperometric sensors

They use synthetic substrates (thiocholine or indoxylacetate esters), transformed upon catalytic hydrolysis in products able to be easily oxidized, as for example:

$$\text{R}'\text{-thiocholine} + H_2O \xrightarrow{\text{ChE}} \text{thiocholine} + \text{R}'\text{COOH} \tag{5}$$

$$\text{thiocholine} \rightarrow \text{dithio-bis-choline} + 2H^+ + 2e^- \tag{6}$$

However, R'-thiocholine is a subject of a spontaneous non-enzymatic hydrolysis. Although slight, it can produce an increase of the anodic current response. Thiocholine oxidation provoking a passivation of the platinum anodes, because of their interaction with the sulfur containing compounds (Nikol'skaya & Evtyugin, 1992) must be taken into consideration, too.

The process of direct thiocholine oxidation occurring at +0.80 V/SCE at conventional metal and graphite transducers (Martorell et al., 1994; Marty et al., 1992; Marty et al., 1993; Marty et al., 1995; Sužnjević et al., 1985) involves the transfer of one electron from the thiol and a dimerization of the intermediate to disulfide (Evtugyn et al., 1999, Liu et al., 2005). The high potential value however causes the appearance of a high background current, as well as electroactive compounds interferences.

Several types of electrodes providing a sensitive electrochemical detection of enzymatically generated thiocholine at low potential were reported, such as the ones chemically modified with phtalocyanines (Harlbert & Baldwin, 1985; Hart & Hartley, 1994; Skladal, 1991), Prussian blue (Ricci et al., 2004), tetracyanoquinodimethane (Kulys & D'Costa, 1991; Martorell et al., 1997) and ferrocene (Evtugyn et al., 1996). However, mediator addition also could provoke interferences.

The alternative route to achieve potential lowering avoiding electrode modification involves acylthiocholine enzymatic hydrolysis (Eq. 5), chemical reduction of the produced thiocholine in solution (Eq. 7), and electrochemical detection of the product of the homogeneous redox reaction (Eq. 8), as suggested by Neufeld (Neufeld et al., 2000) and Ovalle (Ovalle et al., 2009):

$$\text{R}'\text{-thiocholine} + 2[Fe(CN)_6]^{3-} \rightarrow \text{dithio-bis-choline} + 2[Fe(CN)_6]^{4-} \tag{7}$$

$$[Fe(CN)_6]^{4-} \rightarrow [Fe(CN)_6]^{3-} + e^- \tag{8}$$

However, the reported sensitivity of the OPs (chlorofos) determination is lower in comparison to that, attained by direct thiocholine oxidation (Ovalle et al., 2009).

The exploited response-generating reaction in some acylcholinesterase sensors of second generation for OPs quantification is the electrochemical oxidation of the leucoindigo, produced upon enzymatic hydrolysis of indoxylacetate (Kulys, 1989):

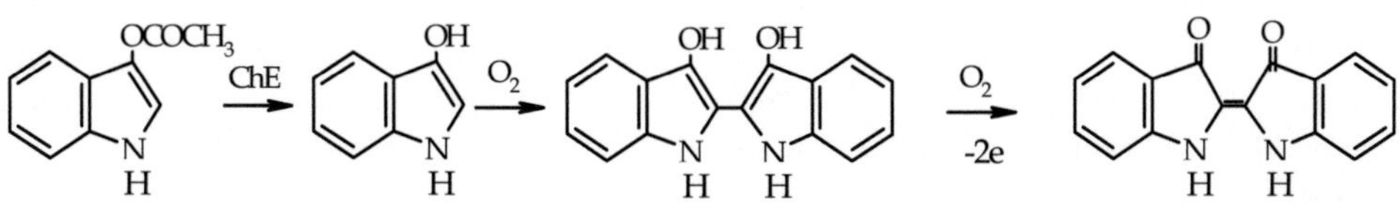

(9)

The disadvantage of the method consists in the fact that the leucoindigo is exposed to a chemical, as well as to electrochemical oxidation involving O_2, which complicates the formation of the analytical signal (Nikol'skaya & Evtyugin, 1992).
The phosphatases inhibition, although reversible (which avoid enzyme reactivation), is rarely applied in the electrochemical biosensors for OPs detection (Danzer & Schwedt, 1996; Mazzei et al., 1996).
The inhibition-based determinations are very sensitive, but indirect. Drawbacks of the method are also the lack of selectivity and the need, in some cases, of enzyme incubation and enzyme reactivation/regeneration. In addition, as shown by Gunaratna (Gunaratna & Wilson, 1990), the cholinesterase is very sensitive to its micro-environment and even small changes provoke significant lost of enzyme activity resulting in decreasing of the sensor sensitivity. An overview of the methods based on enzyme inhibition with emphasis on the non-ideal behavior of the enzyme inhibition-based biosensors and biosensing systems is presented by Luque de Castro (Luque de Castro & Herrera, 2003).
Direct OP pesticides analysis could be achieved applying organophosphorus hydrolase (OPH) electrochemical sensors (Anzai, 2006; Chough et al., 2002; Lei et al., 2007 ; Mulchandani et al., 2001a; Mulchandani et al., 2001b; Prieto-Simón et al., 2006; Rodriguez-Mozaz et al., 2004; Wang et al., 2003). The enzyme OPH demonstrates substrate specificity toward paraoxon, parathion, coumaphos, diazinon, dursban, methyl parathion, etc, and toward some chemical warfare agents (sarin, soman, tabun, VX, etc.) (Dumas et al., 1990; Munnecke, 1980). The detection of parathion is also possible using parathion hydrolase (PH) (Sacks et al., 2000). The enzymatically catalyzed OP substrates hydrolysis involves pH changes and generates electroactive products:

$$\mathrm{RO{-}\overset{\overset{\large O(S)}{\|}}{\underset{\underset{\large OR}{|}}{P}}{-}X} + H_2O \xrightarrow{\text{OPH}} \mathrm{RO{-}\overset{\overset{\large O(S)}{\|}}{\underset{\underset{\large OR}{|}}{P}}{-}OH} + HX \qquad (10)$$

Thus, the detection could be performed in a single step, using potentiometric (pH sensitive) or amperometric transducers (Mulchandani et al., 2001a).
OPH-based systems allow the selective determination of the family of the OP compounds, in contrast to the enzyme inhibition based techniques, but the reported detection limit is higher (Mulchandani et al., 2006). An important drawback represents the complex, long-lasting, and expensive procedure for OPH or PH extraction and purification, performed in specialized microbiological laboratories (to note that these enzymes are not commercially available) (Prieto-Simón et al., 2006).
Some reviews summarize the performances of the enzyme electrochemical sensors for OP pesticides determination and the principles of their operation (Andreescu & Marty, 2006; Anzai, 2006; Jaffrezic-Renault, 2001; Mazzei et al., 1996; Mulchandani et al., 2001a; Noguer et al., 1999; Prieto-Simón et al., 2006; Rodriguez-Mozaz et al., 2004; Solé et al., 2003a; Solé et al., 2003b; Tran-Minh, 1985; Turdean et al., 2002). Selected relevant data, demonstrating the sensitivity of the enzyme sensors are given in Table 1 and Table 2.
The commune disadvantages of this group of biosensors are the instability of the response (due to enzyme leaking or deactivation), the observed interferences at high electrode potentials, the passivation of the electrode surface and the short life-time at ambient temperature.

Enzyme	Target	LOD	Reference
AChE	paraoxon	0.1 nM	Tran-Minh et al., 1990
AChE	malathion	1 nM	Tran-Minh et al., 1990
AChE/BuChE	paraoxon	2.8 ppb	Skladal, 1991
BuChE	diazinon	2 ppb	Budnikov & Evtugyn, 1996
BuChE/ChO/HRP	chlorofos	0.0002 nM	Ghindilis et al., 1996
AChE/BuChE	paraoxon	0.08 ppb	Skladal et al., 1996
AChE	paraoxon	0.5 ppb	Noguer et al., 1999
AChE/ChO	methyl parathion	0.05 μM	Lin et al., 2004

Table 1. LOD of some acylcholinesterase sensors for OPs determination (AChE is the acetylcholinesterase and BuChE is the butyrylcholinesterase).

Enzyme	Target	LOD	Reference
OPH	paraoxon	90 nM	Mulchandani et al., 1999
OPH	methyl parathion	70 nM	Mulchandani et al., 1999
OPH	paraoxon	2 μM	Mulchandani et al., 2001a
OPH	methyl parathion	2 μM	Mulchandani et al., 2001a
OPH	diazinon	2 μM	Mulchandani et al., 2001a
OPH	parathion	15 nM	Chough et al., 2002
OPH	paraoxon	20 nM	Chough et al., 2002
OPH	paraoxon	0.4 μM	Lei et al., 2007

Table 2. LOD of some OPH sensors for OPs determination.

3.2 Bacterial electrochemical sensors

Bacteria-based electrochemical sensors are developed by coupling these microorganisms to electrochemical transducers. Bacteria offer several advantages over the isolated enzymes for biosensor application, as for example: lower cost, because of the elimination of the time-consuming and expensive processes of extraction of the intracellular enzymes and their purification; ability to catalyze sequential reactions involving multiple enzymes; resistance to pH and temperature changes, because of the retention of the enzymes in their natural environment; higher tolerance to toxic substances; enzyme activity recovery in nutrient medium (D'Souza, 1989).

The bacterial electrochemical sensors are less sensitive and less selective than the enzyme ones, and their response time is relatively long, because of the difusional constraints imposed by the bacterial cell wall. However, these drawbacks could be overcome, by genetic engineering and by cell permeabilizing (D'Souza, 1989) respectively, applying various techniques.

Only few bacterial electrochemical sensors for OP pesticides quantification have been developed until now. They include, as biological recognition element, genetically engineered *Moraxella sp.*, *Pseudomonas putida* or *Escherichia coli* with surface-expressed OPH (Mulchandani et al., 1998; Mulchandani et al., 2001c; Mulchandani et al., 2006; Richins et al., 1997). The detection principle is identical to the described above, when employing the isolated and purified enzyme. Recently, microbial sensors based on Clark dissolved oxygen electrode modified with recombinant p-nitrophenol degrading/oxidizing bacteria endowed with OPH activity was reported (Lei et al., 2005; Lei et al., 2006). The surface-displayed OPH catalyzes the hydrolysis of OP pesticides with nitrophenyl substituent to release products, metabolized by the bacteria while consuming oxygen. The oxygen consumption is measured and correlated to the OP concentration.

Ley (Lei et al., 2004) reports the construction of a hybrid biosensor for direct determination of OP pesticides using purified OPH for their initial hydrolysis and *Arthrobacter sp. JS443* for the subsequent oxidation of the released p-nitrophenol to carbon dioxide through electroactive intermediates. The biocatalytic layer is prepared by bacteria and enzyme co-immobilization on a carbon paste electrode. The registered signal is the current of oxidation of the intermediates, function of the OP concentration.

The mentioned microbial and hybrid sensors for direct OP pesticides quantification display long term stability, good reproducibility and accuracy, and relatively short response time. However, the reached LOD is over the OP concentration in environmental samples and higher than that for acylcholinesterases inhibition-based sensors, immunoassays, and gas, liquid and thin layer chromatography (Mulchandani et al., 2006).

Recently, an electrochemical biosensor for OP pesticides trace level concentrations determination was developed and characterized (Stoytcheva et al., 2009). It integrates a hybrid biorecognition element consisting of immobilized *Arthrobacter globiformis* and free acetylcholinesterase (ACh) with a Clark type oxygen probe transducer. The bacteria convert the ACh-generated choline to betaine with oxygen consumption measured as a Clark probe current change. This change, representing the sensor response, correlates to the concentration of the OP pesticides inhibiting the Ach catalyzed acetylcholine hydrolysis to choline.

The conditions for maximal sensor response to choline are optimized according to the methodology of Design of Experiments. The analytical performances of the enzyme substrate determination in a wide concentration range (0.1 μmol dm^{-3} - 20 μmol dm^{-3} of acetylcholine) and different ACh activities are established. It is demonstrated that the biosensor ensures reproducible, accurate and reliable chlorofos quantification reaching a LOD of 1 nmol dm^{-3} and a sensitivity of 0.0252 μA/p(mol dm^{-3}) under optimal experimental conditions.

The biosensor response time is 200 s and the storage stability is t_{L50} = 49 days for the bacterial membrane at ambient temperature. The device is reusable, the bacterial membrane being not affected by OP. The biosensor was applied to chlorofos determination in contaminated milk.

The proposed approach combines the advantages of the bacterial sensors with those of the cholinesterases inhibition-based ones, namely: stable response and long life-time at ambient temperature, because of the conservation of the enzyme system of the bacteria in its natural environment; reproducible characteristics ensured controlling the bacterial charge and the bacterial activity; high sensitivity. In addition, it provides reliable, free of interferences measurement of the dissolved oxygen reduction current, the polymer membrane of the oxygen probe being permeable only for gases. The biosensor fabrication is simple and cost-effective, enzyme extraction and purification or genetic engineering being avoided.

The biosensor is suitable for general toxicity screening or for determining the concentration of isolated OP pollutants.

Some comparative data are presented in Table 3.

Microorganism	Target	LOD	Reference
Recombinant *P. coli*	paraoxon	2 μM	Mulchandani et al., 1998
Recombinant *P. coli*	methyl parathion	2 μM	Mulchandani et al., 1998
Recombinant *P. coli*	diazinon	5 μM	Mulchandani et al., 1998
Recombinant *Moraxella*	methyl parathion	1 μM	Mulchandani et al., 2001c
Recombinant *Moraxella*	paraoxon	0.2 μM	Mulchandani et al., 2001c
Recombinant *P. putida*	paraoxon	55 ppb	Lei et al., 2005
Recombinant *P. putida*	methyl paraoxon	53 ppb	Lei et al., 2005
Recombinant *P. putida*	parathion	58 ppb	Lei et al., 2005
Recombinant *P. putida*	fenitrothion	277 ppb	Lei et al., 2006
Recombinant *P. putida*	EPN	1.6 ppm	Lei et al., 2006
Recombinant *Moraxella*	paraoxon	0.1 μM	Mulchandani et al, 2006
Arthrobacter globiformis	chlorofos	1 nM	Stoytcheva et al., 2009

Table 3. LOD of some bacterial electrochemical sensors for OPs determination

4. Conclusion

Despite of the still limited application of the electrochemical biosensors for OPs quantification in real samples, their analytical potential is obvious. Thus, current efforts are axed on biosensors' performance improvement, development of compact and portable or disposable devices for *in-field* analysis and their commercialization. Promising opportunities offer the nanomaterials transducers modification, permitting the sensitive OPs monitoring at low electrode potential (Periasamy et al., 2009) and the genetic engineering of the biological recognition elements leading to selectivity increase (Campàs et al., 2009).

5. References

Andreescu, S. & Marty, J.-L. (2006). Twenty years research in cholinesterase biosensors:from basic research to practical applications. Biomol. Eng., 23, 1, (March, 2006) 1-15, ISSN: 13890344

Anzai, J. (2006). Use of biosensors for detecting organophosphorus agents. *Yakugaku Zasshi*, 126, 12, (December, 2006) 1301-1308, ISSN: 0031-6903, EISSN: 1347-5231

Aprea, C.; Colosio, C.; Mammone, T.; Minoia, C. & Maroni, M. (2002). Biological monitoring of pesticide exposure: a review of analytical methods. *J. Chromatogr.* B, 769, 2, (April 2002) 191–219, ISSN: 1570-0232

Budnikov, H. V. & Evtugyn, G. A. (1996). Electrochemical biosensors for inhibitor determination: selectivity and sensitivity control. *Electroanalysis*, 8, 8-9, (August-September, 1996) 817-820, ISSN: 1040-0397, ESSN: 1521-4109

Campàs, M; Prieto-Simón, B. & Marty J.-L. (2009). A review of the use of genetically engineered enzymes in electrochemical biosensors. *Seminars in Cell & Developmental Biology*, 20, 1, (February 2009) 3-9, ISSN: 1084-9521

CDC, *Third national report on human exposure to environmental chemicals* (2005). Centers for Disease Control and Prevention (CDC), Atlanta

Chough, S. H.; Mulchandani, A.; Mulchandani, P.; Chen, W.; Wang, J. & Rogers, K. R. (2002). Organophosphorus hydrolase-based amperometric sensor: modulation of sensitivity and substrate selectivity. *Electroanalysis,* 14, 4, (February, 2002) 273-276, ISSN: 1040-0397, EISSN: 1521-4109

Corbett, J. R.; Wright, K. & Baillie, A. C. (1984). *The biochemical mode of action of pesticides,* 2nd ed., Academic press, ISBN 0-12-187860-0, ISBN-13: 978-0-12-187860-3, London

Danzer, T. & Schwedt, G. (1996). Chemometric methods for the development of a biosensor system and the evaluation of inhibition studies with solutions and mixtures of pesticides and heavy metals. Part I. Development of an enzyme electrodes system for pesticides and heavy metal screening using selected chemometric methods. *Anal. Chim. Acta,* 318, 3, (January, 1996) 275-286, ISSN: 0003-2670

D'Souza, S., F. (1989). Immobilized cells: techniques and applications. *Indian J. Microbiol.,* 29, 2, (June, 1989) 83-117, ISSN: 0046-8991, EISSN: 0973-7715

Dumas, D. P.; Durst, H. D.; Landis, W. G.; Raushel, F. M. & Wild, J. R. (1990). Inactivation of organophosphorus nerve agents by the phosphotriesterase from *Pseudomonas diminuta. Arch. Biochem. Biophys.,* 227, 1, (February, 1990) 155-159, ISSN: 0003-9861

Edmundson, R. S. (1988). *Dictionary of organophosphorus compounds,* Chapman & Hall, ISBN 10: 0-412-25790-4, ISBN-13: 978-0-412-25790-2, London

Eto, M. (1974). *Organophosphorus pesticides: organic and biological chemistry,* CRS Press, ISBN-10: 0-87819-023-6, ISBN-13: 978-0-87819-023-2, Cleveland

Evtugyn, G.; Budnikov, H.; Galyametdinov, Yu. & Suntsov E. (1996). Amperometric determination of thiocholine esters in the presence of butyrylcholinesterase. *Zh. Anal. Khim.,* 51, 4, 391-393, ISSN: 0044-4502

Evtugyn, G.; Ivanov, A.; Gogol, E.; Marty, J.-L. & Budnikov, H. (1999). Amperometric flow-through biosensor for the determination of cholinesterase inhibitors. *Anal. Chim. Acta,* 385, 1-3, (April, 1999) 13-21, ISSN: 0003-2670

Fukuto, R. (1990). Mechanism of action of organophosphorus and carbamate insecticides. *Environmental Health Perspectives,* 87, (July 1990) 245-254, ISSN: 00916765, EISSN 15529924

Ghindilis, A.; Morzunova, H.; Barmin, A. & Kurochkin, I. (1996). Potentiometric biosensors for cholinesterase inhibitor analysis based on mediatorless bioelectrocatalysis. *Biosens. Bioelectr.,* 11, 9, 873-880, ISSN: 0956-5663

Gunaratna, C. & Wilson, G. (1990). Optimization of multienzyme flow reactors for determination of acetylcholine, *Anal. Chem.,* 62, 4, (February, 1990) 402–407, ISSN: 0003-2700, EISSN: 1520-6882

Gupta, R. C. (Ed.) (2005). *Toxicology of organophosphate & carbamate compounds,* 1st ed., Elsevier Academic Press ISBN-10: 0-12-088523-9, ISBN-13: 978-0-12-088523-7, London

Hayes, W. J. (1991). *Handbook of pesticide toxicology,* Academic Press, ISBN-10: 0-12-334160-4, ISBN-13: 978-0-12-334160-0, San Diego

Harlbert, M. & Baldwin, R. (1985). Electrocatalytic and analytical response of cobalt phthalocyanine containing carbon paste electrodes toward sulfhydryl compounds. *Anal. Chem.,* 57, 3, (March, 1985) 591-595, ISSN: 0003-2700, EISSN: 1520-6882

Hart, J. & Hartley, I. (1994). Voltammetric and amperometric studies of thiocholine at a screen-printed carbon electrode chemically modified with cobalt phthalocyanine: studies towards a pesticide sensor. *Analyst,* 119, 2, 259-265, ISSN: 0003-2654

Hassall, K. A. (1982). *The chemistry of pesticides. Their metabolism, mode of action and uses in crop protection,* Verlag Chemie, ISBN-10: 3527259694, ISBN-13: 9783527259694, Weinheim, Deerfield Beach, Florida, Basel, 1982

Jaffrezic-Renault, N. (2001). New trends in biosensors for organophosphorus pesticides. *Sensors*, 1, 2, (July, 2001) 60-64, ISSN: 1424-8220

Jeannot, R. & Dagnac, T. (2006). In: *Chromatographic analysis of the environmental*. 3rd edition, Nollet L. (Ed.), 841-889, CRC Press, Boca Raton, London, New York

Kulys, J. (1989). Amperometric enzyme electrodes in analytical chemistry, *Frez. J. Anal. Chem.*, 335, 1, (January 1989) 86-91, ISSN: 0937-0633; EISSN: 1432-1130

Kulys, J. & D'Costa, E. J. (1991). Printed amperometric sensor based on TCNQ and cholinesterase. *Biosens. Bioelectron.*, 6, 2, 109-115, ISSN: 0956-5663

Larson, S. J.; Capel, P. D. & Majewski, M. S. (1997). *Pesticides in surface waters: distribution, trends, and governing factors*, CRC Press, ISBN-10: 1-57504-006-9, ISBN-13: 978-1-57504-006-6

Lee, H. S.; Kim, Y. A.; Chao, Y. A. & Lee, Y. T. (2002). Oxidation of organophosphorus pesticides for the sensitive detection by a cholinesterase-based biosensor. *Chemosphere*, 46, 4, (January, 2002) 571-576, ISSN: 0045-6535

Lei, Y.; Mulchandani, P.; Chen, W.; Wang J. & Mulchandani, A. (2004). Whole cell-enzyme hybrid amperometric biosensor for direct determination of organophosphorous nerve agents with p-nitrophenyl substituent. *Biotechnol. Bioeng.*, 85, 7, (March, 2004) 706-713, ISSN: 0006-3592, EISSN: 1097-0290.

Lei, Y.; Mulchandani, P.; Chen, W. & Mulchandani, A. (2005). Direct determination of p-nitrophenyl substituent organophosphorus nerve agents using a recombinant *Pseudomonas putida* JS444-modified Clark oxygen electrode. *J. Agric. Food Chem.*, 53, 3, (February, 2005) 524-527, ISSN: 0021-8561, EISSN: 1520-5118

Lei, Y.; Mulchandani, P.; Chen, W. & Mulchandani, A. (2006). Biosensor for direct determination of fenitrothion and EPN using recombinant *Pseudomonas putida* JS444 with surface expressed organophosphorus hydrolase. 1. Modified Clark oxygen electrode. *Sensors* 6, 4, (April, 2006) 466-472, ISSN: 1424-8220

Lei, C., Valenta, M., Sapiralli, K. P. & Ackerman, E. J. (2007). Biosensing paraoxon in simulated environmental samples by immobilized organophosphorus hydrolase in functionalized mesoporous silica. *J. Environ. Qual.*, 36, 1, (January-February, 2007) 233-238, ISSN: 0047-2425, EISSN: 1537-2537

Lin, Y. H., Lu, F. & Wang, J. (2004). Disposable carbon nanotube modified screen-printed biosensor for amperometric detection of organophosphorus pesticides and nerve agents. *Electroanalysis*, 16, 1-2, (January, 2004) 145-149, ISSN: 1040-0397, EISSN: 1521-4109

Liu, G.; Riechers, S.; Mellen, M. & Lin, Y. (2005). Sensitive electrochemical detection of enzymatically generated thiocholine at carbon nanotube modified glassy carbon electrode. *Electrochem. Commun.*, 7, 11, (November, 2005) 1163-1169, ISSN: 1388-2481

Luque de Castro M. D. & Herrera, M. C. (2003). Enzyme inhibition-based biosensors and biosensing systems: questionable analytical devices. *Biosens. Bioelectron.*, 18, 2-3, (March, 2003) 279-294, ISSN: 0956-5663

Majewski M. S. & Capel, P. D. (1995). *Pesticides in the atmosphere: distribution, trends, and governing factors*, CRC Press, ISBN-10: 1-57504-004-2, ISBN-13: 978-1-57504-004-2

Martorell, D.; Céspedes, F.; Martínez-Fàbregas, E. & Alegret, S. (1994). Amperometric determination of pesticides using a biosensor based on a polishable graphie-epoxy biocomposite. *Anal. Chim. Acta*, 290, 3, (May, 1994) 343-348, ISSN: 0003-2670

Martorell, D.; Céspedes, F.; Martínez-Fàbregas, E. & Alegret, S. (1997). Determination of organophosphorus and carbamate pesticides using a biosensor based on a polishable, 7,7,8,8-tetracyanoquino – dimethane - modified, graphite - epoxy biocomposite. *Anal. Chim. Acta,* 337, 3, (January, 1997) 305-313, ISSN: 0003-2670

Marty, J.-L.; Mionetto, N. & Rouillon, R. (1992). Entrapped enzymes in photocrosslinkable gel for enzyme electrodes. *Anal. Lett.,* 25, 8, 1389-1398, ISSN: 0003-2719, EISSN: 1532-236X

Marty, J.-L.; Mionetto, N.; Noguer, T.; Ortega, F. & Roux, C. (1993). Enzyme sensors for the detection of pesticides. *Biosens. Bioelectron.,* 8, 6, 273-280, ISSN: 0956-5663

Marty, J.-L.; Mionetto, N.; Lacorte, S. & Barceló, D. (1995). Validation of an enzymatic biosensor with various liquid chromatographic techniques for determining organophosphorus pesticides and carbaryl in freeze-dried waters. *Anal. Chim. Acta,* 311, 3, (August, 1995) 265-271, ISSN: 0003-2670

Matsumura, F. (1980). *Toxicology of insecticides,* Plenum Press, ISBN-10: 0-306-30787-1, ISBN-13: 978-0-306-30787-4, New York

Mazzei, F.; Botré, F. & Botré, C. (1996). Acid phosphatase/glucose oxidase-based biosensors for the determination of pesticides. *Anal. Chim. Acta,* 336, 1-3, (December, 1996) 67-75, ISSN: 0003-2670

Mulchandani, A.; Mulchandani, P.; Kaneva, I. & Chen, W. (1998). Biosensor for direct determination of organophosphate nerve agents using recombinant *Escherichia coli* with surface-expressed organophosphorus hydrolase. 1. Potentiometric microbial electrode. *Anal. Chem.,* 70, 19, (October, 1998) 4140-4145, ISSN: 0003-2700, EISSN: 1520-6882

Mulchandani, A.; Mulchandani, P.; Chen, W.; Wang, J. & Chen, L. (1999). Amperometric thick-film strip electrodes for monitoring organophosphate nerve agents based on immobilized organophosphorus hydrolase. Anal. Chem., 71, 11, (June, 1999) 2246-2249, ISSN: 0003-2700, EISSN: 1520-6882

Mulchandani, A.; Chen, W.; Mulchandani, P.; Wang, J. & Rogers, K. R. (2001a). Biosensors for direct determination of organophosphate pesticides. *Biosens. Bioelectron.,* 16, 4-5, (June, 2001) 225-230, ISSN: 0956-5663

Mulchandani, P.; Chen, W. & Mulchandani, A. (2001b). Flow injection amperometric enzyme biosensor for direct determination of organophosphate nerve agents. *Environ. Sci. Technol.,* 35, 12, (June, 2001) 2562-2565, ISSN: 0013-936X, EISSN: 1520-5851

Mulchandani, P.; Chen, W.; Mulchandani, A.; Wang, J. & Chen, L. (2001c). Amperometric microbial biosensor for direct determination of organophosphate pesticides using recombinant microorganism with surface expressed organophosphorus hydrolase. *Biosens. Bioelectron.,* 16, 7-8, (September, 2001) 433-437, ISSN: 0956-5663

Mulchandani, P.; Chen, W. & Mulchandani, A. (2006). Microbial biosensor for direct determination of nitrophenyl-substituted organophosphate nerve agents using genetically engineered Moraxella sp. *Anal. Chim. Acta,* 568, 1-2, (May, 2006) 217-221, ISSN: 0003-2670

Munnecke, D. M. (1980). Enzymatic detoxification of waste organophosphate pesticides. *J. Agric. Food Chem.,* 28, 1, (January, 1980) 105-111, ISSN: 0021-8561, EISSN: 1520-5118

Nikol'skaya, E. B. & Evtyugin, G. A. (1992). Cholinesterases application in analytical chemistry. *Zh. Anal. Khim.,* 47, 8, 1358–1378, ISSN: 1061-9348, EISSN: 1608-3199

Neufeld, T; Eshkenazi, I; Cohen, E. & Rishpon, J. (2000). A micro flow injection electrochemical biosensor for organophosphorus pesticides. *Biosens. Bioelectr.*, 15, 5-6, (August, 2000) 323-329, ISSN: 0956-5663

Noguer, T.; Leca, B.; Jeanty, G. & Marty, J.-L. (1999). Biosensors based on enzyme inhibition: Detection of organophosphorus and carbamate insecticides and dithiocarbamate fungicides. *Field Anal. Chem. Technol.*, 3, 3, 171-178, ISSN: 1086-900X, EISSN: 1520-6521

Ovalle, M.; Stoytcheva, M.; Zlatev, R. & Valdez, B. (2009). Electrochemical study of rat brain acetylcholinesterase inhibition by chlorofos: kinetic aspects and analytical applications. *Electrochimica acta*, DOI 10.1016/j.electacta.2009.09.008, (in press), ISSN: 0013-4686

Periasamy, A. P.; Umasankar Y. & Chen S.-M. (2009). Nanomaterials-acetylcholinesterase enzyme matrices for organophosphorus pesticides electrochemical sensors: a review. *Sensors*, 2009, 9, (September, 2009) 4034-4055; ISSN 1424-8220

Prieto-Simón, B.; Campàs, M.; Andreescu, S. & Marty, J.-L. (2006). Trends in flow-based biosensing systems for pesticide assessment. *Sensors*, 6, 10, (October, 2006) 1161-1186, ISSN: 1424-8220

Quin, L. D. (2000). *A guide to organophosphorus chemistry*, Wiley-Interscience, ISBN-10: 0-471-31824-8, ISBN-13: 978-0-471-31824-8

Ricci, F.; Arduini, F.; Amine, A.; Moscone, D. & Palleschi, G. (2004). Characterisation of Prussian blue modified screen-printed electrodes for thiol detection. *J. Electroanal. Chem.*, 563, 2, (March, 2004) 229-237, ISSN: 0022-0728

Richins, R.; Kaneva, I.; Mulchandani, A. & Chen, W. (1997). Biodegradation of organophosphorus pesticides by surface-expressed organophosphorus hydrolase. *Nature Biotechnol.*, 15, 10, (October, 1997) 984-987, ISSN: 1087-0156, EISSN: 1546-1696

Rodriguez-Mozaz, S.; Marco, M.-P.; Lopez de Alda M. J. & Barceló, D. (2004). Biosensors for environmental applications: future development trends. *Pure Appl. Chem.*, 76, 4, 723-752, ISSN: 0033-4545, EISSN: 1365-3075

Sacks, V.; Eshkenazi, I.; Neufeld, T.; Dosoretz, C. & Rishpon, J. (2000). Immobilized parathion hydrolase: An amperometric sensor for parathion. *Anal. Chem.*, 72, 9, (May, 2000) 2055-2058, ISSN: 0003-2700, EISSN: 1520-6882

Schlecht, P. C. & O'Connor, P. F., (Eds.) (1994). *NIOSH manual of analytical methods*, 4th ed., DHHS (NIOSH) Publication 94-113

Skladal, P. (1991). Determination of organophosphate and carbamate pesticides using a cobalt phthalocyanine-modified carbon paste electrode and a cholinesterase enzyme membrane. *Anal. Chim. Acta*, 252, 1-2, (November, 1991) 11, ISSN: 0003-2670

Skladal, P.; Fiala, M. & Krejcí, J. (1996). Detection of pesticides in the environment using biosensors based on cholinesterases. *Intern. J. Environ. Anal. Chem.*, 65, 1-4, 139-148, ISSN: 0306-7319

Solé, S.; Merkoçi, A. & Alegret, S. (2003a). Determination of toxic substances based on enzyme inhibition. Part I. Electrochemical biosensors for the determination of pesticides using batch procedures. *Crit. Rev. Anal. Chem.*, 33, 2, 89-126, ISSN: 1040-8347, EISSN: 1547-6510

Solé, S.; Merkoçi, A. & Alegret, S. (2003b). Determination of toxic substances based on enzyme inhibition. Part I. Electrochemical biosensors for the determination of pesticides using flow procedures. *Crit. Rev. Anal. Chem.*, 33, 2, 127-143, ISSN: 1040-8347, EISSN: 1547-6510

Stoytcheva, M.; Zlatev, R.; Velkova, Z.; Valdez, B.; Ovalle, M. & Petkov, L. (2009). Hybrid electrochemical biosensor for organophosphorus pesticides quantification. Electrochimica Acta, 54, 6, (February, 2009) 1721-1727, ISSN: 0013-4686

Sužnjević, D. Ž.; Veselinović, D. S.; Vukelić, N. S.; Pavlović, D. Ž. & Nikolić, A. V. (1985). Investigation of the system butyrylthiocholineiodide-butyrocholinesterase by cyclovoltammetry and chronopotentiometry using inert working electrodes. *J. Serb. Chem. Soc.*, 50, 2, 83-88, ISSN: 0352-5139

Thévenot, D. R.; Tóth, K.; Durst, R. A. & Wilson, G. S. (1999). Electrochemical biosensors: recommended definitions and classification. *Pure Appl. Chem.*, 71, 12, 2333-2348, ISSN: 0033-4545, EISSN: 1365-3075

Tran-Minh, C. (1985). Immobilized enzyme probes for determining inhibitors. *Ion-Selective Electrode Rev.*, 7, 41-75, ISBN-10: 0-08-033201-3, ISBN-13: 978-0-08-033201-7

Tran-Minh, C.; Pandey, P. C. & Kumaran, S. (1990). Studies on acetylcholine sensor and its analytical application based on the inhibition of cholinesterase. *Biosens. Bioelectron.*, 5, 6, 461-471, ISSN: 0956-5663

Turdean, G.; Popescu, I. C. & Oniciu, L. (2002). Biocapteurs ampérométriques a cholinestérases pour la détermination des pesticides organophosphorés. *Can. J. Chem.*, 80, (March, 2002) 315-331, ISSN: 1480-3291

Van Emon, J. M., (Ed.) (2006). *Immunoassay and other bioanalytical techniques*, CRC Press, ISBN-10: 0-8493-3942-1, ISBN-13: 978-0-8493-3942-4, Boca Raton, London, New York

Vighi, M. & Funari, E. (1995). *Pesticide risk in groundwater*, CRC Press, ISBN-10: 0-87371-439-3, ISBN-13: 978-0-87371-439-6

Wang, J.; Krause, R.; Block, K.; Musameh, M.; Mulchandani, A. & Schöning, M. J. (2003). Flow injection amperometric detection of OP nerve agents based on an organophosphorus–hydrolase biosensor detector. *Biosens. Bioelectron.*, 18, 2-3, (March, 2003) 255-260, ISSN: 0956-5663

WHO/IPCS. (1986). *Organophosphorus insecticides: a general introduction (Environmental health criteria Series No 63)*, ISBN-10: 92-4-154263-2, ISBN-13: 978-92-4-154263-0, Geneva

Worthing, C. R. & Hance, R. J. (Eds). (1991). *The pesticide manual: A world compendium*, 9th ed., British Crop Protection, ISBN-10: 0948404426, ISBN-13: 9780948404429, Surrey UK

12

Neuropathy Target Esterase Biosensor

Devesh Srivastava[1], Neeraj Kohli[1], Rudy J. Richardson[2], Robert M. Worden[1], and Ilsoon Lee[1]
[1]*Department of Chemical Engineering and Materials Science, School of Engineering, Michigan State University,*
[2]*Toxicology Program, Department of Environmental Health Sciences, University of Michigan*
United States of America

1. Introduction

Neuropathy Target Esterase (NTE), is a membrane-bound protein found in neurons of vertebrates (Glynn, 1999; Atkins & Glynn, 2000; van Tienhoven et al., 2002; Li et al., 2003; Makhaeva et al., 2003; Kropp et al., 2004), has been shown to be necessary for embryonic development in mice, and is believed to be involved in cell-signaling pathways and lipid trafficking (Glynn, 1999).

NTE has serine esterase activity and can hydrolyze ester, peptide, and amide bonds. The nucleophilic serine residue (active site) of NTE attacks the carbonyl carbon atom of the substrate, forming a covalent acyl-enzyme intermediate, which is subsequently hydrolyzed. A consequence of this reaction mechanism is that the esterase activity of NTE is susceptible to covalent inhibition by organophosphorus esters (OPs) with which it forms an analogous phosphyl-enzyme intermediate.

Irreversible binding of some OP compounds to the active serine site results in a debilitating neural disease known as OP-induced delayed neuropathy (OPIDN) (Glynn, 1999). Signs of OPIDN include flaccid paralysis of the lower limbs, which becomes evident two to three weeks after exposure to neuropathic OPs. Recovery from this disease is usually poor, and there is no specific treatment. In addition, mutations in the NTE gene have been linked to motor neuron disease (Rainier et al., 2008).

Because NTE plays a central role in both chemically induced and spontaneously occurring neurological diseases, approaches that can help measure its esterase activity and inhibition are of tremendous scientific and commercial importance. Because NTE is difficult to produce for research purposes, research to study its esterase activity is typically done using a fragment of the NTE protein that contains the esterase activity and can be more easily produced. One such fragment, known as NEST, (Atkins & Glynn, 2000; Forshaw et al., 2001; Kropp et al., 2004) reacts with esters and inhibitors in a manner very similar to NTE.

Conventionally, the esterase activity of NTE (or NEST) is measured using two distinct steps. In the first step, a solution containing phenyl valerate is brought into contact with NEST or NTE protein solution, whose esterase activity reacts with a portion of the artificial substrate phenyl valerate to form phenol. In the second step, the concentration of phenol in the solution is determined either colorimetrically, in the presence of 4-amino antipyrine

(Kayyali et al., 1991), or electrochemically, in the presence of tyrosinase enzyme (Sigolaeva et al., 2001; Sokolovskaya et al., 2005). Tyrosinase converts phenol first to catechol and then to *o*-quinone, which can be measured electrochemically at an electrode (Makhaeva et al., 2003). The current generated by the electrode increases with the amount of *o*-quinone present, thus giving an indirect measurement of the amount of NTE esterase activity present during the first step. To test for esterase inhibition, this procedure is repeated both in the absence and presence of a putative inhibitor (e.g., an OP compound). A reduced signal indicates inhibition of the esterase activity. This method has the disadvantages of being slow, and requiring two steps, making it unsuitable for some important applications, such as high-throughput screening of compounds for NTE inhibition and continuous, on-line, environmental monitoring to detect chemical warfare agents that target NTE (Richardson et al., 2009). The present chapter reviews and extends our work on the first continuous, electrochemical biosensor for real-time, rapid measurement of NEST (or NTE) esterase activity. The biosensor was fabricated by co-immobilizing NEST protein and tyrosinase enzyme on an electrode using the layer by layer assembly approach by Decher (Decher, 1997). To our knowledge, this is the first time NEST has been immobilized in an active conformation on an electrode. Potential applications of this sensor include detecting the presence of chemical weapons that target NTE, screening industrial and agricultural OP compounds for NTE inhibition, studying the fundamental reaction kinetics of NTE, and investigating the effect of NTE mutations found in motor neuron disease patients on NTE's enzymatic properties. The same approach can be used for activitiy measurements of other serine hydrolases, such as acetylcholinesterase (AChE) and butyrylcholinesterase (BChE) (Kohli et al., 2007).

2. Experimental section

Materials

Thioctic acid, poly-L-lysine (PLL) (molecular weight ~ 15,000), tyrosinase (Tyr), sodium phosphate (monobasic and dibasic), ethylenediaminetetraacetic acid (EDTA), sodium chloride, 3-[(3-cholamidopropyl) dimethylammonio]-1-propanesulfonate (CHAPS) and isopropyl thiogalactoside (IPTG) were obtained from Sigma (St. Louis, MO). Ultrapure water (18.2MΩ) was supplied by a Nanopure-UV four-stage purifier (Barnstead International, Dubuque, IA); the purifier was equipped with a UV source and a final 0.2 μm filter.

NEST expression and purification

NEST was expressed and purified according to published procedures (Atkins & Glynn, 2000). Briefly, a DNA fragment encoding NEST was cloned into pET-21b vector, and the resulting expression vector was transformed into *E. coli* BL21 (DE3). An overnight culture of transformed *E. coli* was inoculated with M9 media containing ampicillin and grown in a fermentor. IPTG was added to the resulting cell culture after a day to induce the expression of NEST. The resulting cells were collected 4 h after induction by centrifugation and subjected to protein expression techniques. Briefly, 5 g of cell paste was suspended in 30 ml of PEN buffer (50mM sodium phosphate/0.3 M NaCl/0.5 mM EDTA, pH 7.8) containing 2% (w/v) CHAPS and tip sonicated four times. The cell lysate was centrifuged at 2000*g* for 30 min at 4°C, the supernatant was collected, and about 7 mL of supernatant was added to a mini column (volume 10 mL) containing 3 mL of Ni-nitrilotriacetic acid (NTA) resin. The mini column was rotated at room temperature for 20 min, centrifuged at 2000*g* for 20 sec and then the top solution was drawn off. The histidine-tagged NEST was eluted from the Ni-NTA resin using 10 mL of PEN buffer containing 0.3% (w/v) CHAPS and 0.3 M imidazole. The protein purity was determined using SDS-PAGE and protein concentration was determined using BioRad Dc protein assay kit. For long term storage, 25% (v/v) glycerol was added to the protein solution, which was then stored at -20°C.

Preparation of gold electrode for NEST biosensor

Tyrosinase is a copper-containing oxidase (Forzani et al., 2000; Coche-Guerente et al., 2001), which possesses two different activities, as illustrated in reaction 1.

$$\textbf{phenol} \rightarrow \textbf{catechol} \rightarrow \textit{o}\textbf{-quinone} + \mathbf{H_2O} \qquad (1)$$

The first step is referred to as the enzyme's hydroxylase activity (also known as cresolase activity) where phenol is hydroxylated by the aid of molecular oxygen to produce catechol. In the second step, known as the catecholase activity, the enzyme oxidizes catechol to o-quinone and is simultaneously oxidized by oxygen to its original form, with the production of water. The reaction product, o-quinone, is electrochemically active and can be reduced back to the catechol form at low applied potentials, as illustrated in reaction 2.

$$\textit{o}\textbf{-quinone} + \mathbf{2H^+} + \mathbf{2e^-} \rightarrow \textbf{catechol} \qquad (2)$$

We exploited these characteristics of tyrosinase to fabricate a NEST biosensor, capable of measuring the NEST's esterase activity and its inhibition, by co-immobilizing NEST and tyrosinase on a gold electrode using the layer by layer assembly approach.
The molecular architecture of the biosensor interfaces are shown schematically in Figure 1 (a) & (b). Two molecular self-assembly approaches, (a) layer-by-layer (LBL) assembly (Decher, 1997) and (b) tethered lipid bilayer membranes (tBLM) (Kohli et al., 2006), were utilized in constructing nanostructured NEST biosensors. Gold electrodes cleaned in piranha solution were dipped in a 5 mM solution of thioctic acid in ethanol for 30 min. The electrodes were washed with ethanol, dried under nitrogen and dipped in PLL solution for 45 min. The PLL solution was prepared by adding 12 mg of PLL in 50 mL of 20 mM phosphate buffer (pH 8.5). The electrodes were then rinsed with water and dipped in an aqueous solution of tyrosinase (Tyr) (0.2 mg/ml) for 1 h. The last two steps were repeated varying number times to create PLL-Tyr bilayers with PLL being the topmost layer. The electrodes were washed with water and dipped in a solution of NEST protein (0.1 mg/ml) in 100 mM phosphate buffer, pH (7.0) for 1 h. The electrodes were then washed with water, dried under nitrogen and dipped in phosphate buffer (0.1 M, pH 7.0) for testing.

Preparation of phenyl valerate solution

To prepare phenyl valerate solution, 15 mg of phenyl valerate was dissolved in 1 mL of dimethylformamide (DMF), and 15 mL of water containing 0.03% (w/v) Triton-X100 was added slowly under vigorous stirring. For potential step voltammetry experiments, small aliquots of the resulting phenyl valerate micellar solution (5.286 mM nominal concentration) were added to the phosphate buffer to obtain the desired apparent concentrations.

Ellipsometry

Ellipsometric measurements were obtained with a rotating analyzer ellipsometer (model M-44; J.A. Woollan Co. Inc., Lincoln, NE) using WVASE32 software. The thickness values for

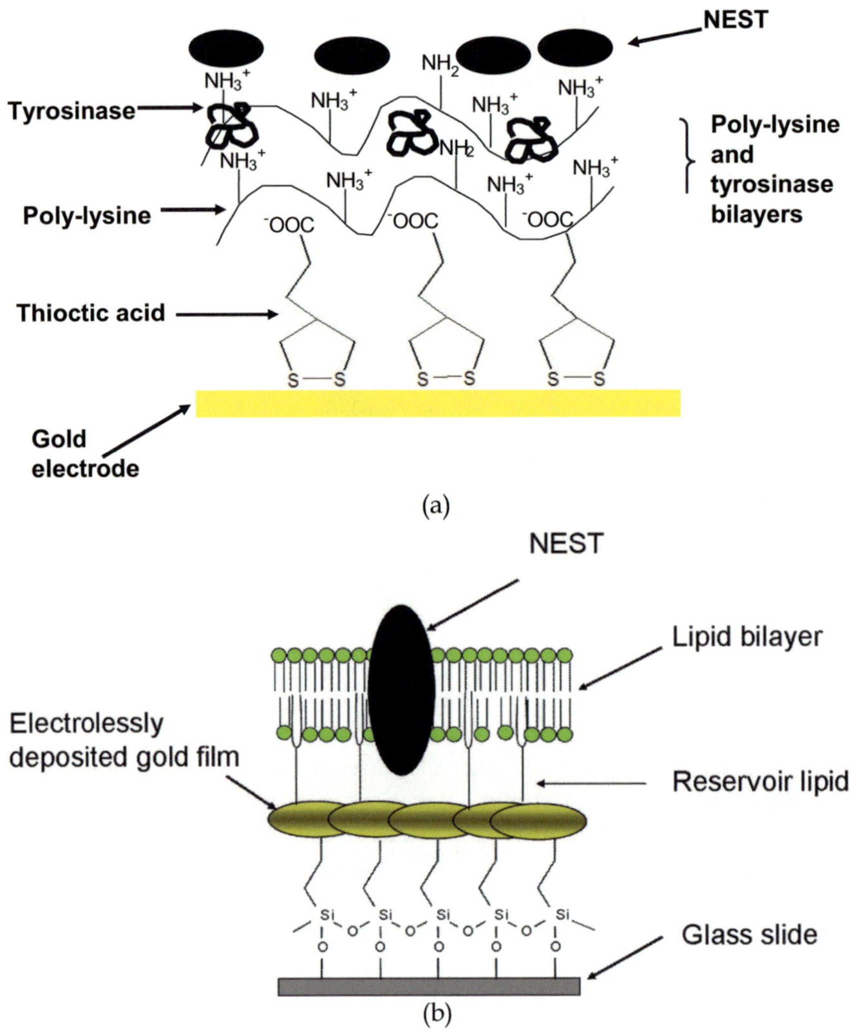

Fig. 1. Molecular architecture of the nanostructured NEST biosensors via (a) layer-by-layer (LBL) deposition scheme as adapted/reproduced with permission from (Kohli et al., 2007; Srivastava, 2008), and (b) tethered lipid bilayer membranes (tBLM) adapted with permission from (Kohli et al., 2006).

dried films were determined using 44 wavelengths between 414.0 and 736.1 nm. The angle of incidence was 75° for all experiments. Refractive indices of films containing PLL and proteins was assumed to be n=1.5, k=0. These optical constants compare well with those determined for 4 bilayer films consisting of poly-L-lysine and tyrosinase using ellipsometry.

Potential step voltammetry and other measurements

The electrodes (sensors) were maintained at a potential of -100 mV (vs Ag/AgCl reference electrode) using a BAS CV-50W electrochemical analyzer. The esterase activity of the NEST biosensor was monitored by measuring the output current for a variety of phenyl valerate concentrations, under stirred conditions. The NEST protein converts phenyl valerate to phenol, which gets converted to *o*-quinone by tyrosinase. The *o*-quinone gets reduced at the electrode's surface, resulting in the generation of current. The electroreduction of *o*-quinone produces catechol, which again gets converted to *o*-quinone by tyrosinase, thus amplifying the signal.

To measure inhibition of the esterase activity, a known quantity of phenyl valerate was added to the phosphate buffer (pH 7.0), under stirred conditions. After the stabilization of current, a known amount of NEST inhibitor was added, and the resulting drop in current was measured.

3. Results and discussion

We have tested both LBL assembly and tBLM methods to fabricate novel nanostructured NEST biosensors, as schemed in Figure 1 (a) & (b) (Kohli et al., 2006; Kohli et al., 2007; Srivastava, 2008). In this Chapter, we will focus on the former approach. The latter is briefly summarized as below. The phenyl valerate assay was used to confirm whether tBLMs could immobilize NEST in a functional conformation. Incubation of phenyl valerate with NEST-containing BLMs on gold resulted in the production of about 2 ± 0.19 nmol/min of phenol over an area of 1 cm^2. Incubation of phenyl valerate with NEST-DOPC liposomes in solution resulted in the production of 40 ± 1.2 nmol/min of phenol per μg of NEST protein. This result suggests the immobilization of approximately 50 ng/cm^2 of active NEST in tBLMs. To our knowledge, this is the first time NEST has been immobilized in an active conformation on a surface (Kohli et al., 2006).

3.1 Ellipsometry

Ellipsometry were used to confirm the deposition of different layers that make up the NEST biosensor. As shown in Figure 2, the thickness increase following the addition of the first

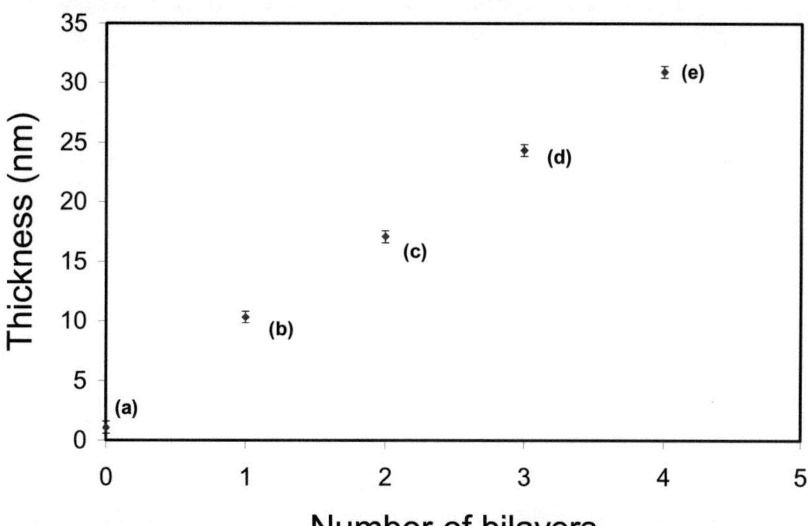

Fig. 2. Ellipsometric thicknesses after the successive addition of following layers: thioctic acid (point a), PLL-Tyr first bilayer (point b), PLL-Tyr second bilayer (point c), PLL-Tyr third bilayer (point d), and PLL and NEST final bilayer (point e). Reproduced with permission from (Kohli et al., 2007).

PLL and Tyr bilayer was approximately 9.3 ± 0.4 nm. The thickness increase for the next two PLL-Tyr bilayers was approximately the same and equal to 7.2± 0.3 nm. The thickness increase following the addition of final PLL-NEST bilayer was approximately 6.6 ± 0.3 nm.

3.2 Dependence of current response on working potential and pH

The various experimental parameters (such as pH and applied potential), which can affect the amperometric determination of phenyl valerate, were optimized. The effect of applied potential on the amperometric response of the sensor was tested in the range between 0.05

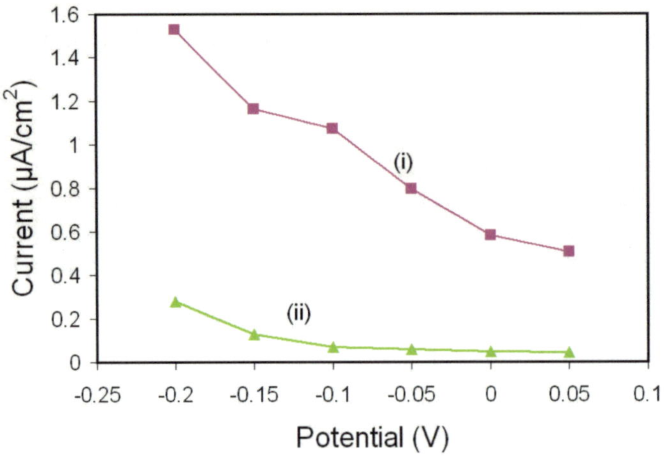

(a)

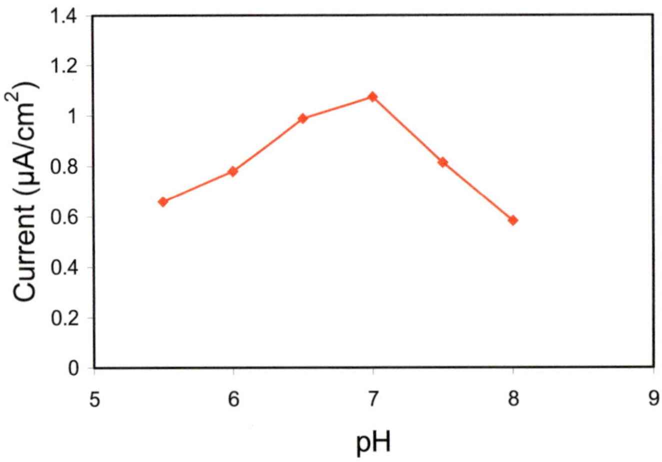

(b)

Fig. 3. (a) Effect of working potential on the response current of the enzyme electrode in 0.1 M phosphate buffer (pH 7.0) with (i) and without (ii) 12 µM phenyl valerate solution, in 0.1 M phosphate buffer at an applied potential of -0.1 V (vs Ag/AgCl). (b) Effect of pH on the response current of the electrode, in the presence of 12 µM phenyl valerate solution, in 0.1 M phosphate buffer at an applied potential of -0.1V (vs Ag/AgCl). Rreproduced with permission from (Kohli et al., 2007).

and -0.20 V. Figure 3a illustrates the signal and background for the whole range. The highest signal-to background ratio, was obtained at -0.1 V. At a working potential more negative than -0.1 V, higher signals were obtained, but the background current also increased distinctly. Therefore, a working potential of -0.1 V was used for further studies. The effect of pH was also studied in the pH range 5.5 to 8.0 in 0.1 M phosphate buffer at working potential of -0.1 V. As shown in Figure 3b, the response current attained a maximum value at pH 7.0. This pH was used for further studies.

3.3 Measurement of esterase activity using NEST biosensor

Figure 4a displays a typical current-time response under the optimal experimental conditions after the successive addition of aliquots of 4 μM phenyl valerate to the phosphate

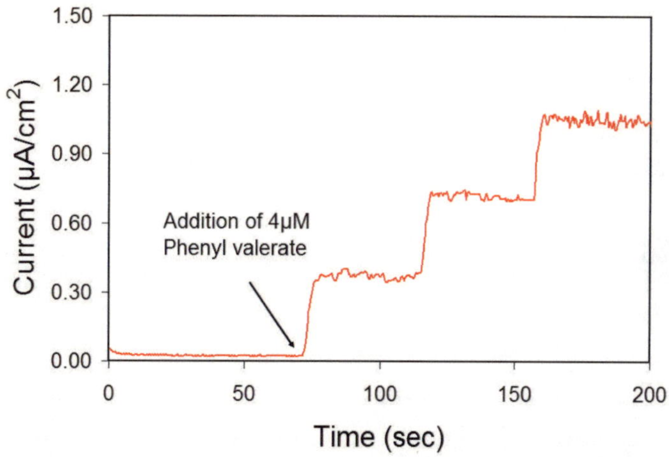

(a)

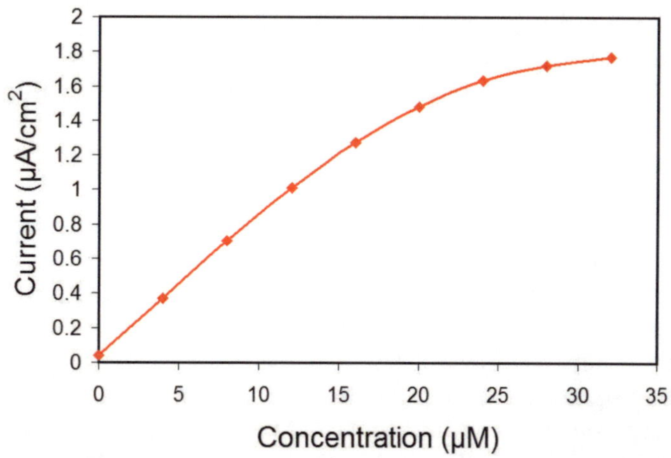

(b)

Fig. 4. (a) Current time response of the NEST biosensor to the addition of aliquots of 4 μM phenyl valerate, in 0.1 M phosphate buffer, pH 7.0, at an applied potential of -0.1V (vs Ag/AgCl). (b) Calibration plot. Reproduced with permission from (Kohli et al., 2007).

buffer. A well defined reduction current, proportional to the amount of phenyl valerate, was observed. The response time of the electrode was less then 20 seconds, due to the nano-scale thickness of the interface. The response to phenyl valerate was linear (r=0.991) in the range 0.5 μM to 12 μM, and it reached saturation at approx. 30 μM (Figure 4b). The limit of detection was 0.5 μM at a signal-to-noise ratio of 3. The reproducibility of the sensor was investigated at a phenyl valerate concentration of 4 μM; the mean current was approximately 348 nAcm-2, with a relative standard deviation of 9.9%. Figure 5 shows a control experiment which was done on an electrode containing only poly-L-lysine and tyrosinase bilayers. As expected, a relatively very small rise in steady state current was observed on the addition of phenyl valerate. The small rise can be attributed to the presence of a small amount of phenol produced due to auto-hydrolysis of phenyl valerate solution.

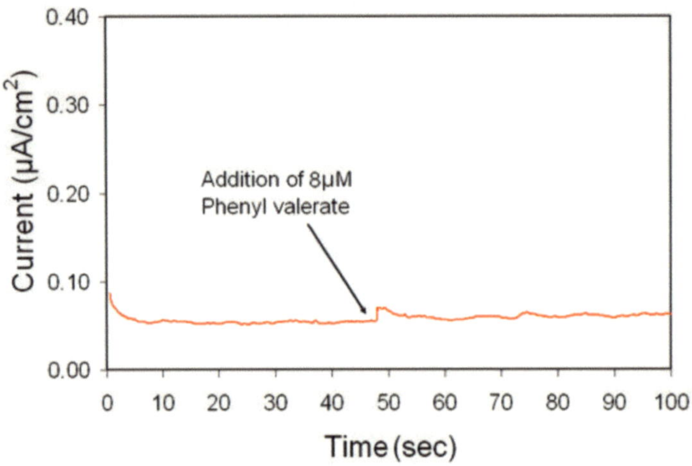

Fig. 5. Control experiment: Current time response on an electrode containing only tyrosinase. The electrode was assembled in exactly the same way as NEST biosensor, except that the final NEST layer was not deposited. The Reproduced with permission from (Kohli et al., 2007).

3.4 Inhibition of esterase activity

To measure inhibition of the esterase activity, an aliquot of phenyl valerate was added to the phosphate buffer. After a steady biosensor signal was obtained, a known quantity of phenylmethylsulfonyl fluoride (PMSF), a non-neuropathic compound previously shown to inhibit NEST (or NTE) esterase activity, was added to the phosphate buffer solution, and the resulting drop in current was measured. At very low concentration there was not an appreciable drop in signal as shown in Figure 6. As shown in Figure 7, however, a 20% (± 3%) decrease in response on the addition of 100 μM PMSF and a 70% (± 4%) decrease on the addition of 1000 μM PMSF was observed as shown in Figure 8. PMSF inhibition of NEST esterase activity reduces the amount of phenol and subsequently *o*-quinone produced. Therefore, less *o*-quinone gets reduced at the electrode surface, leading to a drop in current. These results suggest that the NEST biosensor can be used for concentration-dependent detection of NEST inhibitors.

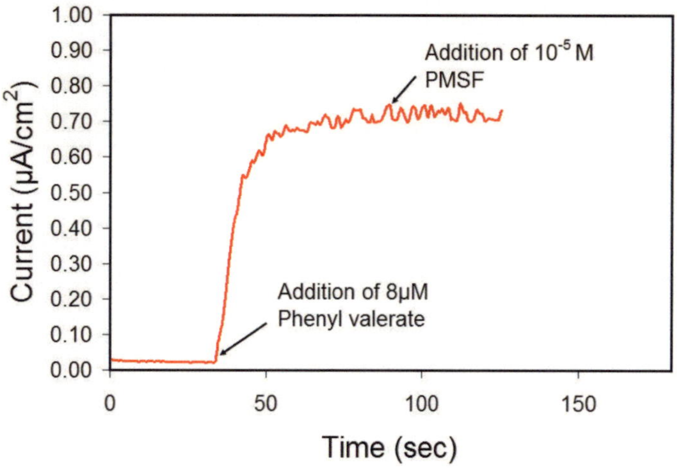

Fig. 6. Current time response of NEST biosensor to the addition of phenyl valerate in phosphate buffer (0.1 M, pH 7.0) to obtain a final phenyl valerate concentration of 8 μM followed by the addition of NEST inhibitor PMSF to obtain a final PMSF concentration of 10 μM. Reproduced with permission from (Kohli et al., 2007).

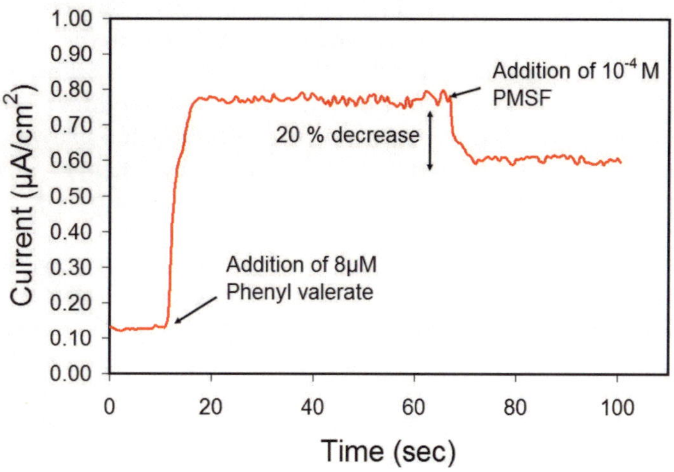

Fig. 7. Current time response of NEST biosensor to the addition of phenyl valerate in phosphate buffer (0.1 M, pH 7.0) to obtain a final phenyl valerate concentration of 8 μM followed by the addition of NEST inhibitor PMSF to obtain a final PMSF concentration of 100 μM. Reproduced with permission from (Kohli et al., 2007).

3.5 Higher-sensitivity NEST biosensor

NEST biosensor sensitivity could be increased by increasing the number of bilayers of PLL-Tyr to six. As discussed by Kohli et. al (Kohli et al., 2007) in the mathematical model developed for the NEST biosensor, the sensitivity can be improved more efficiently by increasing the amount of tyrosinase immobilized on the surface rather than increasing the

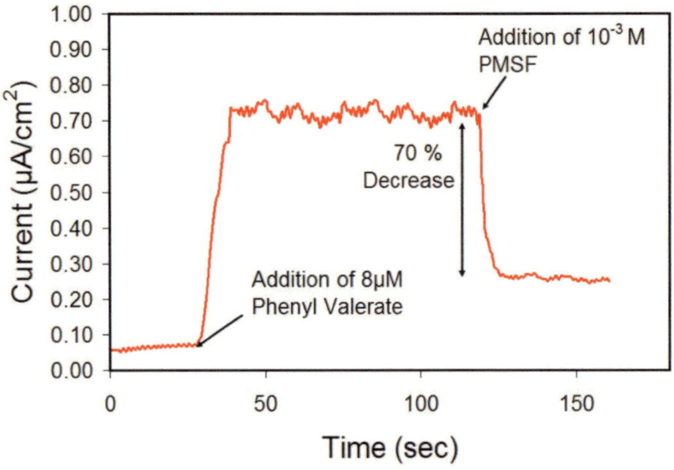

Fig. 8. Current versus time response of the NEST biosensor to the addition of phenyl valerate in phosphate buffer (0.1 M , pH 7.0) to obtain a final phenyl valerate concentration of 8 μM followed by the addition of the NEST inhibitor PMSF to obtain a final PMSF concentration of 1000 μM. Reproduced with permission from (Kohli et al., 2007).

amount of NEST. Hence, we developed a higher-sensitivity sensor by increasing the bilayers to six as the sensitivity of the catechol sensor was maximized with 6 bilayers (Srivastava, 2008). The same procedure used previously for the NEST biosensor was followed to fabricate the higher-sensitivity biosensor. The gold electrode was first modified with thioctic acid followed by the deposition of PLL-Tyr bilayers. After addition of 6 bilayers a layer of NEST was added. The sensor was tested for NEST activity by phenyl valerate assay. The sensitivity went up to 847 ± 158 nA cm-2μM-1 for the addition of phenyl valerate. The plot for phenyl valerate is shown in Figure 9. NEST inhibition was also done by addition of 100 μM and 1mM of PMSF. The decrease in current was the same as observed with 3 bilayers of NEST. The plots for inhibition of NEST on 6 bilayers of PLL-Tyr are shown in Figures 10 and 11 for PMSF concentrations of 100 μM and 1 mM, respectively. There was no remarkable decrease in current with 10 μM addition of PMSF (data not shown). Hence, a higher-sensitivity NEST biosensor can be obtained by increasing the amount of tyrosinase on the interface. It also implies that better sensors can be prepared with marginal increment to cost as tyrosinase is commercially available and can be easily deposited onto the electrode by using LBL deposition.

3.6 Significance of NEST biosensor

This new biosensor approach to measuring NEST esterase activity and its inhibition can in principle easily be extended to full length NTE. The approach offers several advantages over the old two step method. First, it requires only a single step to measure NEST (or NTE) esterase activity. Because the NEST esterase activity is co-immobilized with tyrosinase on the sensor interface, the presence of phenyl valerate triggers sequential reactions that result in an electrical signal. Second, the nanometer-scale thickness of layers in the sensing interface provides a very short diffusion path giving a rapid response time (less than 10 seconds). Third, the biosensor is suitable for continuous, real-time measurements of esterase

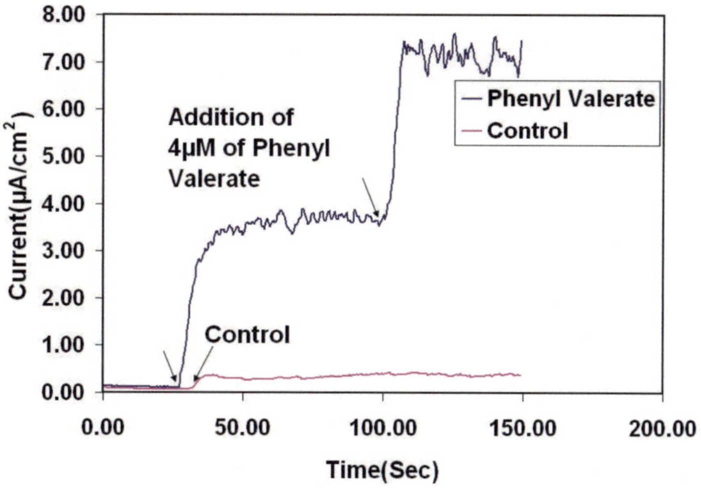

Fig. 9. Current versus time response of the higher-sensitivity NEST biosensor with 6 bilayers of PLL-Tyr underneath the NEST layer. The sensor was tested in phosphate buffer (0.1M) with electrode maintained -0.1V vs Ag/AgCl reference electrode. For the control the electrode was prepared in exactly the same manner but the NEST layer was not added. Reproduced with permission from (Srivastava, 2008).

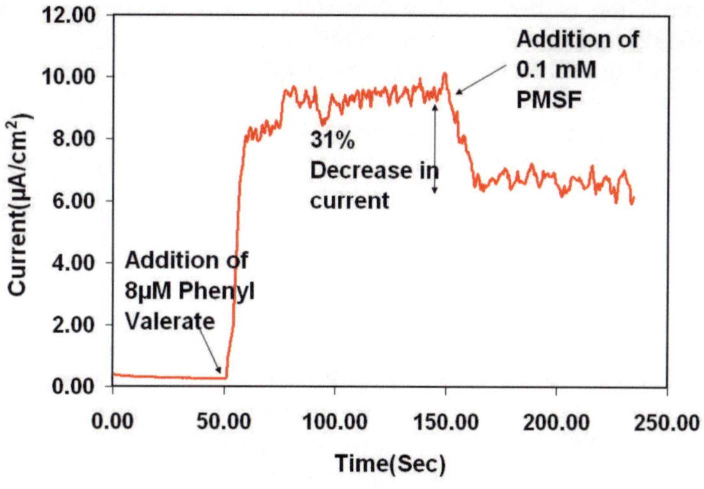

Fig. 10. Current response of the higher-sensitivity NEST biosensor with 6 layers of PLL-Tyr followed by inhibition of NEST by addition of 0.1 mM PMSF. First phenyl valerate was added to get the final substrate concentration of 8 µM in bulk solution. The current response was allowed to achieve steady state before addition of an aliquot of PMSF to get a final inhibitor concentration of 0.1 mM. Reproduced with permission from (Srivastava, 2008).

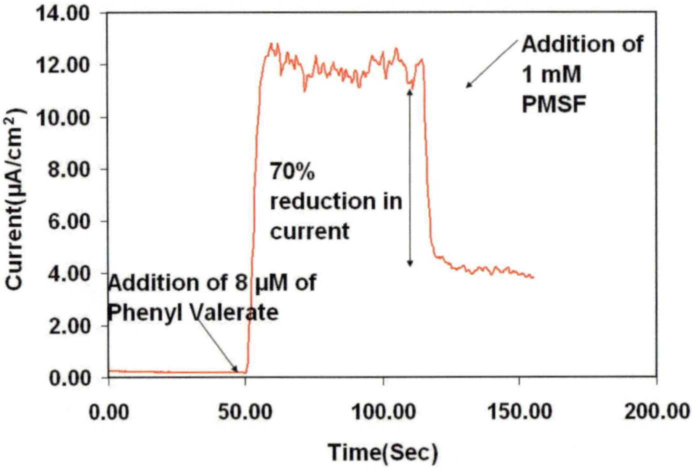

Fig. 11. Current response of the higher-sensitivity NEST biosensor with 6 layers of PLL-Tyr and followed by inhibition of NEST by addition of 1 mM PMSF. First phenyl valerate was added to get the final substrate concentration of 8 μM in bulk solution. The current response was allowed to achieve steady state before addition of an aliquot of PMSF to get a final inhibitor concentration of 1 mM. Reproduced with permission from (Srivastava, 2008).

activity. Fourth, the biosensor is designed to achieve signal amplification via recycling of *o*-quinone to catechol, thus increasing the sensitivity of the sensor. Fifth, the biosensor interface is generated by flexible, layer-by-layer (LBL), molecular self-assembly methods that would allow it to be assembled on electrodes inside microfluidic channels, thus enabling the production of high-density biosensor arrays consisting of various esterases (e.g., AchE and BchE) for high-throughput applications.

This combination of desirable properties makes this interface well suited for important applications, including studying the kinetic properties of esterases such as NEST protein, high-throughput screening of compounds for NEST (or NTE) inhibition and continuous, on-line, environmental monitoring to detect chemical warfare agents that target NEST (or NTE) and other esterases.

4. Conclusions

A biosensor has been developed that allows the activity of NEST to be measured continuously. The biosensor was fabricated by a layer-by-layer assembly approach to co-immobilize NEST and tyrosinase on a gold electrode. Ellipsometry provided evidence for the sequential assembly of the multiple layers that make up the interface. Constant potential voltammetry allowed NEST enzyme activity to be measured with a rapid response time ($<$ 10 s). The biosensor gave a concentration-dependent response to a known non-neuropathic (PMSF) NEST inhibitor.

5. Acknowledgment

This work was funded in part by the National Science Foundation (0609164, 0756703, and 0832730), the U.S. Army Research Office (DAAD19-02-1-0388), the University Research Corridor, and the MSU Foundation.

6. References

Atkins, J. & Glynn, P. (2000). Membrane association of and critical residues in the catalytic domain of human neuropathy target esterase. *Journal of Biological Chemistry* 275, 32, 24477-24483.

Coche-Guerente, L.; Labbe, P. & Mengeaud, V. (2001). Amplification of amperometric biosensor responses by electrochemical substrate recycling. 3. Theoretical and experimental study of the phenol-polyphenol oxidase system immobilized in Laponite hydrogels and layer-by-layer self-assembled structures. *Analytical Chemistry* 73, 14, 3206-3218.

Decher, G. (1997). Fuzzy nanoassemblies: Toward layered polymeric multicomposites. *Science* 277, 5330, 1232-1237.

Forshaw, P. J.; Atkins, J.; Ray, D. E. & Glynn, P. (2001). The catalytic domain of human neuropathy target esterase mediates an organophosphate-sensitive ionic conductance across liposome membranes. *Journal of Neurochemistry* 79, 2, 400-406.

Forzani, E. S.; Solis, V. M. & Calvo, E. J. (2000). Electrochemical behavior of polyphenol oxidase immobilized in self-assembled structures layer by layer with cationic polyallylamine. *Analytical Chemistry* 72, 21, 5300-5307.

Glynn, P. (1999). Neuropathy target esterase. *Biochemical Journal* 344, 625-631.

Kayyali, U. S.; Moore, T. B.; Randall, J. C. & Richardson, R. J. (1991). Neurotoxic Esterase (Nte) Assay - Optimized Conditions Based on Detergent-Induced Shifts in the Phenol/4-Aminoantipyrine Chromophore Spectrum. *Journal of Analytical Toxicology* 15, 2, 86-89.

Kohli, N.; Hassler, B. L.; Parthasarathy, L.; Richardson, R. J.; Ofoli, R. Y.; Worden, R. M. & Lee, I. (2006). Tethered lipid bilayers on electrolessly deposited gold for bioelectronic applications. *Biomacromolecules* 7, 12, 3327-3335.

Kohli, N.; Srivastava, D.; Sun, J.; Richardson, R. J.; Lee, I. & Worden, R. M. (2007). Nanostructured biosensor for measuring neuropathy target esterase activity. *Analytical Chemistry* 79, 14, 5196-5203.

Kropp, T. J.; Glynn, P. & Richardson, R. J. (2004). The mipafox-inhibited catalytic domain of human neuropathy target esterase ages by reversible proton loss. *Biochemistry* 43, 12, 3716-3722.

Li, Y.; Dinsdale, D. & Glynn, P. (2003). Protein domains, catalytic activity, and subcellular distribution of neuropathy target esterase in mammalian cells. *Journal of Biological Chemistry* 278, 10, 8820-8825.

Makhaeva, G. F.; Sigolaeva, L. V.; Zhuravleva, L. V.; Eremenko, A. V.; Kurochkin, I. N.; Malygin, V. V. & Richardson, R. J. (2003). Biosensor detection of neuropathy target esterase in whole blood as a biomarker of exposure to neuropathic organophosphorus compounds. *Journal of Toxicology and Environmental Health-Part A* 66, 7, 599-610.

Rainier, S.; Bui, M.; Mark, E.; Thornas, D.; Tokarz, D.; Ming, L.; Delaney, C.; Richardson, R. J.; Albers, J. W.; Matsunami, N.; Stevens, J.; Coon, H.; Leppert, M. & Fink, J. K. (2008). Neuropathy target esterase gene mutations cause motor neuron disease. *American Journal of Human Genetics* 82, 3, 780-785.

Richardson, R. J.; Worden, R. M. & Makhaeva, G. F. (2009). Biomarkers and biosensors of delayed neuropathic agents. *Handbook of Toxicology of Chemical Warfare Agents* R. C. Gupta. Amsterdam, Academic Press/Elsevier: 859-876.

Sigolaeva, L. V.; Makower, A.; Eremenko, A. V.; Makhaeva, G. F.; Malygin, V. V.; Kurochkin, I. N. & Scheller, F. W. (2001). Bioelectrochemical analysis of neuropathy target esterase activity in blood. *Analytical Biochemistry* 290, 1, 1-9.

Sokolovskaya, L. G.; Sigolaeva, L. V.; Eremenko, A. V.; Gachok, I. V.; Makhaeva, G. F.; Strakhova, N. N.; Malygin, V. V.; Richardson, R. J. & Kurochkin, I. N. (2005). Improved electrochemical analysis of neuropathy target esterase activity by a tyrosinase carbon paste electrode modified by 1-methoxyphenazine methosulfate. *Biotechnology Letters* 27, 16, 1211-1218.

Srivastava, D. (2008). Fabrication of nanostructures and nanostructure based interfaces for biosensor application. *PhD Dissertation*, Michigan State University, East Lansing, MI.

van Tienhoven, M.; Atkins, J.; Li, Y. & Glynn, P. (2002). Human neuropathy target esterase catalyzes hydrolysis of membrane lipids. *Journal of Biological Chemistry* 277, 23, 20942-20948.

13

Amperometric Enzyme-based Biosensors for Lowering the Interferences

Po-Chin Nien, Po-Yen Chen and Kuo-Chuan Ho
National Taiwan University
Taiwan

1. Introduction

1.1 Glucose, enzymes and mediators

Glucose becomes more and more important and popular research topics for medicine and biochemistry that monitoring biomarkers of chronic diseases, such as glucose to diabetes, bilirubin to jaundice and creatinine to kidney disease. Among many biomarkers, glucose is a common and an important biological species of human blood, found out normally in the range of about 4~8 mM. According to statistical information system of World Health Organization (WHO), the number of people with diabetes is estimated more than 180 million worldwide and it is likely to more than double by 2030. Besides, it is also estimated that 9% of all deaths worldwide are due to diabetes. Most notably, diabetes deaths are projected to increase by over 80% in upper-middle income countries between 2006 and 2015. Therefore, it is necessary to develop an efficient glucose biosensor for monitoring the glucose level of diabetics.

Glucose is an attractive target, because it is not only an important biomarker for diabetes but also a kind of fuel for biofuel cells. In other words, the glucose biosensor can work for detecting the glucose level and for the anode of the biofuel cell. The biofuel cells were intended to power cardiac assist devices, such as artificial hearts or cardiac pacemakers (Rao & Richter, 1974; Rao et al., 1974). For getting a good specific property, enzymes are widely applied as recognized molecules. Two kinds of enzymes with different redox potentials and electron transfer pathways are usually used to catalyze the glucose. One is the glucose oxidase (GOD) (Franke & Deffner, 1939) from *Aspergillus niger* and the other is glucose dehydrogenases (GDH) from *Acinetobacter calcoaceticus*. For GOD catalyst, the cofactor is flavin adenine dinucleotide (FAD) with a strong bond to apo-GOD, but the cofactor can be nicotinamide adenine dinucleotide (NAD) (Boguslavsky et al., 1995), FAD (Tsujimura et al., 2006) and pyrrole quinoline quinone (PQQ) (Duine et al., 1979) for GDH. As an example, the FAD-GOD was selected in this chapter as the recognized molecule. The FAD-GOD has an apparent formal redox potential of -0.048 V *vs.* standard hydrogen electrode (SHE) (Kulys et al., 2006) and it has a catalyzed rate of 5×10^3 glucose molecules per second (Willner et al., 2007a). The series catalytic mechanisms in a solution with oxygen are shown in Eqs. (1) and (2) (Warburg & Christian, 1932).

$$\text{glucose} + \text{FAD-GOD (oxidized, yellow)} \rightarrow \text{gluconic acid} + \text{FADH}_2\text{-GOD (reduced, colorless)} \quad (1)$$

$$\text{FADH}_2\text{-GOD (reduced, colorless)} + O_2 \rightarrow \text{FAD-GOD (oxidized, yellow)} + H_2O_2 \quad (2)$$

$$H_2O_2 \rightarrow 2H^+ + O_2 + 2e^- \quad (3)$$

$$H_2O_2 + 2H^+ + 2I^- \rightarrow 2H_2O + I_2 \quad (4)$$

$$2H_2O_2 + \text{4-aminoantipyrine} + \text{phenol} \xrightarrow{\text{peroxidase}} 4H_2O + \text{quinoneimine} \quad (5)$$

$$\text{FADH}_2\text{-GOD} + \text{mediator (oxidized)} \rightarrow \text{FAD-GOD} + \text{mediator (reduced)} \quad (6)$$

The glucose concentrations can be determined indirectly by the consumption of O_2 or the further reaction of H_2O_2. For example, the amperometric current can be collected by the oxidation of H_2O_2 directly (shown in Eq. (3)) (Chaubey & Malhotra, 2002), the reaction of H_2O_2 and I^- gave a I^-/I_2 potentiometry (shown in Eq. (4)) (Malmstadt & Pardue, 1961), and a spectrum change of the red dye (quinoneimine) was observed based on the reaction of Eq. (5) (Nien et al., 2008). However, the above sensing signals are sensitive to ambient oxygen concentration by any detection methods, so mediators are added into the system as shown by Eq. (6) instead of Eq. (2). The electron transfer from the redox center of $FADH_2$ to an electrode is very sluggish and hard, because the $FADH_2$ is embedded inside GOD by glycoprotein at a distance of about 1.3-1.5 nm (Hecht et al., 1993). The mediators not only facilitate the electron transfer from $FADH_2$ to electrodes but also lower the sensing potential, so the choice of the mediator is very important to the sensing performance. Cyclic voltammogram is a good electro-analytical method to obtain the properties of mediators and to find suitable mediators (Gilmartin & Hart, 1995; Nakaminami et al., 1997). The most used mediators for GOD with their formal potentials *vs.* standard calomel electrode (SCE) are partially listed in Table 1 (Chaubey & Malhotra, 2002). Generally speaking, the mediators can be classified into three kinds, including organic, inorganic and metal-organic (Heller & Feldman, 2008). In the organic mediators, methylene blue (Karyakin et al., 1993; Willner et al., 2007a; Willner et al., 2007b), quinone and its derivatives (Battaglini et al., 1994; Bourdillon et al., 1986; Cenas et al., 1983; Cosnier et al., 1998; Williams et al., 1970) have been studied for a long time. In the second kind, the main inorganic mediators are the hexacyano-complexes of iron (Dubinin et al., 1991; Jaffari & Turner, 1997; Shulga et al., 1994), cobalt and ruthenium, especially $Fe(CN)_6^{4-}$ is widely used in commercial glucose strips. In the final category, the metal-organic mediators cover ferrocene (Hendry et al., 1993; Luong et al., 1994), ferrocenemethanol (Bourdillon et al., 1995; Yang et al., 2003; Zhang et al., 2005; Zhang et al., 2006b; Zhao & Wittstock, 2005), ferrocenecarboxylic acid (Chen et al., 2002; Kohma et al., 2007; Tian & Zhu, 2002), Os-complex (Mano et al., 2005; Mao et al., 2003; Zakeeruddin et al., 1992) and so on. Besides, Wang et al. reported that the multi-walled carbon nanotubes

Mediators	Formal potentials (mV *vs.* SCE)
1,1-dimethyl ferrocene	100
ferrocene	165
ferrocene carboxylic acid	275
hydroxyl methyl ferrocene	185
benzoquinone	39
$[Fe(CN)_6]^{4-}$	180

Table 1. A partial list of the commonly used mediators for GOD.

(MWCNTs) can disturb the secondary structure of GOD and get close to its redox center to pass the electron directly without mediators (Wang et al., 2009).

1.2 The immobilization of enzymes and mediators

Among various detection methods, the amperometric enzyme-based biosensor probably is the best choice for biochemical analysis due to its good selectivity, high sensitivity, rapid response, convenient measurement, miniature size, and reproducible results (Hamdi et al., 2006). In order to reuse the expensive recognized biomolecules, the enzyme has to be immobilized on the electrode. In 1972, the company of Yellow Spring Instrument in America manufactured the first commercial glucose biosensor according to the prototype of the enzyme-immobilized electrode reported by Clark and Lyons (Clark & Lyons, 1962). In the following decades, the immobilization of enzyme became a key issue in developing the enzyme-based biosensor. Generally speaking, the immobilized methods (Cunningham, 1998) of enzyme include adsorption (Chu et al., 2007; Ekanayake et al., 2007), entrapment (Ngounou et al., 2007; Seo et al., 2007), cross-linking (Akyilmaz & Yorganci, 2007) and covalent bonding (Lin et al., 2007a; Seo et al., 2007). For adsorption, the enzyme was attached on the electrode by the attractive force of hydrogen bonds or opposite charges, such as nylon (Gamati et al., 1991) and ion exchange resin (Zhujun & Seitz, 1986), but it did not form a good adhesive force between biomolecules and a transducer. The enzyme also can be entrapped in a matrix, such as sol-gel (Lin et al., 2007b), Nafion® (Bogdanovskaya et al., 1997) and a conducting polymer (Brahim et al., 2001; Singh et al., 2004). The cross-linking and covalent bonding methods must be carried out by specific functional groups to link together, such as $-NH_2$ and $-COOH$ groups (Battaglini et al., 2000; Tamiya et al., 1990) or cross-linking agents (Tamiya et al., 1990). In addition, there are other methods used to immobilize the enzyme on the electrodes by thermal inkjet printing (Setti et al., 2005) or by enzyme-linked-immunosorbent-assay (ELISA) (Sehr et al., 2001). Among all methods, entrapment is considered to be one of the most attractive and popular methods to grasp the biomolecules. The electrochemical devices made by different conducting polymers entrapping recognized biomolecules have been reported extensively (Habermuller & Schuhmann, 1998; Rahman et al., 2004; Selampinar et al., 1997), because their major advantages (Cosnier, 1999) are that polymer film can be polymerized with immobilizing enzyme in one step, and the film thickness can be controlled easily by adjusting capacity. The most common polymers used as matrixes to entrap enzyme are polyaniline (Borole et al., 2004), polythiophene, polypyrrole and its derivatives (Trojanowicz et al., 1995).

In addition to enzymes, the mediators should be immobilized in the same matrix for biosensors or biofuel cells. However, the immobilization of mediators is more difficult than that of enzyme, because the mediators usually suffer from the leakage of small molecules, water-insoluble. In the literatures reported, the covalent method is a more effective way to stabilize the mediators on the electrode. For example, the mediators were linked on the MWCNTs (Qiu et al., 2009), the polymer matrix (Himuro et al., 2009) or even the enzyme directly (Wu et al., 2008). Moreover, the mediator was linked with the electrode and the redox center of enzyme for increasing the efficiency of electron transfer from enzymes to the external circuit through mediators (Zayats et al., 2008). Qiu et al. (Qiu et al., 2007) proposed that the small molecules, mediators, were linked on the large molecules, Fe_3O_4@SiO_2 nanoparticles, and afterward the matrix entrapped the enzyme and the nanoparticles at the same time.

1.3 Challenges

In the aspect of clinical diagnosis, the selectivity is the most major concern. For the amperometric enzyme-based biosensor which is the subject of this chapter, the challenges are how to lower the interference signals and get a precise value of glucose level in real samples. There are many oxidation-favored species in whole blood resulting in extra amperometric sensing signals, and it is a major problem of selectivity especially for electrochemical sensing.

In order to eliminate this factor, a cationic exchange membrane (Nafion®) was the most common and easy way to put outside the electrode and this can prevent the negatively-charged interfering species, such as ascorbic acid, from reaching the surface of the electrode (Chen et al., 2009; Mailley et al., 2000; Wu et al., 2002; Zhang et al., 1994). But, the Nafion® film raised the resistance of ion-transport, in which, the response time may be increased. Another way to eliminate the interference effect is to set a pre-reaction zone on the upstream of the major sensing section. For example, L-ascorbate oxidase was immobilized in the front section of the channel (Kurita et al., 2002) to catalyze the ascorbic acid, but the other interferences passing to the electrode may still result in noises. Besides, for an electrochemical system, a new way to decrease the interferences is by means of applying different potentials for targets and interfered species. In previous study (Yuan et al., 2005), two different potentials were applied at the two working electrodes attached to scanning electrochemical microscopy (SECM) system where one was at low potential (0.5 V) on the substrate of glucose oxidase modified electrode and the other was at high potential (0.7 V) on the tip of bare platinum. Therefore, the oxidation-favored species reacted on the substrate electrode at low potential and the glucose can be catalyzed by the enzyme-modified electrode to produce hydrogen peroxide. Afterward, the H_2O_2 was oxidized again on the tip of the electrode when the gap between tip and substrate electrodes was small (11 µm). Based on the similar idea, Jia et al. (Jia et al., 2008; Jia et al., 2007) proposed the probe-in-tube microdevice for eliminating the interference by the tube and detecting the target by the enzyme immobilized probe.

2. Reviews and motivations

In the past decade, the technique of Micro-Electro-Mechanical-Systems (MEMS) has become more and more popular for fabricating sensor chips. Due to the recent development in biotechnology, bio-MEMS is widely incorporated into the microfluidic devices in biosensors with the recognized biomolecules. The sensing chips integrate the steps of sampling, reaction, separation and detection on a chip (Richter et al., 2002). Nevertheless, they miniature the size and have the properties of fast response, less sample and low cost (Auroux et al., 2002) and this kind of sensing chip is also called Lab-on-a-chip. For example, the biosensors based on the field effect transistor (FET) made by MEMS immobilize anti-PSA on the carbon nanotubes (CNTs) (Kojima et al., 2005), liquid-chromatography-based biochip detects peptide mixture (Xie et al., 2005), and the biochip combines PCR-based DNA amplification and electrochemical detection (Lee et al., 2003) have been reported. Other few examples include antibody-based chips for determining protein isoform (Loonberg & Carlsson, 2006), liquid-chromatography-based chips for detecting peptide mixture (Xie et al., 2005), and electrophoresis-based chips for sensing catechol and dopamine (Schoning et al., 2005). Moreover, there are many choices for the materials of the microchannel, such as poly(dimethylsiloxane) (PDMS) (McDonald et al., 2000), poly(methyl-methacrylate)

(PMMA) (Ford et al., 1998) and polycarbonate (PC) (Liu et al., 2001) … etc. Among this, PDMS offers many advantages, including outstanding elasticity, pervious to light, good bio-compatible, good mechanical stability and convenient to be fabricated, and it can be used not only for the channel stamp but also for the gas-pump (Unger et al., 2000) and gas-valve (Hosokawa & Maeda, 2000). The PDMS stamp of channel is prepared with an air section between two layers. By filling and releasing gas to the air sections inside, the lower PDMS layer of channel can close and open the fluidic way in the micro-channel as a valve. Further, the fluid can be moved by gas-pump which is operated by three or more air sections in series filled and released continuously.

In the aspect of the electrodes on the MEMS-based biochip, the interdigitated ultramicroelectrode arrays (IDUAs) are usually used as they offer several advantages, including low ohmic drop (iR drop), high response time, enhanced sensitivity and increased signal-to-noise ratio (S/N ratio). The redox cycle of the species in IDUA was proposed by Bard et al. in 1986 (Bard et al., 1986). Further applications using IDUA (Fiaccabrino et al., 1998; Sheppard et al., 1996) and the search for the parameters of IDUA (Min & Baeumner, 2004) also have been reported. Additionally, there is another new way to increase the sensitivity up to 50 times by nanopores (Muller et al., 2007). The metal-insulator-metal electrode was created with many porous caves formed by nanoparticles then etched these caves to form cylindrical holes by plasma in CF4, so the porous electrode can achieve electrochemical redox cycles in each hole vertically.

Yamato et al. (Yamato et al., 1995), firstly demonstrated that a polythiophene derivative, poly(3,4-ethylenedioxythiophene) (PEDOT), has a better long-term electrochemical stability than that of polypyrrole, and the good stability of the PEDOT was also confirmed by other researchers (Kros et al., 2005; Lerch et al., 1998). They all show that the PEDOT is a suitable material for electrochemical biosensor, so it was mainly acted as the matrix to entrap the enzyme in the studies. According to the literatures, PEDOT film not only can entrap glucose oxidase (Fabiano et al., 2002; Nien et al., 2006) or polyphenol oxidase (Vedrine et al., 2003) to fabricate a specific biosensor, but also detect single strand DNA directly (Krishnamoorthy et al., 2004).

In this chapter, two systems were reviewed to cover a good interference-independent glucose biosensor. One (system A) was designed that a three-electrode pattern was fabricated on the glass substrate by combining the technique of MEMS and covering a microchannel by the PDMS to form a sensing chip, thus the biochip worked in a flow system with the advantages of miniature, reuse, less injecting sample and continuous operation. Based on the electrochemical method, the recognized biomolecules, glucose oxidase, was immobilized by the conducting polymer, PEDOT, on the working electrode of the biochip for determining the glucose concentration. The enzyme-immobilized working electrode directly senses the catalyzed product, H_2O_2, according to Eqs. (1)-(3). Besides, a second working electrode of bare platinum, which is located in the near front of the first enzyme-immobilized working electrode, is designed for eliminating the oxidation-favored interferences near the surface of electrode before the fluid in microchannel reaching the enzyme-immobilized working electrode by applying the same potential. The schematic of the whole microfluidic sensing system, both the lateral and vertical views, is illustrated in Fig. 1.

The other (system B) is that the all-in-one electrodes, which co-immobilize with the enzymes and the mediators based on layer by layer structure shown in Fig. 2. The first layer, the carbon paste which was coated on the flexible substrate of stainless steel (ssteel), was acted as an adsorbent layer for the mediator, p-benzoquinone (BZQ), by the hydrophobic force. The BZQ and GOD were drop-coated on the electrode in order and the entrapped matrix, PEDOT, was electropolymerized on the outer layer to prevent the leakage of mediators and enzymes. The all-in-one electrode has the advantages of flexible, workable in oxygen-independent solution, convenient, reusable, lower sensing potential and lower interference effect.

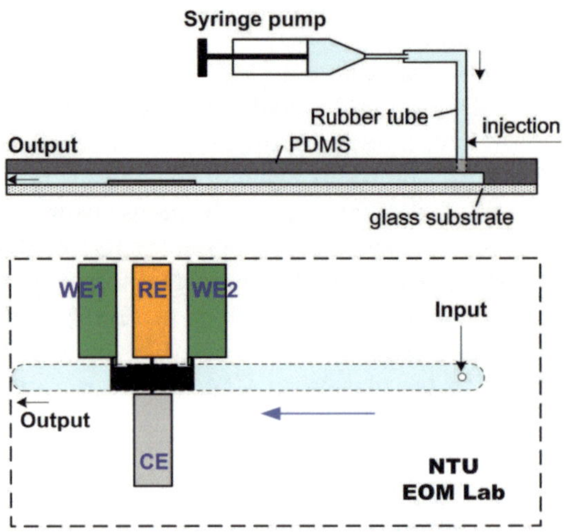

Fig. 1. The schematic of the whole system in operation for system A. (Nien et al., 2008)

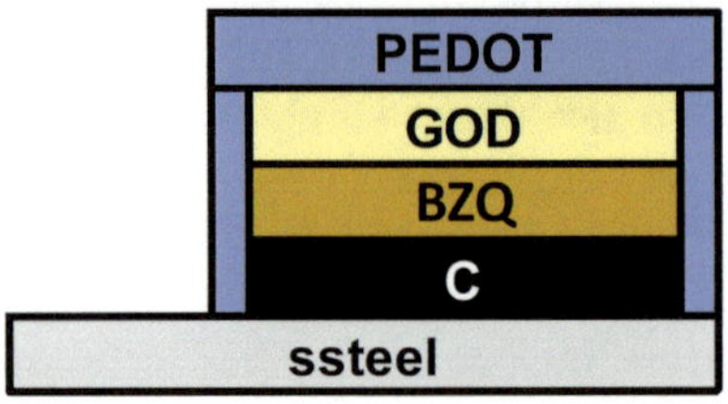

Fig. 2. The schematic of the layer by layer structure for system B.

3. Experimental

3.1 Chemicals and instruments

The target (or fuel), D-(+)-glucose, and the interferences, ascorbic acid (AA) (> 99%), uric acid (UA) (> 99%), dopamine hydrochloride (DA) and acetaminophen (AP) (> 99%), were purchased from Sigma. For the enzymes, glucose oxidase (GOD) (EC 1, 1, 3, 4) type VII-S from *Aspergillus niger*, and laccase (Lac) (EC 1, 10, 3, 2) from *Trametes versicolor* were purchased from Sigma and Fluka, respectively. For the mediators, p-benzoquinone (~ 98%, reagent grade) 2,2-Azino-bis(3-ethylbenzothiazoline-6-sulfonic acid) (ABTS) diammonium salt were purchased from and Aldrich and Sigma, respectively. The monomer, 3,4-ethylenedioxythiophene (EDOT), surfactant, polyethylene glycol (PEG, MW=20,000) and bacteriostat, sodium azide (>99.5%) were purchased from Aldrich, Merck and Sigma, respectively. The phosphate buffer containing monosodium phosphate monohydrate, disodium phosphate heptahydrate and potassium chloride (99.0~100.5%), were all purchased from Sigma. Besides, in system A, the positive photoresist, FH-6400, and the developer, FHD-5, were purchased from Fujifilm. The pre-polymer PDMS (Sylgard 184) and curing agent were from Dow Corning. The photolithographic equipments in clean-room are following: UV mask aligner (EVG 620) and inductively coupled plasma-reactive ion etching (ICP-RIE). The solution in the channel was pumped by a syringe pump (KdScientific, model 100). In system B, the flexible substrate was stainless steel SUS 301 and the membrane for biofuel cell was Nafion® 117 (thickness is 0.007 in). The de-ionized water (DIW) was used throughout the experiments. All electrochemical experiments, including CV and amperometric measurements were performed with a potentiostat/galvanostat (CHI 440 and CHI 900).

3.2 Fabrication of system A

First, the film mask with a resolution of 10,000 dpi was made by Taiwan Kong King Company according to the self-designed electrode shown in Fig. 3. All of the following steps were done by silicon planar technology in a clean-room environment. The glass wafer with a diameter of 4 in and a thickness of 1 mm was cleaned by acetone, water and N_2-purge orderly. For enhancing the adhesive force between photoresist and glass wafer, the wafer was coated with hexamethyldisilazane (HMDS) in advance by vapor priming. Then the glass wafer was covered with chemical positive photoresist (FH-6400) by spin-coating at 1,500 rpm for 30 s and hardened at 90 °C for 90 s on a hot plate. After soft baking, the wafer was selectively exposed through a UV mask aligner to UV light (12 s, 10 mJ/cm^2) with the first mask, and removed photoresist in the developer soup (FHD-5) for 12 s to form the pattern of the reference electrode. For the reference electrode, the metal layers of Cr, Au and Ag were deposited by sputtering in order, and the thicknesses of those are about 30, 90 and 360 nm, respectively. The layers of Cr and Au are served as buffer layers to enhance the adhesive force of silver on glass. The unnecessary metal layers were lifted off completely in the acetone solution by ultrasonic method. In the same process, the patterns of working and counter electrodes with the metal layers, 30 nm Cr and 100 nm Pt, were fabricated by the second mask. The working and counter electrodes are the designation of IDA with the same width (50 μm) of fingers and gaps, as shown in the insert of Fig. 3. The real geometric surface areas of working, counter, and reference electrode are 4.5, 9.75 and 1.3 mm^2 respectively.

The channel stamp was made by PDMS according to the mother mold of the silicon wafer. First, the silicon substrates were washed with acetone and sulfuric acid to remove any organic contaminants. All the substrates were then dried under a N_2 stream and used immediately after cleaning. Silicon wafers were coated with a 2 μm thick positive photoresist (FH-6400) by using a spin coater. They were pre-baked on a hot plate with a temperature of 90 °C for 90 s. The light exposure was followed for 12 s and developed for 12 s. Finally, silicon wafer was dry-etched by ICP-RIE for 100 μm deep and the patterns were transferred to the silicon mold. A fully mixed viscous precursor of PDMS and curing agent in the ratio of 10:1, was poured into the silicon master, pumped in a vacuum for a period of time to remove all bubbles, and then thermally cured at 60 °C in an oven for 3 hrs. After curing, the PDMS stamp could be peeled off from the silicon master. Finally, the PDMS and the glass wafer were bombarded by oxygen plasma at 50 W for 3 min to modify their functional groups of surfaces from hydrophobic to hydrophilic temporarily. Then the channel of the PDMS was covered and glued on the glass to form a sensor chip.

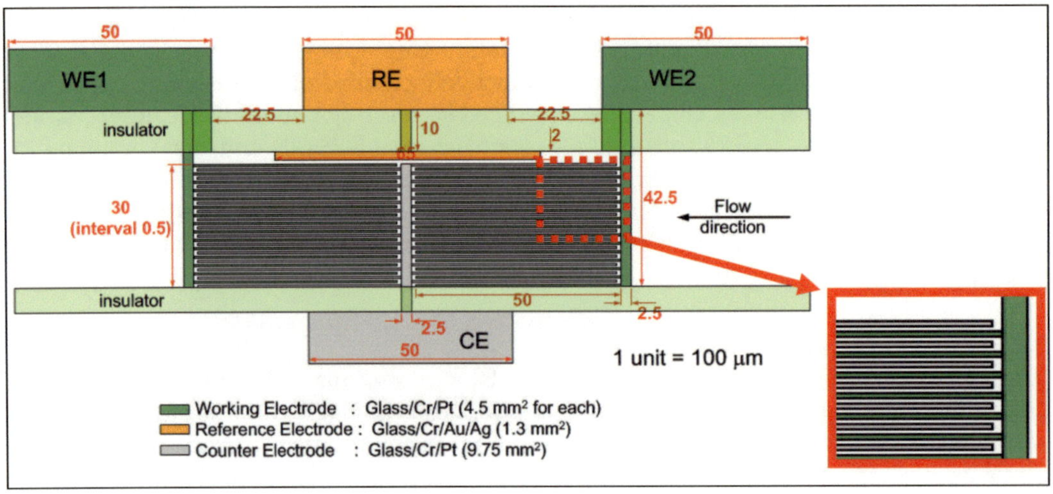

Fig. 3. The schematic of the microelectrode.

For the purpose of getting a more stable reference, the silver surface of reference electrode was modified to Ag/AgCl by chemical deposition. According to Eq. (7), the Ag surface was oxidized to form a thin layer of AgCl in 0.1 M $FeCl_3$ solution spontaneously for 1 hr. For the enzyme-modified working electrode, the conducting polymer, PEDOT, was prepared in a flow system and the other conditions are the same as described in our previous work (Nien et al., 2006). The PEDOT film was obtained by electropolymerization of EDOT with the sweeping potential from 0.2 to 1.2 V for 20 cycles at a flow rate of 5 ml/hr and it was used as a matrix to entrap the glucose oxidase for immobilization on "WE1" (in Fig. 3) in a 0.02 M PBS electrolyte containing 2,000 U/ml glucose oxidase and 0.3 M KCl. After electropolymerization, the 0.02 M PBS solution was allowed to flow in the channel for some time to wash out the residuals. The sensing chip was stored at 4 °C when not use.

$$Ag + Cl^- + Fe^{3+} \rightarrow AgCl + Fe^{2+} \qquad E^0_{reaction} = 0.55\ V \qquad (7)$$

3.3 Fabrication of system B

The substrate, ssteel, was cleaned in the alcohol and water by supersonic wave to remove the organic matter. Then the carbon paste was roll coated on the substrate with constant spacer and area of 1 x 1 cm^2, which is a large area comparing to literatures, and thermally cured in the oven at 130 °C for 2 hr to remove solvent. Afterward, the mediator, BZQ (50 mM) dissolved in dimethylformamide (DMF), and the GOD dissolved in water (5000 U/ml) were both dropped a volume of 40 μl on the ssteel/C electrode to dry in order. At last, the conducting polymer, PEDOT was electropolymerized on the outer layer of the prepared ssteel/C/BZQ-GOD electrode to prevent the leakage of GOD, in a pH 7 phosphate buffer solution containing 10 mM EDOT monomer and 0.1 mM non-ionic surfactant, PEG, by applying a constant potential of 1.2 V vs. Ag/AgCl/sat'd KCl for 50 s. Afterward, the ssteel/C/BZQ-GOD/PEDOT electrode was stored in a pH 7 PBS at 4 °C when not in use.

4. Results and discussions of system A

4.1 The sensing chip

In each 4-in glass wafer, two pieces of sensing chips (70 mm × 35 mm) were cut by a diamond cutter. The microelectrode arrays can be divided into four sections (mentioned in section 3.2) and the surface metal layer of the working, reference and counter electrodes are platinum, silver and platinum, respectively. The SEM pictures (not shown) indicated that the dimension of the interdigitated array was the same as that of the designed pattern. Finally, by covering the PDMS with a microfluidic channel of 100 μm height, the sensing chip was fabricated. Moreover, for getting a better stability of long-term operation, the surface of reference electrode was modified as Ag/AgCl by chemical deposition. The open circuit voltage (V_{oc}) of the Ag/AgCl is about 95 mV vs. SCE (commercial model) in the electrolyte of 0.3 M KCl and the variation between the two electrodes is less than 5 mV for a period of 2,500 s. It was approximately corresponding to the theoretical value of 102.9 mV based on the electrochemical theory.

When the potential of the first working electrode (WE1) was cycled between a potential range of 0.2 ~ 1.2 V at a scan rate of 0.1 V/s, the current for the first cycle increased at around 0.7 V due to the oxidation of the EDOT monomer. On electrooxidation, a radical cation of EDOT is produced which is transformed to a polymeric species via several follow-up reactions. However, the anodic current at higher potential (0.9-1.2 V) decreased with the cycle number, because the high potential may result in the partial degradation (Fabiano et al., 2002) or overoxidation of PEDOT film. In the 15th to 20th cycles, the CVs of polymerization were almost the same and this implies that the polymer film was not growing due to the resistance of polymer film. During the polymerization process, the PEDOT possesses positive charges, so the negatively charged glucose oxidase (pI=4.2) would migrate to the PEDOT surface at pH=7.4 (PBS) and be grabbed by the growing polymer chains. Besides, it is also an advantage of CV method that the enzyme has more time to diffuse to the polymer surface when the applied potential was swept to the cathodic direction in which the EDOT can't be polymerized. The immobilized enzyme was quantified as about 0.101 U/cm^2 by UV spectrophotometer after series chemical reactions in previous work (Nien et al., 2008).

4.2 The sensing performance

In Fig. 4, the flow injection data were obtained by applying 0.7 V at a flow rate of 10 ml/hr and each current pulse was resulted from different concentrations with an injecting volume of 30 μl. Besides, both the peak current and the charge capacity of each pulse can be collected as the sensing signal. However, the reproducibility in the peak currents was not good and hence the charge capacities were used for recording the sensing signal instead of current. The relationship obtained between the net charge capacities and the different glucose concentrations by applying a voltage of 0.7 V vs. Ag/AgCl on PEDOT modified enzyme electrode (WE1) with the same injecting volume of 30 μl at different flow rates is shown in Fig. 5. The linear regression falls from 1 to 10 mM, which includes the range of normal human blood, with a sensitivity of 157 μC cm^{-2} mM^{-1} (4.6 μA cm^{-2} mM^{-1} in current plot, which is not shown). The sampling time, the time taken from each injection of the sample to the pulse current returning approximately to the background level, was within 180, 100, 70 and 30 s at a flow rate of 5, 10, 20 and 50 ml/hr, respectively. Operating at a high flow rate had a faster response, but lost another important parameter, sensitivity. Hence the

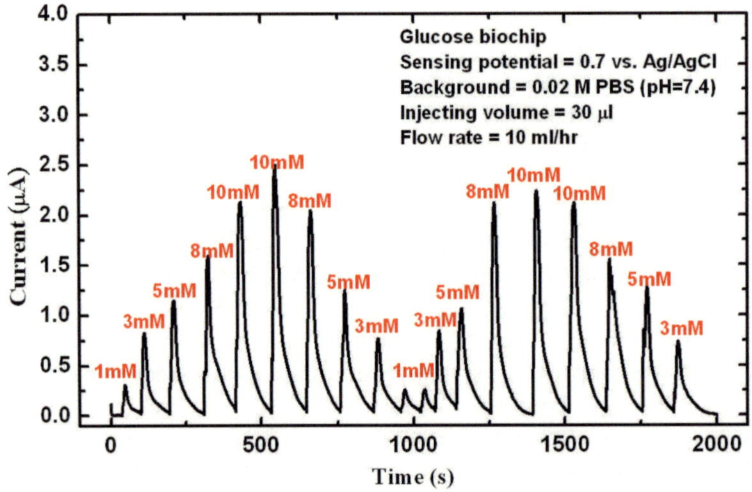

Fig. 4. The sensing signals of the biosensor in response to various glucose concentrations using flow injection analysis.

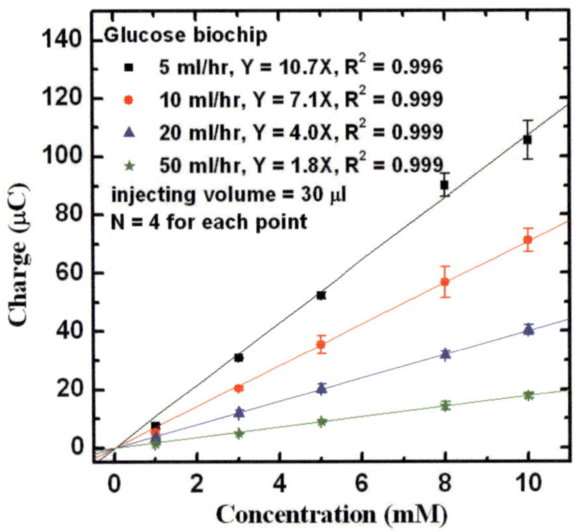

Fig. 5. The calibration curve based on charge at different flow rates.

proper flow rate was selected as 10 ml/hr by considering the performance. The response time and the recovery time, defined as the time taken for the current reaching of 95% of the steady-state level, are about 15 s and 35-75 s, respectively. For different concentrations of the samples, the response time is almost the same, but the recovery time varies with the concentration. The higher concentration of sample leads to longer recovery time, since the larger driving force of mass transport results in a broader concentration profile. Additionally, the limit of detection (LOD) based on signal to noise ratio equaling to 3 is 0.15 mM at 10 ml/hr.

Table 2 is a partial list of the amperometric GOD-based glucose sensors, obtained from the literatures based on PDMS chips. They used capillary electrophoresis to separate the interferences (Liu et al., 2006; Zhang et al., 2006a) and immobilized lactate oxidase to catalyst the ascorbic acid on the upstream (Kurita et al., 2002). Besides, the sensing chip (Huang et al., 2007) can not only detect glucose concentrations but also inject insulin automatically. In the aspect of sensing performance, the linear ranges almost covered the normal human range (3.5-8 mM), but system A provided fast response and recovery times. However, the limit of the detection was not as low as the others, and hence the applications may have some limitations.

References	Immobilized method	Sensitivity (μA cm^{-2} mM^{-1})	Linear range (mM)	Response time (s)	Recovery time (s)	LOD (μM)
(Zhang et al., 2006a)	adsorption	---	0-30	10	15	6.5
(Liu et al., 2006)	adsorption	0.0312	0.01-5	---	---	5
(Yamaguchi et al., 2002)	entrapment	8.67	0-20	50	---	-
(Kurita et al., 2002)	entrapment	0.0025	0.01-1	120	---	2.3
(Huang et al., 2007)	entrapment	0.0076	2-30	50	---	---
System A	entrapment	4.6	1-10	15	35-75	150

Table 2. Partial literatures of the amperometric GOD-based glucose sensors on PDMS chips.

4.3 The interferences effect and the monitoring of real sample

One of the most important problems to tackle for any practical application of amperometric biosensors is to minimize the effect of interfering substances possibly present in a real sample. For oxidase-based systems, reductants are the most severe interferences and among these ascorbate and uric acid (Navera et al., 1993; Vasantha & Chen, 2006) are two of the most considered. Moreover, well-separated voltammetric peaks were observed for dopamine and ascorbate anion at the PEDOT modified electrodes at 0.21 and 0.08 V, respectively (Matuszewski et al., 1990). Although the linear range covers the glucose level of normal human, the oxidation-favored interferences in blood, such as ascorbic acid (AA) and uric acid (UA), still raise the sensing currents at a high voltage of 0.7 V. To solve this, the pre-reaction section, "WE2" in Fig. 3, was designed to reduce the interference effect in this microsystem. Here, the bi-potential was applied simultaneously to both WE1 and WE2 by the bi-potentiostat of CHI 900. In the flow injecting analysis, when the samples were injected, the oxidation-favored substances near the boundary layer were oxidized at 0.7 V (vs. Ag/AgCl) on WE2. Consequently, the interferences near the boundary layer were partially eliminated to some extent before the analyte arriving to WE1. The electrode gap between WE1 and WE2 (0.25 mm) is designed to be very close so as to avoid the solution diffusing from the outside boundary layer into the inside layer. For a single-potential test on WE1, both 0.08 mM AA sample and a blend of 0.08 mM AA plus 10 mM glucose sample reached 31.3% and 145.5% of the sensing current obtained for 10 mM glucose, respectively. AA contributes a significant current to the total current on the PEDOT enzyme-modified electrode. In contrast, the sensing current of the blend sample reached 99.6% that of 10 mM glucose response in a bi-potential test. The result shows that the concentration of the oxidation-favored species in the sample was reduced appreciably. Therefore, it is concluded that the bi-potential configuration can reduce the interferences in a flow injection system and thereby improving the selectivity and specificity of an enzyme modified electrode towards glucose oxidation.

For the real sample test, three different methods were used to monitor the glucose concentration of the human blood. One was determined by a hospital, another was obtained by a handheld commercial product (EasiCheck blood glucose test strips) and the third was detected by this sensing chip. After the oxidation of the interferences on WE2, the reduced concentration of the interferences in the boundary layer can enhance the accuracy of glucose sensing for WE1. The results obtained from the three methods are shown in Table 3 and the percentages of the detecting error were calculated according to the value obtained from hospital as a standard. Moreover, the bias of the bi-potential (+13.6%) was much lesser than that of single-potential (+141%), and this confirms that the WE2 helps to eliminate the interference. For the commercial product, the average concentration of three tests was 4.77 mM and the bias was about +5% which is within the bias range (±20%) of the product prescription. Although the error of the bi-potential was acceptable grudgingly, it may be lowered further by increasing the active area of WE2.

<table>
<tr><th>Glucose biochip</th><th>Commercial product</th><th>NTU Hospital</th></tr>
<tr><td>Single-potential = 10.99 mM
(Bias = +141%)</td><td rowspan="2">4.77 mM
(Bias = +4.6%)</td><td rowspan="2">4.56 mM
(as a standard)</td></tr>
<tr><td>Bi-potential = 5.18 mM
(Bias = +13.6%)</td></tr>
</table>

Table 3. A summary of the detecting errors for a real sample tested against different methods.

5. Results and discussion of system B

5.1 The enzyme electrode

For the stable test of BZQ adsorbed inside the electrodes, it was under the sweeping potentials between -0.6 and 0.8 V for 100 cycles. With increasing cycle numbers, the peak currents of redox reaction were decreased to stable values after about 50 cycles (not shown). This implied that the electrodes can reach to a stable situation after the leakage of the weakly-adhesive BZQ. It showed that the first layer, carbon, was a good substrate for the adsorption of BZQ. For the third layer, the GOD dry-coated on the electrode may dissolve into the electrolyte while the step of electropolymerization. As a result, the immobilized amount of GOD can be quantified by the absorbance change of the electrolyte before and after polymerization. According to the UV spectrum (not shown) of the electrolyte at 280 nm, which is the maximum absorbent wavenumber for GOD, the leakage of GOD in the electrolyte was calculated to be about 132 U and the entrapped efficiency was about 33% for the electrode B. The immobilized amount of GOD by this method is about 68 U/cm^2 which is higher than 0.101 U/cm^2 of the GC electrode by entrapping enzyme and polymerizing PEDOT at the same time reported in the previous work (Nien et al., 2006).

5.2 The sensing performance

For glucose biosensors, the prepared electrode worked in the nitrogen purged glucose solutions at a stiring rate of 100 rpm by applying a sensing potential of 0.3 V to record the oxidation sensing current of BZQ. The calibration curve of the electrode was shown in Fig. 6

and the sensitivity was 2.21 mA M^{-1} cm^{-2} with a R^2 value of 0.993. Besides, the other performances including linear range, response time and limit of detection were 1.1-15 mM (human range included), 95-105 s and 1.1 mM, respectively. Comparing to the previous works of co-immobilization of GOD and mediators, the sensitivity is better than 0.79 (Himuro et al., 2009), 0.111 (Crespilho et al., 2008) and 1.86 (Qiu et al., 2007) mA M^{-1} cm^{-2} In the first work, the GOD was linked on the mediator-based copolymer backbone, poly(vinylferrocene-co-2-hydroxyethyl methacrylate), and polyamidoamine particle linked by GOD was co-immobilized with the gold nanoparticles modified by cobalt hexacyanoferrate (mediator) on conducting glass in the second work. In the last work, the GOD and ferrocene monocarboxylic acid-modified Fe_3O_4 nanoparticles were both entrapped on carbon paste electrode. In addition, only the linear range of the first literature (1.4-8.9 mM) covered the normal human range.

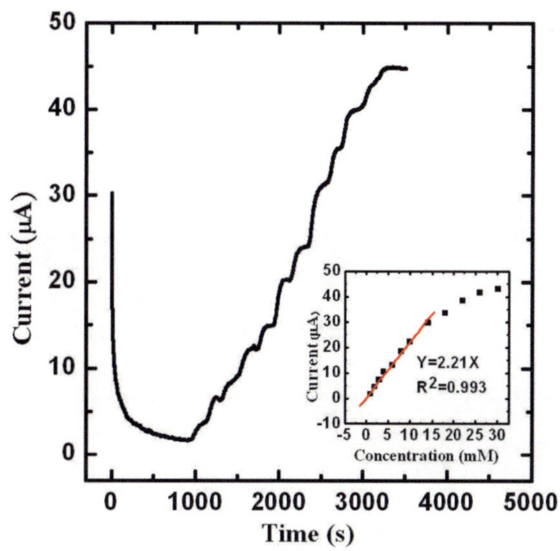

Fig. 6. The current response with increasing glucose concentrations and the calibration curve (inset) for system B.

5.3 The interferences effect and monitoring of real sample

For simulating the real sample, the most common interferences including AA, DA, UA and AP were applied in this system, and their formal potentials are about 0.2 V, 0.3 V, 0.5V and 0.3 V vs. Ag/AgCl/sat'd KCl, respectively. Besides, the normal ranges of those four species in blood are 34-80 μM, <1 μM, 178-416 μM and 130-150 μM, respectively. The current responses of the interferences were shown in Fig. 7 based on the sensing current of 6 mM glucose as 100%. In Fig. 7, there is almost no current response for UA owing to the insufficient overpotential. However, the sensing current of DA was higher than that of AA which has a lower oxidized potential. It is because some carbons on the polymer backbone was over-oxidized and transformed into carboxylic groups at a high potential when polymerization (Cosnier, 2003; Vidal et al., 2001). In the literature (Palmisano et al., 1995), the carboxylic groups on the over-oxidized conducting polymer, polypyrrole, were proved by X-ray photoelectron spectroscopy (XPS). In other words, the charge of PEDOT polymer chain changed to partial negative from positive, so the PEDOT film preferred to attract positive DA (pK=8.87) than negative AA (pK=4.1) in the PBS of pH 7. Additionally, the AP with positive charge resulted in 3% current response owing to the same way stated above. Finally, the whole blood from human beings was also monitored in a batch system and it shows an bias of +3.6% according to the standard glucose concentration of 4.94 mM obtained from National Taiwan University Hospital. As a result, the modified electrode presents a good performance for real samples detections in an oxygen-independent system.

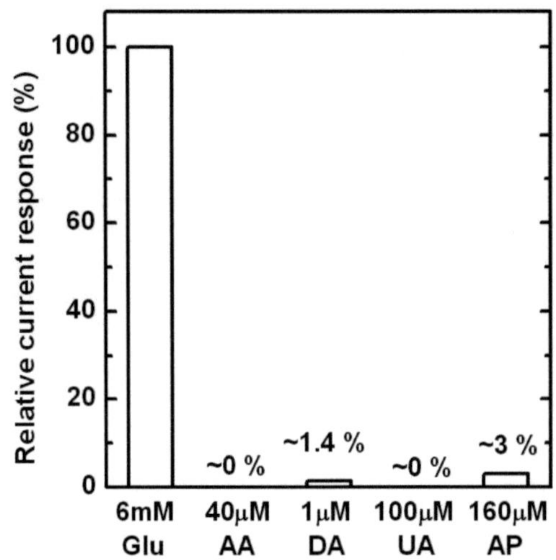

Fig. 7. The relative current response of the common interferences in human blood.

5.4 The application of biofuel cell

The modified electrode was employed for not only as a glucose biosensor but also as an anode for biofuel cell. In the following biofuel cell system proposed, the anode was the modified electrode immobilized BZQ and GOD, and the cathode was the platinum electrode in the ABTS and Lac solution. Figure 8 shows the I-V curves obtained by sweeping potentials from open circuit voltage (V_{oc}) to 0 V and power curves in 0 M and 0.1 M glucose solution at room temperature and body temperature, which means 25 ^{o}C and 37 ^{o}C, respectively. In the Fig. 8A, the V_{oc} increased to 0.6 V from 0.52 V and the cell current had an obvious enhancement after adding 0.1 M glucose. It implied that the glucose biofuel cell was workable and sensitive to glucose concentration. Based on Fig. 8A, the power curves shown in Fig. 8B can be calculated from the current multiplied by cell voltage. In Fig. 8B, the cell power of the 0 M glucose solution was 7 μW/cm^2 and the cell acted as a non-regenerated cell by the redox reactions of the mediators in each compartments. Besides, the maximum power of 22.5 μW/cm^2 (at V_{cell}=0.235 V and I=95.8 μA) at body temperature was slightly higher than that of 18.9 μW/cm^2 (at V_{cell} =0.212 V and I=89.1 μA) at room temperature. It is because the power at 37 ^{o}C is affected by the higher catalytic activity of enzyme and the lower fuel solubility of oxygen in cathode.

In this system, the anode was assigned as the rate-determining electrode to optimize the amount of BZQ and GOD. Thus, the catholyte always contains sufficient ABTS and Lac comparing to anodic electrolyte and the maximum reaction rate of cathode was much higher

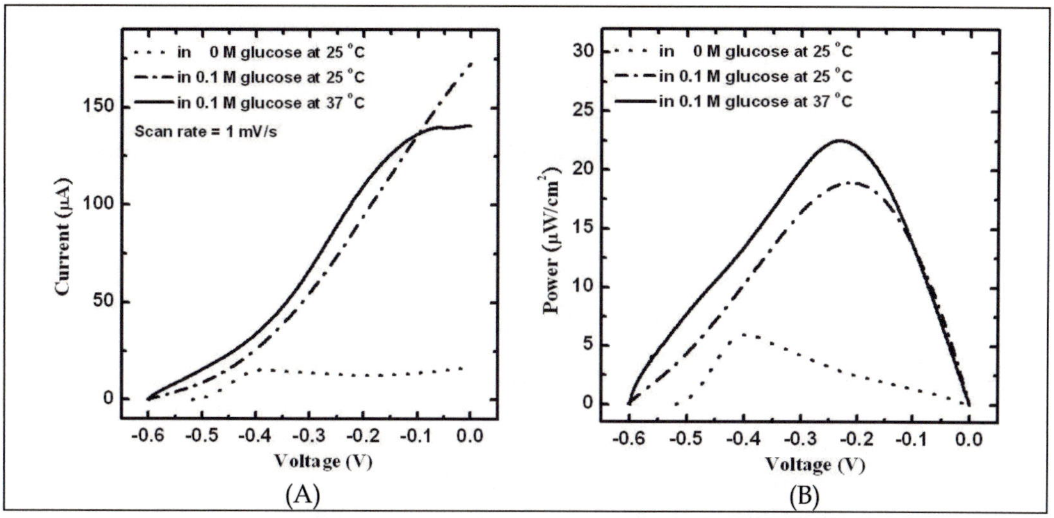

Fig. 8. (A) The I-V curve and (B) the power curve of the biofuel cell at 25 °C and 37 °C.

than that of anode. Figure 9 shows the maximum powers of the cell with the anodes prepared by different amounts of BZQ and GOD at 25 °C. The maximum powers were only varied with the amount of BZQ but GOD in Fig. 9. However, the immobilized content of BZQ was much high according to its redox peak current, and the mole ratio of that to the quantitative GOD (mole of BZQ/mole of GOD) was much larger than 10. It may be due to the poor contact between the BZQ with hydrophobic property and GOD with hydrophilic property. In other words, the electron-transfer reaction may be only carried out in the near-interface of BZQ and GOD layers, so it also resulted in lower sensing current and cell power. Besides, the powers of the electrode prepared by 80 μl BZQ were almost the same as that by 40 μl BZQ, so the optimal condition was 40 μl BZQ and GOD.

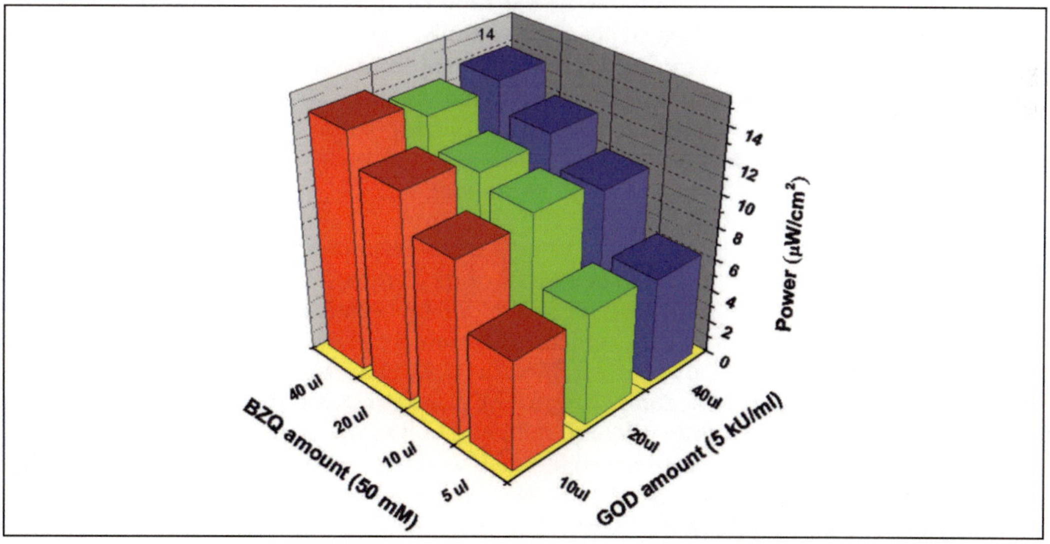

Fig. 9. The maximum cell powers using different anodes prepared by various amounts of BZQ and GOD at 25 °C

Table 4 shows a partial list of the literatures for the biofuel cells immobilized GOD and Lac by physical immobilized methods, such as adsorption and entrapment. In the first three references (Nos. 1-3), the cells with the mediators dissolved in electrolytes were carried out in membrane systems. However, the mediators were immobilized on the electrodes for the last two references (Nos. 4-5). According to Table 4, this system can provide a largest V_{oc} and the maximum power is better than that of some references (Nos. 1, 3, 4).

No.	Reference	Immobilized Method	V_{oc} (V)	Power (μW/cm²)	
				23 °C	37 °C
1	(Yan et al., 2007)	Lipid based	0.45	3.2	---
2	(Liu & Dong, 2007a)	Gel	0.4	29	---
3	(Liu & Dong, 2007b)	Gel	0.25	10	---
4	(Habrioux et al., 2007)	Adsorption	0.3	---	16
5	(Brunel et al., 2007)	Adsorption	0.3	---	29
6	System B (Nien et al., 2009)	Entrapment	0.6	18.9	22.5

Table 4. A partial list of literatures on the power output of biofuel cells with glucose oxidase and laccase which were immobilized by adsorption and entrapment.

6. Conclusions and future works

In system A, the PEDOT-modified electrode was used as a matrix to entrap glucose oxidase and was integrated in a flow system of sensing chip successfully. The optimal injecting volume and flow rate were 30 μl and 10 ml/hr, respectively. The performances of sensitivity, linear range, response time, recovery time and limit of detection were 157 μC cm^{-2} mM^{-1}, 1-10 mM, 15 s, 35-75 s and 0.15 mM at a flow rate of 10 ml/hr, respectively. With an applied potential of 0.7 V on WE2, it can reduce the interference current of WE1. Since the interferences in the flow channel near the surface of the first electrode (WE2) had been pre-reacted electrochemically, and the interference-free sensor can be achieved at the second electrode (WE1). In the real sample test, the bias of bi-potential was +13.6%, which is lower than that of single-potential. In system B, the proposed electrode fabricated by multilayer structures successfully works as a glucose biosensor in the oxygen-independence solution, and the anode of the biofuel cell by adding not only glucose solution but also the real blood of human beings. The electrode prepared by BZQ/DMF, shows a sensitivity of 2.21 mA M^{-1} cm^{-2}, a linear concentration range of 1.1~15 mM (including the human blood range) and a response time of 100 s at a sensing potential of 0.3 V. Besides, the current responses of the common interferences in blood were much lower than that of 6 mM glucose because of the low sensing potential and the patially negative charged polymer film. As the glucose/O_2 biofuel cell, the V_{oc} can reach to 0.6 V and the maximum power was 22.5 μW/cm² at 37 °C in 0.1 M glucose solution. For the real blood tests, the bias was about +3.6% comparing to the standard value from hospital in glucose sensing and the cell power was 25 μW/cm² in biofuel cell at 25 °C.
Nowadays, most of diabetes check their glucose level by the commercial glucose test strips at home and inject insulin if they need. However, hemoglobin A1c, Hb_{A1c}, recommended by the American Diabetes Association (ADA) provides an average blood glucose level during 60-90 days. It is a more accurate biomarker for long-term monitoring without external factors. In literatures, fructosyl valine (FV), which exists after protein digestion of Hb_{A1c}, was

monitored by enzyme-based electrochemical biosensor (Fang et al., 2009) or molecular-imprinting biosensor (Chuang et al., 2009). The recent challenge in Hb_{A1C} part is still how to lower the interference signal, especially the effect of heme in our experiment. Heme also exists along with FV in sample after protein digestion, so this matter will be an issue for future study.

7. Acknowledgement

This work was partially sponsored by a grant received from the Ministry of Economics, Taiwan. Some instruments used in this study were supported by the National Research Council of Taiwan.

8. References

Akyilmaz, E. & Yorganci, E. (2007). Construction of an amperometric pyruvate oxidase enzyme electrode for determination of pyruvate and phosphate. *Electrochimica Acta*, 52, 28, Nov 2007, 7972-7977.

Auroux, P.A.; Iossifidis, D.; Reyes, D.R. & Manz, A. (2002). Micro total analysis systems. 2. Analytical standard operations and applications. *Analytical Chemistry*, 74, 12, Jun 2002, 2637-2652.

Bard, A.J.; Crayston, J.A.; Kittlesen, G.P.; Shea, T.V. & Wrighton, M.S. (1986). Digital-simulation of the measured electrochemical response of reversible redox couples at microelectrode arrays - consequences arising from closely spaced ultramicroelectrodes. *Analytical Chemistry*, 58, 11, Sep 1986, 2321-2331.

Battaglini, F.; Bartlett, P.N. & Wang, J.H. (2000). Covalent attachment of osmium complexes to glucose oxidase and the application of the resulting modified enzyme in an enzyme switch responsive to glucose. *Analytical Chemistry*, 72, 3, Feb 2000, 502-509.

Battaglini, F.; Koutroumanis, M.; English, A.M. & Mikkelsen, S.R. (1994). Targeting glucose oxidase at aspartate and glutamate residues with organic 2 electron redox mediators. *Bioconjugate Chemistry*, 5, 5, Sep 1994, 430-435.

Bogdanovskaya, V.A.; Kuznetsova, L.N. & Tarasevich, M.R. (1997). Bioelectrocatalysis by immobilized peroxidase: The effects caused by the carbon black surface coverage with the enzyme and by the enzyme-Nafion composition on the activity in the hydrogen peroxide reduction. *Russian Journal of Electrochemistry*, 33, 10, Oct 1997, 1087-1091.

Boguslavsky, L.I.; Geng, L.; Kovalev, I.P.; Sahni, S.K.; Xu, Z. & Skotheim, T.A. (1995). Amperometric thin-film biosensors based on glucose dehydrogenase and toluidine-blue-o as catalyst for NADH electroxidation. *Biosensors & Bioelectronics*, 10, 8, Fal 1995, 693-704.

Borole, D.D.; Kapadi, U.R.; Mahulikar, P.P. & Hundiwale, D.G. (2004). Glucose oxidase electrodes of polyaniline, poly(o-toluidine) and their copolymer as a biosensor: a comparative study. *Polymers for Advanced Technologies*, 15, 6, Jun 2004, 306-312.

Bourdillon, C.; Demaille, C.; Moiroux, J. & Saveant, J.M. (1995). Catalysis and mass transport in spatially ordered enzyme assemblies on electrodes. *Journal of the American Chemical Society*, 117, 46, Nov 1995, 11499-11506.

Bourdillon, C.; Laval, J.M. & Thomas, D. (1986). Enzymatic electrocatalysis - controlled potential electrolysis and cosubstrate regeneration with immobilized enzyme modified electrode. *Journal of the Electrochemical Society*, 133, 4, Apr 1986, 706-711.

Brahim, S.; Narinesingh, D. & Guiseppi-Elie, A. (2001). Amperometric determination of cholesterol in serum using a biosensor of cholesterol oxidase contained within a polypyrrole-hydrogel membrane. *Analytica Chimica Acta*, 448, 1-2, Dec 2001, 27-36.

Brunel, L.; Denele, J.; Servat, K.; Kokoh, K.B.; Jolivalt, C.; Innocent, C.; Cretin, M.; Rolland, M. & Tingry, S. (2007). Oxygen transport through laccase biocathodes for a membrane-less glucose/O-2 biofuel cell. *Electrochemistry Communications*, 9, 2, Feb 2007, 331-336.

Cenas, N.K.; Pocius, A.K. & Kulys, J.J. (1983). Electron exchange between flavin-containing and heme-containing enzymes and electrodes modified by redox polymers. *Bioelectrochemistry and Bioenergetics*, 11, 1, Jan 1983, 61-73.

Chaubey, A. & Malhotra, B.D. (2002). Mediated biosensors. *Biosensors & Bioelectronics*, 17, 6-7, Jun 2002, 441-456.

Chen, L.Q.; Zhang, X.E.; Xie, W.H.; Zhou, Y.F.; Zhang, Z.P. & Cass, A.E.G. (2002). Genetic modification of glucose oxidase for improving performance of an amperometric glucose biosensor. *Biosensors & Bioelectronics*, 17, 10, Oct 2002, 851-857.

Chen, P.-Y.; Vittal, R.; Nien, P.C. & Ho, K.C. (2009). Enhancing dopamine detection using a glassy carbon electrode modified with MWCNTs, quercetin and Nafion. *Biosensors & Bioelectronics*, 24, May 2009, 3504-3509.

Chu, X.; Duan, D.X.; Shen, G.L. & Yu, R.Q. (2007). Amperometric glucose biosensor based on electrodeposition of platinum nanoparticles onto covalently immobilized carbon nanotube electrode. *Talanta*, 71, 5, Mar 2007, 2040-2047.

Chuang, S.W.; Rick, J. & Chou, T.C. (2009). Electrochemical characterisation of a conductive polymer molecularly imprinted with an Amadori compound. *Biosensors & Bioelectronics*, 24, 10, Jun 2009, 3170-3173.

Clark, L.C. & Lyons, C. (1962). Electrode systems for continuous monitoring in cardiovascular surgery. *Annals of the New York Academy of Sciences*, 102, 1, Apr 1962, 29-33.

Cosnier, S. (1999). Biomolecule immobilization on electrode surfaces by entrapment or attachment to electrochemically polymerized films. A review. *Biosensors & Bioelectronics*, 14, 5, May 1999, 443-456.

Cosnier, S. (2003). Biosensors based on electropolymerized films: new trends. *Analytical and Bioanalytical Chemistry*, 377, 3, Oct 2003, 507-520.

Cosnier, S.; Lepellec, A.; Guidetti, B. & Rico-Lattes, I. (1998). Enhancement of biosensor sensitivity in aqueous and organic solvents using a combination of poly(pyrrole-ammonium) and poly(pyrrole-lactobionamide) films as host matrices. *Journal of Electroanalytical Chemistry*, 449, 1-2, Jun 1998, 165-171.

Crespilho, F.N.; Ghica, M.E.; Gouveia-Caridade, C.; Oliveira, O.N. & Brett, C.M.A. (2008). Enzyme immobilisation on electroactive nanostructured membranes (ENM): Optimised architectures for biosensing. *Talanta*, 76, 4, Aug 2008, 922-928.

Cunningham, A.J. (1998). *Introduction to Bioanalytical Sensors*, John Wiley & Sons Inc., New York.

Dubinin, A.G.; Li, F.C.; Li, Y.R. & Yu, J.T. (1991). A solid-state immobilized enzyme polymer membrane microelectrode for measuring lactate ion concentration. *Bioelectrochemistry and Bioenergetics*, 25, 1, Feb 1991, 131-135.

Duine, J.A.; Frank, J. & Vanzeeland, J.K. (1979). Glucose dehydrogenase from acientobacter calcoaceticus quinoprotein. *Febs Letters*, 108, 2, Feb 1979, 443-446.

Ekanayake, E.; Preethichandra, D.M.G. & Kaneto, K. (2007). Polypyrrole nanotube array sensor for enhanced adsorption of glucose oxidase in glucose biosensors. *Biosensors & Bioelectronics*, 23, 1, Aug 2007, 107-113.

Fabiano, S.; Tran-Minh, C.; Piro, B.; Dang, L.A.; Pham, M.C. & Vittori, O. (2002). Poly 3,4-ethylenedioxythiophene as an entrapment support for amperometric enzyme sensor. *Materials Science & Engineering C-Biomimetic and Supramolecular Systems*, 21, 1-2, Sep 2002, 61-67.

Fang, L.; Li, W.; Zhou, Y. & Liu, C.C. (2009). A single-use, disposable iridium-modified electrochemical biosensor for fructosyl valine for the glycoslated hemoglobin detection. *Sensors and Actuators B-Chemical*, 137, 1, Mar 2009, 235-238.

Fiaccabrino, G.C.; de Rooij, N.F. & Koudelka-Hep, M. (1998). On-chip generation and detection of electrochemiluminescence. *Analytica Chimica Acta*, 359, 3, Feb 1998, 263-267.

Ford, S.M.; Kar, B.; McWhorter, S.; Davies, J.; Soper, S.A.; Klopf, M.; Calderon, G. & Saile, V. (1998). Microcapillary electrophoresis devices fabricated using polymeric substrates and X-ray lithography. *Journal of Microcolumn Separations*, 10, 5, 1998, 413-422.

Franke, W. & Deffner, M. (1939). On the knowledge of the so-called glucose oxidase II. *Justus Liebigs Annalen Der Chemie*, 541, Nov 1939, 117-150.

Gamati, S.; Luong, J.H.T. & Mulchandani, A. (1991). A microbial biosensor for trimethylamine using pseudomonas-aminovorans cells. *Biosensors & Bioelectronics*, 6, 2, Feb 1991, 125-131.

Gilmartin, M.A.T. & Hart, J.P. (1995). Development of one-shot biosensors for the measurement of uric acid and cholesterol. *Analytical Proceedings*, 32, 8, Aug 1995, 341-345.

Habermuller, K. & Schuhmann, W. (1998). A low-volume electrochemical cell for the deposition of conducting polymers and entrapment of enzymes. *Electroanalysis*, 10, 18, Dec 1998, 1281-1284.

Habrioux, A.; Sibert, E.; Servat, K.; Vogel, W.; Kokoh, K.B. & Alonso-Vante, N. (2007). Activity of platinum-gold alloys for glucose electrooxidation in biofuel cells. *Journal of Physical Chemistry B*, 111, 34, Aug 2007, 10329-10333.

Hamdi, N.; Wang, J.J.; Walker, E.; Maidment, N.T. & Monbouquette, H.G. (2006). An electroenzymatic L-glutamate microbiosensor selective against dopamine. *Journal of Electroanalytical Chemistry*, 591, 1, Jun 2006, 33-40.

Hecht, H.J.; Kalisz, H.M.; Hendle, J.; Schmid, R.D. & Schomburg, D. (1993). Crystal structure of glucose oxidase from aspergillus niger refined at 2 3 angstrom resolution. *Journal of Molecular Biology*, 229, 1, Jan 1993, 153-172.

Heller, A. & Feldman, B. (2008). Electrochemical glucose sensors and their applications in diabetes management. *Chemical Reviews*, 108, 7, Jul 2008, 2482-2505.

Hendry, S.P.; Cardosi, M.F.; Turner, A.P.F. & Neuse, E.W. (1993). Polyferrocenes as mediators in amperometric biosensors for glucose. *Analytica Chimica Acta*, 281, 3, Sep 1993, 453-459.

Himuro, Y.; Takai, M. & Ishihara, K. (2009). Poly(vinylferrocene-co-2-hydroxyethyl methacrylate) mediator as immobilized enzyme membrane for the fabrication of amperometric glucose sensor. *Sensors and Actuators B-Chemical*, 136, 1, Feb 2009, 122-127.

Hosokawa, K. & Maeda, R. (2000). A pneumatically-actuated three-way microvalve fabricated with polydimethylsiloxane using the membrane transfer technique. *Journal of Micromechanics and Microengineering*, 10, 3, Sep 2000, 415-420.

Huang, C.J.; Chen, Y.H.; Wang, C.H.; Chou, T.C. & Lee, G.B. (2007). Integrated microfluidic systems for automatic glucose sensing and insulin injection. *Sensors and Actuators B-Chemical*, 122, 2, Mar 2007, 461-468.

Jaffari, S.A. & Turner, A.P.F. (1997). Novel hexacyanoferrate(III) modified graphite disc electrodes and their application in enzyme electrodes. *Biosensors & Bioelectronics*, 12, 1, Mar 1997, 1-9.

Jia, W.Z.; Hu, Y.L.; Song, Y.Y.; Wang, K. & Xia, X.H. (2008). Highly selective amperometric glucose microdevice derived from diffusion layer gap electrode. *Biosensors & Bioelectronics*, 23, 6, Jan 2008, 892-898.

Jia, W.Z.; Wang, K.; Song, Y.Y. & Xia, X.H. (2007). Diffusion layer based probe-in-tube microdevice for selective analysis of electroactive species. *Electrochemistry Communications*, 9, 7, Jul 2007, 1553-1557.

Karyakin, A.A.; Strakhova, A.K.; Karyakina, E.E.; Varfolomeyev, S.D. & Yatsimirsky, A.K. (1993). The electrochemical polymerization of methylene blue and bioelectrochemical activity of the resulting film. *Synthetic Metals*, 60, 3, Oct 1993, 289-292.

Kohma, T.; Hasegawa, H.; Oyamatsu, D. & Kuwabata, S. (2007). Utilization of AC impedance measurements for electrochemical glucose sensing using glucose oxidase to improve detection selectivity. *Bulletin of the Chemical Society of Japan*, 80, 1, Jan 2007, 158-165.

Kojima, A.; Hyon, C.K.; Kamimura, T.; Maeda, M. & Matsumoto, K. (2005). Protein sensor using carbon nanotube field effect transistor. *Japanese Journal of Applied Physics Part 1-Regular Papers Short Notes & Review Papers*, 44, 4A, Apr 2005, 1596-1598.

Krishnamoorthy, K.; Gokhale, R.S.; Contractor, A.Q. & Kumar, A. (2004). Novel label-free DNA sensors based on poly(3,4-ethylenedioxythiophene). *Chemical Communications*, 7, Apr 2004, 820-821.

Kros, A.; Sommerdijk, N. & Nolte, R.J.M. (2005). Poly(pyrrole) versus poly (3,4-ethylenedioxythiophene): implications for biosensor applications. *Sensors and Actuators B-Chemical*, 106, 1, Apr 2005, 289-295.

Kulys, J.; Tetianec, L. & Ziemys, A. (2006). Probing Aspergillus niger glucose oxidase with pentacyanoferrate(III) aza- and thia-complexes. *Journal of Inorganic Biochemistry*, 100, 10, Oct 2006, 1614-1622.

Kurita, R.; Hayashi, K.; Fan, X.; Yamamoto, K.; Kato, T. & Niwa, O. (2002). Microfluidic device integrated with pre-reactor and dual enzyme-modified microelectrodes for monitoring in vivo glucose and lactate. *Sensors and Actuators B-Chemical*, 87, 2, Dec 2002, 296-303.

Lee, T.M.H.; Carles, M.C. & Hsing, I.M. (2003). Microfabricated PCR-electrochemical device for simultaneous DNA amplification and detection. *Lab on a Chip*, 3, 2, Apr 2003, 100-105.

Lerch, K.; Jonas, F. & Linke, M. (1998). Properties and applications of Baytron (PEDT). *Journal De Chimie Physique Et De Physico-Chimie Biologique*, 95, 6, Jun 1998, 1506-1509.

Lin, C.L.; Shih, C.L. & Chau, L.K. (2007a). Amperometric L-Lactate sensor based on sol-gel processing of an enzyme-linked silicon alkoxide. *Analytical Chemistry*, 79, 10, May 2007a, 3757-3763.

Lin, T.Y.; Wu, C.H. & Brennan, J.D. (2007b). Entrapment of horseradish peroxidase in sugar-modified silica monoliths: Toward the development of a biocatalytic sensor. *Biosensors & Bioelectronics*, 22, 2007b, 1861-1867.

Liu, A.L.; Zhou, T.; He, F.Y.; Xu, J.J.; Lu, Y.; Chen, H.Y. & Xia, X.H. (2006). Off-line form of the Michaelis-Menten equation for studying the reaction kinetics in a polymer microchip integrated with enzyme microreactor. *Lab on a Chip*, 6, 6, Jun 2006, 811-818.

Liu, Y. & Dong, S.J. (2007a). A biofuel cell harvesting energy from glucose-air and fruit juice-air. *Biosensors & Bioelectronics*, 23, 4, Nov 2007a, 593-597.

Liu, Y. & Dong, S.J. (2007b). A biofuel cell with enhanced power output by grape juice. *Electrochemistry Communications*, 9, 7, Jul 2007b, 1423-1427.

Liu, Y.J.; Ganser, D.; Schneider, A.; Liu, R.; Grodzinski, P. & Kroutchinina, N. (2001). Microfabricated polycarbonate CE devices for DNA analysis. *Analytical Chemistry*, 73, 17, Sep 2001, 4196-4201.

Loonberg, M. & Carlsson, J. (2006). Lab-on-a-chip technology for determination of protein isoform profiles. *Journal of Chromatography A*, 1127, 1-2, Sep 2006, 175-182.

Luong, J.H.T.; Masson, C.; Brown, R.S.; Male, K.B. & Nguyen, A.L. (1994). Monitoring the activity of glucose oxidase during the cultivation of aspergillus niger using novel amperometric sensor with 1,1'-dimethylferricinium as a mediator. *Biosensors & Bioelectronics*, 9, 8, Oct 1994, 577-584.

Mailley, P.; Cosnier, S. & Coche-Guerente, L. (2000). Amperometric glucose biosensors based on composite polymeric structures to prevent interferences. *Analytical Letters*, 33, 9, Sep 2000, 1733-1753.

Malmstadt, H. & Pardue, H.L. (1961). Quantitative analysis by an antomatic potentimetric reaction rate method - specific enzymatic determination of glucose. *Analytical Chemistry*, 33, 8, Aug 1961, 1040-1045.

Mano, N.; Mao, F. & Heller, A. (2005). On the parameters affecting the characteristics of the "wired" glucose oxidase anode. *Journal of Electroanalytical Chemistry*, 574, 2, Jan 2005, 347-357.

Mao, F.; Mano, N. & Heller, A. (2003). Long tethers binding redox centers to polymer backbones enhance electron transport in enzyme "wiring" hydrogels. *Journal of the American Chemical Society*, 125, 16, Apr 2003, 4951-4957.

Matuszewski, W.; Trojanowicz, M. & Lewenstam, A. (1990). Elimination of interferences in flow-injection amperometric determination of glucose in blood-serum using immobilized glucose-oxidase. *Electroanalysis*, 2, 8, Nov 1990, 607-615.

McDonald, J.C.; Duffy, D.C.; Anderson, J.R.; Chiu, D.T.; Wu, H.K.; Schueller, O.J.A. & Whitesides, G.M. (2000). Fabrication of microfluidic systems in poly(dimethylsiloxane). *Electrophoresis*, 21, 1, Jan 2000, 27-40.

Min, J.H. & Baeumner, A.J. (2004). Characterization and optimization of interdigitated ultramicroelectrode arrays as electrochemical biosensor transducers. *Electroanalysis*, 16, 9, May 2004, 724-729.

Muller, U.; Nisch, W.; Pawlak, M.; Gierke, B.; Breisch, S.; Burkhardt, C.; Rudorf, R.; Neugebauer, S.; Schuhmann, W.; Linke, S.; Kaczor, M.; Lohmuller, T.; Spatz, J.; Motz, M.; Sorsa, J.; Hecke, S.; Hartwich, G. & Stelzle, M. (2007). A novel nano-porous electrode system to enhance Biosensor sensitivity., *Proceedings of NSTI-Nanotech 2007*, pp. 206-209, Santa Clara, May and 2007, Nano Science and Technology Institute.

Nakaminami, T.; Kuwabata, S. & Yoneyama, H. (1997). Electrochemical oxidation of cholesterol catalyzed by cholesterol oxidase with use of an artificial electron mediator. *Analytical Chemistry*, 69, 13, Jul 1997, 2367-2372.

Navera, E.N.; Suzuki, M.; Tamiya, E.; Takeuchi, T. & Karube, I. (1993). Nafion-coated carbon-fiber for acetylcholine and choline sensors. *Electroanalysis*, 5, 1, Jan 1993, 17-22.

Ngounou, B.; Aliyev, E.H.; Guschin, D.A.; Sultanov, Y.M.; Efendiev, A.A. & Schuhmann, W. (2007). Parallel synthesis of libraries of anodic and cathodic functionalized electrodeposition paints as immobilization matrix for amperometric biosensors. *Bioelectrochemistry*, 71, 1, Sep 2007, 81-90.

Nien, P.C.; Huang, M.C.; Chang, F.Y. & Ho, K.C. (2008). Integrating an enzyme-entrapped conducting polymer electrode and a prereactor in a microfluidic system for sensing glucose. *Electroanalysis*, 20, 6, Mar 2008, 635-642. Copyright Wiley-VCH Verlag GmbH & Co. KGaA. Reproduced with permission.

Nien, P.C.; Tung, T.S. & Ho, K.C. (2006). Amperometric glucose biosensor based on entrapment of glucose oxidase in a poly(3,4-ethylenedioxythiophene) film. *Electroanalysis*, 18, 13-14, Jul 2006, 1408-1415.

Nien, P.C.; Wang, J.Y.; Chen, P.Y.; Chen, L.C. & Ho, K.C. (2009). Co-immobilization of benzoquinone and glucose oxidase in a PEDOT: Application to oxygen-independent glucose sensors and glucose/O_2 biofuel cells, submitted to *Biosensors and Bioelectronics*.

Palmisano, F.; Malitesta, C.; Centonze, D. & Zambonin, P.G. (1995). Correlation between permselectivity and chemical structure of overoxidized polypyrrole membranes used in electroproduced enzyme biosensors. *Analytical Chemistry*, 67, 13, Jul 1995, 2207-2211.

Qiu, H.; Peng, H. & Liang, R. (2007). Ferrocene-modified Fe_3O_4@SiO_2 magnetic nanoparticles as building blocks for construction of reagentless enzyme-based biosensors. *Electrochemistry Communications*, 9, 11, Nov 2007, 2734-2738.

Qiu, J.D.; Zhou, W.M.; Guo, J.; Wang, R. & Liang, R.P. (2009). Amperometric sensor based on ferrocene-modified multiwalled carbon nanotube nanocomposites as electron mediator for the determination of glucose. *Analytical Biochemistry*, 385, 2, Feb 2009, 264-269.

Rahman, A.; Park, D.S. & Shim, Y.B. (2004). A performance comparison of choline biosensors: anodic or cathodic detections of H_2O_2 generated by enzyme immobilized on a conducting polymer. *Biosensors & Bioelectronics*, 19, 12, Jul 2004, 1565-1571.

Rao, J.R. & Richter, G. (1974). Implantable bioelectrochemical power sources. *Naturwissenschaften*, 61, 5, May 1974, 200-206.

Rao, J.R.; Richter, G.; Sturm, F.V.; Weidlich, E. & Wenzel, M. (1974). Metal-oxygen and glucose-oxygen cells for implantable devices. *Biomedical Engineering*, 9, 3, Mar 1974, 98-103.

Richter, T.; Shultz-Lockyear, L.L.; Oleschuk, R.D.; Bilitewski, U. & Harrison, D.J. (2002). Bi-enzymatic and capillary electrophoretic analysis of non-fluorescent compounds in microfluidic devices - Determination of xanthine. *Sensors and Actuators B-Chemical*, 81, 2-3, Jan 2002, 369-376.

Schoning, M.J.; Jacobs, M.; Muck, A.; Knobbe, D.T.; Wang, J.; Chatrathi, M. & Spillmann, S. (2005). Amperometric PDMS/glass capillary electrophoresis-based biosensor microchip for catechol and dopamine detection. *Sensors and Actuators B-Chemical*, 108, 1-2, Jul 2005, 688-694.

Sehr, P.; Zumbach, K. & Pawlita, M. (2001). A generic capture ELISA for recombinant proteins fused to glutathione S-transferase: validation for HPV serology. *Journal of Immunological Methods*, 253, 1-2, Jul 2001, 153-162.

Selampinar, F.; Akbulut, U.; Ozden, M.Y. & Toppare, L. (1997). Immobilization of invertase in conducting polymer matrices. *Biomaterials*, 18, 17, Sep 1997, 1163-1168.

Seo, K.D.; Lee, K.P.; Gopalan, A.I.; Chung, S.J.; Lim, Y.T. & Choi, S.H. (2007). Horseradish peroxidase (HRP) immobilized poly(aniline-co-m-aminophenol) film electrodes-fabrication and evaluation as hydrogen peroxide sensor. *Sensors*, 7, 5, May 2007, 719-729.

Setti, L.; Fraleoni-Morgera, A.; Ballarin, B.; Filippini, A.; Frascaro, D. & Piana, C. (2005). An amperometric glucose biosensor prototype fabricated by thermal inkjet printing. *Biosensors & Bioelectronics*, 20, 10, Apr 2005, 2019-2026.

Sheppard, N.F.; Mears, D.J. & GuiseppiElie, A. (1996). Model of an immobilized enzyme conductimetric urea biosensor. *Biosensors & Bioelectronics*, 11, 10, Dec 1996, 967-979.

Shulga, A.A.; Koudelkahep, M.; Derooij, N.F. & Netchiporouk, L.I. (1994). Glucose-sensitive enzyme field-effect transistor using potassium ferricyanide as an oxidizing substrate. *Analytical Chemistry*, 66, 2, Jan 1994, 205-210.

Singh, S.; Chaubey, A. & Malhotra, B.D. (2004). Amperometric cholesterol biosensor based on immobilized cholesterol esterase and cholesterol oxidase on conducting polypyrrole films. *Analytica Chimica Acta*, 502, 2, Jan 2004, 229-234.

Tamiya, E.; Sugiura, Y.; Akiyama, A. & Karube, I. (1990). Ultramicro-H_2O_2 electrode for fabrication of the invivo biosensor. *Annals of the New York Academy of Sciences*, 613, Dec 1990, 396-400.

Tian, F.M. & Zhu, G.Y. (2002). Bienzymatic amperometric biosensor for glucose based on polypyrrole/ceramic carbon as electrode material. *Analytica Chimica Acta*, 451, 2, Jan 2002, 251-258.

Trojanowicz, M.; Geschke, O.; Krawczyk, T.K.V. & Cammann, K. (1995). Biosensors based on oxidases immobilized in various conducting polymers. *Sensors and Actuators B-Chemical*, 28, 3, Sep 1995, 191-199.

Tsujimura, S.; Kojima, S.; Kano, K.; Ikeda, T.; Sato, M.; Sanada, H. & Omura, H. (2006). Novel FAD-dependent glucose dehydrogenase for a dioxygen-insensitive glucose biosensor. *Bioscience Biotechnology and Biochemistry*, 70, 3, Mar 2006, 654-659.

Unger, M.A.; Chou, H.P.; Thorsen, T.; Scherer, A. & Quake, S.R. (2000). Monolithic microfabricated valves and pumps by multilayer soft lithography. *Science*, 288, 5463, Apr 2000, 113-116.

Vasantha, V.S. & Chen, S.M. (2006). Electrocatalysis and simultaneous detection of dopamine and ascorbic acid using poly(3,4-ethylenedioxy)thiophene film modified electrodes. *Journal of Electroanalytical Chemistry*, 592, 1, Jul 2006, 77-87.

Vedrine, C.; Fabiano, S. & Tran-Minh, C. (2003). Amperometric tyrosinase based biosensor using an electrogenerated polythiophene film as an entrapment support. *Talanta*, 59, 3, Mar 2003, 535-544.

Vidal, J.C.; Garcia-Ruiz, E. & Castillo, J.R. (2001). Design of a multilayer cholesterol amperometric biosensor for preparation and use in flow systems. *Electroanalysis*, 13, 3, Mar 2001, 229-235.

Wang, Z.G.; Wano, Y.; Xu, H.; Li, G. & Xu, Z.K. (2009). Carbon Nanotube-Filled Nanofibrous Membranes Electrospun from Poly(acrylonitrile-co-acrylic acid) for Glucose Biosensor. *Journal of Physical Chemistry C*, 113, 7, Feb 2009, 2955-2960.

Warburg, O. & Christian, W. (1932). On a new oxidation enzyme and its absorption spectrum. *Biochemische Zeitschrift*, 254, Jul 1932, 438-458.

Williams, D.L.; Doig, A.R. & Korosi, A. (1970). Electrochemical-enzymatic analysis of blood glucose and lactate. *Analytical Chemistry*, 42, 1, Jan 1970, 118-123.

Willner, I.; Baron, R. & Willner, B. (2007a). Integrated nanoparticle-biomolecule systems for biosensing and bioelectronics. *Biosensors & Bioelectronics*, 22, 9-10, Apr 2007a, 1841-1852.

Willner, I.; Willner, B. & Katz, E. (2007b). Biomolecule-nanoparticle hybrid systems for bioelectronic applications. *Bioelectrochemistry*, 70, 1, Jan 2007b, 2-11.

Wu, F.H.; Zhao, G.C. & Wei, X.W. (2002). Electrocatalytic oxidation of nitric oxide at multi-walled carbon nanotubes modified electrode. *Electrochemistry Communications*, 4, 9, Sep 2002, 690-694.

Wu, X.M.; Du, P.; Wu, P. & Cai, C.X. (2008). Effects of 1-butyl-3-methylimidazolium tetrafluoroborate on the oxidation of glucose catalyzed by glucose oxidase. *Electrochimica Acta*, 54, 2, Dec 2008, 738-743.

Xie, J.; Miao, Y.N.; Shih, J.; Tai, Y.C. & Lee, T.D. (2005). Microfluidic platform for liquid chromatography-tandem mass spectrometry analyses of complex peptide mixtures. *Analytical Chemistry*, 77, 21, Nov 2005, 6947-6953.

Yamaguchi, A.; Jin, P.; Tsuchiyama, H.; Masuda, T.; Sun, K.; Matsuo, S. & Misawa, H. (2002). Rapid fabrication of electrochemical enzyme sensor chip using polydimethylsiloxane microfluidic channel. *Analytica Chimica Acta*, 468, 1, Sep 2002, 143-152.

Yamato, H.; Ohwa, M. & Wernet, W. (1995). Stability of polypyrrole and poly(3,4-ethylenedioxythiophene) for biosensor application. *Journal of Electroanalytical Chemistry*, 397, 1-2, Nov 1995, 163-170.

Yan, Y.M.; Su, L. & Mao, L.Q. (2007). Multi-walled carbon nanotube-based glucose/O_2 biofuel cell with glucose oxidase and laccase as biocatalysts. *Journal of Nanoscience and Nanotechnology*, 7, 4-5, Apr-May 2007, 1625-1630.

Yang, X.H.; Hall, S.B. & Tan, S.N. (2003). Electrochemical reduction of a conjugated cinnamic acid diazonium salt as an immobilization matrix for glucose biosensor. *Electroanalysis*, 15, 10, Jul 2003, 885-891.

Yuan, J.H.; Wang, K. & Xia, X.H. (2005). Highly ordered platinum-nanotubule arrays for amperometric glucose sensing. *Advanced Functional Materials*, 15, 5, May 2005, 803-809.

Zakeeruddin, S.M.; Fraser, D.M.; Nazeeruddin, M.K. & Gratzel, M. (1992). Towards mediator design - characterization of tris-(4,4'-substituted-2,2'-bipyridine) complexes of iron(II), ruthenium(II) and osmium(II) as mediators for glucose oxidase of aspergillusniger and other redox proteins. *Journal of Electroanalytical Chemistry*, 337, 1-2, Oct 1992, 253-283.

Zayats, M.; Willner, B. & Willner, I. (2008). Design of amperometric biosensors and biofuel cells by the reconstitution of electrically contacted enzyme electrodes. *Electroanalysis*, 20, 6, Mar 2008, 583-601.

Zhang, Q.; Xu, J.J. & Chen, H.Y. (2006a). Glucose microfluidic biosensors based on immobilizing glucose oxidase in poly(dimethylsiloxane) electrophoretic microchips. *Journal of Chromatography A*, 1135, 1, Nov 2006a, 122-126.

Zhang, S.X.; Wang, N.; Niu, Y.M. & Sun, C.Q. (2005). Immobilization of glucose oxidase on gold nanoparticles modified Au electrode for the construction of biosensor. *Sensors and Actuators B-Chemical*, 109, 2, Sep 2005, 367-374.

Zhang, S.X.; Yang, W.W.; Niu, Y.M.; Li, Y.C.; Zhang, M. & Sun, C.Q. (2006b). Construction of glucose biosensor based on sorption of glucose oxidase onto multilayers of polyelectrolyte/nanoparticles. *Analytical and Bioanalytical Chemistry*, 384, 3, Feb 2006b, 736-741.

Zhang, Y.N.; Hu, Y.B.; Wilson, G.S.; Moattisirat, D.; Poitout, V. & Reach, G. (1994). Elimination of the acetaminophen interference in an implantable glucose sensor. *Analytical Chemistry*, 66, 7, Apr 1994, 1183-1188.

Zhao, C. & Wittstock, G. (2005). Scanning electrochemical microscopy for detection of biosensor and biochip surfaces with immobilized pyrroloquinoline quinone (PQQ)-dependent glucose dehydrogenase as enzyme label. *Biosensors & Bioelectronics*, 20, 7, Jan 2005, 1277-1284.

Zhujun, Z. & Seitz, W.R. (1986). Optical sensor for oxygen based on immobilized hemoglobin. *Analytical Chemistry*, 58, 1, Jan 1986, 220-222.

14

Carbon Fiber-based Microelectrodes and Microbiosensors

Dénes Budai
University of Szeged
Hungary

1. Introduction

The chemically relatively inert carbon fiber (CF) has outstanding mechanical and electrical properties and provides an excellent base electrode for electrophysiological, electrochemical and biosensor applications on a micrometer or perhaps even on a submicrometer scale. CF microelectrodes have been used to record neuronal action potentials (spikes) since 1979 (Armstrong-James & Millar, 1979). The CFs are graphite monofilaments about 7 μm in diameter. In microelectrodes, they have outstanding extracellular recording qualities similar to those of the best tungsten electrodes.

The CF microelectrodes have been demonstrated to be very suitable for *in vivo* electrochemical detection of catecholamines (Ponchon et al., 1979) and other oxidizable biological species including nitric oxide (NO) (Malinski & Taha, 1992). Since the early times in CF applications for biorecording, a great variety of enzyme-modified CF microbiosensors has been introduced for the *in situ* determination of glucose, acetylcholine, choline, lactate, glutamate and other important compounds. The immobilization of DNA molecules (Millan & Mikkelsen, 1993) or carbon nanotubes (CNTs) (Zhang et al., 2007) onto CF microelectrodes has opened up new avenues in electrochemical detection of biologically significant species.

A basic CF microelectrode is an elementary carbon filament built in a mechanically supportive and electrically insulating borosilicate glass or plastic sheathing. The uninsulated carbon tip protruding from the sheathing by 10 to 100 μm provides a conductive surface for picking up spikes from the near vicinity of neurons and/or surface for electron transfer in microbiosensor applications. In the latter case, the carbon tip is covered with biological sensing elements such as an enzyme, receptor protein, antobody or nucleic acid immobilized in a conducting polymer matrix.

This chapter will discuss the fabrication of single- and multibarrel CF microelectrodes, the covalent modifications of the carbon surface as well as the applications of CF microelectrodes in recording spikes from neurons, electrochemical or biosensor signals from the nervous or other tissues. Attention will primarily be focused on microelectrodes containing CFs that have diameters no greater than 30 μm. A novel use of CF microelectrodes as oxigen detectors usable *in vitro* and *in vivo* will also be described for the first time.

2. Construction of CF microelectrodes

During the fabrication of CF microelectrodes, individual carbon fibers are inserted into borosilicate glass capillary tubing and single or multibarrel electrode blanks can easily be assembled. Because of the great tensile strength of the carbon fibers, they do not break when blanks are pulled to microelectrodes. After the pulling, the microelectrode is left with several centimeters of carbon fiber protruding from the glass tip. The simplest way to trim the end of the carbon fiber to the correct tip length (10-30 µm) is to cut off the excess with microscissors under a microscope. This is a difficult operation even for an experienced worker with steady hands, and the glass tip can easily be damaged. Another method of trimming the carbon fiber is electrochemical etching in dilute chromic acid or saline by applying a few tenths of a mA of alternating current. A third technique is spark etching, which allows the best control of tip length and shape for selective extracellular unit recording or electrochemical measurements (Budai & Molnár, 2001).

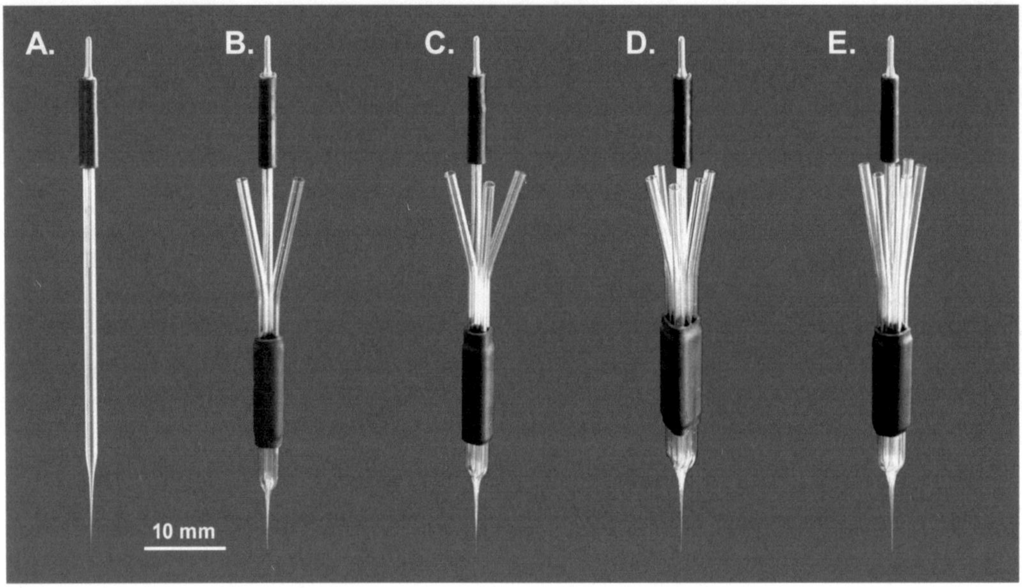

Fig. 1. View of CF microelectrodes. The base, single-barrel type (A) recording microelectrode can be completed with a varying number of micropipette barrels (B-E) used for drug delivery by means of iontophoresis or pressure or for reference/auxiliary electrodes. Tip ultrastructures are shown in Fig. 2. Courtesy of Kation Scientific.

CF microelectrodes are fabricated using 1.5 mm diam. borosilicate glass capillary tubings. Single-barrel, recording only, CF electrodes are made from standard borosilicate glass capillaries with no internal glass filament (Fig. 1A). Multi-barrel, recording and iontophoresis combination electrodes (Fig. 1, B-E) are constructed from the appropriate number of thin-wall glass tubings glued together before pulling. The CF containing recording barrel has no inner filament, whereas the iontophoresis barrels are made from glass tubings with a solid inner glass filament fused to the inner wall, which accelerates the filling of the barrels. A 10 cm long individual CF with a diameter of about 7 µm is glued to a piece of tin-plated copper wire with conductive paint or silver-filled epoxy glue. One end of the wire has previously been soldered into a gold plated male connector pin. Beginning at

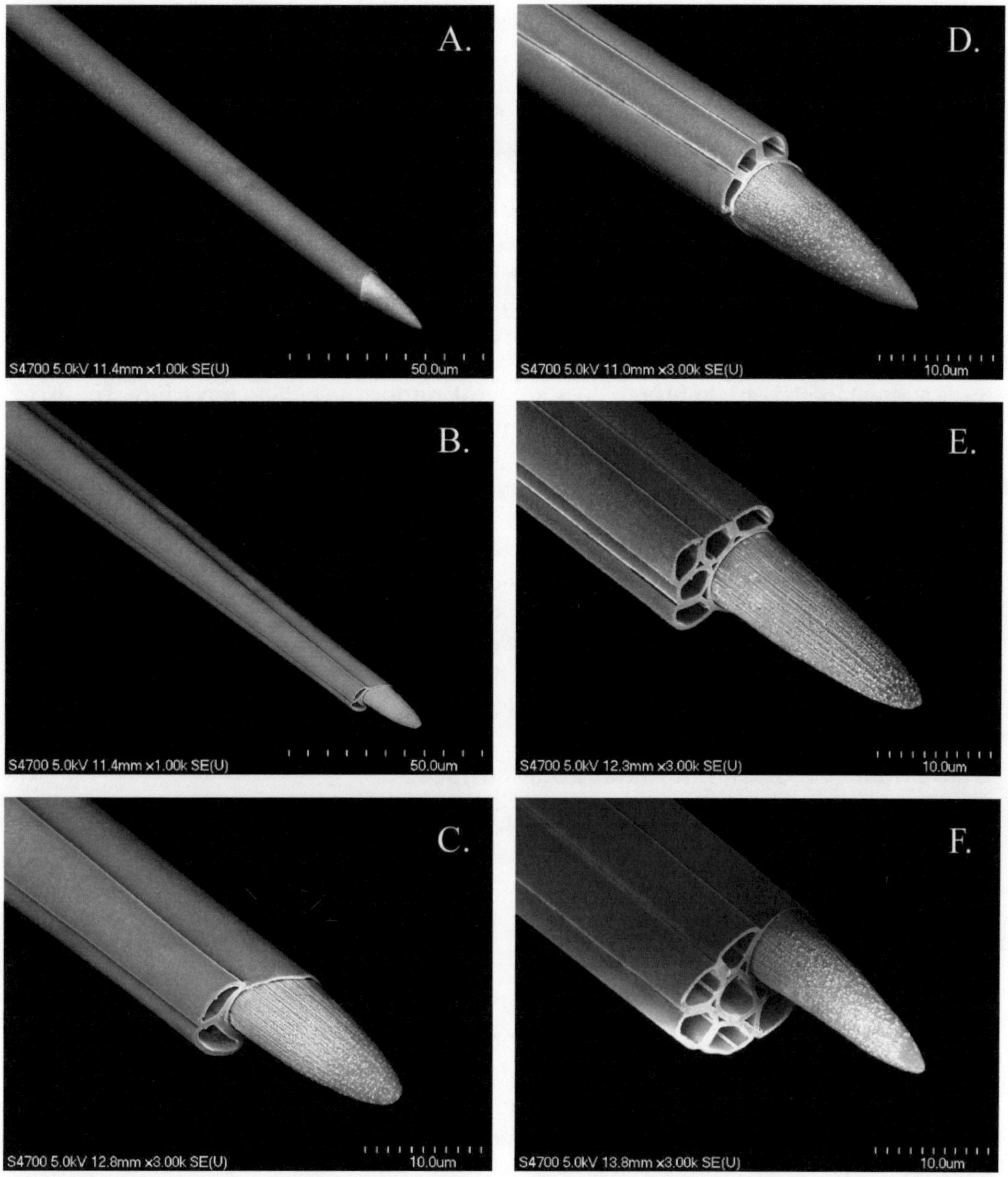

Fig. 2. Scanning electron micrographs of tips of CF microelectrodes shown in Fig. 1. Single-barrel microelectrodes are consisted of a conical carbon tip protruding from the borosilicate glass insulation (A). A varying number of micropipettes can be attached to the recording carbon fiber containing barrel (B-F) for delivering drugs by microiontophoresis or pressure. Filling of the drug barrels is facilitated by inner glass microfilaments fused to the inner wall of the microcapillaries (for example, see panel F). Courtesy of Kation Scientific.

its free end, the carbon fiber is sucked into the glass capillary tubing by gentle vacuum. The connector pin is then fixed onto the end of the glass tubing by heat-shrinkable plastic tubing.

For single-barrel electrodes, this assembly is ready to be pulled. For multi-barreled arrays, the appropriate number of inner filament-containing capillary tubes are attached to the recording barrel with two-component epoxy glue at both ends of the arrays. The glued portions of the arrays are covered with heat-shrinkable plastic tubings at both ends to provide further stability for the assembly and suitable locations for keeping the multi-barrel blanks in place during pulling and later in the electrode holder. The two ends of the electrode blank are then held by the chucks of a vertical electrode puller and the heating coil is used to soften the glass gently in the central portion of the assembly. As the glass is beginning to soften, the lower chuck is slowly rotated by one-half to two-thirds of a full circle while the electrode blank is pulled slowly by gravity only. This rotation and pulling cause the lengths of tubing to fuse together. The combination of the current supply to the heating coil and the degree and timing of the pull may be varied to produce pipettes of different lengths and diameters. Due to the very high tensile strength of the carbon fiber, it does not break during the pulling procedure. The excess fiber protruding from the tip of the glass assembly is shortened with fine scissors to about 5 mm. The exposed carbon fiber is finally trimmed by spark etching under a light microscope. Sparks are generated by a high voltage of about 800 V using a piece of polished gold wire as counter electrode. Finally, the free ends of the glass tubings in the multi-barrel electrode are heated up and bent out radially from the center to facilitate access and to reduce cross-contamination between barrels during filling. The finished single- and multi-barrel CF microelectrodes are shown in Fig. 1. Scanning electron micrographs of tips of the same electrode types are shown in Fig. 2. Using etching in chromic acid, longer tips ending in submicrometer size can also be achieved (Fig. 3). This type of carbon tip is recommended for enzyme-modifie CF microbiosensors. See also Fig. 9.

3. Modifications of CF microelectrode surfaces

Modifications of carbon surfaces are of great importance in electrochemistry and material science. Most of the procedures used for modifying the carbon surface involve oxidation leading to the formation of carboxylic, quinonic, ketonic or hydroxylic groups that can be covalently coupled with molecules of further interest.

3.1 Unmodified CF microelectrodes

Unmodified or bare carbon tips are used in extracellural spike recordings (Fig. 4) or in simple electrochemical measurements of electroactive biomolecules by voltammetry or amperometry. However, oxidation of the carbon surface may occur when these electrodes are manufactured using electrochemical, flame or spark etching (Strand & Venton, 2008). Similarly to more complex biosensor CF microelectrodes, carbon surfaces of microelectrodes made for voltammetry or amperometry are covered with Nafion, a sulphonated polymer which repels anions but is selectively permeable to cations.

3.2 Nafion coating

Nafion film coating has been widely used for surface modification of CF microelectrodes for sensitive and selective determination of biological species such as domapine in the presence of ascorbic acid. However, Nafion coating may significantly increase the electrode response time. Nafion coating is usually formed by simple dipping the electrode several times in 5% Nafion solution in aliphatic alcohol followed by drying at room temperature or in an oven at 170 °C (Gerhardt et al., 1984).

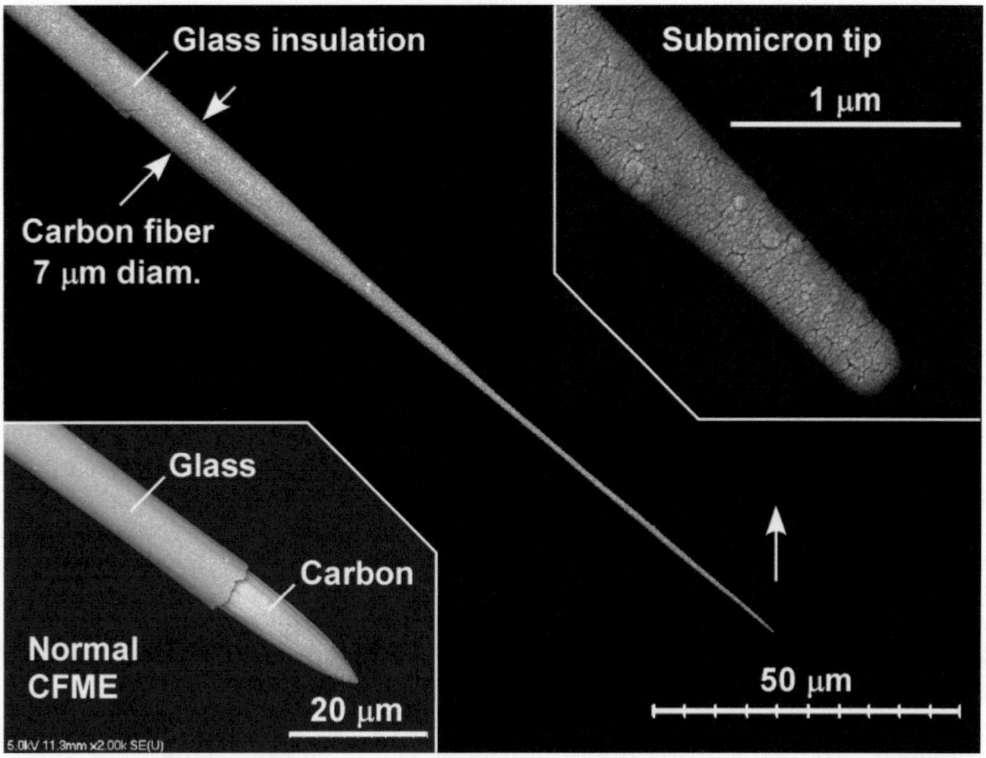

Fig. 3. Scanning electron micrograph of a single-barrel CF microelectrode with tip etched to a submicron size. Courtesy of Kation Scientific.

3.3 Covalent modifications of carbon electrodes using electrochemical methods

Using electrochemical procedures, primary and secondary amines may be covalently coupled to CF surfaces via oxidation of the amine in anhydrous ethanol or acetonytrile electrolyte solutions. One-electron reduction of aryl diazonium salts at carbon electrodes leads to grafting of aryl groups to the surface. Oxidation of arylacetates in acetonitrile may result in a monolayers of freely rotating naphtyl and anthryl groups. Formation of a covalently attached layer of alkyl groups has been described when high positive potential was applied to carbon electrodes in anhydrous solution of primary aliphatic alcohol. The robust linkage between the carbon surface and the modifier makes the initial covalently attached monolayer very suitable for functionalization of CF microelectrodes. For reviews, see (Downard, 2000; Pinson & Podvorica, 2005).

Recent research has shown that CF microelectrodes modified electrochemically with 4-sulfobenzene showed inreased sensitivity and selectrivity for catecholamines. The sulfonate group can provide a cation exchange site similar to Nafion but with a thinner grafted layer that is covalently attached to the electrode surface (Hermans et al., 2006).

Electrically conductive polymer layers of pyrrole or thiophene derivatives with immobilized anionic or cationic groups have recently been electrodeposited onto 7 μm carbon fibers (Sarac et al., 2008; Sarac et al., 2009). Insulating poly(oxyphenylene) polymer layers may also be deposited by electrochemical means onto CF microelectrodes (El-Deen et al., 2006; Budai et al., 2007).

3.4 Carbon nanotubes-modified CF microelectrodes

The carbon nanotube (CNT) with attractive physicochemical property has become a material of great interest for the neuro-electronic or biosensor interface. By growing CNTs on CF microelectrodes, the nanostructure of CNTs inherently increases the effective interfacial area between microelectrode and neuron (Yeh et al., 2009). Cyclic voltammetry results indicate that the prepared multi-walled CNT-modified CF microelectrodess possess a marked electrocatalytic activity toward ascorbic acid oxidation and can be used for its selective measurement in the presence of other kinds of electroactive species coexisting in rat brain (Zhang et al., 2007). Application of single-walled CNTs on a CF microdisk electrode dramatically increased the sensitivity of CF microelectrode for nitric oxide (NO) as the detection limit proved to be about 10 times lower for NO than that of the bare carbon surface (Du et al., 2008).

4. *In vivo* applications

4.1 Extracellular neuronal spike recording and microiontophoresis

Bare or Nafion-treated carbon tips of 7 μm carbon fibers protruding from the borosilicate glass insulation of CF microelectrodes provide excellent tools for extracellular recordings (Fig. 4). Electric current flows in the tissue around the neurons during action potentials can be detected by means of extracellular microelectrodes as extracellular 'spikes'. Extracellular spike potentials recorded from the mammalian central nervous system have a duration of between 0.2 and 20 ms. Their amplitudes are typically a few hundred microvolts depending on the type of neuron and the quality of the recording system. The greatest advantage of extracellular recording is that the activity of neurons can be recorded without having to impale and damage them. For this reason, most *in vivo* neuronal spike detection is done with extracellular recording. Signals picked up by extracellular electrodes need to be amplified to be able to be processed in more conventional electronic devices such as oscilloscopes or computers. The usual degree of amplitude amplification in extracellular amplifiers is around 10,000. The main difficulty with extracellular recording is the electrical "noise" which may result from external interference from electrical sources in the vicinity of the recording set-up and from the intrinsic properties of the substances making up the electrode and electrical circuit (thermal noise) used to amplify electrode signals.

In extracellular recordings and in terms of noise, CF microelectrodes are superior to tungsten microelectrodes used for the same purpose. This is due to the roughly 10 times less electrical resistance of CF microelectrodes as compared to that of tungstens. If the measured noise voltages are squared and the mean square is computed, the fluctuations of both signs contribute positively. The square root of this mean (RMS) is the usual way of expressing the magnitude of noise voltages. The RMS of the thermal (Johnson) noise is $(4kTR\Delta f)^{1/2}$, where k is the Boltzmann constant (1.38×10^{-23} JK^{-1}), T is the absolute temperature in Kelvin, R is the resistance of the microelectrode in ohm, and Δf is the noise bandwidth in Hz. If Δf is 5 KHz, this formula gives 5.6 μV RMS for thermal noise in the case of carbon fiber electrodes with a resistance of 0.4 MΩ when the temperature is 20 °C= 293 °K. In a good-quality recording system, CF microelectrodes used *in vivo* exhibit a total peak-to-peak noise level of about 25 μV which corresponds to about 6 μV RMS (Budai, 2004).

Microiontophoresis is the technique whereby ions and charged molecules can be ejected in very small amounts from solutions contained in glass micropipettes. Microiontophoresis is most often used for: (1) deposition of dyes and neural transport tracers for histological

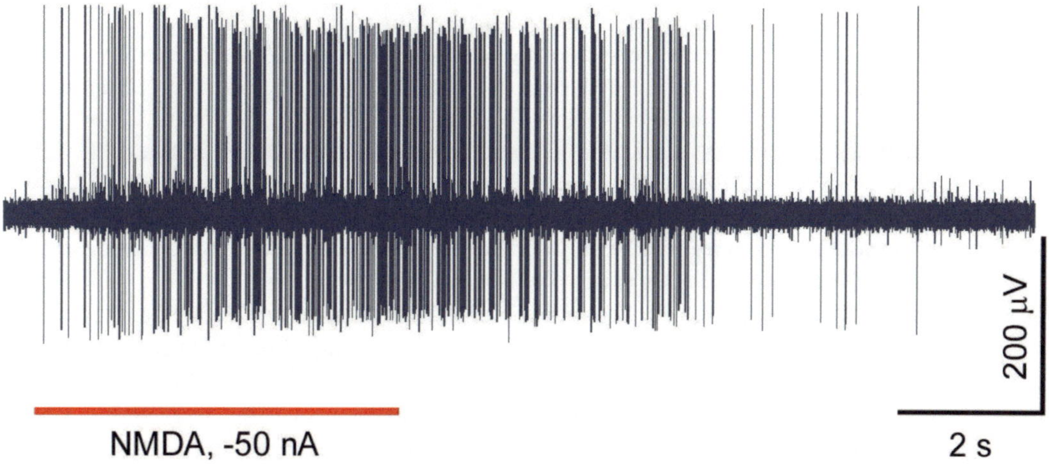

Fig. 4. Extracellularly recorded spikes from a hippocampal CA1 neuron stimulated by iontophoretic application of N-methyl-D-aspartate, NMDA. Spike recordings and microiontophoresis were performed using a Kation Scientific-made six-barreled CF microelectrode (see Figs. 1D and 2E). Courtesy of Dr. Viktor Szegedi, University of Szeged, Hungary.

examination or (2) for administration of neuroactive compounds (*e.g.* neurotransmitters, modulators, drugs or hormones) by microiontophoresis to examine their effects on firing parameters of single neurons *in vivo* (Fig. 4). Microiontophoretic ejection is accomplished by applying a voltage across the micropipette and causing it to become polarized. If a voltage is applied to a solution, ions and charged molecules will migrate toward and away from the source of the imposed electrical field depending upon the sign of their net charge. If the pipette is positioned close to a neuron, drugs may be ejected and their pharmacological effects inferred by resulting changes in the rate or pattern of firing. Typically, this neuropharmacological technique is used to determine the effects of various substances upon firing parameters of neurons. A chief advantage of the microiontophoretic method is that it is possible to examine the effects of drugs upon single neurons without affecting the whole of the nervous system such as may occur when drugs are administered systemically.

4.2 *In vivo* voltammetry

In voltammetry, voltage is applied to a working electrode and information about an electroactive analyte is obtained by measuring the current as the potential is varied. In a classical, three-electrode voltammeric system the redox reaction (electron transfer) of interest takes place at the surface of the working electrode at applied potentials and measured relative to the reference electrode which is kept at a constant potential and through which no currents flow. The current circuit is completed by an auxiliary (counter or ground) electrode to which sufficient potential is applied to balance the current produced at the working electrode. For picoampere currents produced by ultramicro working electrodes, voltammetry can be performed successfully using two-electrode configurations without significant disturbance of the reference potential.

In vivo voltammetry involves the electrochemical detection of oxidisable substances in the central nervous system. The technique now benefits from ultraminiature and more sensitive and selective working electrodes than ever before, allowing high temporal and spatial resolutions. In *in vivo* voltammetry, the commonly used reference electrodes are the sodium-saturated calomel (SSCE), Ag/AgCl pellet (Kruk et al., 1998) or a piece of chlorided silver wire while the indifferent auxiliary electrode can be made of platinum, chromalloy (Kawagoe et al., 1993), stainless steel or it is simply a brass screw attached to the skull. When CF containing multi-barrel microelectrodes are used to record electrochemical signals, many times along with neuronal spikes in a 'time-shared' manner, the Ag/AgCl reference electrode (chlorided silver wire) is placed in one of the electrolyte filled barrels (Armstrong-James et al., 1980; Armstrong-James et al., 1981).

Small diameter (5-30 μm) carbon fibers have been used for working electrodes since 1979 when Pujol and colleagues first used them to measure oxidation of neurotransmitters including dopamine, norepinephrine and serotonin. (Ponchon et al., 1979). Ever since, a great number of surface treatments, chemical modifications and film coatings have been developed to improve the sensitivity, selectivity and temporal resolution of CF working microelectrodes used in electrochemistry *in vitro* or *in vivo*. Due to their physicochemical properties and biocompatible nature, CF microelectrodes can be used for working electrode in all forms of voltammetry used *in vivo* including chronoamperometry, linear potential scanning (*e.g.* cyclic voltammetry, Fig. 5) or pulsed voltammetry techniques as wells as in constant potential amperometry (Fig. 6).

The extracellular fluid in the central nervous system contains a variety of electroactive organic species that oxidize at similar potential on the carbon surface of a CF working microelectrode. These include ascorbic acid (AA); neurotransmitter cathecholamines such as dopamine (DA) and norepinephrine (NE), as well as their metabolites, 3,4-dihydroxyphenylacetic acid (DOPAC) , 3-methoxytyramine (3MT), and homovanillic acid (HVA); the 5-hydroxyindole neuromediator 5-hydroxytriptamine (serotonine, 5-HT) and its metabolite 5-hydroxyindoleacetic acid (5HIAA); and the purine metabolite uric acid (UA).

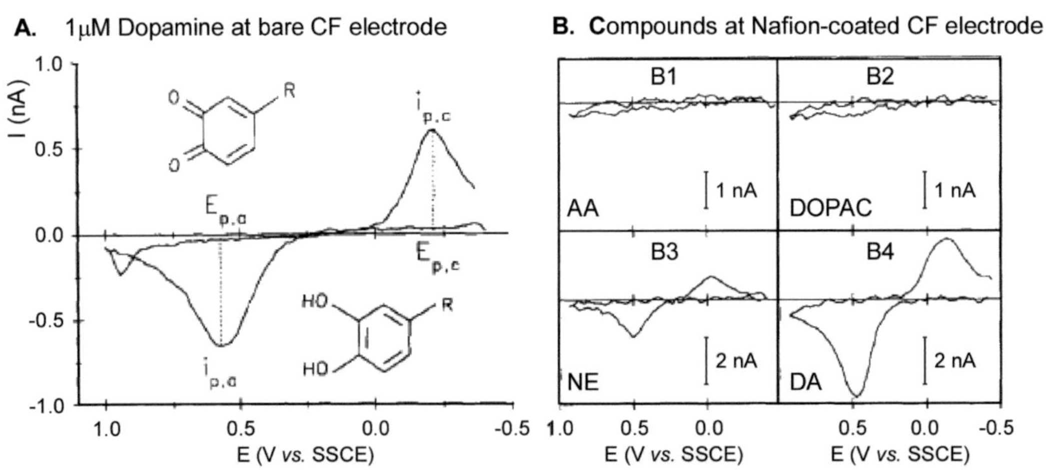

Fig. 5. Cyclic voltammograms of electroactive biological compounds. Compounds in panel B are: B1, ascorbic acid (AA), 200 μM; B2, DOPAC, 200 μM; B3, norepinephrin (NE), 10 μM and B4, dopamine (DA), 10 μM. Adapted with permission from Kawagoe *et al.*, 1993.

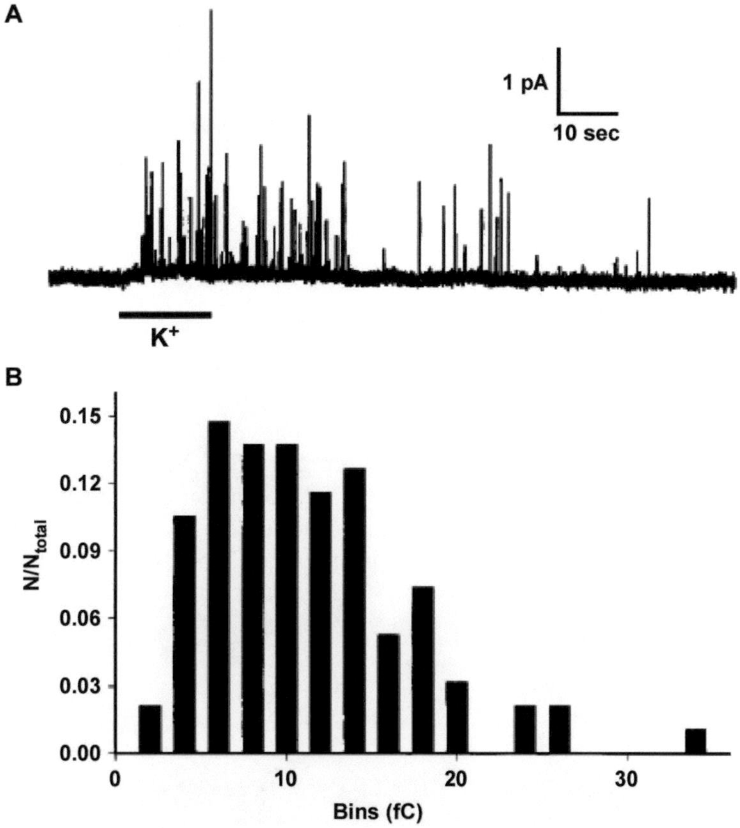

Fig. 6. Exocytotic current spikes from a dopaminergic amacrine cell stimulated with potassium (K^+). Recording was taken by constant potential amperometry using a 5 μm diameter CF microelectrode (A). Panel B shows charge distribution from the spikes in panel A. Reprinted with permission from Hochstetler *et al.*, 2000.

One way of increasing the selectivity of CF working electrodes between these species is using discriminative measurement techniques including chrono- or constant potential amperometry, linear sweep- , cyclic-, fast cyclic- staircase-, differential pulse- or differential normal pulse voltammetry. For review, see (O'Neill et al., 1998). The other possibility is to apply a coating like Nafion to repel unwanted species or to chemically change the carbon surface by modifying the carbon surface with 4--sulfobenzene (Hermans et al., 2006) or using flame etching (Strand & Venton, 2008).

4.3 Monitoring nitric oxide (NO)

Nitric oxide (NO) is a gaseous signaling molecule known to influence a great variety of physiological and pathological events in all vertabrate species including humans. NO has a lifetime of a few seconds, diffuses freely across cell mambranes and quite easily reacts with other biological components such as superoxide, oxygen or thiols. Electrochemical detection of NO (mostly amperometry) is the most suitable technique sensitive enough to measure concentrations of NO in biological tissues in real time without significant interference

caused potentially by other species such as nitrite, nitrate, dopamine, ascorbate and L-arginine. For review, see (Barbosa et al., 2008). The first amperometric NO electrode based on a classical Clark electrode design and consisted of a fine platinum wire as the working electrode and a separate silver wire used for reference electrode (Shibuki, 1990).
Oxidation of NO at solid electrodes, which is usually used to measure NO, takes place via an electrochemical reaction (electron transfer to the electrode):

$$NO - e^- > NO^+ \quad (1)$$

followed by a chemical reaction:

$$NO^+ + OH^- > HNO_2 \quad (2)$$

Carbon fiber NO microelectrodes can be made on the micro- and nanoscale allowing extreme spatial and temporal resolutions and they cause minimal damage when inserted in a living tissue. Early CF NO microelectrodes were covered a variety of porphyrins and Nafion to increase selectivity by repelling interfering species (Malinski & Taha, 1992). Later, to circumvent some of the problems with porphyrin coatings (Lantoine et al., 1995; Nagase et al., 1997) phthalocyanins were used instead to modify CF microelectrode surfaces (Vilakazi & Nyokong, 2001). A great variety of different CF microelectrode coatings for NO sensors have also been reported. For review, see (Davies & Zhang, 2008).

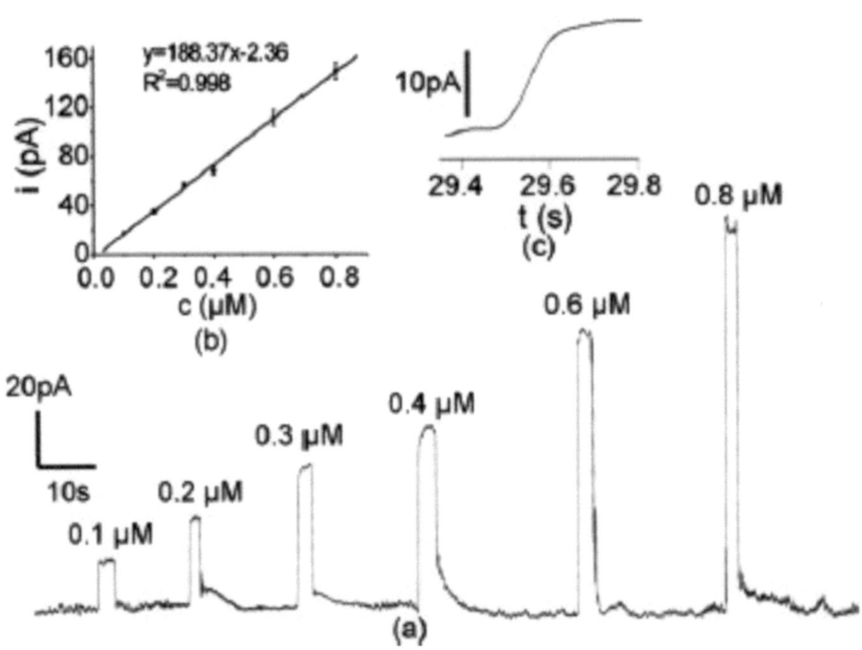

Fig. 7. (a) Typical amperometric response of a carbon microdisk electrode modified with carbon nanotubes to increasing concentrations of NO using a calibration system. (b) The calibration curve based on data shown in panel a. (c) An amperometric curve illustrating the sensor's response time to NO. Reprinted with permission from Du *et al.*, 2008.

As a new approach, combination CF-based NO sensors with micron or submicron size tip diameters have been developed by Zhang and co-workers. These sensors combine a CF working electrode with an integrated Ag/AgCl reference electrode and both coated with a proprietary NO-selective membrane. The electrode is operated as the platinum wire-based Clark-type NO sensor (Zhang et al., 2001; Zhang et al., 2002).

Surface variations among types of carbon fibers made by different companies seem to influence the characteristics of their NO sensitivity and selectivity when coated with Nafion and *o*-phenylenediamine. The 30 μm Textron CF showed high selectivity for NO against ascorbate, nitrite and dopamine than fibers from other makers. This may be due to the strong adhesion or more uniform coating of Nafion to the smooth surface of the Textron fiber (Santos et al., 2008).

A novel NO microsensor has recently been reported using a single-walled carbon nanotubes (SWNTs) attached to the surface of a CF microdisk (cross-cut area of a 7 μm carbon fiber) and covered with a Nafion membrane (Du et al., 2008). Application of carbon nanotubes dramatically increased the sensitivity of CF microelectrode as the detection limit proved to be about 10 times lower for NO (4.3 nM) than that of the bare carbon surface and lower than most electrochemical sensors reported before (Fig. 7). The Nafion layer provided a good barrier to some of the interferents without decreasing the response speed to NO. The microsensor has been successfully applied to the measurement of NO release from single isolated endothelium cells.

4.4 A novel use of CF microelectrodes; sensing tissue oxigen levels

In its simplest form, a polarographic oxygen sensor consists of two electrodes, between which a negative polarization voltage is applied. Oxygen is chemically reduced at the cathode according to the following reaction:

$$O_2 + 2H_2O + 4e^- > 4OH^- \quad (3)$$

Typically, a Ag/AgCl reference electrode is used for the anode, providing the following half-reaction:

$$4Ag^+ + 4Cl^- > 4AgCl + 4e^- \quad (4)$$

The amount of current flowing through the sensor is proportional to the concentration of oxygen at the surface of the cathode. Polarographic oxygen sensors of various designs have been used for over 60 years to measure changes in oxygen tension within the brain.

The CF microelectrodes can be converted into amperometric oxygen sensors by applying a negative polarization voltage between the carbon tip (cathode) and an external Ag/AgCl reference electrode. Polarization between the anode and cathode is set to the center of the plateau region in the current voltage curve. The center of the plateau region is empirically determined for each electrode, and is consistently found to be between -0.8 and -0.95 V (Fig. 8). Within this region, the sensor current is determined by the diffusion of oxygen at the cathode and is relatively insensitive to small changes in the applied voltage. Measurements with the novel sensor are highly similar to the spontaneous and stimulus-induced oxygen responses obtained with a conventional Clark-style oxygen electrode (Allen, 2008). However, the ultraminiature barrel size and extended carbon tip make CF microelectrodes superior for combined transcranial magnetic stimulation and electrophysiology investigations (Allen et al., 2007). Multi-barreled configuration of the CF microelectrode represents a further advantage as the built-in microcapillaries can be used for recording neuronal extracellular spikes and/or applying various drugs of interest by iontophoresis or pressure.

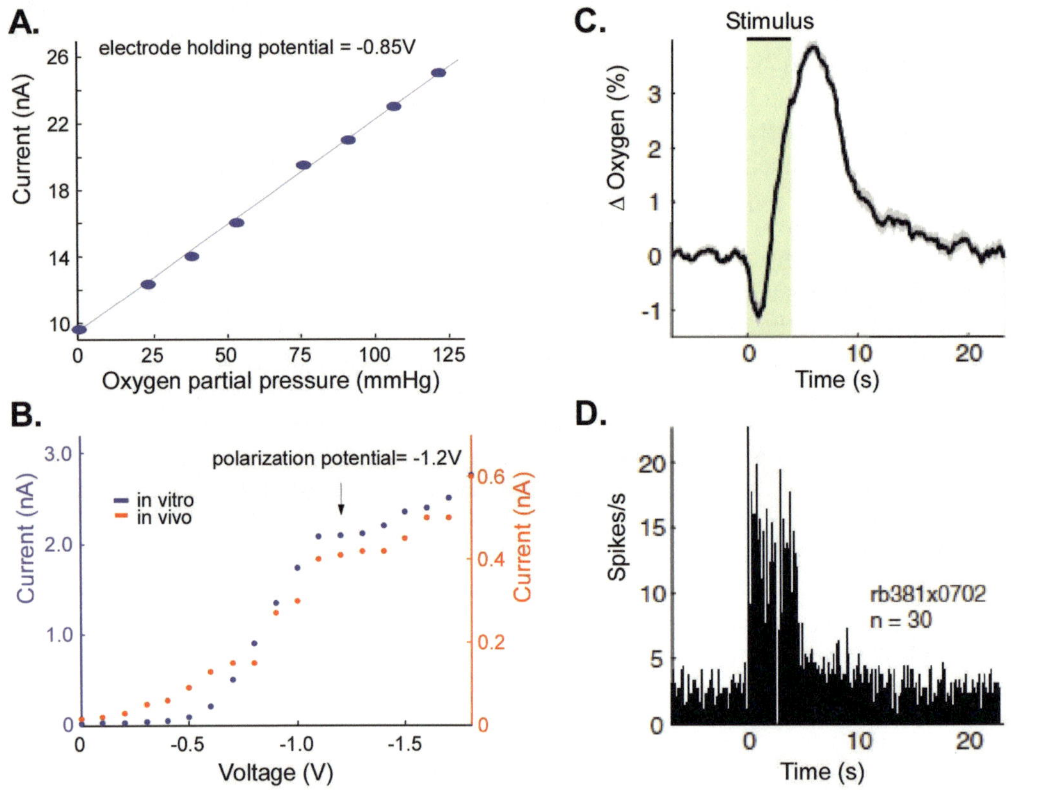

Fig. 8. Responses of CF microelectrodes to oxigen *in vitro* (A, B) and *in vivo* (C, D). A typical calibration curve for the CF oxygen sensor is shown in panel A. Note CF current plateau nearly identical in the *in vitro* and *in vivo* conditions (B) Visually evoked oxygen responses (C) and co-localized multi-unit neural activity (D) recorded from the lateral geniculate nucleus. Recordings were taken using a Kation Scientific-made seven-barreled CF microelectrode (see Figs. 1E and 2F). Reprinted with permission from the dissertation of E.A. Allen (Allen, 2008).

4.5 Enzyme-based CF biosensors

The enzyme-linked microelectrode is the fundamental component of amperometric bisosensors. Physicochemical change produced by specific interactions between a target analyte (substrate) and the biorecognition element (enzyme) is detected and measured by a transducer. The transducer converts the biochemical signal into an electrical signal which can be further processed using more conventional electronic devices.

The enzyme is selected based upon the type of reaction being used to determine the analyte of interest. The most frequently used redox enzymes are: alcohol dehydrogenase, aldehyde dehydrogenase, glucose oxidase, glutaminase, horse radix peroxidase, catalase, xanthine oxidase, choline oxidase, urease, billirubin oxidase and lactate oxidase. In addition to redox enzymes, hydrolytic enzymes like lipases or esterase are also used along with the redox enzymes for added specificity or to sense a substrate where no oxidoreductase is known. For review, see (Sarma et al., 2009).

The supporting electrode material is selected based upon the electrical conductivity and hardness of the material and is conventionally made of solid supports, such as gold, platinum or carbon. To establish electrical communication between redox proteins and electrode surface, the insulating effect of the immobilized protein layer must be transformed into a charge transport matrix. Immobilization of enzymes in conducting polymers or functionalized polymers, application of composite materials, composites of metal complexes, carbon nanotubes or other nanomaterials are used to overcome this obstacle.

Carbon fibers of 7 to 30 μm in diameter are widely used for supporting base microelectrodes in fabricating enzyme-based electrochemical sensors. Dehyrogenase enzymes have been immobilized onto CF microelectrode via avidin-biotin technology and a covalently linked hydrophilic tether to detect neurotransmitters including glutamate (Pantano & Kuhr, 1993; Hayes & Kuhr, 1999). CF microelectrodes have been coated with cross-linked redox polimer hydrogel containing glutamate oxidase (Figs. 9 and 10), horse radix peroxidase and ascorbate oxidase to monitor glutamate and ascorbate levels in extracellular space (Kulagina et al., 1999; Oldenziel & Westerink, 2005; Oldenziel et al., 2006).

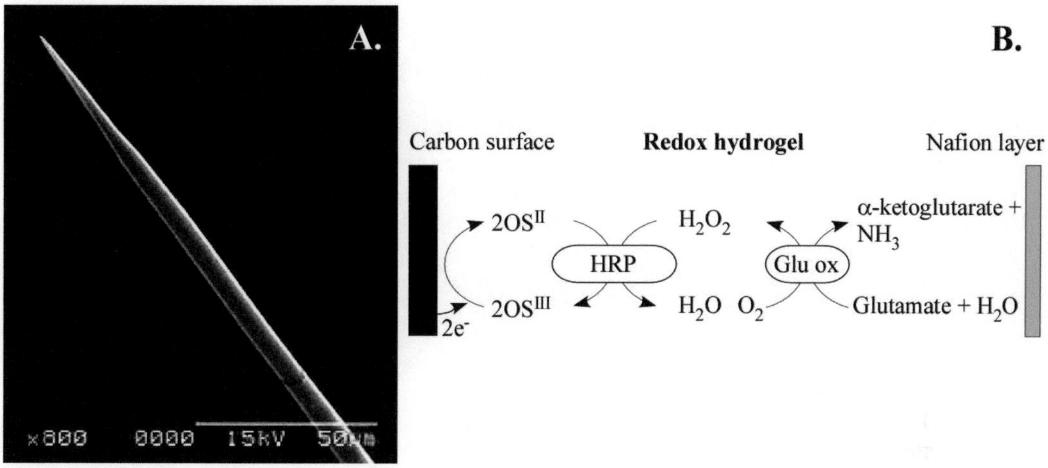

Fig. 9. (A) Scanning electron micrograph of a CF glutamate microbiosensor. Note the 7 μm carbon fiber ends in submicron tip and protrudes from the glass insulation by about 100 μm (courtesy of Kation Scientific). (B) Schematic of electrochemical detection of glutamate using osmium and oxidase-peroxidase enzymes containing redox hydrogel. Abbreviations: HRP, horse-radix peroxidase; Glu-ox, glutamate oxidase; OS, osmium.

Acetylcholine and choline microbiosensors were developed using acetylcholinesterase and choline oxidase immobilized onto CF microelectrodes (Navera et al., 1991; Tamiya & Karube, 1992; Karube et al., 1993; Garguilo & Michael, 1994; Garguilo & Michael, 1996; Cui et al., 2001; Schuvailo et al., 2005). Lactate oxidase or superoxide dismutases were immolized on CF microelectrodes to detect lactate in rat brain (Shram et al., 1998) or superoxide anions (Tian et al., 2005), respectively. In the latter case, a third-generation biosensor was implemented by electro-deposition of gold nanoparticles on the 10 μm CF microelectrode and then modification of the gold nanoparticles by cysteine followed by immobilization of superoxide dismutase. For review on electrical contacting of redox proteins by nanotechnological means, see (Willner et al., 2006; Willner et al., 2007).

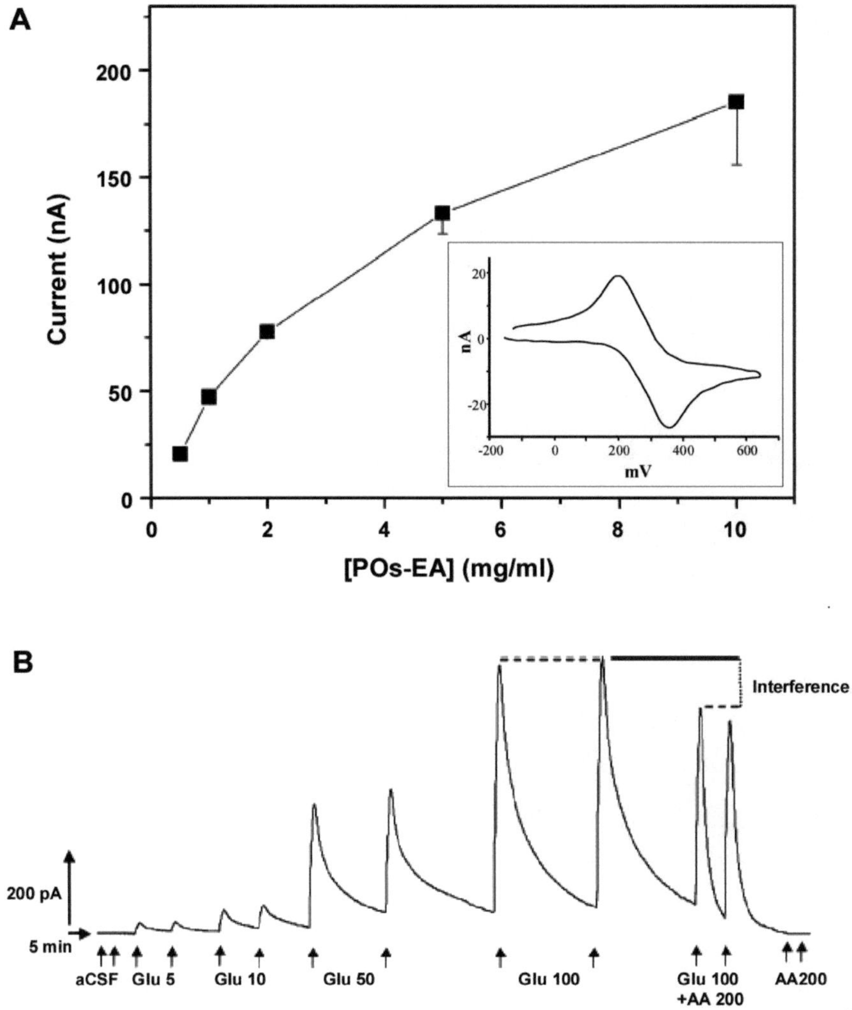

Fig. 10. Performance of a CF microelectrode-based glutamate microsensor. (A) Correlation between the concentration of the glutamate oxidase containing redox polymer (Pos-EA) and current quantified by cycliy voltammetry. A typical example of the cyclic voltammogram is shown in the inset. (B) Amperometric calibration of the glutamate microsensor. Concentration is shown in μM. Abbreviations: aCSF, artificial cerebrospinal fluid; Glu, glutamate; AA, ascorbic acid. Reprinted with permission from Oldenziel and Westerink, 2005.

Carbon fiber-based glucose microbiosensors were made by immobilization of glucose oxidase on the carbon surface using various methods (Nakayama & Matsuda, 1992; Karube et al., 1993; Furbee et al., 1994; Netchiporouk et al., 1996; Wipf et al., 2000; Cui et al., 2001) Recenly, single-walled carbon nanotubes and platinum nanoparticles (Hrapovic et al., 2004), osmium redox polymer/enzyme composite film (Fei et al., 2005) or electrochemical electrometallization and electropolymerisation of phenylene diamine film with covalently bound enzymes (Schuvailo et al., 2006) were introduced to improve selectivity and sensitivity of CF glucose biosensors. An inplantable version of these glucose biosensors has also been reported (Ahmad et al., 2007).

4.6 DNA biosensors on CF microelectrodes

A tremendous progress has been made in the field of DNA bisoensors since Mikkelsen and colleagues first reported an electrochemical DNA hybridisation biosensor (Millan & Mikkelsen, 1993; Millan et al., 1994). There have been two main approaches to the electrochemical transduction of DNA hybridisation, which can be broadly referred to as labelled methods and label-free methods. Labelled methods use redox active molecules (*e.g.* $Co(Phen)_3^{3+}$, methylene blue or AQMS that bind to DNA and give different electrochemical signals depending on whether the DNA is double- or single-stranded. Label-free methods rely on either changes to the electrical characteristics of the DNA-modified interface upon hybridisation or on the natural electroactivity of DNA. For turorial review, see (Odenthal & Gooding, 2007). A further advantage of DNA deposition on biosensing surfaces is the ability to greatly increase the effective surface area. In comparison with Nafion film coatings, the DNA sensing layer also display some affinity toward cationic species and repelling ability toward anionic species. Equally important that the DNA layer exhibits adsorption, insertion and interchelating abilities with many bioactive species.

DNA can directly be deposited on the carbon surface of highly oriented pyrolitic graphite, carbon fiber or carbon disk microelectrodes under controlled DC potentials. Using a labelled method, the covalently bound DNA deposition resulted in a 500 to 1000-fold increase in the effective surface area and similarly enlarged voltammetric response to $Co(Phen)_3^{3+}$(Lin et al., 2005).

In a label-free method, double-stranded DNA was attached to the carbon surface via gold nanoparticles and was aplied to determine dopamine, serotonine and ascorbic acid using cyclic or differential pulse voltammetry (Lu et al., 2004). Simultaneous differential pulse voltammetry determination of dopamine and serotonine could be achieved in the presence of 1 mM ascorbic acid.

An overoxidized microporous polypyrrole film could serve as template for directing DNA immobilization on the surface of CF microelectrodes. The formed DNA-polypyrrole biocomposite layer exhibited more effective rejection of anionic ascorbate or uric acid and more preferential collection of the cationic dopamine and epinephrine than pure polypyrrole or DNA coatings. The electrochemical signal from ascorbic acid could be totally suppressed at concentrations lower than 20 mM (Fig. 11). The selectivity factors of dopamine/ascorbate and epinephrine/ascorbate were 5000 and 2000, respectively. Unfortunately, responses of dopamine and epinephrine superposed one another with no adequate separation (Jiang & Lin, 2005).

5. Conclusion

In this chapter, the fabrication, main properties and a great deal of applications of CF microelectrodes have extensively been reviewed. It has been shown that, taking advantages of the unique and biocompatible physicochemical properties of carbon fibers, even submicron CF microelectrodes can be made for *in vivo* applications. This allows an unprecedented spatial and temporal resolution in understanding basic signalling mechanisms of dopamine and other neurostransmitters. The ever increasing sensitivity and selectivity of CF microelectrodes will facilitate detection of even lower concentrations of analytes and the number of detectable and biologically important species will probably increase.

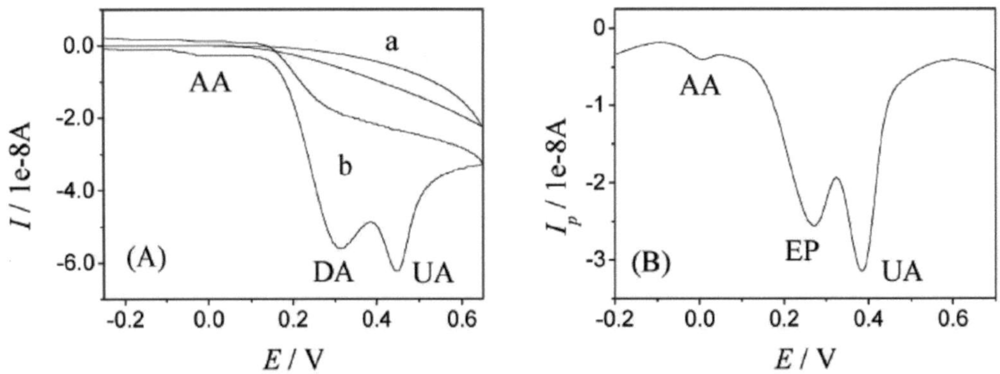

Fig. 11. (A) Cyclic voltammograms of 0.5 mM uric acid (UA), 0.1 mM dopamine (DA) and 25 mM ascorbic acid (AA) at (a) bare CF microelectrode and (b) DNA-polypyrrole covered CF microelectrode. (B) Square wave voltammogram of 0.5 mM uric acid, 0.1 mM epinephrine (EP) and 25 mM ascorbic acid using a DNA-polypyrrole CF microelectrode. Reprinted with permission from Jiang & Lin, 2005.

Despite the relative chemical inertness of CFs, their surface can be functionalized using vigorous oxidation methods. The strong bound between the carbon surface and the modifiers (carboxylic, quinonic, ketonic, hydroxylic, aryl, naphtyl, anthryl or alkyl groups, primary and secondary amines) makes the initial covalently attached layer very suitable for further functionalization of CF microelectrodes. Electrically conducting polymer matrices deposited onto the carbon surface provide means to electrically connect redox enzymes with the electrodes. Non-conducting polymer layers allow an ultrathin electrical insulation on portions of CF microelectrodes where needed.

Reports on attaching DNA or carbon nanotubes (or functionalized CNTs) onto CF microelectrodes signals the coming of a new and even more intriguing era of sensing biomolecules of interest *in situ* and in real time. Both procedures greatly extend not only the sensing surfaces of CF microelectrodes but the number of detectable organic compounds, too.

6. Acknowledgement

This work was supported by the National Office for Research and Technology, Hungary (grant no.: GVOP 3.3.1-0141/3.0) and Kation Scientific, Minneapolis, MN USA. Scanning electron microscopy is gratefully thanked to Dr. Zsolt Tóth, University of Szeged, Hungary.

7. References

Ahmad, F., Christenson, A., Bainbridge, M., Yusof, A.P. & Ab Ghani, S. (2007). Minimizing tissue-material interaction in microsensor for subcutaneous glucose monitoring. *Biosens Bioelectron,* Vol. 22, No. 8, pp. 1625-32.

Allen, E.A. (2008). Explorations of the function of the central visual pathway with visual and electrical stimulation. *Ph.D. Dissertation, University of California, Berkeley.*

Allen, E.A., Pasley, B.N., Duong, T. & Freeman, R.D. (2007). Transcranial magnetic stimulation elicits coupled neural and hemodynamic consequences. *Science,* Vol. 317, No. 5846, pp. 1918-21.

Armstrong-James, M., Fox, K., Kruk, Z.L. & Millar, J. (1981). Quantitative ionophoresis of catecholamines using multibarrel carbon fibre microelectrodes. *J Neurosci Methods,* Vol. 4, No. 4, pp. 385-406.

Armstrong-James, M. & Millar, J. (1979). Carbon fibre microelectrodes. *J Neurosci Methods,* Vol. 1, No. 3, pp. 279-87.

Armstrong-James, M., Millar, J. & Kruk, Z.L. (1980). Quantification of noradrenaline iontophoresis. *Nature,* Vol. 288, No. 5787, pp. 181-3.

Barbosa, R.M., Lourenco, C.F., Santos, R.M., Pomerleau, F., Huettl, P., Gerhardt, G.A. & Laranjinha, J. (2008). In vivo real-time measurement of nitric oxide in anesthetized rat brain. *Methods Enzymol,* Vol. 441, pp. 351-67.

Budai, D. (2004). Ultralow-noise headstage and main amplifiers for extracellular spike recording. *Acta Biol Szeged,* Vol. 48, No. 1-4, pp. 13-17.

Budai, D., Horváth, K. & Szabó, A. (2007). Polymer insulation of ultramicro carbon fiber electrodes for electrophysiological, electrochemical and biosensor applications. *Acta Biol Szeged,* Vol. 51, No. 2, pp. 81-85.

Budai, D. & Molnár, Z. (2001). Novel carbon fiber microelectrodes for extracellular electrophysiology. *Acta Biol Szeged,* Vol. 45, No. 1, pp. 65-73.

Cui, J., Kulagina, N.V. & Michael, A.C. (2001). Pharmacological evidence for the selectivity of in vivo signals obtained with enzyme-based electrochemical sensors. *J Neurosci Methods,* Vol. 104, No. 2, pp. 183-9.

Davies, I.R. & Zhang, X. (2008). Nitric oxide selective electrodes. *Methods Enzymol,* Vol. 436, pp. 63-95.

Downard, A.J. (2000). Electrochemically assisted covalent modification of carbon electrodes. *Electroanalysis,* Vol. 12, No. 14, pp. 1085-1096.

Du, F., Huang, W., Shi, Y., Wang, Z. & Cheng, J. (2008). Real-time monitoring of NO release from single cells using carbon fiber microdisk electrodes modified with single-walled carbon nanotubes. *Biosens Bioelectron,* Vol. 24, No. 3, pp. 415-21.

El-Deen, E., El-Giar, M. & Wipf, D.O. (2006). Preparation of tip-protected poly(oxyphenylene) coated carbon-fiber ultramikroelectrodes. *Electroanalysis,* Vol. 18, No. 23, pp. 2281-2289.

Fei, J., Wu, K., Wang, F. & Hu, S. (2005). Glucose nanosensors based on redox polymer/glucose oxidase modified carbon fiber nanoelectrodes. *Talanta,* Vol. 65, No. 4, pp. 918-24.

Furbee, J.W., Jr., Kuwana, T. & Kelly, R.S. (1994). Fractured carbon fiber-based biosensor for glucose. *Anal Chem,* Vol. 66, No. 9, pp. 1575-7.

Garguilo, M.G. & Michael, A.C. (1994). Quantitation of choline in the extracellular fluid of brain tissue with amperometric microsensors. *Anal Chem,* Vol. 66, No. 17, pp. 2621-9.

Garguilo, M.G. & Michael, A.C. (1996). Amperometric microsensors for monitoring choline in the extracellular fluid of brain. *J Neurosci Methods,* Vol. 70, No. 1, pp. 73-82.

Gerhardt, G.A., Oke, A.F., Nagy, G., Moghaddam, B. & Adams, R.N. (1984). Nafion-coated electrodes with high selectivity for CNS electrochemistry. *Brain Res,* Vol. 290, No. 2, pp. 390-5.

Hayes, M.A. & Kuhr, W.G. (1999). Preservation of NADH voltammetry for enzyme-modified electrodes based on dehydrogenase. *Anal Chem,* Vol. 71, No. 9, pp. 1720-7.

Hermans, A., Seipel, A.T., Miller, C.E. & Wightman, R.M. (2006). Carbon-fiber microelectrodes modified with 4-sulfobenzene have increased sensitivity and selectivity for catecholamines. *Langmuir,* Vol. 22, No. 5, pp. 1964-9.

Hochstetler, S.E., Puopolo, M., Gustincich, S., Raviola, E., & Wightman, R.M. (2000). Real-time amperometric measurements of zeptomole quantities of dopamine released from neurons. *Anal Chem,* Vol. 72, No.3, pp. 489–496.

Hrapovic, S., Liu, Y., Male, K.B. & Luong, J.H. (2004). Electrochemical biosensing platforms using platinum nanoparticles and carbon nanotubes. *Anal Chem,* Vol. 76, No. 4, pp. 1083-8.

Jiang, X. & Lin, X. (2005). Immobilization of DNA on carbon fiber microelectrodes by using overoxidized polypyrrole template for selective detection of dopamine and epinephrine in the presence of high concentrations of ascorbic acid and uric acid. *Analyst,* Vol. 130, No. 3, pp. 391-6.

Karube, I., Yokoyama, K. & Tamiya, E. (1993). Microbiosensors for acetylcholine and glucose. *Biosens Bioelectron,* Vol. 8, No. 3-4, pp. 219-28.

Kawagoe, K.T., Zimmerman, J.B. & Wightman, R.M. (1993). Principles of voltammetry and microelectrode surface states. *J Neurosci Methods,* Vol. 48, No. 3, pp. 225-40.

Kruk, Z.L., Cheeta, S., Milla, J., Muscat, R., Williams, J.E. & Willner, P. (1998). Real time measurement of stimulated dopamine release in the conscious rat using fast cyclic voltammetry: dopamine release is not observed during intracranial self stimulation. *J Neurosci Methods,* Vol. 79, No. 1, pp. 9-19.

Kulagina, N.V., Shankar, L. & Michael, A.C. (1999). Monitoring glutamate and ascorbate in the extracellular space of brain tissue with electrochemical microsensors. *Anal Chem,* Vol. 71, No. 22, pp. 5093-100.

Lantoine, F., Trevin, S., Bedioui, F. & Devynck, J. (1995). Selective and sensitive electrochemical measurement of nitric-oxide in aqueous-solution: Discussion and new results. *J. Electroanal. Chem.,* Vol. 392, pp. 85-89.

Lin, X., Jiang, X. & Lu, L. (2005). DNA deposition on carbon electrodes under controlled dc potentials. *Biosens Bioelectron,* Vol. 20, No. 9, pp. 1709-17.

Lu, L., Wang, S. & Lin, X. (2004). Attachment of DNA to the carbon fiber microelectrode via gold nanoparticles for simultaneous determination of dopamine and serotonin. *Anal Sci,* Vol. 20, No. 8, pp. 1131-5.

Malinski, T. & Taha, Z. (1992). Nitric oxide release from a single cell measured in situ by a porphyrinic-based microsensor. *Nature,* Vol. 358, No. 6388, pp. 676-8.

Millan, K.M. & Mikkelsen, S.R. (1993). Sequence-selective biosensor for DNA based on electroactive hybridization indicators. *Anal Chem,* Vol. 65, No. 17, pp. 2317-23.

Millan, K.M., Saraullo, A. & Mikkelsen, S.R. (1994). Voltammetric DNA biosensor for cystic fibrosis based on a modified carbon paste electrode. *Anal Chem,* Vol. 66, No. 18, pp. 2943-8.

Nagase, S., Ohkoshi, N., Ueda, A., Aoyagi, K. & Koyama, A. (1997). Hydrogen peroxide interferes with detection of nitric oxide by an electrochemical method. *Clin Chem,* Vol. 43, No. 7, pp. 1246.

Nakayama, Y. & Matsuda, T. (1992). Surface fixation of hydrogels. Heparin and glucose oxidase hydrogelated surfaces. *Asaio J,* Vol. 38, No. 3, pp. M421-4.

Navera, E.N., Sode, K., Tamiya, E. & Karube, I. (1991). Development of acetylcholine sensor using carbon fiber (amperometric determination). *Biosens Bioelectron,* Vol. 6, No. 8, pp. 675-80.

Netchiporouk, L.I., Shram, N.F., Jaffrezic-Renault, N., Martelet, C. & Cespuglio, R. (1996). In vivo brain glucose measurements: differential normal pulse voltammetry with enzyme-modified carbon fiber microelectrodes. *Anal Chem,* Vol. 68, No. 24, pp. 4358-64.

Odenthal, K.J. & Gooding, J.J. (2007). An introduction to electrochemical DNA biosensors. *Analyst,* Vol. 132, No. 7, pp. 603-10.

Oldenziel, W.H., Dijkstra, G., Cremers, T.I. & Westerink, B.H. (2006). Evaluation of hydrogel-coated glutamate microsensors. *Anal Chem,* Vol. 78, No. 10, pp. 3366-78.

Oldenziel, W.H. & Westerink, B.H. (2005). Improving glutamate microsensors by optimizing the composition of the redox hydrogel. *Anal Chem,* Vol. 77, No. 17, pp. 5520-8.

O'Neill, R.D., Lowry, J.P. & Mas, M. (1998). Monitoring brain chemistry in vivo: voltammetric techniques, sensors, and behavioral applications. *Crit Rev Neurobiol,* Vol. 12, No. 1-2, pp. 69-127.

Pantano, P. & Kuhr, W.G. (1993). Dehydrogenase-modified carbon-fiber microelectrodes for the measurement of neurotransmitter dynamics. 2. Covalent modification utilizing avidin-biotin technology. *Anal Chem,* Vol. 65, No. 5, pp. 623-30.

Pinson, J. & Podvorica, F. (2005). Attachment of organic layers to conductive or semiconductive surfaces by reduction of diazonium salts. *Chem Soc Rev,* Vol. 34, No. 5, pp. 429-39.

Ponchon, J.L., Cespuglio, R., Gonon, F., Jouvet, M. & Pujol, J.F. (1979). Normal pulse polarography with carbon fiber electrodes for in vitro and in vivo determination of catecholamines. *Anal Chem,* Vol. 51, No. 9, pp. 1483-6.

Santos, R.M., Lourenco, C.F., Piedade, A.P., Andrews, R., Pomerleau, F., Huettl, P., Gerhardt, G.A., Laranjinha, J. & Barbosa, R.M. (2008). A comparative study of carbon fiber-based microelectrodes for the measurement of nitric oxide in brain tissue. *Biosens Bioelectron,* Vol. 24, No. 4, pp. 704-9.

Sarac, A.S., Gencturk, A., Gilsing, H.D., Schulz, B. & Turhan, C.M. (2009). Effect of electrolyte on the electropolymerization of 2,2-dibutyl-3,4-propylenedioxythiophene on carbon fiber microelectrodes. *J Nanosci Nanotechnol,* Vol. 9, No. 5, pp. 2877-86.

Sarac, A.S., Sezgin, S., Ates, M. & Turhan, C.M. (2008). Electrochemical impedance spectroscopy and morphological analyses of pyrrole, phenylpyrrole and methoxyphenylpyrrole on carbon fiber microelectrodes. *Surface and Coatings Technology,* Vol. 202, No. pp. 3997-4005.

Sarma, A.K., Vatsyayan, P., Goswami, P. & Minteer, S.D. (2009). Recent advances in material science for developing enzyme electrodes. *Biosens Bioelectron,* Vol. 24, No. 8, pp. 2313-22.

Schuvailo, O.M., Soldatkin, O.O., Lefebvre, A., Cespuglio, R. & Soldatkin, A.P. (2006). Highly selective microbiosensors for in vivo measurement of glucose, lactate and glutamate. *Anal Chim Acta,* Vol. 573-574, pp. 110-6.

Schuvailo, O.N., Dzyadevych, S.V., El'skaya, A.V., Gautier-Sauvigne, S., Csoregi, E., Cespuglio, R. & Soldatkin, A.P. (2005). Carbon fibre-based microbiosensors for in vivo measurements of acetylcholine and choline. *Biosens Bioelectron,* Vol. 21, No. 1, pp. 87-94.

Shibuki, K. (1990). An electrochemical microprobe for detecting nitric oxide release in brain tissue. *Neurosci Res,* Vol. 9, No. 1, pp. 69-76.

Shram, N.F., Netchiporouk, L.I., Martelet, C., Jaffrezic-Renault, N., Bonnet, C. & Cespuglio, R. (1998). In vivo voltammetric detection of rat brain lactate with carbon fiber microelectrodes coated with lactate oxidase. *Anal Chem,* Vol. 70, No. 13, pp. 2618-22.

Strand, A.M. & Venton, B.J. (2008). Flame etching enhances the sensitivity of carbon-fiber microelectrodes. *Anal Chem,* Vol. 80, No. 10, pp. 3708-15.

Tamiya, E. & Karube, I. (1992). Ultramicrobiosensors for monitoring of neurotransmitters. *Ann N Y Acad Sci,* Vol. 672, pp. 272-7.

Tian, Y., Mao, L., Okajima, T. & Ohsaka, T. (2005). A carbon fiber microelectrode-based third-generation biosensor for superoxide anion. *Biosens Bioelectron,* Vol. 21, No. 4, pp. 557-64.

Vilakazi, S.L. & Nyokong, T. (2001). Voltammetric determination of nitric oxide on cobalt phthalocyanine modified microelectrodes. *J. Electroanal. Chem.,* Vol. 512, pp. 56-63.

Willner, B., Katz, E. & Willner, I. (2006). Electrical contacting of redox proteins by nanotechnological means. *Curr Opin Biotechnol,* Vol. 17, No. 6, pp. 589-96.

Willner, I., Baron, R. & Willner, B. (2007). Integrated nanoparticle-biomolecule systems for biosensing and bioelectronics. *Biosens Bioelectron,* Vol. 22, No. 9-10, pp. 1841-52.

Wipf, D.O., Ge, F., Spaine, T.W. & Baur, J.E. (2000). Microscopic measurement of pH with iridium oxide microelectrodes. *Anal Chem,* Vol. 72, No. 20, pp. 4921-7.

Yeh, S.-R., Chen, Y.-C., Su, H.-C., Yew, T.-R., Kao, H.-H., Lee, Y.-T., Liu, T.-A., Chen, H., Chang, Y.-C., Chang, P. & Chen, H. (2009). Interfacing Neurons both Extracellularly and Intracellularly Using Carbon Nanotube Probes with Long-Term Endurance. *Langmuir,* Vol. 25, No. 13, pp. 7718-7724. 0743-7463.

Zhang, M., Liu, K., Xiang, L., Lin, Y., Su, L. & Mao, L. (2007). Carbon nanotube-modified carbon fiber microelectrodes for in vivo voltammetric measurement of ascorbic acid in rat brain. *Anal Chem,* Vol. 79, No. 17, pp. 6559-65.

Zhang, X.J., Cardoso, L., Broderick, M., Fein, H. & Lin, J. (2001). An integrated nitric oxide sensor based on carbon fiber coated with selective membranes. *Electroanalysis,* Vol. 12, No. pp. 1113-1117.

Zhang, X.J., Kislyak, Y., Lin, J., Dickson, A., Cardoso, L., Broderick, M. & Fein, H. (2002). Nanometer size electrode for nitric oxide and S-nitrosothiols measurement. *Electrochem. Commun.,* Vol. 4, pp. 11-16.

15

The Microbial Cell Based Biosensors

Reshetilov A.N., Iliasov P.V. and Reshetilova T.A.
Institute of Biochemistry & Physiology of Microorganisms,
Russian Academy of Sciences
Russian Federation

1. Introduction

The typical feature of the advancement of knowledge as a whole is initiation of novel interdisciplinary trends and divisions of science. They usually appear as a result of joint creative work of specialists of different profiles, which is conditioned by widening of the scope of scientific problems, interests, objects and methods of research. One of these trends is biosensor research (biosensorics), the branch of biotechnology that originated in the second half of the 20th century at the interfaces between biology, biophysics, chemistry, physics, electronics, and informatics.

The essence of this trend may be defined as follows: biosensor studies pursue the construction of analytic systems, i.e. biosensors, the primary function of which is express analysis for sought-for substance detection. The main "character" in biosensor analyzer is biological material: it provides sensitivity of instrument to sought-for substance.

The analysis of events resulting in the development of biosensorics as a research trend shows that the author of biosensor conception and the first biosensor developer is USA biochemist L. C. Clark, Jr. In 1962, Clark and Lyons introduced the term "enzyme electrode" into practice (Turner, 1996). For manufacture of this device, a minor quantity of glucose oxidase was applied onto the surface of platinum electrode and covered with cellophane. The platinum was at positive potential to relative to silver electrode. The system did not react to dissolved oxygen but generated current in the presence of hydrogen peroxide. L. Clark showed that the electrode current quickly increased at addition of glucose to the solution and was proportional to its concentration (Clark, 1993).

The formalization and specification of terminology related to electrochemical biosensors but extendable to biosensors of other types was carried out by recommendation of the International Union of Pure and Applied Chemistry (IUPAC). It gives recommendations for researchers, editorial boards of journals, and publishers on application of concepts such as biosensor and its parameters: sensitivity, general and linear concentration measurement range, detection limit, selectivity, life time, etc. (Thevenot et al., 2001).

Quite a number of publications show the stages of development and state-of-the-art of biosensor studies. So the question of efficiency of biosensor analysis of the environment is considered in papers (Rodriguez-Mozaz et al., 2006); general problems of the analytical aspects of biosensors are presented in review (Pearson et al., 2000); specific problems of electrochemical biosensor measurement are presented in review (Mehrvar & Abdi, 2004); the aspects of the functioning of biosensors based on ion-selective field transistors are described in paper (Yuqing et al., 2003). The analysis of application of whole cells in biosensors can be found in reviews (Bousse, 1996; Ziegler, 2000; Bentley et al., 2001). Review (Murphy, 2006) presents the analysis of advantages of biosensors (DNA-, immunosensors, enzyme sensors with direct charge transfer, etc.) constructed with application of nanomaterials. The use of microbial cells in receptor elements of biosensors is described in works (D'Souza, 2001b; Riedel et al., 1989; Racek, 1995).

The microbial cells based biosensors are considered in the present chapter.

2. Microbial biosensors design and characteristics

2.1 Biosensor design

The first microbial biosensor as indicated in the review (Turner, 1996) was described in 1975 by Divies and was based on the use of *Acetobacter xylinum* and oxygen electrode. The work became the foundation of the investigations devoted to the development of microbial biosensors for application in biotechnology and environmental monitoring.

Taking a biomaterial type in the bioreceptor as a basis it is possible to pick out the class of cell based biosensors (Thevenot et al., 2001). They can incorporate the plant or animal isolated cells or subcellular structures as well as the microbial cells. The most of the cell based biosensors developed to date fall into the subclass of microbial biosensors (D'Souza, 2001b; Bousse, 1996). This is due to the simplicity of the microorganisms' cultivation, the rich analytical prospects of the microbial cells (Racek, 1995) and their reliability when using as the base of the immobilized biocatalysts (Cassidy et al., 1996).

The appearance of the microbial sensors was the logical extension of the enzyme electrodes' development. The signal generation mechanism is analogous in general terms for both of the microbial and enzyme biosensors. In either case the biocatalytic reaction following the enzyme kinetics statements takes place. According to the model used in the work (Ikeda et al., 1996) the microbial cell is treated as the "bag of enzymes". The representation is unconditionally primitive and do not take into the account the complexity of the cell's structural organization and homeostatic system of intracellular biochemical processes but from the standpoint of the biosensorics in its elementary form the microbial cell could really be considered as an integrated biocatalyst that is analogous to the enzyme preparation in many ways.

The scheme of the intracellular metabolic processes underlying the background of microbial biosensors could be represented as follows. The analyte enters the cell and is converted using the intracellular enzymes. As a result, the co-substrates are consumed and the reaction products that could also be electrochemically active are generated. The registration of the oxygen level, medium ionic composition and other parameters in the immobilized cells' layer can be used as the indicators of the cells' metabolic state and the background for the electrochemical determination of biologically active compounds.

The selection of the microorganism for the use in a biosensor is a milestone of the development process. The key factors of the problem are the substrate specificity and the sensitivity of detection. Thus, the study of a number of *Gluconobacter* strains allowed to predict the cells' specificity to carbohydrates, alcohols, and organic acids using the potentiometric and amperometric transducers (Reshetilov et al., 1997a).

The bioreceptor of the typical microbial biosensor is represented by a membrane or gel strip containing the immobilized microorganisms fixed onto the working area of a transducer. The immobilization of cells ensures small (~10-100 mg) biomaterial consumption, high assay rate and allows the multiple measurements without the bioreceptor replacement. The choice of the immobilization technique is determined by the criteria of the sensor stability and measurement rate (i.e. the diffusion characteristics of a support). The immobilization methods have been improved with the time (D'Souza, 2001a); the most common of them have been considered in the manuscript (D'Souza, 2001b). In the most of cases the cells' immobilization in the bioreceptor have been carried out by the sorption or inclusion into the gel or polymer matrixes.

Generally, the immobilization techniques could be divided into active and passive. The natural adhesive ability of microorganisms can be used for their passive immobilization. On the other hand, the active immobilization supposes the use of chemical and physical methods for cell fixing. The choose of the most efficient technique is determined by the type of supposed assay and cells' features. The inventory of the microorganisms immobilization includes the same approaches as for the enzyme immobilization (Thevenot et al., 2001). These approaches are described below in short form.

Inclusion into a gel or polymer matrix. This method ensures the retention of cells in the spatial network formed by a polymer. The key advantage of the method is the improved (over against the adsorbed cells) sensor stability (Racek, 1991). Furthermore, it is known that in a number of cases the polysaccharide gels reduce the toxic effect of aromatics on the microbial cells (Fedorov et al., 1999) that is the important factor during the development of the sensors for environmental needs. Agar, Ca-alginate, carrageenan, gelatin and collagen gels and PVA are widely used in microbial sensors. Although the polymerization of these materials arises in the stress conditions they ensure high cells' viability and reproducibility of analysis. The polyacrylamide gel is also every so often used in microbial sensors (Wollenberger et al., 1980) in spite of its toxicity. The PVA cryogels (Philp et al., 2003) and photo-crosslinked polymers like ENT/ENTP (a composite mixture polymerizing under near UV light) or modified PVA (Fukui & Tanaka, 1984), poly(carbamoyl sulfonate) and polyurethane (Konig et al., 1998), sol-gel matrixes based on alumina or composite polymers (Jia et al., 2003), latex-type polymers based on acrylic and methacrylic acids (D'Souza, 2001a), redox hydrogels like $[Os(bpy)_2Cl]^{+/2+}$ also should be mentioned among the high-used carriers. Generally, the inclusion have been used in microbial biosensorics approximately as often as the adsorption and essential in the case of high cells' desorption from the support.

Adsorption. The common supports for adsorption include various membranes, a filter paper, carbon materials and other carriers possess the high absorbance; sometimes the cells have been adsorbed directly onto the electrode surface. The review (D'Souza, 2001b) describes the immobilization by the simultaneous adhesion of viable and unviable cells on the different materials including the glass, cotton, and polymer carriers. The specific for microorganisms technique is the flocculation - the aggregation of cells and sorption of the aggregates on the support (Cassidy et al., 1996). One of the major advantages of the adsorption is its simplicity; also, the adsorption is a "soft" method with minimal damaging action. The stability of the sensors with adsorbed cells is rather high; it have been observed that such biosensors retain the activity within several weeks and even months (Rechnitz et al., 1977; Karube et al., 1980; Matsunaga et al., 1984). These factors make the adsorption one of the most preferable approaches for microbial biosensors development.

Covalent attachment. This approach supposes the use of cross-linking agents like glutaraldehyde, carbodiimide, titanium oxide that linked to molecules exposed on the microbial cell wall and with functional groups on the surface of the carrier or transducer. The obtained film has been fixed on the transducer. The approach is widely used with the enzyme electrodes but rarely with microbial sensors because the cross-linking in the most of cases leads to the loss of the viability or decrease of the cells' catalytic activity.

The immobilization on the membrane is not the only possible design of a bioreceptor. A number of biosensors described in works (Alkasrawi et al., 1999; Gu & Gil, 2001) used the receptors represented by reactors with displacement and continuous or pulse substrate feed. The transducer in this case have been installed at the output of the reactor that allow to control the changes of biochemical activity of the immobilized biomass under the substrate feed. The cells immobilization in a bioreactor may be carried out by means of adsorption on a granular carrier or by inclusion into a gel. In the case when the substrate conversion is accompanied by the generation of compounds that could be analyzed using a biosensor an efficient approach consists in a creation of a hybrid sensor by means of installation of a such biosensor at the output of the reactor (Damgaard et al., 2001). However, the reactor based biosensors have been utilized infrequently due to labor content of the reactor exploitation over against the membrane-based sensors as well as high consumption of the biomass for the receptor formation.

One of the reactor biosensor designs is the case when the cells are suspended in the solution of a measuring cuvette (i.e. the biosensor is represented by a transducer placed into the cuvette with the cell suspension or with the suspension of a dispersed carrier). The design is similar to a fuel cell and is known as "fuel-cell-type sensor". The essential disadvantages of the approach consist in the high consumption of a biomaterial, impossibility or difficulty of the continuous measurements. However, in spite of these reasons, the approach have been exploited from time to time in model biosensor studies (Kim et al., 2003; Chang et al., 2004; Vais et al., 1989; Guliy et al., 2003).

2.2 Comparative characteristics of microbial and enzyme biosensors.

The belonging of the electrochemical and calorimetric enzyme or microbial biosensors to the group of catalytic sensors determines their properties and, in particular, the range of detectable concentrations. For the most of models reported to date it lies within 10^{-6}-10^{-2} M. The exception are the optical microbial sensors whose signal is not based directly on catalytic transformation of the analyte; they are characterized by lower limit of detection about 10^{-9}-10^{-7} M. In spite of the similarity of the operating principles of the microbial and enzyme sensors the use of whole microbial cells have particular advantages and disadvantages in contrast to the enzyme utilization (D'Souza, 2001b; Racek, 1995; Riedel et al., 1987; Bousse, 1996). The advantages include:

a) the absence of need in obtaining and exploitation of pure enzymes, i.e. reduction of labor content and prime cost of analysis; b) some enzymes may inactivate during isolation or immobilization if these processes disarrange their molecular structure. The use of whole cells minimizes this obstacle; c) the microbial cells can be genetically modified that makes it possible to obtain recombinant organisms with determined biocatalytic properties; d) the enzymes within the cells are in naturally occurring, evolutionary optimized environment that ensures high stability of a number of microbial sensors. Also, the cells contain coenzymes and activators of biochemical pathways that eliminates the need in their addition in the medium; e) the utilization of microorganisms allows the realization of sequential biochemical processes that in the case of an enzyme sensor would be artificially designed; f) the receptor of microbial sensor can be regenerated by conditioning the cell growth.

The important reason for the utilization of the whole cells in analytical devices is the fact that only the use of living cell allow the obtaining of the functional information, i.e. determining how the factor affects the organism in vivo (Bousse, 1996). The examples supposing the obtaining of functional information include the questions:
a) does the compound affect the cell metabolism and how; b) is the compound agonist or antagonist of the particular receptor (the question is essential for the pharmaceutics and drug development); c) is the sample or substance toxic. The question is directly related to objectives of biosensorics, at the same time the influence of the environment on the organisms in a general sense is related to functional information. The microbial biosensors have been applied for the such investigation over a long period of time. The studies include the evaluation of BOD, total toxicity, genotoxicity, i.e. the parameters that are inherently related to functional state of organisms.
The most common disadvantages of microbial sensors include the decreased rate of signal generation and the low selectivity. The cell based receptor carries out the analyte conversion slower in contrast to the enzyme based one due to presence the cell wall that acts as a diffusion barrier. An efficient approach for solving the problem consists in the exploitation of permeabilized cells (D'Souza, 2001b). Another method allowing to reduce the sensor's reaction time suppose the application of genetic engineering technique in order to ensure the exposing of the particular enzymes on the outer surface of cell wall; in this case the diffusion obstacles are eliminated. Thus, in (Rainina et al., 1996; Mulchandani et al., 1998) the recombinant *Escherichia coli* strain containing the surface-expressed organophosphate hydrolase had been utilized. The cells carried out the substrate degradation with higher rate over the cells with the intracellular expression of the enzyme.

2.3 Hybrid biosensors

The bioreceptor of hybrid biosensors contain two or more different biocatalysts. As applied to the microbial sensors the term "hybrid" usually supposes that the sensor contain a mixed culture of two or more strains or "cells + enzyme" type composite. Both of the biomaterials must catalyze the coupled reactions. In hybrid biosensors' design, two major schemes of the bioreceptor have been utilized - a) the biocatalysts are separated from each other by a membrane allowing the substrate diffusion or b) the biocatalysts are mixed together. The hybrid biosensors with coupling the membrane and reactor bioreceptors have also been reported.
The major advantages of hybrid biosensors are the enhanced selectivity and the possibility to analyze compounds that could not be determined by single-component sensors. On the other hand, the labor content of hybrid biosensors' development and exploitation higher in contrast to the single-component ones. Maybe this explains the small amount of hybrid microbial sensors described to date. The hybrid sensor containing *Bacillus subtilis* cells in combination with the glucoamylase for the evaluation of α-amylase activity was reported in (Renneberg et al., 1984). The hybrid biosensor analyzer using the combination of the enzymes and bacterial cells and the column-type reactor with the membrane receptor was presented in publication (Reiss et al., 1998). The authors utilized two reactors containing α-amylase and amyloglucosidase coupled with a commercial BOD biosensor (Prüfgerätewerk Medingen) based on the immobilized *Trichosporon cutaneum* cells. The results of BOD evaluation in starch-containing wastes agreed well to the data of conventional BOD assay.
Hybrid microbial biosensors based on Clark type electrode and containing *Gluconobacter oxydans* in combination with *Saccharomyces cerevisiae* or *G. oxydans* combining with the

permeabilized *Kluyveromyces marxianus* cells were used for determination of sucrose and lactose, respectively (Svitel et al., 1998). The approach based on the attachment of glucose oxidase to microbial cell surface by concanavalin A or polyethyleneimine was applied for the development of sensors for sucrose and lactose detection; the carrier cells contained induced invertase and β-galactosidase (D'Souza, 1989).
The hybrid biosensors coupling different microorganisms in the bioreceptor have been widely used for BOD index evaluation. Thus, the simultaneous immobilization of *T. cutaneum* and *Bacillus licheniformis* expanded the analyzer's substrate specificity due to differences in metabolic activity of the cultures (Suriyawattanakul et al., 2002). Simultaneous immobilization of yeast strain *T. cutaneum* and bacterial culture *B. subtilis* (Jia et al., 2003) made it possible the creation of a BOD sensor with enhanced long-term stability.

2.4 Substrate specificity of microbial sensors and its improvement

The term "selectivity" usually means the sensor's ability to generate signals in response to the analyte appearance along with the minimal sensitivity to other compounds in the sample. It can be quantitative assessed using two ways. The first one expresses the selectivity as the ratio of the analyte-induced response to responses to the analogous concentration of the interfering substances. The second approach consists in addition of the interfering substances in the medium that already contains the analyte; the selectivity in this case is expressed as the percentage of the signal increment after the interfering compound addition. The second way is more simple but allows to evaluate the selectivity more particularly (Thevenot et al., 2001).
The broad substrate specificity (low selectivity) of microbial biosensors is due to the variety of the intracellular enzyme systems. There is rather small amount of microbial sensor models possessing the sensitivity only to analytes - as a rule, due to the good choice of the strain and/or detection principle or measurement mode optimization. Most of the microbial sensors are characterized by sensitivity to a wide number of substances that can significantly hamper the analysis of complex samples (Riedel et al., 1990b). A number of approaches directed to the improving of microbial sensors' selectivity have been reported. These approaches will be considered below.
In the review (Racek, 1995) several ways of the sensors' selectivity improving have been described. Thus, it has been noted that one of the efficient methods consists in isolating the bioreceptor or transducer from the medium using an additional membrane impermeable for the interfering compounds. For example, the use of cellulose acetate membrane in a biosensor based on the *G. oxydans* cells made it possible the 60-fold increase of the response to ethanol in contrast with the response to glucose. In addition, the authors revealed the effect of culture age on the selectivity. Bacteria collected after 10 and 16 hours of cultivation varied in the ethanol to glucose sensitivity ratio approximately by a factor of 3 (Tkac et al., 2003). In the case when the analyte is volatile it is appropriate to use a gas-permeable membrane isolating the electrode from the medium. The approach is simple and reliable; at the other hand, the covering membrane may be an additional diffusion barrier for the analyte and decrease the rate of analysis.
Another approach that could be related to this section consists in the sample pretreatment in order to eliminate the interfering compounds. The particular case of such pretreatment is the introducing of the enzyme solution into the measuring cell or addition of a membrane containing the immobilized enzyme that carries out the conversion of the interfering substances into inactive products (Park et al., 1991). The approach has been utilized in a

hybrid sensor for sucrose detection. The sensor contained *Zymomonas mobilis* bacteria and invertase. The elimination of glucose initially presented in a sample has been carried out by glucose oxidase.

One of the simplest ways to increase the microbial sensor selectivity is based on the choice of microorganism able to use only the analyte as the carbon and/or energy source. In particular, this approach was used in a works directed to the development of a methane sensor (Karube et al., 1982b). However, it should be noted that this method is not an universal tool for enhancing the selectivity. Even in the case when the organism is able to utilize only one substrate it's metabolic pathway for the most part includes several steps and the pathway intermediates are also expected to induce the biosensor signal. Besides, the inability of the cells to utilize the substrate as the source of carbon does not exclude the sensitivity of sensor to this compound. Thus, *G. oxydans* bacterium can not to utilize glucose as the carbon source due to metabolic peculiarities but the sensors based on the culture possess high sensitivity to glucose due to ability of the cells to convert glucose into ketogluconic acid accompanied by oxygen consumption and acidification of the medium.

In a number of cases a choice of a transducer or measurement mode is also important for the selectivity. The time of response to interfering compounds can differ from the time of response to the analyte due to variation in the rate of their diffusion through cell wall or metabolic processes. If the difference is significant it could be used for the selectivity improving (Racek, 1995). Thus, the use of *G. suboxidans* in a mediator sensor demonstrated a steady level of signal within 30 s and 15 min for ethanol and glucose, respectively (Ikeda et al., 1992). The effect can be used for selective determination of the substances in a mixed sample.

One of the most common ways of the microbial sensor selectivity improving consists in the cultivation of the biomass at a later stage used in a bioreceptor with the expected analyte as a sole source of carbon and energy or as a co-substrate (Simonian et al., 1992; Renneberg et al., 1984). The approach does not eliminate the ability of a sensor to respond to a wide spectrum of substances. It only allows to selectively increase (Renneberg et al., 1984) the sensor sensitivity to the analyte as a result of the induction and expression of the enzymes responsible for its conversion. The popular modification of the approach is the case when the biosensor or biomass after cultivation has been incubated with the analyte (Racek & Musil, 1987a; Riedel et al., 1990b). It is obvious that the efficiency of the approach is extremely high when the enzymes of the analyte metabolism are inducible and the analyte acts as the inductor. The metabolic activation of cells were utilized in a number of studies directed to the development of sensors for determination of carbohydrates, organic acids, sterols, amino acids, phenol etc. Thus, the application of the approach to biomass cultivation allowed to change the selectivity of the sensor based on yeast cells *Pichia angusta* VKM Y-2518. By means of growing the cells on various substrate it was possible to shift the cells' selectivity to ethanol or methanol several times (Voronova et al., 2008).

The similar technique is related to metabolic inhibition of undesirable pathways or their individual steps during the biomass cultivation or after it (Riedel & Scheller, 1987). In contrast to previous, this approach do not affect on the absolute value of the sensitivity to analyte but allows the elimination or reducing the signals to interfering compounds. For the further selectivity improving, it can be combined with the metabolic induction of analyte conversion enzymes. The common drawback of these approaches in the possibility of reducing and even total disappearance of the induction or inhibition effects after long-term downtime or operating of the sensor under the presence of interfering compounds (Racek & Musil, 1987a). The attempts to solve the problem by means of incubation of the sensor between measurements in the solution of inductor or inhibitor are known (Kobos et al., 1979; Suzuki et al., 1992) but this can cause a contamination of the culture and altering the analytical characteristics of the sensor.

A promising approach is related to genetic manipulations allowing to enhance the expression of genes responsible to an analyte conversion or eliminate or block the genes of interfering compounds metabolism (Korpan et al., 1993; Mulchandani et al., 1998). The modification ensures actually the same result as in the case of metabolic activation or inhibition but eliminates the possibility of reverting the initial activity of enzymes after inductor or inhibitor removal. Besides, the biochemical altering of the cells' catalytic activity may affect on a number of enzymes while the genetic approach modifies the particular locus, i.e. is more specific. Also, the application of genetic engineering tools makes it possible to impart the principally new abilities to the cells – for example, such modification are often used for insertion of luciferase loci in the operon encoding the enzymes metabolizing the analyte in order to develop a bioluminescent sensor (Kurittu et al., 2000; Thouand et al., 2003).

Thus, the biosensor based on recombinant *Hansenula polymorpha* strains are described (Korpan et al., 1993). This yeast utilizes methanol to CO_2 and water through formaldehyde and formate. One of the strains was formate dehydrogenase-deficient that led to formate accumulation and acidification of medium during the methanol transformation. In the second case the recombinant strain did not contain two enzymes - alcohol oxidase and formate dehydrogenase. The sensor based on this strain was insensitive to methanol and formate and made it possible for selective determination of formaldehyde.

A special case of cell's genetic modification is the transformation or elimination of a plasmid harboring reporter genes or genes encoding the enzymes of analyte metabolism. The use of plasmids allows to obtain a pair of strains for differential detection system (D'Souza, 2001b). Thus, the high selectivity of biosensor for sulphoaromatic compounds detection was ensured using the strain *Comamonas testosteroni* BS1310 harboring the arylsulphonate degradation plasmid pBS1010. The sensitivity of the eliminant strain based sensor to *p*-toluene sulphonate was reduced 10-fold, in addition this sensor possess the decreased sensitivity to catechol, benzene sulphonate, sulphobenzoate. The results obtained supposed the possibility of selectivity improving using differential measurement principle (Makarenko et al., 1999).

The hybrid biosensor creation is also related to a number of methods of selectivity improving (Renneberg et al., 1984). In this case only one of simultaneously immobilized biocatalysts carries out the reaction registered by a transducer; actually, it's selectivity determines the total selectivity of a system. The second biocatalyst serves for the conversion of an initial analyte to compound recognizable by the detecting component and so ensures the system's sensitivity to analyte.

Another way to improve selectivity is based on the development of differential analyzers and sensor arrays (Racek, 1991; Held et al., 2002). The such analyzer includes two or more sensors that are differs only by the sensitivity to analyte(s). The differential analyzer based on *H. anomala* cells was developed for analysis of glucose in urine (Racek, 1991); the reference electrode contained cells with thermally inactivated glycolysis enzymes. Another example of a differential biosensor system is represented by the sensor of genotoxicity described in (Karube et al., 1982a) and based on the use of two *E. coli* or *Salmonella* strains one of which lacks the SOS reparation system.

The result of this approach development is the case when the sensor array includes a number of low-selective sensors measuring different parameters. The application of chemometrics for processing of the array signals makes it possible to carry out the selective quantitative assay of components in a complex sample. Thus, the differences in the maximal rate of signal changes in response to various substrates allowed to analyze components of mixtures of organic acids with the measurement error less than 10% (Slama et al., 1996; Plegge et al., 2000).

The possibility of selective analysis of a substrate mixture by a system including various combinations of sensors was studied in a number of works (Reshetilov et al., 1998; Lobanov et al., 2001). The system containing an enzyme sensor for glucose determination and a microbial (*Gluconobacter* cell based) sensor sensitive to glucose and ethanol was used for selective ethanol quantification in presence of glucose (Reshetilov et al., 1998). At the next step the authors exploited a system containing microbial sensors based on *G. oxydans* and *P. methanolica* cells (Lobanov et al., 2001). The possibility of selective analysis of both ethanol and glucose in the substrate mixture have been demonstrated. In another work the possibility of identification of glucose, xylose and ethanol in their mixture was shown by means of three microbial sensors based on *G. oxydans, H. polymorpha* and *E. coli* cells. The data were processed using cluster analysis and artificial neural network.

None of the above approach of the selectivity improving is universal. However, their individual or combined application in the most of cases allows to reach the acceptable analysis parameters. To top it all, there are situations when high selectivity is not necessary or even undesirable. These situations, in particular, take place in the field of environmentally oriented sensors. Thus, the analysis of wastes supposes not so much that the determination of particular pollutant as the assessment of a group of compounds or total content of organics indirectly determined through the BOD index (Chee et al., 1999; Kim & Park, 2001). In these conditions the use of sensors sensitive to a wide range of substances is essentially efficient (Lehmann et al., 1999; Suriyawattanakul et al., 2002).

3. Transducers in microbial biosensors

3.1 Amperometric transducers

Among the advances of biosensorics, three generations of amperometric bioelectrodes have been developed (Albery & Craston, 1987). Each of the generations acts according the principles of transformation of the biochemical reaction into the electric current.

The background of the first generarion bioelectrodes operating is the registration of consumption of a co-substrate (usually oxygen) during the analyte oxidation or generation of reaction product. The most typical design is based on the oxygen Clark-type electrode and bears a name "respiratory electrode" (Racek, 1995). As the major part of aerobes' metabolism is accompanied by the oxygen consumption the approach can be used for development of biosensors for determination of a wide number of compounds (Held et al., 2002; Svitel et al., 1998; Karube et al., 1980; Beyersdorf-Radeck et al., 1998). Biosensors of this type are also used for determination of compounds suppressing the microbial activity (Campanella et al., 2001; Okochi et al., 2004) or possessing antibacterial or antimicotic activity. In this case the registering parameter is represented by the decreasing of background respiratory activity of biomass.

The amperometric first generation electrodes registering the products of biochemical reactions (for example, hydrogen peroxide), are widely used in enzyme biosensors but rather rarely in microbial ones (Gonchar et al., 1998). So, the first generation electrodes among the microbial sensors are almost solely represented by the Clark type electrode.

In the second generation amperometric biosensors the registration of the biochemical activity has been carried out using the electron transfer mediators. The phenolic and quinoid compounds, ferricyanide, $NAD^+/NADH$, tetrathiafulvalen (TTF), the derivatives of ferrocene, pyridine, imidazol, complex metal-containing polymers and other substances have been used as mediators in enzyme biosensors (Chaubey & Malhotra, 2002). Sometimes the carrier for biomass immobilization (Tkac et al., 2007; Timur et al., 2007) or the electrode material (McNeil et al., 1992) possess mediatory characteristics - such electrodes belong to third generation able to intercept the electrons from redox enzymatic reaction directly (Shleev et al., 2005).

The major advantage of the 2nd and 3rd generation electrodes is the elimination of the dependence of the sensor signal on a dissolved oxygen concentration. Also, the transducer of mediator sensors is often represented by screen-printed electrodes that allows to reduce the assay cost and facilitates the unification of the sensors' characteristics. At the same time, this approach requires additional expenses for the mediator obtaining. In relation to microbial sensors it can be realized only if the analyte conversion involves the easily accessible cell surface-localized enzymes or if the cell wall and membrane are permeable for mediator in both directions. To date, all types of charge transfer are reported for cell based biosensors including the utilization of various mediators (Katrlik et al., 2007; Tkac et al., 2002; Bhatia et al., 2003), direct charge transfer in biofuel cells (Chaudhuri & Lovley, 2003), and also the immobilization using the conducting carriers (Vostiar et al., 2004; Timur et al., 2007).

The coupling of enzyme and electrochemical reactions on the conducting materials made it possible for the development of a large number of microbial biosensors for carbohydrates and alcohols detection (Ikeda et al., 2004). The amperometric microbial sensors can also be used for determination of a wide spectrum of pollutants; the backgrounds of the method are described in the review (Paitan et al., 2003).

3.2 Potentiometric transducers

In the cases when the biochemical reaction leads to alteration of ionic composition of the medium it can be registered using potentiometric ion-selective electrodes (ISE). If ISE is placed into the medium containing the expected ion an electric potential appears on the electrode's membrane. The ISE most often used in biosensorics is the pH-electrode. Protonation/deprotonation of a bioreceptor due to biochemical reaction results in a potential generation on the electrode membrane.

The development of ion-selective field effect transistors (ISFETs) were started in 70s by P. Bergveld team (University of Twente, The Netherlands). In general, the developments were directed to the creation of pH-selective ISFETs that soon after became compete with glass pH-electrodes (Bergveld, 2003).

The detailed description of ISFETs related studies and their application in biosensorics is presented in a number of reviews (Domansky et al., 1993; Bergveld, 2003; Yuqing et al., 2003). To present, the ISFETs for evaluation of various ions as well as concentration of oxygen and carbon dioxide have been reported. At the same time, the amount of publications devoted to microbial sensors based on ISE is rather small (Mulchandani et al., 1998; Rechnitz & Ho, 1990).

Seeking for the improving the quality of biosensoric analysis is a motivation of new transducer types development. The light-addressable potentiometric sensors (LAPS) was created as a result of the development of the concept related to control of the processes in semiconductor material using applied external electrical field. One of the important characteristics of LAPS is the fact that the photo-generated current reflects the chemical processes at the irradiation point. This lays the background for development of multichannel sensors by means of successive irradiation of the points.

Two major fields of LAPS application are the development of affine biosensors and microphysiometers. The latter's purpose is the evaluation of intracellular metabolic processes in vivo. The majority of to-date reported microphysiometers were used for the studies of metabolism of homoeothermic animal cells. The first paper related to this subject was published in 1989 (Parce et al., 1989). The LAPS based device ensured the possibility of detection the receptor-ligand interaction, assessment of the sensitivity of tumor cells to drugs and evaluation of the toxic action of various factors on the cells (Bousse, 1996). The study of bacterial cells metabolism using LAPS has been presented in paper (Baxter et al., 1994) that is related to evaluation of cells' sensitivity to antibacterial agents.

Thus, it should be conclude that the most important characteristics of LAPS as a biosensor transducer are high reliability and simple design, as well as the possibility to evaluate the metabolic processes in microbial and animal cells in vivo. The LAPS-based multichannel sensors could easily be designed without complex procedures that are necessary during development a multichannel FET-based device.

3.3 Conductometric sensors

Conductometric biosensors register the bioreceptor activity by the changes of the solution conductivity caused by biochemical reactions. The typical design of a conductometric sensor includes interpenetrating electrodes on a dielectric support covered by a biomaterial film. The enzyme conductometric sensors for detection of ethanol, urea, penicillin etc. have been described. An important drawback of conductometric sensors is the susceptibility to unspecific factors associated with biochemical reactions, so the measurements are usually carried out by a pair of sensors for error minimization. The application of conductometry for development of microbial sensors is limited.

Several examples of toxic compounds determination using a conductometric sensor have been reported. Microbial biosensor based on whole *Rhodococcus ruber* cells has been created for express analysis of acrylonitrile (Roach et al., 2003). A sensor based on *Chlorella vulgaris* cells and conductometric transducer has been developed for evaluation of activity of intracellular alkaline phosphatase and cadmium and zinc ions. The cells were immobilized in bovine serum albumin by cross-linking with glutaraldehyde. (Chouteau et al., 2004).

The conductometric microbial sensors for alcohol analysis are also known. Detection of ethanol in beverages has been carried out using a conductometric yeast-based biosensor; the results of analysis correlated well to the gas chromatography data (Korpan et al., 1994).

3.4 Microbial calorimetric sensors

Microcalorimetry is one of the conventional techniques of the cell metabolism assessment. The majority of enzyme reaction have been accompanied by heat emission; their molar enthalpies are in the range of 25-100 kJ/mole (Turner et al., 1987). The heat measurement is the operating principle of the calorimetric or thermal biosensors. The first enzyme thermal sensor also known as "enzyme thermistor" was developed in early 1970s (Mosbach & Danielsson, 1974). The typical calorimetric sensor includes a receptor designed as a reactor heat-insulated from the environment. The temperature measurements have been carried out at the input and output of the reactor. To improve the measurement precision and minimize errors a two-channel differential measurement system has been utilized.

The thermal biosensors advantages include the possibility of continuous measurements, high long-term stability, insensitivity to electrical or optical interferences, the absence of interfering action of the reaction products, high reproducibility and rapid responses. At the other hand, the restrictions are related to necessity of some samples pretreatment and the possibility of the system contamination as a result of continuous measurement of the untreated samples (Ramanathan et al., 1999).

One of the first microbial thermistors has been described in (Mattiasson et al., 1977). The authors mentioned that the sensor could be used for the analysis of a wide spectrum of compounds. However, to date only a small amount of the microbial thermal sensor related studies have been reported in spite of the fact that the heat emission during the microbial conversion of a substrate is similar to that during the enzyme oxidation. The author of review (Schugerl, 2001) notes that the microcalorimetric approach could be used for real-time monitoring of the biomass cultivation processes.

3.5 Optical microbial sensors

The important requirements specified for the environmentally oriented analyzers intended for evaluation of the pollutants in situ include their operational efficiency and specificity. The development of bioluminescent microbial sensors based on the optical transducers allows to obtain analytical devices satisfying all the wants. The detailed review of this subject can be found in reviews (D'Souza, 2001b; Hansen & Sorensen, 2001). It is possible to select two characteristic versions of this approach. The realization of the first one involved the fusion of reporter genes to the operon controlled by the analyte-inducible promoter; the common reporters include bacterial and firefly luciferase components as well as green fluorescent protein (GFP) from the jellyfish *Aequorea victoria* or sea pen *Renilla reniformis* (Daunert et al., 2000). Thus, the appearance of the analyte results in the bioluminescence enhancement that is registered by a transducer; the approach could potentially be realized for detection of almost any compound involved into the cell metabolism. The special case is the technique that is consisted in the insertion of a reporter to one of loci responsible to DNA reparation; thus, any DNA damaging factor induces the biosensor signal that makes it possible the total genotoxicity assessment (Afanassiev et al., 2000; Mitchell & Gu, 2004).

The second version of the bioluminescent sensors related approach supposes the employment of recombinant or wild-type luminescent strains for control of non-specific factors reducing the microorganisms viability. In this case the reporter genes are controlled by constitutive promoters and the sensor's operating principle is based on the registration of background luminescence decrease due to reduction of the living cells amount caused by the effect of an analyte (Philp et al., 2003; Ritchie et al., 2001). This version of the bioluminescent sensor has been realized in the total toxicity evaluation system MICROTOX™ (Ribo & Kaiser, 1987).

The bioluminescence related approach ensures high selectivity of analysis and in a number of cases allows significant (in several orders) enhancement of the detection sensitivity over the biocatalytic sensors (Billard & DuBow, 1998). Its drawbacks include the low rate of analysis and increased labor content due to the need in genetic manipulations. To present, at

least several hundreds of bioluminescent microbial sensors tailored to determination of antimicrobial drugs, pollutants, genotoxicity and total toxicity have been reported (Anko et al., 2002; Applegate et al., 1998; Gu & Chang, 2001; Min et al., 2000).
The original optical microbial sensor based on the employment of surface plasmon resonance device reported in (Kononov et al., 2007). The authors demonstrated the possibility of obtaining the signal reflecting the metabolic state of microorganisms in real time, in spite of high thickness of the cells. The results obtained indicate that the cyclic generation of gas due to metabolic processes leads to reversible alteration of bacterial cells properties in the immobilized cells monolayer.

4. Analytes and application of microbial biosensors

4.1 Determination of carbohydrates.

Carbohydrates are the most common analytes of enzyme and microbial sensors. It suffice to say that the first microbial sensor was tailored to glucose determination and in spite of a plenty of investigations carried out within several dozens of years the determination of carbohydrates and their employment as the model substrates remains a widely used direction of biosensorics. As related to microbial sensors, this circumstance is due to the high bioavailability of carbohydrates and also by practical significance of their analysis for biotechnology, food industry and medicine. The most often reported "carbohydrate" sensors are glucose and lactose analyzers; at the other hand, a large number of microbial biosensor models for detection of other mono- and disaccharides and even polymeric carbohydrates have been described. Thus, in one of characteristic studies a microbial sensor for glucose determination based on *Pseudomonas fluorescens* and oxygen electrode has been developed (Karube et al., 1979). The similar work described three models of microbial sensors for detection of glucose, sucrose and lactose based on *G. oxydans*, co-immobilized *G. oxydans* and *S. cerevisiae* and co-immobilized *G. oxydans* and *K. marxianus* cells, respectively (Svitel et al., 1998). In the publication (Held et al., 2002) a sensor array including a number of oxygen electrodes with immobilized *E. coli* strains lacking the transfer systems of various mono- and disaccharides has been created. Several models of low-selective sensors able to determine the total carbohydrate content are known; they include, for example, the mediator biosensor based on *G. oxydans* cells and tailored to determination of total carbohydrate content in lignocellulose hydrolyzate (Tkac et al., 2000).
It should be noted that among the microbial carbohydrate analyzers there is rather large amount of mediator sensors. Besides of the sensor mentioned in (Tkac et al., 2000) the examples include the sensor based on *G. oxydans* and carbon paste electrode (Takayama et al., 1993), the glucose sensor based on *E. coli* cells and carbon paste electrode modified by benzoquinone and PQQ (Ito et al., 2002) and the glucose biosensor based on *Aspergillus niger* and carbon paste electrode. The ferricyanide and ferrocene were utilized as the mediators. The sensor was exploited for glucose monitoring during biotechnological processes (Katrlik et al., 1997).
The hybrid sensors are also often used for carbohydrate detection. The approach is especially appropriate for di- and polysaccharides analysis; in this case, one of the biocatalysts carries out the glycoside bond hydrolysis while the other determines the generated monomers. Two hybride carbohydrate sensors were mentioned above (Svitel et al., 1998); besides them the hybrid sensors for sucrose determination based on invertase and *Z. mobilis* cells (Park et al., 1991) and for detection of lactose in dairy products based on

glucose oxidase and *E. coli* cells (Svorc et al., 1990) have also been reported. The same approach was used for determination of α-amylase activity using co-immobilized *B. subtilis* and glucoamylase (Renneberg et al., 1984). Another manuscript describes an automated system based on a reactor containing the immobilized cells of *Rhodococcus erythropolis* and *Isaatchenkia orientalis* and screen printed oxygen electrodes (Heim et al., 1999).

In work (Nandakumar & Mattiasson, 1999) the microbial sensor for glucose detection based on psychrophilic bacteria *Deinococcus radiodurans* and oxygen electrode. Other carbohydrates could interfere with the analysis. Sensor was able to determine the analyte under 5 °C, the receptor remained 90% from the initial activity after 45 days from the start of exploitation.

Starch detection is actual for biotechnology and food industry. In (Kitova et al., 2004) microbial and enzyme sensors for detection of the glucose generated by the amylase have been considered. The high correlation of biosensor analysis results with the polarimetric starch determination in wheat and rye flour was obtained.

4.2 Detection of alcohols and organic acids.

Biosensoric determination of alcohols and organic acids is also reported rather often by virtue of the same reason as for the carbohydrate detection. The methodical ware, and in a number of cases the microorganisms employed are also similar to ones utilized in carbohydrate sensors. It should be noted that the microbial cells possessing high selectivity are often used in biosensors for alcohol detection along with the enzymes. The methylotrophic yeast belonging to *Hansenula, Pichia, Candida* genera that are characterized by high intracellular content of alcohol oxidase and substrate specificity alterable by means of biochemical or genetic manipulations seem to be especially promising for this purpose (Voronova et al., 2008; Korpan et al., 1993). Thus, in manuscript (Gonchar et al., 1998) two microbial alcohol sensors based on recombinant *H. polymorpha* cells have been described. The first of the sensors utilized the cells with highly active alcohol oxidase immobilized on an oxygen electrode while the second one was based on catalase-deficient cells and involved a peroxide electrode as a transducer. The sensors were highly stable and insensitive to glucose and glycerol.

The original development consisted in the creation of an alcohol sensor based on *Agaricus bisporus* fungus tissue homogenate. The biomass immobilized in gelatin and cross-linked by glutaraldehyde was fixed on a Clark type electrode. The electrode current linearly depended on the ethanol concentration within the range 0.2 – 20 mM (Akyilmaz & Dinckaya, 2000).

The analysis of lactate in blood plasma and whole blood was carried out by the sensor based on *H. anomala* cells. The sensor possess high reproducibility, stability and rate of analysis. The analysis results agreed with the data obtained using conventional spectrophotometric technique and lactate dehydrogenase based enzyme sensor (Racek & Musil, 1987b). The similare work was intended to the development of a microbial sensor for fatty acids detection based on an oxygen electrode and *Arthrobacter nicotianae* cells immobilized into Ca-alginate gel (Schmidt et al., 1996). In the framework of another study a sensor for detection of tannic acid (a mixture of polygalloyl–glucose esters) from *Rhus chinensis* based on *Aspergillus ustus* cells and oxygen electrode. The analyte detection range made up about 10^{-4} - 10^{-3} M. An evaluation of temperature and pH effects on the sensor response has been carried out (Zhao et al., 1998).

As in the case of carbohydrate analysis the oxygen electrode is not the only transducer employed in the microbial sensors for alcohols and organic acids determination. A microbial ethanol biosensor based on ISFET and *Acetobacter aceti* cells was described (Kitagawa et al.,

1987). A conductometric microbial sensor for ethanol based on alginate-immobilized yeast cells has also been described (Korpan et al., 1994).

PQQ-dependent dehydrogenases of *Gluconobacter* bacteria are characterized by a wide spectrum of substrates. In this connection the enzymes as well as whole *Gluconobacter* cells represent a promising base for biosensor development. In publication (Tkac et al., 2003) a microbial sensor for ethanol detection based on *G. oxydans* cells and glassy carbon electrode modified by ferricyanide was described. The selectivity of the sensor was higher over enzyme sensors due to the application of a membrane barrier for glucose. The biosensor was employed for real-time ethanol monitoring during periodical fermentation of glucose by immobilized yeast.

An original approach was used in the study related to development of a biosensor based on *Chlorella* cells and oxygen electrode for detection of volatile compound vapors. The characteristic feature of the approach was the registration of the oxygen produced by the cells has been employed. Methanol was used as the model analyte. The sensor retained 50% of initial activity after 10 days from the start of operating (Naessens & Tran-Minh, 1998a).

4.3 Environmental application of biosensors - common state

The analysis of pollutants makes specific demands for the characteristics of developed biosensors. One of these demands is high detection sensitivity, which is determined by low MPC values of most xenobiotics. Catalytic sensors can provide the lower limit of target compound detection at a level of 10^{-7} M at best, which in most cases is insufficient. Therefore, among microbial sensors for the analysis of toxic compounds and pollutants there is a lot of bioluminescent sensors providing highly selective detection at a level of 10^{-9} - 10^{-7} M (in some cases, up to 10^{-12} M). Nevertheless, biocatalytic sensors are also used for detection of compounds with relatively low MPC values (phenol, naphthalene, SAS, some ions, etc.) and BOD. The characteristics of some biosensors potentially fit for environmental monitoring and similar nature-conservative measures will be considered in this subsection.

4.4 BOD detection

The methods and equipment for quick and sensitive assessment of the degree of water source pollution are relevant for providing high-performance measures of environmental control and decontamination. One of the most widely used indices for aquatic environment control is biological/biochemical oxygen demand (BOD). At present, the routine BOD analysis is performed mainly by the method of BOD_5 taking five days for completing. The quicker methods of BOD detection are associated with biosensor analyzers usually based on microorganisms that can metabolize the wide range of organic compounds. Although BOD values obtained by these methods are not identical to the values of BOD_5, in most cases it is possible to achieve an acceptable correlation between biosensor readings and the values of conventional methods.

The first work on construction of such sensor was published in 1977 (Karube et al., 1977); microorganisms from the active sludge of water treatment facilities were used as biomaterial. By now, quite a number of laboratory models and several commercial BOD biosensor analyzers are known. Such analyzers provide for BOD detection in the mean range of 5-300 mg/l for about a few minutes.

The sensor similar to the first BOD sensor model is described in (Liu et al., 2000). Its bioreceptor also included active sludge microorganisms. Sensor readings had satisfactory reproducibility and correlated well with BOD_5 values. BOD sensors based on mixed cultures are also reported in (Jia et al., 2003; Li et al., 1994; Suriyawattanakul et al., 2002). The BOD sensor based on a biofuel cell (BFC) containing active sludge is described in the work (Chang et al., 2004).

Although mixed cultures broaden the spectrum of biodegradable compounds (and, consequently, provide more profound BOD detection), the wrong side of this approach in most cases is lower stability and reproducibility of results associated with the ratio dynamics of cultures in bioreceptor. Therefore, pure bacterial and fungal cultures with broad substrate specificity are used in BOD sensors in parallel with active sludge and other microbial mixtures. The examples of such sensors are descirbed in the works (Yang et al., 1997; Kim & Park, 2001; Chee et al., 1999) etc. The list of the microorganisms most frequently used in BOD sensors includes *T. cutaneum, Arxula adeninovorans, E. coli, Bacillus* and *Pseudomonas* species and other microorganisms with broad specificity. Thus, different authors have published no less than ten works on construction of *T. cutaneum*-based BOD sensors; besides, it is used in some of the commercial BOD analyzers. The example of such sensor is described in the work (Yang et al., 1996).

Most of the BOD sensors are based on amperometric oxygen transducers (as a rule, Clark-type electrodes), but this is not the only possible way of constructing BOD sensors. The paper (Trosok et al., 2001) describes a mediator BOD sensor based on yeast cells and a glass-carbon electrode. The authors investigated the possibility of using 10 mediators for BOD detection; among them, ferricyanide was the most effective for detection of glucose-glutamate mixture. The sensor detected BOD in the range of 2-100 mg/l.

The new type of oxygen microsensor measures the level of oxygen using organically modified silicon and oxygen-sensitive dye tris(4,7-diphenyl-1,10-phenanthroline)ruthenium (II) chloride. The bacterial culture of *Stenotrophomonas maltophilia* was used. Measurement time was 20 min. Satisfactory coincidence with the data of standard BOD_5 method was obtained (Pang et al., 2007).

The work (Chee et al., 2000) describes the BOD sensor based on an oxygen optrode and *Pseudomonas putida* cells. The sensor detected BOD in the range of 1-10 mg/l and was insensitive to chlorides and heavy metal ions. Sensor readings correlated well with the BOD_5 data. The sensor was used for the analysis of river water samples.

Bioluminescent BOD sensor was based on the recombinant *E. coli* strain bearing fragments of *V. fisheri lux*-operon (Sakaguchi et al., 2003). Sensor readings correlated well with the BOD_5 data. The sensor was used for assessment of organic pollution in different wastewater samples.

One more approach to BOD detection is based on registration of temperature changes caused by microbiological destruction of organic compounds using calorimetric transducers; the biosensor based on such transducer is described in paper (Mattiasson et al., 1977).

In most cases, the BOD index is supposed to display the total quantity of organic compounds in a sample; accordingly, BOD sensors are constructed, as has been mentioned above, on the basis of microorganisms with broad substrate specificity. However, in some cases, BOD measurement is associated with the presence of specific compounds in the medium, which compels one to correct the choice of biocatalyst. So, the work (Konig et al., 1999) describes the sensor for detection of BOD at nitrification (N-BOD) and the degree of nitrification inhibition in wastewater. The bioreceptor of this sensor included a mixed culture of nitrifying microorganisms isolated from water treatment facilities. Nitrification inhibition was assessed in the presence of allylthiourea. The sensor had a high correlation with the standard method of N-BOD detection and was used for the analysis of wastewater samples.

One more example of biosensor detection of BOD determined by the presence of particular compounds in wastewater samples is described in paper (Reiss et al., 1998). In this case, the sensor was designed for BOD detection in starch-polluted waters. The device was based on a commercial biosensor BOD analyzer (Prüfgerätewerk Medingen) including the cells of *T. cutaneum*. The sensor was additionally equipped with two enzyme reactors containing immobilized α-amylase and amyloglucosidase for starch hydrolysis. Sensor readings were close to the standard BOD_5 data.

The functioning of BOD sensors may be influenced by various factors, including the chemical composition of analyzed samples. In particular, the presence of compounds toxic for cells may partially or completely inactivate the sensor or reduce its lifetime. The work (Qian & Tan, 1999) pursued the study of the effect of heavy metal ions on the BOD sensor based on *B. subtilis* cells killed by heating. This sensor was characterized by rather high sensitivity and stability of readings, in spite of nonviability of the biomaterial. The sensor allowed to estimate the effect of various metal ions on BOD determination.

It should be noted that the biosensor approach usually accounts only for easily utilized organic phase in measured samples and its results may not always correspond to the BOD_5 test. The correlation between biosensoric and conventional BOD measurements was assessed in the work (Liu et al., 2003). It was shown that the high correlation of biosensor and BOD_5 results was observed only for the samples that contained no organic polymers; in the presence of the latter, biosensor estimates were lower. The new approach to enhancement of the correlation between the biosensor method of measurement and traditional BOD_5 is presented in papers (Chee et al., 2005; Chee et al., 2001). The authors have proposed the method of photocatalytic pretreatment of water samples by means of their irradiation with the UV light for decomposition of large organic molecules into smaller ones. It has been shown that such scheme of analysis enhances biosensor sensitivity and increases the degree of correlation between the biosensor data and BOD_5. The analogous work on BOD measurement in river water was carried out at a stopped-flow plant using ozone treatment. After ozone treatment, the biosensor signal increased 1.6-fold (Chee et al., 2007).

One of the problems of BOD biosensors operation is the short time of their functioning because of membrane pollution. Besides, a pure culture based BOD sensor not always has sufficiently broad substrate specificity that would allow more complete estimation of BOD. The application of mediator-less biofuel cell (BFC) was a new approach to creation of analytical system for BOD assessment. In (Kim et al., 2003), the authors presented the experience of 5-year application of mediator-less BFC for BOD monitoring. The main parameters of this system, providing its high practical value, are stability and long (5 years) period of functioning without maintenance and the high correlation of results with the BOD_5 index.

The prevalence and importance of BOD biosensor related studies have naturally resulted in commercialization and industrial production of a number of the most promising models. The first commercial BOD biosensor analyzer was manufactured by Nisshin Denki (Electric) Co. Ltd. in 1983. Later on, similar analyzers were manufactured by some European companies (Riedel, 1998). At present, a number of biosensor systems for the control of biological oxygen demand are produced by European, Japanese and USA manufacturers.

Thus, biosensor BOD detection is a rather well-developed trend of analytical biotechnology. Biosensor BOD analyzers are reliable, simple and inexpensive analytical instruments, which are successfully used for the monitoring of water ecosystems together with the conventional methods of BOD detection.

4.5 Surfactant detection

Surface-active substances (SAS) are widely used both in life and in various fields of economic activity. In spite of the relatively low toxicity of SAS to warm-blooded animals, they facilitate concentration of other toxic substances, thus intensifying their effect on living organisms. Biosensor systems are developed for express detection of SAS. Particular attention is paid to application of microorganisms with this purpose, because the cells growing on SAS-containing medium prove to be adapted to their oxidation. The studies performed in the work (Reshetilov et al., 1997b) have shown that the cells of *P. rathonis* are highly sensitive to anionic and nonionogenic SAS. The comparative data on application of bacteria from the genera *Pseudomonas* and *Achromobacter* in the amperometric biosensor for SAS detection are presented. The substrate specificity of several strains towards a wide range of compounds has been assessed (Taranova et al., 2002; Taranova et al., 2004).

The microbial biosensor based on a column reactor containing activated sludge bacteria oxidizing linear alkylbenzene sulfonates was used for SAS analysis in river water. Biosensor signals linearly depended on SAS concentration up to 6 mg/l. Response time was no more than 15 min (Nomura et al., 1994; Nomura et al., 1998).

The detailed analysis of the problem of development of electrochemical sensors for SAS detection can be found in the work (Sak-Bosnar et al., 2004a). Nonelectrochemical sensors (opto-chemical and piezoelectric) are described in the work (Sak-Bosnar et al., 2004b).

4.6 Pesticides detection

A biosensor for direct detection of organophosphorous neurotoxins has been proposed. The biosensor is based on *E. coli* recombinant bacteria expressing organophosphate hydrolase and immobilized on a pH-electrode. The developed biosensor can be used for detection of a wide range of organophosphorous pesticides and chemical warfare agents (Rainina et al., 1996). A nearly identical sensor was described two years later by a group of USA authors (Mulchandani et al., 1998).

The possibility of quantitative determination of organophosphorous nitroaromatic insecticides (metaphos, sumithion) and the product of their hydrolysis, *p*-nitrophenol, based on the respiratory activity of microbial cells of *P. putida*. The possibility of construction of a microbial sensor system for detection of metaphos, sumithion, and *p*-nitrophenol in aqueous media has been considered (Ignatov et al., 2002).

4.7 Determination of hydrocarbons and their derivatives

Considerations as concerns the specificity of requirements to the parameters of biosensors for xenobiotic detection, which are presented in the beginning of "Environmental application of biosensors" section, relate in full measure to the biosensor analysis of aromatic compounds. On the one hand, the most of monoaromatic compounds and naphthalene are relatively low-toxic and the sensitivity of biocatalytic sensors is quite sufficient for their practical detection (although there are works on their bioluminescent analysis). On the other hand, polynuclear aromatic hydrocarbons (PAH) and, in particular, their chlorine derivatives belong to super toxicants and can exert toxic effect even in trace concentrations, so they can be detected only by highly sensitive analyzers (i.e., in this case, bioluminescent sensors or, as conventional techniques, chromatography, mass spectrometry and immunoassay).

Electrochemical microbial biosensor systems for detection of a wide range of xenobiotics have been described (Riedel et al., 1993; Riedel et al., 1991). For example, an amperomteric biosensor for detection of monoaromatics was based on *Rhodococcus* cells and their extract (Riedel et al., 1991). The microbial biosensor for benzene detection based on an oxygen electrode and *P. putida* cells was described. The sensor is supposed to be used for analyzing industrial wastewater and groundwater (Tan et al., 1994). The microbial biosensor for naphthalene detection based on an oxygen electrode and *Sphingomonas* sp. and *Pseudomonas fluorescens* strains was presented in the work (Konig et al., 1996). The lower limit of naphthalene detection was about 0.01 mg/l. The sensor maintained its activity for 20 days.

The column-type biosensor for amperometric detection of 2,4-dinitrophenol (2,4-DNP) based on the bacterium *Rhodococcus erythropolis* HL PM-1 was developed. The effect of carriers on analysis time and stability was studied (Kitova et al., 2002). The biosensor for amperometric detection of *p*-toluene sulfonate was constructed of immobilized *Comamonas testosteroni* BS1310 (pBS1010) cells and the Clark-type oxygen electrode. The lower detection limit was 5 μM (Makarenko et al., 1999).

Some of the microbial biosensor models based on the Clark-type electrode and strains-destructors of different compounds belonging to the genera *Pseudomonas, Sphinomonas, Rhodococcus,* and *Ralstonia* were described in the work (Beyersdorf-Radeck et al., 1998). In contrast to most of the works on biosensor application, the objective of this study was the screening of degrading capacity of the above strains in relation to polychlorobiphenyls, dibenzofuranes and similar compounds. It has been shown that the biosensor approach may considerably expedite the solution of such problems as compared with the conventional microbiological methods.

As has been mentioned above, the development of bioluminescent sensors for assessment of the presence and concentration of pollutants of different nature is a prospective approach providing much higher sensitivity and selectivity as compared with biocatalytic sensors. It explains the considerable number of publications of this kind since the middle 90s till now. It is known about bioluminescent microbial sensors for detection of naphthalene and salicylate (Heitzer et al., 1994; Matrubutham et al., 1997), chlorophenols (Sinclair et al., 1999), and PAH (Gu & Chang, 2001; Reid et al., 1998). The paper (Willardson et al., 1998) presents characteristics of a bioluminescent sensor based on the *E. coli* strain transformed by a plasmid bearing the firefly luciferase gene under the control of a promoter cut out of the toluene degradation plasmid. The sensor was sensitive to monoaromatic compounds. The analogous biosensors are reported in (Layton et al., 1998; Applegate et al., 1998).

The paper by Sticher et al. describes the microbial bioluminescent sensor based on the recombinant strain of *E. coli* for detection of middle-chain alkanes. The sensitivity to alicyclic and aromatic hydrocarbons was absent. The sensor was used for detection of middle-chain alkanes in groundwater samples (Sticher et al., 1997).

The bioluminescent bacterial sensor for detection of halogenated organic acids was based on a transgenic *E. coli* strain, where the reporter *luxCDABE* genes from *Photorhabdus luminescens* were under the control of promoter DL-2 from the strain *Pseudomonas* DL-DEX. The luminescence increased by 50% in the presence of 100 mg/l of 2-chloropropionic acid. The sensor was highly specific; measurement time was no more than 60 min (Tauber et al., 2001).

Some organic pollutants with low water solubility are characterized by the high value of "air-water" distribution coefficient, so they can be measured more effectively in the gas phase than in the water phase. The works (Werlen et al., 2004; Kononenko & Lukashev, 1995) describe application of a bioluminescent biosensor for the measurement of organic pollutants in the gas and water phases. The employed principle of measurement in combination with the developed biosensor design brought down the low limit of naphthalene detection 10 times. The presented results are further evidence of the efficiency of recombinant microorganisms as a basis of biosensors for highly sensitive detection of pollutants.

4.8 Detection of metal ions and inorganic acids

The subjects of this and the following sections are microbial biosensors that have become widespread in the recent decade and based mainly on genetically modified microorganisms and optical detection. Construction of microbial bioluminescent and catalytic sensors for detection of heavy metal and inorganic acids ions is a rather widespread approach in biosensor analysis; so, the work (Ramanathan et al., 1997) is a survey of bacterial biosensors for detection of heavy metals. The approach is based on genetic modification of bacteria by DNA fusion bearing the regulatory region of the metal-resistance operon and reporter genes. As a particular example, we can instance the bioluminescent sensor based on recombinant *E. coli* strains for the measurement of toxicity of arsenic compounds (Cai & DuBow, 1997).

The optical bacterial biosensor for zinc and copper detection in soil samples was based on the consortium containing the reporter bioluminescent *Rhizobium leguminosarum* biovar *trifolii* and *E. coli* strains. Bacterial suspension was used for registration. It was shown that EC_{25} (concentration that lowered the sensor signal by 25%) for zinc ions in the samples under study was 0.3 mg/l (Chaudri et al., 2000).

In the recombinant strain constructed for bioavailable mercury detection in soil samples, the activity of the *luxCDABE* operon was regulated due to the promoter-operator system of the mer-operon providing cell resistance to mercury. The lower detection limit of such biosensor was around 20 ng of mercury/g of soil (Rasmussen et al., 2000).

The microbial sensor for cyanide detection was based on *S. cerevisiae* cells and an oxygen electrode. The principle of detection was registration of decrease of response to glucose in the presence of cyanide - i.e., the approach typical of toxicity sensors (Nakanishi et al., 1996).

The models of microbial biosensors for nitrite detection based on the bacteria from the genera *Paracoccus* and *Nitrobacter* were described. The microbial biosensor for nitrite detection presented in the work (Karube et al., 1982c) was based on the strain of *Nitrobacter* sp. isolated from the active sludge of food plant treatment facilities. Compartment structure was complicated and included two chambers separated by a gas-permeable membrane; considerable inconvenience of this sensor was associated with the very slow growth of microorganisms. The analogous microbial sensor was constructed for the analysis of gaseous NO_2 on the basis of nitrite-oxidizing bacteria isolated from active sludge of the treatment facilities of food plant (Okada et al., 1983). One more example of potential nitrite and nitrate analyzer is a microbial mediator electrode based on *Paracoccus denitrificans* cells and a carbon electrode. Dihydroquinone was used as a mediator (Takayama et al., 1996). The electrochemical microbial biosensor system for ammonia detection was described as well (Riedel et al., 1990a).

The microbial biosensor for sulfate detection was developed on the basis of *Thiobacillus ferrooxidans* and oxygen electrode. The possibility of using this sensor for sulfate detection in rain water was shown (Sasaki et al., 1997).

The bioluminescent sensor based on recombinant cyanobacteria *Synechococcus* was used for detection of bioavailable phosphorus in water reservoirs (actually, the probability of "bloom" was assessed). The developed model was named as CyanoSensor and provided phosphate assessment in the concentration range of 0.3 – 8 μM. The results correlated with the chemical methods of total phosphorus estimation (Schreiter et al., 2001).

4.9 Assessment of general toxicity and genotoxicity

This subsection presents the most typical examples of sensors for genotoxicity and general toxicity. The approach, which is most frequently used at biosensor assessment of genotoxicity, is associated with application of SOS-promoters that are induced at massive DNA damages. Genetic constructions on their basis can be used for creation of biosensor strains for nonspecific registration of any genotoxic compounds and factors. In the work (Rettberg et al., 1999), luminescence of an *E. coli* strain carrying the plasmid with the *lux*-operon of *Photobacterium leiognathi* under the control of SOS promoter gradually depended on the dose of genotoxicant. The bioluminescent sensor for genotoxic factors estimation was based on the *E. coli* cells bearing a plasmid with the *lux*-operon built-in under the promoter of SOS-reparative locus. The biosensor sensitivity was comparable to that for the standard procedures of mutagenicity detection (Ptitsyn et al., 1997).

The general toxicity sensors also assess nonspecific toxic impacts of different nature; however, the principle of their action is associated with registration of attenuation of vital functions (bioluminescence, background respiration, etc.). The microbial sensor on the basis of luminescence bacteria was designed for detection of glucose and toxic compounds (Lee et al., 1992). Analogous models include a bioluminescent sensor based on the recombinant strain *R. leguminosarum* biovar *trifolii* for detection of general toxicity of the medium (Paton et al., 1997) and a bioluminescent sensor based on *E. coli* cells bearing the *lux*-genes of *V. fischeri* under the promoter of the operon of heat stress proteins (Rupani et al., 1996).

General toxicity can be detected using algae with chlorophyll fluorescence changing under the action of a toxic agent. The optical biosensor based on immobilized cells of the *Scenedesmus subspicatus* alga was described (Frense et al., 1998). The biosensor detected atrazine in a concentration of 1 to 1000 ppb. The paper (Vedrine et al., 2003) presents an optical biosensor based on the microalgae *Chlorella vulgaris* designed for detection of herbicides in the water phase. Similarly, biosensors based on bacterial cells can be effective for detection of antibiotics. Genetically modified luminescent *E. coli* bacteria were used for development of optical biosensors for aminoglycoside antibiotics detection (Vlasova et al., 2004).

Development of electrochemical microbial toxicity sensors is a rather widespread approach as well. As an example of such analyzers, one can mention the sensors based on an oxygen electrode and yeast cells (Campanella et al., 1995) and microscopic algae (Campanella et al., 2001), differential system for detection of genotoxic impacts described in (Karube et al., 1981), etc. In the recent decade, the a number of commercial biosensor toxicity analyzers have been constructed (Bentley et al., 2001; Ribo & Kaiser, 1987).

4.10 Volatile compounds. Miscellaneous

The analysis of concentrations of volatile organic compounds is an important analytical problem. Its relevance is associated with development of the methods of express analysis of abused drugs and explosives, foodstuff quality assessment, detection of toxic gases at chemical plants, air quality assessment in public places, etc. Development of biosensor analytical methods suggests new pathways and methods of solution of the problems of detection of specific organic compounds in the gas phases. The concept and basic principles of application of biological material for construction of "bioelectron nose" systems are stated in the works (Gopel et al., 1998; Gopel, 2000). The described types of biosensors are based on the principles of optical and electrochemical detection. In optical biosensors, it was genetically modified bacteria with bioluminescence depending on the presence of oxidizable compound in the gas phase. The transducer in electrochemical biosensors was the Clark-type oxygen electrode.

The recombinant *E. coli* strain bearing the lux-operon was immobilized in agar and used for detection of toxic compounds present in the gas phase. Benzene was selected as a model volatile compound. The biosensor can be used as an analyzer for measurement of toxic components at workplaces of chemical plants (Gil et al., 2000). Cyanide destructor *P. fluorescens* NCIMB 11764 was used in the microbial biosensor for detection of hydrocyanic acid vapor. The bacteria consumed oxygen at cyanide degradation, and the Clark-type electrode could be used for reaction registration (Lee & Karube, 1996).

The measurement of methane profile in a 3.5-mm sludge layer by microbial sensor is described in paper (Damgaard et al., 2001). The sensor was based on methane-oxidizing bacteria. They were immobilized on the surface of oxygen microelectrode. Oxygen was shown to have an insignificant effect of methane generation. The developed biosensor provided for the study of the effect of inhibitors (nitrates and sulfates) on methanogenesis.

The biosensor based on the cells of *Chlorella* microalgae and direct registration of oxygen production by these cells was used for perchloroethylene aerosol detection in the gas phase. Introduction of perchloroethylene resulted in the increase of released oxygen amount (Naessens & Tran-Minh, 1999). The analogous sensor based on *C. vulgaris* microalgae was used for methanol vapor detection (Naessens & Tran-Minh, 1998b).

5. Conclusion.

While considering the position of microbial biosensors in the series of biosensors constructed by now it should be noted that microbial biosensors undoubtedly form their own niche. Their properties in many respects are analogous to the properties of enzyme biosensors. First of all, it concerns detection range, which in both cases is determined by the K_M value of immobilized biocatalyst and for most of the enzyme and microbial biosensors does not go beyond 10^{-5} – 10^{-2} M. There is no doubt that microbial biosensors are less selective as compared with enzyme sensors. It is due to the nature of microbial cells containing a broad set of enzymes. At the same time, this feature can be effectively used in analytical systems such as BOD assessment. Besides, this disadvantage can be overcome by applying different approaches.

While defining the prospects of analytical application of microorganisms, one can predict their wide use in biosensors for the control of biotechnological processes and monitoring of environmental objects. One can also mention the application of microorganisms in biofuel cells. It seems that in the nearest future we should anticipate considerable progress in creation of effective microbial biofuel cells. To a large extent, the success of extensive application of microbial sensors will be associated with development of high-tech and simple methods of immobilization of microorganisms on the surface of transducers providing the maximum level of vital capacity and stability of cells.

As a whole, based on the analysis of particular data describing the properties of whole-cell sensors it is possible to conclude that the listed advantages and disadvantages of microbial sensors are typical of biosensors based on any other types of cells. The prospects of using cell biocatalysts for analytical purposes are the motive force of investigations on development of novel microbial biosensors and improvement of their parameters.

6. Acknowledgment

This study was supported partially by Federal Task Program "Scientific brainpower and research and educational personnel in innovative Russia" for the period of 2009-2013 (Project NK-37(4), Agreement P258).

7. References

Afanassiev, V.; Sefton, M.; Anantachaiyong, T.; Barker, G.; Walmsley, R. & Wolfl, S. (2000). Application of yeast cells transformed with GFP expression constructs containing the RAD54 or RNR2 promoter as a test for the genotoxic potential of chemical substances. *Mutat. Res.*, Vol. 464, No. 2, pp. 297-308

Akyilmaz, E. & Dinckaya, E. (2000). A mushroom (*Agaricus bisporus*) tissue homogenate based alcohol oxidase electrode for alcohol determination in serum. *Talanta*, Vol. 53, pp. 505-509

Albery, W. J. & Craston, D. H. (1987). Amperometric enzyme electrodes: theory and experiment. In: *Biosensors. Fundamentals and Applications*, Turner, A. P. F.; Karube, I & Wilson, G.S. (Eds.), pp. 180-210, Oxford University Press, New York

Alkasrawi, M.; Nandakumar, R.; Margesin, R.; Schinner, F. & Mattiasson, B. (1999). A microbial biosensor based on *Yarrowia lipolytica* for the off-line determination of middle-chain alkanes. *Biosensors and Bioelectronics*, Vol. 14, No. 8-9, pp. 723-727

Anko, M. L.; Kurittu, J. & Karp, M. (2002). An *Escherichia coli* biosensor strain for amplified and high throughput detection of antimicrobial agents. *J. Biomol. Screen.*, Vol. 7, No. 2, pp. 119-125

Applegate, B. M.; Kehrmeyer, S. R. & Sayler, G. S. (1998). A chromosomally based tod-*luxCDABE* whole-cell reporter for benzene, toluene, ethybenzene, and xylene (BTEX) sensing. *Applied and Environmental Microbiology*, Vol. 64, No. 7, pp. 2730-2735

Baxter, G. T.; Bousse, L. J.; Dawes, T. D.; Libby, J. M.; Modlin, D. N.; Owicki, J. C. & Parce, J. W. (1994). Microfabrication in silicon microphysiometry. *Clin. Chem.*, Vol. 40, No. 9, pp. 1800-1804

Bentley, A.; Atkinson, A.; Jezek, J. & Rawson, D. M. (2001). Whole cell biosensors--electrochemical and optical approaches to ecotoxicity testing. *Toxicol. In Vitro*, Vol. 15, No. 4-5, pp. 469-475.

Bergveld, P. (2003). Thirty years of ISFETOLOGY. What happened in the past 30 years and what may happen in the next 30 years. *Sensors and Actuators B: Chemical*, Vol. 88, pp. 1-20

Beyersdorf-Radeck, B.; Riedel, K.; Karlson, U.; Bachmann, T. T. & Schmid, R. D. (1998). Screening of xenobiotic compounds degrading microorganisms using biosensor techniques. *Microbiol. Res.*, Vol. 153, No. 3, pp. 239-245

Bhatia, R.; Dilleen, J. W.; Atkinson, A. L. & Rawson, D. M. (2003). Combined physico-chemical and biological sensing in environmental monitoring. *Biosensors and Bioelectronics*, Vol. 18, No. 5-6, pp. 667-674

Billard, P. & DuBow, M. S. (1998). Bioluminescence-based assays for detection and characterization of bacteria and chemicals in clinical laboratories. *Clinical Biochemistry*, Vol. 31, No. 1, pp. 1-14

Bousse, L. (1996). Whole cell biosensors. *Sensors and Actuators B: Chemical*, Vol. 34, pp. 270-275

Cai, J. & DuBow, M. S. (1997). Use of a luminescent bacterial biosensor for biomonitoring and characterization of arsenic toxicity of chromated copper arsenate (CCA). *Biodegradation*, Vol. 8, No. 2, pp. 105-111

Campanella, L.; Favero, G. & Tomassetti, M. (1995). Immobilised yeast cells biosensor for total toxicity testing. *Sci. Total Environ.*, Vol. 171, No. 1-3, pp. 227-234

Campanella, L.; Cubadda, F.; Sammartino, M. P. & Saoncella, A. (2001). An algal biosensor for the monitoring of water toxicity in estuarine environments. *Water Research*, Vol. 35, No. 1, pp. 69-76.

Cassidy, M. B.; Lee, H. & Trevors, J. T. (1996). Environmental applications of immobilized microbial cells: a review. *Journal of Industrial Microbiology*, Vol. 16, pp. 79-101

Chang, I. S.; Jang, J. K.; Gil, G. C.; Kim, M.; Kim, H. J.; Cho, B. W. & Kim, B. H. (2004). Continuous determination of biochemical oxygen demand using microbial fuel cell type biosensor. *Biosensors and Bioelectronics*, Vol. 19, No. 6, pp. 607-613

Chaubey, A. & Malhotra, B. D. (2002). Mediated biosensors. *Biosensors and Bioelectronics*, Vol. 17, No. 6-7, pp. 441-456

Chaudhuri, S. K. & Lovley, D. R. (2003). Electricity generation by direct oxidation of glucose in mediator-less microbial fuel cells. *Nature Biotechnology*, Vol. 21, No. 10, pp. 1229-1232

Chaudri, A. M.; Lawlor, K.; Preston, S.; Paton, G. I.; Killham, K. & McGrath, S. P. (2000). Response of a *Rhizobium*-based luminescence biosensor to Zn and Cu in soil solutions from sewage sludge treated soils. *Soil Biology and Biochemistry*, Vol. 32, pp. 383-388

Chee, G.-J.; Nomura, Y. & Karube, I. (1999). Biosensor for the estimation of low biochemical oxygen demand. *Analytica Chimica Acta*, Vol. 379, pp. 185-191

Chee, G. J.; Nomura, Y.; Ikebukuro, K. & Karube, I. (2000). Optical fiber biosensor for the determination of low biochemical oxygen demand. *Biosensors and Bioelectronics*, Vol. 15, No. 7-8, pp. 371-376.

Chee, G.-J.; Nomura, Y.; Ikebukuro, K. & Karube, I. (2001). Biosensor for the evaluation of biochemical oxygen demand using photocatalytic pretreatment. *Sensors and Actuators B: Chemical*, Vol. 80, pp. 15-20

Chee, G. J.; Nomura, Y.; Ikebukuro, K. & Karube, I. (2005). Development of photocatalytic biosensor for the evaluation of biochemical oxygen demand. *Biosensors and Bioelectronics*, Vol. 21, No. 1, pp. 67-73

Chee, G. J.; Nomura, Y.; Ikebukuro, K. & Karube, I. (2007). Stopped-flow system with ozonizer for the estimation of low biochemical oxygen demand in environmental samples. *Biosensors and Bioelectronics*, Vol. 22, No. 12, pp. 3092-3098, ISSN 0956-5663

Chouteau, C.; Dzyadevych, S.; Chovelon, J. M. & Durrieu, C. (2004). Development of novel conductometric biosensors based on immobilised whole cell *Chlorella vulgaris* microalgae. *Biosensors and Bioelectronics*, Vol. 19, No. 9, pp. 1089-1096

Clark, L. C., Jr. (1993). How the first enzyme electrode was invented [editorial]. *Biosensors and Bioelectronics*, Vol. 8, No. 1, pp. iii-vii

D'Souza, S. F. (2001a). Immobilization and stabilization of biomaterials for biosensor applications. *Appl. Biochem. Biotechnol.*, Vol. 96, No. 1-3, pp. 225-238.

D'Souza, S. F. (2001b). Microbial biosensors. *Biosensors and Bioelectronics*, Vol. 16, No. 6, pp. 337-353.

D'Souza, S. E. (1989). Potentials of co-immobilizates in biochemical processing: the current state of the art. *J. Microbiol. Biotechnol.*, Vol. № 4, pp. 63-73

Damgaard, L. R.; Nielsen, L. P. & Revsbech, N. P. (2001). Methane microprofiles in a sewage biofilm determined with a microscale biosensor. *Water Research*, Vol. 35, No. 6, pp. 1379-1386.

Daunert, S.; Barrett, G.; Feliciano, J. S.; Shetty, R. S.; Shrestha, S. & Smith-Spencer, W. (2000). Genetically engineered whole-cell sensing systems: coupling biological recognition with reporter genes. *Chem. Rev.*, Vol. 100, pp. 2705-2738

Domansky, K.; Janata, J.; Josowicz, M. & Petelenz, D. (1993). Present state of fabrication of chemically sensitive field effect transistors. *Analyst*, Vol. 118, No. 4, pp. 335-340

Fedorov, A.; Volchenko, E. B.; Singirtsev, I. N.; Korzhenevich, V. I. & Shub, G. M. (1999). [Protective effects of agar during immobilization of strains capable to degrade aromatic compounds]. *Prikl. Biokhim. Mikrobiol.*, Vol. 35, No. 2, pp. 165-172, ISSN 0555-1099

Frense, D.; Muller, A. & Beckmann, D. (1998). Detection of environmental pollutants using optical biosensor with immobilized algae cells. *Sensors and Actuators B: Chemical*, Vol. 51, pp. 256-260

Fukui, S. & Tanaka, A. (1984). Application of biocatalysts immobilized by prepolymer methods. *Adv. Biochem. Eng. Biotechn.*, Vol. 29, pp. 2-33

Gil, G. C.; Mitchell, R. J.; Chang, S. T. & Gu, M. B. (2000). A biosensor for the detection of gas toxicity using a recombinant bioluminescent bacterium. *Biosensors and Bioelectronics*, Vol. 15, No. 1-2, pp. 23-30

Gonchar, M. V.; Maidan, M. M.; Moroz, O. M.; Woodward, J. R. & Sibirny, A. A. (1998). Microbial O2- and H2O2-electrode sensors for alcohol assays based on the use of permeabilized mutant yeast cells as the sensitive bioelements. *Biosensors and Bioelectronics*, Vol. 13, No. 9, pp. 945-952

Gopel, W.; Ziegler, C.; Breer, H.; Schild, D.; Apfelbach, R.; Joerges, J. & Malaka, R. (1998). Bioelectronic noses: a status report. Part I. *Biosensors and Bioelectronics*, Vol. 13, No. 3-4, pp. 479-493

Gopel, W. (2000). From electronic to bioelectronic olfaction, or: from artificial "moses" to real noses. *Sensors and Actuators B: Chemical*, Vol. 65, pp. 70-72

Gu, M. B. & Chang, S. T. (2001). Soil biosensor for the detection of PAH toxicity using an immobilized recombinant bacterium and a biosurfactant. *Biosensors and Bioelectronics*, Vol. 16, No. 9-12, pp. 667-674.

Gu, M. B. & Gil, G. C. (2001). A multi-channel continuous toxicity monitoring system using recombinant bioluminescent bacteria for classification of toxicity. *Biosensors and Bioelectronics*, Vol. 16, No. 9-12, pp. 661-666

Guliy, O. I.; Ignatov, O. V.; Makarov, O. E. & Ignatov, V. V. (2003). Determination of organophosphorus aromatic nitro insecticides and *p*-nitrophenol by microbial-cell respiratory activity. *Biosensors and Bioelectronics*, Vol. 18, No. 8, pp. 1005-1013

Hansen, L. H. & Sorensen, S. J. (2001). The use of whole-cell biosensors to detect and quantify compounds or conditions affecting biological systems. *Microbial Ecology*, Vol. 42, pp. 483-494

Heim, S.; Schnieder, I.; Binz, D.; Vogel, A. & Bilitewski, U. (1999). Development of an automated microbial sensor system. *Biosensors and Bioelectronics*, Vol. 14, No. 2, pp. 187-193

Heitzer, A.; Malachowsky, K.; Thonnard, J. E.; Bienkowski, P. R.; White, D. C. & Sayler, G. S. (1994). Optical biosensor for environmental on-line monitoring of naphthalene and salicylate bioavailability with an immobilized bioluminescent catabolic reporter bacterium. *Appl. Environ. Microbiol.*, Vol. 60, No. 5, pp. 1487-1494

Held, M.; Schuhmann, W.; Jahreis, K. & Schmidt, H.-L. (2002). Microbial biosensor array with transport mutants of *Escherichia coli* K12 for the simultaneous determination of mono-and disaccharides. *Biosensors and Bioelectronics*, Vol. 17, No. 11-12, pp. 1089-1094, ISSN 0956-5663

Ignatov, O. V.; Gulii, O. I.; Singirtsev, I. N.; Shcherbakov, A. A.; Makarov, O. E. & Ignatov, V. V. (2002). [Effects of *p*-nitrophenol and organophosphorous nitroaromatic insecticides on the respiratory activity of free and immobilized cells of strains S-11 and BA-11 of *Pseudomonas putida*]. *Prikl. Biokhim. Mikrobiol.*, Vol. 38, No. 3, pp. 278-285

Ikeda, T.; Matsuyama, K.; Kobayashi, D. & Matsushita, F. (1992). Whole-cell enzyme electrodes based on mediated bioelectrocatalysis. *Biosci. Biotechnol. Biochem.*, Vol. 56, No. 8, pp. 1359-1360

Ikeda, T.; Kurosaki, T.; Takayama, K.; Kano, K. & Miki, K. (1996). Measurements of oxidoreductase-like activity of intact bacterial cells by an amperometric method using a membrane-coated electrode. *Analytical Chemistry*, Vol. 68, No. 1, pp. 192-198

Ikeda, T.; Tsujimura, S. & Kano, K. (2004). Bioelectrochemical energy conversion systems based on mediated bioelectrocatalysis, *Proceedings of Biosensors 2004*, Granada, Spain

Ito, Y.; Yamazaki, S.; Kano, K. & Ikeda, T. (2002). *Escherichia coli* and its application in a mediated amperometric glucose sensor. *Biosensors and Bioelectronics*, Vol. 17, No. 11-12, pp. 993-998

Jia, J.; Tang, M.; Chen, X.; Qi, L. & Dong, S. (2003). Co-immobilized microbial biosensor for BOD estimation based on sol-gel derived composite material. *Biosensors and Bioelectronics*, Vol. 18, No. 8, pp. 1023-1029

Karube, I.; Matsunaga, T.; Mitsuda, S. & Suzuki, S. (1977). Microbial electrode BOD sensors. *Biotechnol. Bioeng.*, Vol. 19, No. 10, pp. 1535-1547

Karube, I.; Mitsuda, S. & Suzuki, S. (1979). Glucose sensor usind immobilized whole cells of *Pseudomonas fluorescens*. *Eur. J. Appl. Microbiol. Biotechn.*, Vol. 7, No. 4, pp. 343-350

Karube, I.; Suzuki, S.; Okada, T. & Hikuma, M. (1980). Microbial sensors for volatile compounds. *Biochimie*, Vol. 62, No. 8-9, pp. 567-573

Karube, I.; Matsunaga, T.; Nakahara, T.; Suzuki, S. & Kada, T. (1981). Preliminary screening of mutagens with a microbial sensor. *Analytical Chemistry*, Vol. 53, No. 7, pp. 1024-1026

Karube, I.; Nakahara, T.; Matsunaga, T. & Suzuki, S. (1982a). *Salmonella* electrode for screening mutagens. *Analytical Chemistry*, Vol. 54, No. 11, pp. 1725-1727

Karube, I.; Okada, T. & Suzuki, S. (1982b). A methane gas sensor based on oxidizing bacteria. *Analytica Chimica Acta*, Vol. 135, No. 1, pp. 61-67

Karube, I.; Okada, T.; Suzuki, S.; Suzuki, H.; Hikuma, M. & Yasuda, T. (1982c). Amperometric determination of sodium nitrite by a microbial sensor. *European J. Appl. Microbiol. Biotechnol.*, Vol. 15, pp. 127-132

Katrlik, J.; Brandsteter, R.; Svorc, J.; Rosenberg, M. & Miertus, S. (1997). Mediator type of glucose microbial biosensor based on *Aspergillus niger*. *Analytica Chimica Acta*, Vol. 356, pp. 217-224

Katrlik, J.; Vostiar, I.; Sefcovicova, J.; Tkac, J.; Mastihuba, V.; Valach, M.; Stefuca, V. & Gemeiner, P. (2007). A novel microbial biosensor based on cells of *Gluconobacter oxydans* for the selective determination of 1,3-propanediol in the presence of glycerol and its application to bioprocess monitoring. *Anal. Bioanal. Chem.*, Vol. 388, No. 1, pp. 287-295, ISSN 1618-2642

Kim, B. H.; Chang, I. S.; Gil, G. C.; Park, H. S. & Kim, H. J. (2003). Novel BOD (biological oxygen demand) sensor using mediator-less microbial fuel cell. *Biotechnol. Lett.*, Vol. 25, No. 7, pp. 541-545

Kim, M.-N. & Park, K.-H. (2001). *Klebsiella* BOD sensor. *Sensors and Actuators B: Chemical*, Vol. 80, pp. 9-14

Kitagawa, Y.; Tamiya, E. & Karube, I. (1987). Microbial-FET alcohol sensor. *Analytical Letters*, Vol. 20, No. 1, pp. 81-96

Kitova, A. E.; Kuvichkina, T. N.; Il'iasov, P. V.; Arinbasarova, A. & Reshetilov, A. N. (2002). [Biosensor of the reactor type based on *Rhodococcus erythropolis* HL TM-1 cells for determining 2,4-dinitrophenol]. Prikl. Biokhim. Mikrobiol., Vol. 38, No. 5, pp. 585-590

Kitova, A. E.; Alferov, V. A.; Ponamoreva, O. N.; Ashin, V. V.; Kuzmichev, A. V.; Ezhkov, A. A.; Arsenyev, D. V. & Reshetilov, A. N. (2004). Enzyme biosensors for starch, glucose and ethanol concentrations express-analysis, In: *Biotechnology and industry*, Zaikov, G. E. (Ed.), pp. 19-29, Nova Science Publishers, Inc., New York

Kobos, R. K.; Rice, D. J. & Flournoy, D. S. (1979). Bacterial membrane electrode for the determination of nitrate. *Analytical Chemistry*, Vol. 51, No. 8, pp. 1122-1125

Konig, A.; Zaborosch, C.; Muscat, A.; Vorlop, K.-D. & Spener, F. (1996). Microbial sensors for naphthalene using *Sphingomonas* sp. B1 or *Pseudomonas fluorescens* WW4. *Appl. Microbiol. Biotechnol.*, Vol. 45, pp. 844-850

Konig, A.; Riedel, K. & Metzger, J. W. (1998). A microbial sensor for detecting inhibitors of nitrification in wastewater. *Biosensors and Bioelectronics*, Vol. 13, No. 7-8, pp. 869-874

Konig, A.; Bachmann, T. T.; Metzger, J. W. & Schmid, R. D. (1999). Disposable sensor for measuring the biochemical oxygen demand for nitrification and inhibition of nitrification in wastewater. *Appl. Microbiol. Biotechnol.*, Vol. 51, No. 1, pp. 112-117

Kononenko, A. A. & Lukashev, E. P. (1995). Light biosensors based on bacteriorhodopsin and photosynthetic reaction centers, In: *Advances in Biosensors*, Turner, A. P. F. & Yevdokimov, Y. M. (Eds.), pp. 191-211, JAI Press Inc., Greenwich, London

Kononov, M. A.; Nikitin, D. I. & Savranskii, V. V. (2007). [A study of the metabolism of bacterial cells by the method of surface plasmon spectroscopy]. *Biofizika*, Vol. 52, No. 4, pp. 681-686, ISSN 0006-3029

Korpan, Y. I.; Gonchar, M. V.; Starodub, N. F.; Shulga, A. A.; Sibirny, A. A. & Elskaya, A. V. (1993). A Cell biosensor specific for formaldehyde based on ph-sensitive transistors coupled to methylotrophic yeast cells with genetically adjusted metabolism. *Analytical Biochemistry*, Vol. 215, No. 2, pp. 216-222, ISSN 0003-2697

Korpan, Y. I.; Dzyadevich, S. V.; Zharova, V. P. & El'skaya, A. V. (1994). Conductometric biosensor for ethanol detection based on whole yeast cells. *Ukr. Biokhim. Zh.*, Vol. 66, No. 1, pp. 78-82

Kurittu, J.; Karp, M. & Korpela, M. (2000). Detection of tetracyclines with luminescent bacterial strains. *Luminescence*, Vol. 15, No. 5, pp. 291-297.

Layton, A. C.; Muccini, M.; Ghosh, M. M. & Sayler, G. S. (1998). Construction of a bioluminescent reporter strain to detect polychlorinated biphenyls. *Applied And Environmental Microbiology*, Vol. 64, No. 12, pp. 5023-5026

Lee, J. I. & Karube, I. (1996). Development of a biosensor for gaseous cyanide in solution. *Biosensors and Bioelectronics*, Vol. 11, No. 11, pp. 1147-1154

Lee, S.; Sode, K.; Nakanishi, K.; Marty, J. L.; Tamiya, E. & Karube, I. (1992). A novel microbial sensor using luminous bacteria. *Biosensors and Bioelectronics*, Vol. 7, No. 4, pp. 273-277

Lehmann, M.; Chan, C.; Lo, A.; Lung, M.; Tag, K.; Kunze, G.; Riedel, K.; Gruendig, B. & Renneberg, R. (1999). Measurement of biodegradable substances using the salt-tolerant yeast *Arxula adeninivorans* for a microbial sensor immobilized with poly(carbamoyl)sulfonate (PCS). Part II: Application of the novel biosensor to real samples from coastal and island regions. *Biosensors and Bioelectronics*, Vol. 14, No. 3, pp. 295-302

Li, F.; Tan, T. C. & Lee, Y. K. (1994). Effects of pre-conditioning and microbial composition on the sensing efficacy of a BOD biosensor. *Biosensors and Bioelectronics*, Vol. 9, No. 3, pp. 197-205

Liu, J.; Bjornsson, L. & Mattiasson, B. (2000). Immobilised activated sludge based biosensor for biochemical oxygen demand measurement. *Biosensors and Bioelectronics*, Vol. 14, No. 12, pp. 883-893

Liu, J.; Olsson, G. & Mattiasson, B. (2003). Monitoring of two-stage anaerobic biodegradation using a BOD biosensor. *Journal of Biotechnology*, Vol. 100, No. 3, pp. 261-265

Lobanov, A. V.; Borisov, I. A.; Gordon, S. H.; Greene, R. V.; Leathers, T. D. & Reshetilov, A. N. (2001). Analysis of ethanol-glucose mixtures by two microbial sensors: application of chemometrics and artificial neural networks for data processing. *Biosensors and Bioelectronics*, Vol. 16, pp. 1001-1007

Makarenko, A. A.; Balashov, S. V.; Kuvichkina, T. N.; Il'yasov, P. V. & Reshetilov, A. N. (1999). [A biosensor analyzer of sulfoaromatic compounds based on the strain *Comamonas testosteroni* BS1310 (pBS1010)]. *Prikl. Biochem. Microbiol.*, Vol. 35, No. 4, pp. 375-379

Matrubutham, U.; Thonnard, J. E. & Sayler, G. S. (1997). Bioluminescence induction response and survival of the bioreporter bacterium *Pseudomonas fluorescens* HK44 in nutrient-deprived conditions. *Appl. Microbiol. Biotechnol.*, Vol. 47, pp. 604-609

Matsunaga, T.; Toshihiko, S. & Tomoda, R. (1984). Photomicrobial sensors for selective determination of phosphate. *Enzyme Microb. Technol.*, Vol. 6, No. 8, pp. 335-358

Mattiasson, B.; Larsson, P. O. & Mosbach, K. (1977). The microbe thermistor. *Nature*, Vol. 268, No. 5620, pp. 519-520

McNeil, C. J.; Cooper, J. M. & Spoors, J. A. (1992). Amperometric enzyme electrode for determination of theophylline in serum. *Biosensors and Bioelectronics*, Vol. 7, No. 5, pp. 375-380

Mehrvar, M. & Abdi, M. (2004). Recent developments, characteristics, and potential applications of electrochemical biosensors. *Analytical Sciences*, Vol. 20, pp. 1113-1126

Min, J.; Lee, C. W.; Moon, S. H.; LaRossa, R. A. & Gu, M. B. (2000). Detection of radiation effects using recombinant bioluminescent *Escherichia coli* strains. *Radiat. Environ. Biophys.*, Vol. 39, No. 1, pp. 41-45

Mitchell, R. J. & Gu, M. B. (2004). An *Escherichia coli* biosensor capable of detecting both genotoxic and oxidative damage. *Appl. Microbiol. Biotechnol.*, Vol. 64, No. 1, pp. 46-52

Mosbach, K. & Danielsson, B. (1974). An enzyme thermistor. *Biochim. Biophys. Acta*, Vol. 364, pp. 140-145

Mulchandani, A.; Mulchandani, P.; Kaneva, I. & Chen, W. (1998). Biosensor for direct determination of organophosphate nerve agents using recombinant *Escherichia coli* with surface-expressed organophosphorus hydrolase. 1. Potentiometric microbial electrode. *Analytical Chemistry*, Vol. 70, No. 19, pp. 4140-4145

Murphy, L. (2006). Biosensors and bioelectrochemistry. *Curr. Opin. Chemistry & Biology*, Vol. 10, No. 2, pp. 177-184, ISSN 1367-5931

Naessens, M. & Tran-Minh, C. (1998a). Whole-cell biosensor for direct determination of solvent vapours. *Biosensors and Bioelectronics*, Vol. 13, No. 3-4, pp. 341-346

Naessens, M. & Tran-Minh, C. (1998b). Whole-cell biosensor for determination of volatile organic compounds in the form of aerosols. *Analytica Chimica Acta*, Vol. 364, pp. 153-158

Naessens, M. & Tran-Minh, C. (1999). Biosensor using immobilized Chlorella microalgae for determination of volatile organic compounds. *Sensors and Actuators B: Chemical*, Vol. 59, pp. 100-102

Nakanishi, K.; Ikebukuro, K. & Karube, I. (1996). Determination of cyanide using a microbial sensor. *Appl. Biochem. Biotechnol.*, Vol. 60, No. 2, pp. 97-106

Nandakumar, R. & Mattiasson, B. (1999). A low temperature microbial biosensor using immobilised psychrophilic bacteria. *Biotechnology Techniques*, Vol. 13, pp. 683-693

Nomura, Y.; Ikebukuro, K.; Yokoyama, K.; Takeuchi, T.; Arikawa, Y.; Ohno, S. & Karube, I. (1994). A novel microbial sensor for anionic surfactant determination. *Analytical Letters*, Vol. 27, No. 15, pp. 3095-3108

Nomura, Y.; Ikebukuro, K.; Yokoyama, K.; Takeuchi, T.; Arikawa, Y.; Ohno, S. & Karube, I. (1998). Application of a linear alkylbenzene sulfonate biosensor to river water monitoring. *Biosensors and Bioelectronics*, Vol. 13, No. 9, pp. 1047-1053

Okada, T.; Karube, I. & Suzuki, S. (1983). NO2 sensor which uses immobilized nitrite oxidizing bacteria. *Biotechnology and Bioengineering*, Vol. 25, pp. 1641-1651

Okochi, M.; Mima, K.; Miyata, M.; Shinozaki, Y.; Haraguchi, S.; Fujisawa, M.; Kaneko, M.; Masukata, T. & Matsunaga, T. (2004). Development of an automated water toxicity biosensor using *Thiobacillus ferrooxidans* for monitoring cyanides in natural water for a water filtering plant. *Biotechnology and Bioengineering*, Vol. 87, No. 7, pp. 905-911

Paitan, Y.; Biran, D.; Biran, I.; Shechter, N.; Babai, R.; Rishpon, J. & Ron, E. Z. (2003). On-line and in situ biosensors for monitoring environmental pollution. *Biotechnology Advances*, Vol. 22, pp. 27-33

Pang, H. L.; Kwok, N. Y.; Chan, P. H.; Yeung, C. H.; Lo, W. & Wong, K. Y. (2007). High-throughput determination of biochemical oxygen demand (BOD) by a microplate-based biosensor. *Environ. Sci. Technol.*, Vol. 41, No. 11, pp. 4038-4044, ISSN 0013-936X

Parce, J. W.; Owicki, J. C.; Kercso, K. M.; Sigal, G. B.; Wada, H. G.; Muir, V. C.; Bousse, L. J.; Ross, K. L.; Sikic, B. I. & McConnell, H. M. (1989). Detection of cell-affecting agents with a silicon biosensor. *Science*, Vol. 246, No. 4927, pp. 243-247

Park, J. K.; Ro, H. S. & Kim, H. S. (1991). A new biosensor for specific determination of sucrose using an oxidoreductase of *Zymomonas mobilis* and invertase. *Biotechnology and Bioengineering*, Vol. 38, No. 3, pp. 217-223

Paton, G. I.; Palmer, G.; Burton, M.; Rattray, E. A.; McGrath, S. P.; Glover, L. A. & Killham, K. (1997). Development of an acute and chronic ecotoxicity assay using *lux*-marked *Rhizobium leguminosarum* biovar *trifolii*. *Lett. Appl. Microbiol.*, Vol. 24, No. 4, pp. 296-300

Pearson, J. E.; Gill, A. & Vadgama, P. (2000). Analytical aspects of biosensors. *Ann. Clin. Biochem.*, Vol. 37, No. Pt 2, pp. 119-145

Philp, J. C.; Balmand, S.; Hajto, E.; Bailey, M. J.; Wiles, S.; Whiteley, A. S.; Lilley, A. K.; Hajto, J. & Dunbar, S. A. (2003). Whole cell immobilised biosensors for toxicity assessment of a wastewater treatment plant treating phenolics-containing waste. *Analytica Chimica Acta*, Vol. 487, pp. 61-74

Plegge, V.; Slama, M.; Suselbeck, B.; Wienke, D.; Spener, F.; Knoll, M. & Zaborosch, C. (2000). Analysis of ternary mixtures with a single dynamic microbial sensor and chemometrics using a nonlinear multivariate calibration. *Analytical Chemistry*, Vol. 72, No. 13, pp. 2937-2942

Ptitsyn, L. R.; Horneck, G.; Komova, O.; Kozubek, S.; Krasavin, E. A.; Bonev, M. & Rettberg, P. (1997). A biosensor for environmental genotoxin screening based on an SOS lux assay in recombinant *Escherichia coli* cells. *Appl. Environ. Microbiol.*, Vol. 63, No. 11, pp. 4377-4384

Qian, Z. & Tan, T. C. (1999). BOD measurement in the presence of heavy metal ions using a thermally-killed-*Bacillus subtilis* biosensor. *Water Research*, Vol. 33, No. 13, pp. 2923-2928

Racek, J. & Musil, J. (1987a). Biosensor for lactate determination in biological fluids. 2. Interference studies. *Clin. Chim. Acta*, Vol. 167, No. 1, pp. 59-65

Racek, J. & Musil, J. (1987b). Biosensor for lactate determination in biological fluids. I. Construction and properties of the biosensor. *Clin. Chim. Acta*, Vol. 162, No. 2, pp. 129-139

Racek, J. (1991). A yeast biosensor for glucose determination. *Appl. Microbiol. Biotechnol.*, Vol. 34, No. 4, pp. 473-477

Racek, J. (1995). *Cell-based biosensors*, Technomic Publishing Company, Lancaster, Basel

Rainina, E. I.; Efremenco, E. N.; Varfolomeyev, S. D.; Simonian, A. L. & Wild, J. R. (1996). The development of a new biosensor based on recombinant *E. coli* for the direct detection of organophosphorus neurotoxins. *Biosensors and Bioelectronics*, Vol. 11, No. 10, pp. 991-1000

Ramanathan, K.; Rank, M.; Svitel, J.; Dzgoev, A. & Danielsson, B. (1999). The development and applications of thermal biosensors for bioprocess monitoring. *Trends Biotechnol.*, Vol. 17, No. 12, pp. 499-505

Ramanathan, S.; Ensor, M. & Daunert, S. (1997). Bacterial biosensors for monitoring toxic metals. *Trends Biotechnol.*, Vol. 15, No. 12, pp. 500-506

Rasmussen, L. D.; Sorensen, S. J.; Turner, R. R. & Barkay, T. (2000). Application of a *mer-lux* biosensor for estimating bioavailable mercury in soil. *Soil Biology & Biochemistry*, Vol. 32, pp. 639-646

Rechnitz, G. A.; Kobos, R. K.; Riechel, S. J. & Gebauer, C. R. (1977). A bio-selective membrane electrode prepared with living bacterial cells. *Analytica Chimica Acta*, Vol. 94, No. 2, pp. 357-365

Rechnitz, G. A. & Ho, M. Y. (1990). Biosensors based on cell and tissue material. *Journal of Biotechnology*, Vol. 15, No. 3, pp. 201-218

Reid, B. J.; Semple, K. T.; Macleod, C. J.; Weitz, H. J. & Paton, G. I. (1998). Feasibility of using prokaryote biosensors to assess acute toxicity of polycyclic aromatic hydrocarbons. *FEMS Microbiology Letters*, Vol. 169, No. 2, pp. 227-233

Reiss, M.; Heibges, A.; Metzger, J. & Hartmeier, W. (1998). Determination of BOD-values of starch-containing waste water by a BOD-biosensor. *Biosensors and Bioelectronics*, Vol. 13, No. 10, pp. 1083-1090

Renneberg, R.; Riedel, K.; Liebs, P. & Scheller, F. (1984). Microbial and hybrid sensors for determination of α-amylase activity. *Analytical Letters*, Vol. 17, No. 85, pp. 349-358

Reshetilov, A. N.; Iliasov, P. V.; Donova, M. V.; Dovbnya, D. V.; Boronin, A. M.; Leathers, T. D. & Greene, R. V. (1997a). Evaluation of a *Gluconobacter oxydans* whole cell biosensor for amperometric detection of xylose. *Biosensors and Bioelectronics*, Vol. 12, No. 3, pp. 241-247

Reshetilov, A. N.; Semenchuk, I. N.; Iliasov, P. V. & Taranova, L. A. (1997b). The amperometric biosensor for detection of sodium dodecyl sulfate. *Analytica Chimica Acta*, Vol. 347, pp. 19-26

Reshetilov, A. N.; Lobanov, A. V.; Morozova, N. O.; Gordon, S. H.; Greene, R. V. & Leathers, T. D. (1998). Detection of ethanol in a two-component glucose/ethanol mixture using a nonselective microbial sensor and a glucose enzyme electrode. *Biosensors and Bioelectronics*, Vol. 13, No. 7-8, pp. 787-793

Rettberg, P.; Baumstark-Khan, C.; Bandel, K.; Ptitsyn, L. R. & Horneck, G. (1999). Microscale application of the SOS-LUX-TEST as biosensor for genotoxic agents. *Analytica Chimica Acta*, Vol. 387, pp. 289-296

Ribo, J. M. & Kaiser, K. L. E. (1987). *Photobacterium phosphoreum* toxicity bioassay. I. Test procedures and applications. *Toxicity Assessment: An International Quarterly*, Vol. 2, No. 3, pp. 305-323

Riedel, K.; Renneberg, R.; Liebs, P. & Kaiser, G. (1987). Microbial sensors. *Studia Biophysica*, Vol. 119, No. 1-3, pp. 163-166

Riedel, K. & Scheller, F. (1987). Inhibitor-treated microbial sensor for the selective determination of glutamic acid. *Analyst*, Vol. 112, No. 3, pp. 341-342

Riedel, K.; Renneberg, R.; Wollenberger, U.; Kaiser, G. & Scheller, F. W. (1989). Microbial sensors: fundamentals and application for process control. *J. Chem. Tech. Biotechnol.*, Vol. 44, No. 2, pp. 85-106

Riedel, K.; Huth, J.; Kuehn, M. & Liebs, P. (1990a). Amperometric determination of ammonium ions with a microbial sensor. *J. Chem. Tech. Biotechnol.*, Vol. 47, No. 2, pp. 109-116

Riedel, K.; Renneberg, R. & Scheller, F. (1990b). Adaptable microbial sensors. *Analytical Letters*, Vol. 23, No. 5, pp. 757-770

Riedel, K.; Hensel, J. & Ebert, K. (1991). [Biosensors for the determination of phenol and benzoate on the basis of *Rhodococcus* cells and enzyme extracts]. *Zentralbl Mikrobiol.*, Vol. 146, No. 6, pp. 425-434

Riedel, K.; Hensel, J.; Rothe, S.; Neumann, B. & Scheller, F. (1993). Microbial sensors for determination of aromatics and their chloroderivatives. 2. Determination of chlorinated phenols using a *Rhodococcus*-containing biosensor. *Appl. Microbiol. Biotechnol.*, Vol. 38, No. 4, pp. 556-559

Riedel, K. (1998). Application of biosensors to environmental samples, In: *Commercial biosensors: applications to clinical, bioprocess, and environmental samples*, Ramsay, G. (Ed.), pp. 267-294, John Wiley & Sons, Inc.

Ritchie, J. M.; Cresser, M. & Cotter-Howells, J. (2001). Toxicological response of a bioluminescent microbial assay to Zn, Pb and Cu in an artificial soil solution: relationship with total metal concentrations and free ion activities. *Environmental Pollution*, Vol. 114, pp. 129-136

Roach, P. C. J.; Ramsden, D. K.; Hughes, J. & Williams, P. (2003). Development of a conductimetric biosensor using immobilised *Rhodococcus ruber* whole cells for the detection and quantification of acrylonitrile. *Biosensors and Bioelectronics*, Vol. 19, pp. 73-78

Rodriguez-Mozaz, S.; de Alda, M. J. L. & Barceló, D. (2006). Biosensors as useful tools for environmental analysis and monitoring. *Anal. Bioanal. Chem.*, Vol. 386, No. 4, pp. 1025-1041, ISSN 1618-2642

Rupani, S. P.; Gu, M. B.; Konstantinov, K. B.; Dhurjati, P. S.; Van Dyk, T. K. & LaRossa, R. A. (1996). Characterization of the stress response of a bioluminescent biological sensor in batch and continuous cultures. *Biotechnol. Prog.*, Vol. 12, No. 3, pp. 387-392

Sak-Bosnar, M.; Grabaric, Z. & Grabaric, B. S. (2004a). Surfactant sensors in biotechnology. Part 1 - Electrochemical sensors. *Food Technol. Biotechnol.*, Vol. 42, No. 3, pp. 197-206

Sak-Bosnar, M.; Grabaric, Z. & Grabaric, B. S. (2004b). Surfactant sensors in biotechnology. Part 2 - Non-electrochemical sensors. *Food Technol. Biotechnol.*, Vol. 42, No. 3, pp. 207-212

Sakaguchi, T.; Kitagawa, K.; Ando, T.; Murakami, Y.; Morita, Y.; Yamamura, A.; Yokoyama, K. & Tamiya, E. (2003). A rapid BOD sensing system using luminescent recombinants of *Escherichia coli*. *Biosensors and Bioelectronics*, Vol. 19, No. 2, pp. 115-121

Sasaki, S.; Yokoyama, K.; Tamiya, E.; Karube, I.; Hayashi, C.; Arikawa, Y. & Numata, M. (1997). Sulfate sensor using *Thiobacillus ferrooxidans*. *Analytica Chimica Acta*, Vol. 347, pp. 275-280

Schmidt, A.; Standfuss-Gabisch, C. & Bilitewski, U. (1996). Microbial biosensor for free fatty acids using an oxygen electrode based on thick film technology. *Biosensors and Bioelectronics*, Vol. 11, No. 11, pp. 1139-1145

Schreiter, P. P.-Y.; Gillor, O.; Post, A.; Belkin, S.; Schmid, R. D. & Bachmann, T. T. (2001). Monitoring of phosphorus bioavailability in water by an immobilized luminescent cyanobacterial reporter strain. *Biosensors and Bioelectronics*, Vol. 16, No. 9-12, pp. 811-818

Schugerl, K. (2001). Progress in monitoring, modeling and control of bioprocesses during the last 20 years. *Journal of Biotechnology*, Vol. 85, pp. 149–173

Shleev, S.; Tkac, J.; Christenson, A.; Ruzgas, T.; Yaropolov, A. I.; Whittaker, J. W. & Gorton, L. (2005). Direct electron transfer between copper-containing proteins and electrodes. *Biosensors and Bioelectronics*, Vol. 20, No. 12, pp. 2517-2554

Simonian, A. L.; Rainina, E. I.; Lozinsky, V. I.; Badalian, I. E.; Khachatrian, G. E.; Tatikian, S.; Makhlis, T. A. & Varfolomeyev, S. D. (1992). A biosensor for *L*-proline determination by use of immobilized microbial cells. *Appl. Biochem. Biotechnol.*, Vol. 36, No. 3, pp. 199-210

Sinclair, G. M.; Paton, G. I.; Meharg, A. A. & Killham, K. (1999). *Lux*-biosensor assessment of pH effects on microbial sorption and toxicity of chlorophenols. *FEMS Microbiology Letters*, Vol. 174, No. 2, pp. 273-278

Slama, M.; Zaborosc, C.; Wienke, D. & Spener, F. (1996). Simultaneous mixture analysis using a dynamic microbial sensor combined with chemometrics. *Analytical Chemistry*, Vol. 68, No. 21, pp. 3845-3850

Sticher, P.; Jaspers, M. C.; Stemmler, K.; Harms, H.; Zehnder, A. J. & van der Meer, J. R. (1997). Development and characterization of a whole-cell bioluminescent sensor for bioavailable middle-chain alkanes in contaminated groundwater samples. *Appl. Environ. Microbiol.*, Vol. 63, No. 10, pp. 4053-4060

Suriyawattanakul, L.; Surareungchai, W.; Sritongkam, P.; Tanticharoen, M. & Kirtikara, K. (2002). The use of co-immobilization of *Trichosporon cutaneum* and *Bacillus licheniformis* for a BOD sensor. *Appl. Microbiol. Biotechnol.*, Vol. 59, No. 1, pp. 40-44

Suzuki, M.; Lee, S. F., K.; Arikawa, I.; Kubo, I.; Kanagawa, T.; Mikami, E. & Karube, I. (1992). Determination of sulfite ion by using microbial sensor. *Analytical Letters*, Vol. 25, No. 6, pp. 973-982

Svitel, J.; Curilla, O. & Tkac, J. (1998). Microbial cell-based biosensor for sensing glucose, sucrose or lactose. *Biotechnol. Appl. Biochem.*, Vol. 27, No. Pt 2, pp. 153-158

Svorc, J.; Miertus, S. & Barlikova, A. (1990). Hybrid biosensor for the determination of lactose. *Analytical Chemistry*, Vol. 62, No. 15, pp. 1628-1631

Takayama, K.; Kurosaki, T. & Ikeda, T. (1993). Mediated eletrocatalysis at a biocatalyst electrode based on a bacterium, *Gluconobacter industrius*. *J. Electroanal. Chem.*, Vol. 356, pp. 295-301

Takayama, K.; Kano, K. & Ikeda, T. (1996). Mediated electrocatalytic reduction of nitrate and nitrite based on the denitrifying activity of *Paracoccus denitrificans*. *Chemistry Letters*, Vol. 11, pp. 1009-1010

Tan, H. M.; Cheong, S. P. & Tan, T. C. (1994). An amperometric benzene sensor using whole sell *Pseudomonas putida* ML2. *Biosensors and Bioelectronics*, Vol. 9, pp. 1-8

Taranova, L.; Semenchuk, I.; Manolov, T.; Iliasov, P. & Reshetilov, A. (2002). Bacteria-degraders as the base of an amperometric biosensor for detection of anionic surfactants. *Biosensors and Bioelectronics*, Vol. 17, No. 8, pp. 635-640

Taranova, L. A.; Fesai, A. P.; Ivashchenko, G. V.; Reshetilov, A. N.; Winter-Nielsen, M. & Emneus, J. (2004). [*Comamonas testosteroni* strain TI as a potential base for a microbial sensor detecting surfactants]. *Prikl. Biokhim. Mikrobiol.*, Vol. 40, No. 4, pp. 472-477

Tauber, M.; Rosen, R. & Belkin, S. (2001). Whole-cell biodetection of halogenated organic acids. *Talanta*, Vol. 55, pp. 959-964

Thevenot, D. R.; Toth, K.; Durst, R. A. & Wilson, G. S. (2001). Electrochemical biosensors: recommended definitions and classification. *Biosensors and Bioelectronics*, Vol. 16, No. 1-2, pp. 121-131.

Thouand, G.; Horry, H.; Durand, M. J.; Picart, P.; Bendriaa, L.; Daniel, P. & DuBow, M. S. (2003). Development of a biosensor for on-line detection of tributyltin with a recombinant bioluminescent *Escherichia coli* strain. *Appl. Microbiol. Biotechnol.*, Vol. 62, No. 2-3, pp. 218-225

Timur, S.; Anik, U.; Odaci, D. & Gorton, L. (2007). Development of a microbial biosensor based on carbon nanotube (CNT) modified electrodes. *Electrochemistry Communications*, Vol. 9, pp. 1810–1815

Tkac, J.; Gemeiner, P.; Svitel, J.; Benikovsky, T.; Sturdik, E.; Vala, V.; Petrus, L. & Hrabarova, E. (2000). Determination of total sugars in lignocellulose hydrolysate by a mediated *Gluconobacter oxydans* biosensor. *Analytica Chimica Acta*, Vol. 420, pp. 1-7

Tkac, J.; Vostiar, I.; Gemeiner, P. & Sturdik, E. (2002). Monitoring of ethanol during fermentation using a microbial biosensor with enhanced selectivity. *Bioelectrochemistry*, Vol. 56, No. 1-2, pp. 127-129

Tkac, J.; Vostiar, I.; Gorton, L.; Gemeiner, P. & Sturdik, E. (2003). Improved selectivity of microbial biosensor using membrane coating. Application to the analysis of ethanol during fermentation. *Biosensors and Bioelectronics*, Vol. 18, No. 9, pp. 1125-1134

Tkac, J.; Whittaker, J. W. & Ruzgas, T. (2007). The use of single walled carbon nanotubes dispersed in a chitosan matrix for preparation of a galactose biosensor. *Biosensors and Bioelectronics*, Vol. 22, No. 8, pp. 1820-1824, ISSN 0956-5663

Trosok, S. P.; Driscoll, B. T. & Luong, J. H. (2001). Mediated microbial biosensor using a novel yeast strain for wastewater BOD measurement. *Appl. Microbiol. Biotechnol.*, Vol. 56, No. 3-4, pp. 550-554.

Turner, A. P. F.; Karube, I. & Wilson, G. S. (Eds.) (1987). *Biosensors: fundamentals and applications*, Oxford University Press, New York

Turner, A. P. F. (1996) *Biosensors: Past, Present and Future*, http://www.cranfield.ac.uk/health/researchareas/biosensorsdiagnostics/page18795.jsp

Vais, H.; Ardelean, I. & Margineanu, D. G. (1989). Bioelectrical conversion in sensors with living cells. *Physiologie*, Vol. 26, No. 4, pp. 349-353

Vedrine, C.; Leclerc, J. C.; Durrieu, C. & Tran-Minh, C. (2003). Optical whole-cell biosensor using *Chlorella vulgaris* designed for monitoring herbicides. *Biosensors and Bioelectronics*, Vol. 18, No. 4, pp. 457-463

Vlasova, II; Asrieli, T. V.; Gavrilova, E. M. & Danilov, V. S. (2004). New approach for specific determination of antibiotics by use of luminescent *Escherichia coli* and immune serum. *Appl. Environ. Microbiol.*, Vol. 70, No. 2, pp. 1245-1248

Voronova, E.; Iliasov, P. & Reshetilov, A. (2008). Development, investigation of parameters and estimation of possibility of adaptation of Pichia angusta based microbial sensor for ethanol detection. *Analytical Letters*, Vol. 41, № 3, pp. 377-391

Vostiar, I.; Ferapontova, E. & Gorton, L. (2004). Electrical "wiring" of viable *Gluconobacter oxydans* cells with a flexible osmium-redox polyelectrolyte. *Electrochemistry Communications*, Vol. 6, pp. 621–626

Werlen, C.; Jaspers, M. C. & Van Der Meer, J. R. (2004). Measurement of biologically available naphthalene in gas and aqueous phases by use of a *Pseudomonas putida* biosensor. *Appl. Environ. Microbiol.*, Vol. 70, No. 1, pp. 43-51

Willardson, B. M.; Wilkins, J. F.; Rand, T. A.; Schupp, J. M.; Hill, K. K.; Keim, P. & Jackson, P. J. (1998). Development and testing of a bacterial biosensor for toluene-based environmental contaminants. *Appl. Environ. Microbiol.*, Vol. 64, No. 3, pp. 1006-1012

Wollenberger, U.; Scheller, F. & Atrat, P. (1980). Microbial membrane electrode for steroid assay. *Analytical Letters*, Vol. 13, pp. 1201-1210

Yang, Z.; Suzuki, H.; Sasaki, S. & Karube, I. (1996). Disposable sensor for biochemical oxygen demand. *Appl. Microbiol. Biotechnol.*, Vol. 46, No. 1, pp. 10-14

Yang, Z.; Sasaki, S.; Karube, I. & Suzuki, H. (1997). Fabrication of oxygen electrode arrays and their incorporation into sensors for measuring biochemical oxygen demand. *Analytica Chimica Acta*, Vol. 357, pp. 41-49

Yuqing, M.; Jianguo, G. & Jianrong, C. (2003). Ion sensitive field effect transducer-based biosensors. *Biotechnology Advances*, Vol. 21, pp. 527-534

Zhao, Y. B.; Wen, M. L.; Liu, S. Q.; Liu, Z. H.; Zhang, W. D.; Yao, Y. & Wang, C. Y. (1998). Microbial sensor for determination of tannic acid. *Microchemical Journal*, Vol. 60, pp. 201-209

Ziegler, C. (2000). Cell-based biosensors. *Fresenius J. Analytical Chemistry*, Vol. 366, No. 6-7, pp. 552-559

16

A Novel Type of Nucleic Acid-based Biosensors: the Use of PNA Probes, Associated with Surface Science and Electrochemical Detection Techniques

Eva Mateo-Martí[1] and Claire-Marie Pradier[2]
[1]*Centro de Astrobiología (CSIC-INTA) Ctra.Torrejón-Ajalvir Km.4, 28850 -Torrejón de Torrejón de Ardoz-Madrid, Spain*
[2]*Laboratoire de Réactivité de Surface, UMR CNRS 7197, Université Pierre et Marie Curie, 4, Pl Jussieu, 75005-Paris, France*

1. Introduction

DNA biosensors are now recognized as unvaluable tools for detecting target genes responsible for diseases, or pollution, in various fields (Fodor et al., 1991; DeRisi et al., 1997; Landegren et al., 1998). Therefore, detection of DNA hybridisation is of significant scientific and technological importance, as manifest, for example, from the growing interest in chip-based characterisation of gene expression pattern and detection of pathogens. DNA biosensors technologies are currently under intense investigation owing to their great promise for rapid and low-cost detection of specific DNA sequences. These technologies commonly rely on the immobilisation of a single-strand (ss) DNA probe onto optical, electrochemical, or mass-sensitive transducers (Xu et al., 1995; Mikkelsen et al., 1996; Okahata et al., 1992). There is still a crucial need to improve the sensitivity, selectivity and rapidity of the DNA hybridisation detection. Among the possible strategies, a new artificial Peptide Nucleic Acid (PNA), a highly specific probe, combined with the use of surface science techniques to optimise the sensing layer as well as to detect biomolecular recognition, open promising ways to win this biotechnological challenge. This chapter will focus on these two novel aspects of DNA biosensors.

1.1 PNA versus DNA comparison

Peptide Nucleic Acid was first described by Nielsen's group in 1991 (Nielsen et al., 1991). Knowledge of the PNA structure is essential for understanding its remarkable hybridisation behaviour and DNA recognition capacity (Figure 1).
PNA is an analog of DNA in which the entire negatively-charge sugar-phosphate backbone is replaced with a neutral « peptide like » backbone consisting on repeated N-(2-aminoethyl) glycine units linked by amide bonds (Figure 1). The four natural nucleobases (i.e., adenine, cytosine, guanine, and thymine) come off the backbone at equal spacing to the DNA bases.

Methylene carbonyl linkages connect the bases to the central amine of the backbone. Thus, PNA contains the same number of backbone bonds between bases and the same number of bonds between the backbone and the bases, as DNA. Such a structure offers a high biological stability, as it is not prone to degradation by nucleases or proteases (Demidov et al., 1994).
Owing to its neutral backbone and proper interbase spacing, PNA binds to its complementary nucleic acid sequence with higher affinity and specificity compared to traditional oligonucleotides. It was shown (Egholm et al., 1993) that PNA hybridisation to complementary oligonucleotides obeys the Watson-Crick base-pairing rules with the PNA and DNA strands joined via hydrogen bonds (see Figure 1). The neutral backbone also implies a lack of electrostatic repulsion between the PNA and DNA strands (compared to that existing between two negatively-charge DNA oligomers), and hence a higher thermal stability of PNA/DNA duplexes. It was also demostrated that the thermal stability of the resulting PNA/DNA duplex is essentially independent of the salt concentration in the hybridisation solution (Orum et al., 1995; Wang, 1998).
(ss)PNA oligomers exhibit superior hybridisation properties, as well as improved chemical and enzymatic stability, compared to natural nucleic acids. For many applications, the synthetic DNA mimic, PNA, could be advantageously used as a probe molecule, owing to its unique physicochemical and biochemical properties. The unique structure and the resultant hybridisation properties of PNA, open up many important biological and diagnostic applications, not achievable with traditional oligonucleotides. In addition, the different molecular structures of DNA and PNA (see Figure 1), offer a large set of chemical signatures to be detected after hybridisation, thus allowing the use of label-free techniques of detection. The chapter will explain why and how these unique properties of PNA may be applied to DNA specific recognition.

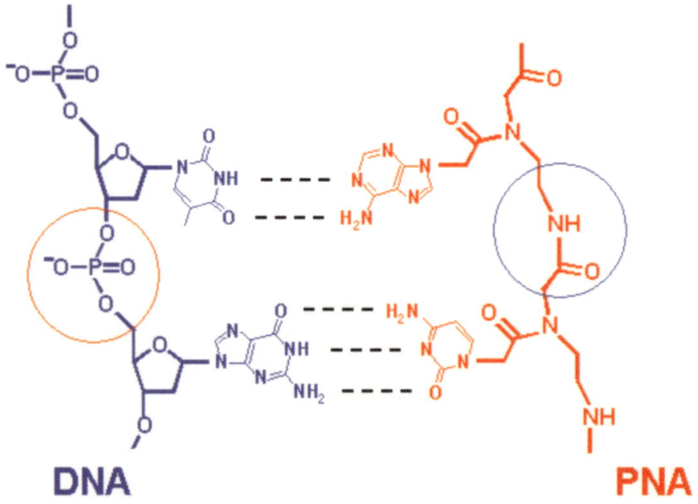

Fig. 1. Schematic chemical model of PNA and DNA molecules, showing the different backbone linkages, (Mateo-Marti et al., 2007).

When searching to optimise biosensors, it is crucial to characterise all steps of their elaboration, as well as to detect, and possibly quantify, with the highest possible sensitivity and specificity, the reaction of molecular recognition onto the receptor. Of course, we are talking about a characterisation at a molecular level, some properties being determining for the biosensor parameters: the surface coverage, the orientation/conformation of the adsorbed molecules, their spatial arrangement and, possibly, their charge. Since this chapter is focused on PNA-DNA systems, most of the time involving rather short oligonucleotides, surface science techniques are particularly well suited, though still rather seldom used in this domain.

1.2 Novel detection techniques for PNA-DNA-based biosensors

The unique properties of ssPNA and its physico-chemical differences with respect to DNA, encourage the use of surface characterisation techniques for the detection of label-free nucleic acid targets in biological samples. Under the term "surface" techniques, we will include electrochemical, gravimetric techniques, Quartz Crystal Microbalance (QCM), as well as specifically surface science characterisation techniques like X-ray Photoelectron Spectroscopy (XPS), Reflection Absorption Infrared Spectroscopy (RAIRS), Surface Plasmon Resonance (SPR), Surface Enhanced Raman Scattering (SERS) and Time-of-Flight Ion Mass Spectrometry (ToF SIMS); for the first time, these techniques, rather original when applied to PNA-DNA detection, will be gathered and compared in one chapter.

Electrochemical detection of DNA binding to DNA or PNA has been widely described in the literature (Liu et al., 2005; Steichen et al., 2007; Fang et al., 2008) Cyclic Voltametry (CV), or more sophisticated, Differential Pulse Voltametry (DPV), Electrochemical Impedance Spectroscopy (EIS), conductivity changes may be used as sensitive transduction techniques. The principles of these electrochemical techniques will be recalled; the advantage of using redox markers or electroactive labels will be considered. Often associated with impedance measurements, QCM, but also SPR, based on the detection of refraction index variations, have been successfully used to identify DNA hybridisation in real time.

Less commonly used for PNA-DNA hybridisation detection, though very sensitive, are the specifically surface science techniques, like XPS and RAIRS. XPS, though not applicable to instant, on line detection, has been applied to the characterisation of PNA, and then PNA + DNA layers, thus bringing valuable chemical information about the density/integrity of these molecular layers at these two steps (Mateo-Marti et al, 2005; Mateo-Marti et al, 2007). Surface infrared, RAIRS, whose sensitivity is enhanced on planar surfaces, is a new, very easy to handle, chemical detection technique.

Major drawbacks of current well-standardized molecular biology techniques are their time requirements for sample processing and amplification, risk of false positives from sample or reagent contamination, heavy instrumentation, laboratory costs and need for labeling of the analytes (Gau 2005). To overcome these drawbacks, a lot of research work is focussed on the development of label-free DNA biosensors, which allow the direct detection, and specific identification of point mutations in genes. Detection methods that avoid labeling of the target molecule to be hybridised usually guarantee a higher accuracy of the measurements (Buetow et al., 2001; Briones et al., 2005).

The PNA biosensor technology holds promises for rapid and cost-effective detection of specific DNA sequences. A single-strand nucleic acid probe is immobilised onto optical, electrochemical, or mass-sensitive transducers to detect the complementary (or mismatch) strand in a sample solution. The response from the hybridisation event is converted into a measurable signal by the transducer. We describe here the use of PNA as a novel probe for

sequence-specific biosensors and highlight some of the advantages of using it as a recognition probe.
This chapter presents a review of recent studies, focussed on PNA-DNA hybridisation detection by using "chemical", or purely "surface science" techniques; the latter provide alternatives for optimizing nucleic acid-based sensors and expanding the range of detection methods available; the conditions of their use for this specific application as well as a comparison of their respective performances will be attempted and, moreover some indications helping to choose the best technique for the best detection, depending on the scientific case, will be suggested, based on the most recent literature survey.

2.Techniques and results

2.1 Surface spectroscopies

2.1.1 X-Ray Photoemission Spectroscopy (XPS)

XPS is one of the most universal techniques used for analysing surfaces from a chemical point of view. The bases of the technique ly in Einstein's discovery of the photoelectric effect, whereby photons can induce electrons emission from a solid provided that the photon energy (hv) is greater than the work function (the work function of a solid is defined as the minimum energy required to remove an electron from the highest occupied energy level in the solid to the vacuum level). The vacuum level may be used as an "energy zero". Surface analysis by XPS is accomplished by irradiating a sample with monoenergetic soft x-rays and analysing the energy of the detected electrons. These photons have a limited penetrating power in a solid of the order of 1-10 micrometers (Moulder, 1992) and, overall, the electron have a free path in solids of the order of 5-10 nm which makes XPS a true surface sensitive technique. They interact with atoms in the surface region, causing electrons to be emitted by the photoelectric effect. The emitted electrons have measured kinetic energies (KE) given by:

$$KE = hv - BE - Qs$$

Where hv is the energy of the photon, BE is the binding energy of the atomic orbital from which the electron originates, and Qs is the spectrometer work function.
The binding energy may be regarded as the energy difference between the initial and final states after the photoelectron has left the atom. Hence it is clear that for a fixed photon energy, photoemission from an atom which well-defined core levels (of particular binding energy) will produce photoelectrons with well-defined kinetic energies varying systematically from one element to another (Attard & Barnes, 1998). Because each element has a unique set of binding energies, XPS can be used to identify and determine the concentration of the elements in the surface layers. Variations in the elemental binding energies (the chemical shift) arise from differences in the chemical potential and polarisability of compounds. These chemical shifts can be used to identify the chemical state of the materials being analysed. XPS is also a probe of the chemical environment or oxidation state of surfaces species. The detection limit for surface impurities in XPS can, in favourable circumstances, be less than 1% of a monolayer.
Structural-chemical differences between PNA and DNA molecule, encourage the use of XPS surface to detect and quantify the hybridisation.
In the following example, ssPNA molecules on gold surfaces, were adsorbed from water, forming a layer stable in the air, and showing efficient and specific ssDNA recognition capability. The quality of the sensing PNA layer, and then, the biological activity of the

SAMs of ssPNA and their interaction with complementary ssDNA have indeed been investigated by XPS. Immobilisation of ssPNA (1μM) on polycrystalline Au layers was performed at 22ºC for 3.5 h in a humid chamber. After immobilisation, the gold samples were rinsed in H_2O at 22ºC; at this optimal concentration, 1μM, PNA molecules realign their molecular axes with the surface normal and form SAMs without the need of co-immobilisation of spacers or other adjuvant molecules molecules (Mateo-Marti et al., 2005). PNA hybridisation with 100μM ssDNA, 2005). Hybridisation with 100μM ssDNA target solution was carried at 54ºC for 1 h, in a buffer pH 7.2. Post-hybridisation washing was performed. Finally, blowing helium gas dried the gold samples.

XPS was also performed to estimate the dynamic range of the recognition process of ssPNA by ssDNA. For PNA concentrations ranging from 0.1 to 1 μM, an average increase of the normalized N1s peak ranging from 2.6 to 3.2 times after hybridisation was observed. The number of N atoms per ssPNA molecule is 64, versus 116 in the complementary DNA. An enhancement of the N signal by a factor of 2.8 may thus be expected from an approximate atom-counting model. A good agreement between the expected and obtained values suggests that, under optimal conditions, the fraction of ssPNA hybridised with DNA target is near 100%. This value is higher than that reported for DNA-DNA hybridisation measured with the same technique (Casero *et al.* 2003, D.Y. Petrovykh *et al.*, 2003). For PNA concentrations higher than approximately 5μM, the surface is completely covered by ssPNA and the photoemission signal does not change after hybridisation, indicating that the bioSAM is not behaving as an active biosensor. It can be concluded that bioSAMs of ssPNA offer optimal biosensor capacity when immobilised at concentrations of up to 1μM, thus forming non dense sensing layers.

The P signal, related to the phosphate groups in the DNA backbone but absent in PNA, together with an increase in the N signal detected after hybridisation, are the fingerprints of the hybridisation of complementary ssDNA to bioSAMs of ssPNA, in the XPS detection (Briones et al., 2004; Mateo-Marti et al., 2007). Moreover, the N(1s) core level peak was analysed at high resolution to search for a chemical shift due to the PNA-DNA hybridisation process. A spectral shift of 0.4 eV to higher binding energies, was indeed observed. The shift of the N (1s) peak to higher energy values has been ascribed to the hydrogen bonds, occurring in the hybridisation process, thus also constituting a fingerprint of the DNA to PNA binding .

Silicon, that represents a remarkable compromise between stability, biocompatibility, and maturity of the semiconductor processing technology, was also used for nucleic acid biosensors, combined with XPS characterisation. Cattani-Scholz et al. reported a stepwise functionalization of SiO_2-terminated Si surface by phosphonate and siloxane films modified with polyethylene glycol (PEG) and PNA as selective probes for DNA. Hybridisation has been characterised by XPS among others techniques; the biofunctional interfaces exhibit good resistance against non specific interactions, having potential applications for PNA/DNA microdevices. (Cattani-Scholz et al., 2008; Cattani-Scholz et al., 2009).

2.1.2 Reflection Absorption Infrared Spectroscopy (RAIRS)

Infrared spectroscopy may also be employed to identify the chemical nature and conformation of molecules adsorbed on surfaces. The fact that infrared spectroscopy provides specific information on the types of bonds present in a molecule, is nondestructive, and does not require Ultra High Vacuum has made it a highly versatile technique for surface analysis. Moreover, the majority of vibrations of functional groups within adsorbed molecules generally occur above 800 cm^{-1}. To characterise adsorption and reaction phenomena occurring at the surface of a metal or of a semi-conductor, transmission experiments are not relevant; they can be advantageously replaced by applying IR spectroscopy in the reflection mode, where the sample is acting as a mirror, reflecting the beam (Attard & Barnes, 1998). RAIRS uses infrared light to excite the internal vibrations of the adsorbed molecules. The frequency of these vibrations can reveal the chemical groups in the adsorbate, the adsorption geometry and the adsorption site occupied by the surface molecule.

Classically, the general infrared selection rule states that ***for a vibration to be infrared active, the electric dipole moment of the molecule must change during the vibration.*** While for a molecule adsorbed on a metal surface, the interaction of the infrared radiation with the adsorbate dipole is influenced by the dielectric behaviour of the metal. This gives rise to the following selection rule for RAIRS:

'ONLY VIBRATIONAL MODES WITH A DIPOLE MOMENT CHANGE NORMAL TO THE SURFACE WILL BE OBSERVED'

An infrared spectroscopy experiment consists in measuring the differences between the light intensity of the incident and transmitted beams of radiation in a particular frequency region; for RAIRS the difference between light reflected on a clean and modified surfaces will be measured. Because of the extremely highly inherent resolution of RAIRS (less than 4 cm^{-1}) inspection of the spectra for simple molecules yields unique information about the chemical state and interactions, H-binding or charge transfer for example.

The different molecular structures of DNA and PNA offer a wide range of chemical signatures to be detected only after hybridisation, thus allowing the use of RAIRS as detection technique. Figure 2 shows, a comparison between PNA and PNA-DNA infrared spectra on gold surfaces, some features are enhanced, and also, the characteristic bands of DNA molecular groups, appear. These findings indicate the possibility to detect a hybridisation process by IR (Mateo-Marti et al., 2007).

The various chemical functional groups present in each molecule, PNA and DNA have been identified and associated to specific infrared features. Vibrational modes associated with nucleobases (heterocyclic) and vibrational features associated with the backbone (CH_2 alkane group, -O-ether functionality, NH-CO amide group). Regarding the nucleic bases, the main features should appear in the following regions (Mantsch, 1996): the in-plane (ip) double bond vibrations of the bases are located at 1780-1500 cm^{-1}, base-deformation motions appear at 1500-1250 cm^{-1}, and out-of-plane (oop) base vibrations at frequencies lower than 1000 cm^{-1} (see Figure 2).

Two features are specific fingerprints of the DNA, as no phosphate groups are present in the PNA molecule. The appearance of two strong absorption bands, assigned to the phosphate vibrations (antisymmetric PO_2^- stretching vibration at 1237 cm^{-1} and symmetric stretching vibrations at 1081 cm^{-1}) can be clearly identified on the spectrum (see Figure 2). They are reliable proofs of the PNA-DNA hybridisation process; phosphates, and their respective infrared signals, should only be present when a nucleic acid has bound to the complementary PNA molecule.

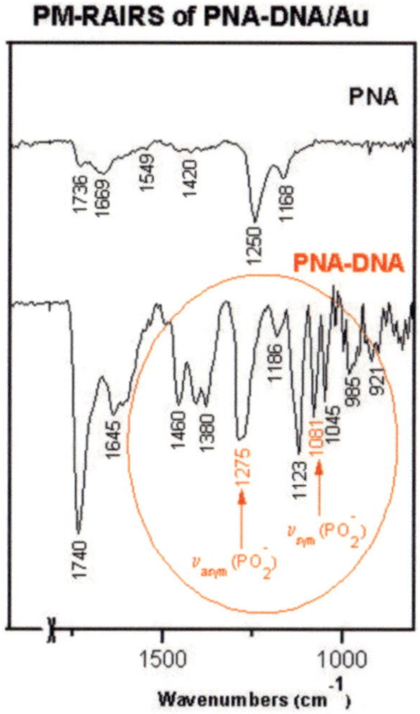

Fig. 2. A comparison PM-RAIRS spectra of PNA and PNA-DNA after hybridisation process (Mateo-Marti et al., 2007).

2.1.3 Surface Enhanced Raman Scattering (SERS)

Surface Enhanced Raman Scattering (SERS) is a particularly sensitive surface analytical technique, taking advantage of the increased local field on nanostructured surfaces; the ideal substrates are typically Au or Ag. Researches using SERS on nanostructured surfaces and/or nanoparticles have given rise to spectacular results, in term of sensitive detection, applied for instance to biosensors; examples of DNA hybridisation are not common due to the difficulty to immobilise these probes on nanostructures in a controlled way.

Detection of DNA by SERS may also take advantage of the electrostatic interactions generated when the oligonucleotides interacts with PNA; this enables the binding of positively charged nanoparticles bearing a SERS reporter molecule for instance. In Fabris et al. study (Fabris et al., 2007), DNA was hybridised to PNA immobilised on slides, leaving a negatively-charged surface; immersion in a solution of positively-charged Ag Nanoparticles (NPs), and then in a solution of rhodamine SERS reporters, leads to intense SERS signal, attributed to the specific PNA-DNA interaction. Note that addition of non-complementary ssDNA, at the initial step, leaves the PNA layer unmodified, thus not binding nanoparticles; a resulting none or quasi no SERS signal has been observed (see Fig. 3).

Another way to detect DNA hybridisation by SERS was recently described by Fang et al. It consisted in using ordered arrays of silicium nanostructures, coated with gold or silver as SERS substrates; the latter were functionnalised with PNA and submitted to target DNA. Thanks to the affinity of the DNA phosphate groups towards Zr^{4+} cations, these oligonucleotides, immersed in zirconide chloride, were bearing Zr cations and this only on PNA-duplex; after incubation in Rhodamine B that reacts with Zr cations, the hybridisation

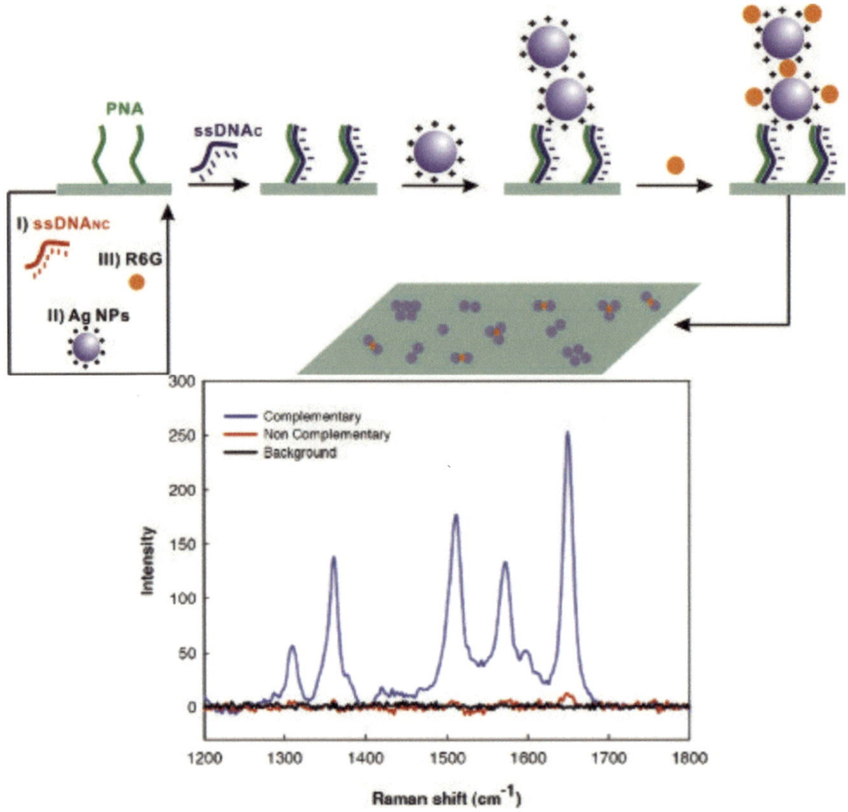

Fig. 3. General scheme of the assay, PNA in green and complementary DNA in blue. SERS signals from PNA slides hybridised with ssDNAc (blue) or ssDNAnc (red) (Fabris et al., 2007).

could be detected by SERS (Fang et al., 2008a), with a detection limit of $1x10^{-12}$ M. Of course, the sensitivity increases with the oligonucleotide length due to the higher amount of phosphate groups. Note that all Raman measurements were obtained in the air, after sample rinsing; this appears not to perturbate the data. The selectivity of this assay was checked by testing a single base mismatched DNA; no signals were observed in that case.

This method, enabling sensitive SERS detection, is applicable to other biological recognition systems, but our purpose is to show here the interest of using neutral PNA as the specific probe for DNA; commercial PNA-slides now even exist (Ujihara et al., 2005).

2.1.4 Time-of-Flight Ion Mass Spectrometry (ToF SIMS)

Worth mentioning are some recent studies, using ToF SIMS, an ultra sensitive surface analysis technique to detect unlabeled DNA targets on PNA microarrays (Arlinghaus & Kwoka, 1997; Brandt et al., 2003). The experiment consists in bombarding the sample with an ion beam that induces molecular fragments and/or ions from the topmost surface layer to desorb. They are then detected by a ToF mass spectrometer. In Arlinghaus et al. work, ToF-SIMS was used to monitor the amount of immobilised PNA on platinum-coated silicon chips, and thus check the sample reproducibility. These chips were then hybridised and analysed for phosphorous signal; a peak was observed in the case of complementary nucleotides and no peaks at the non complementary spot, demonstrating the successful selective hybridisation. The method takes advantage of its great sensitivity to PO_2^- and PO_3^- fragments of the phosphate ions present on DNA (and not on PNA).

2.2 Optical and gravimetric techniques
2.2.1 Surface Plasmon Resonance (SPR)
Surface Plasmon Resonance (SPR) is a surface analysis technique that measures changes in the refractive index that occur upon adsorption on a gold film.

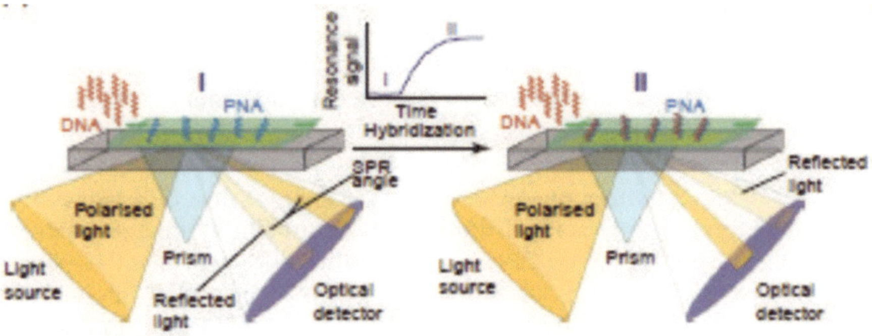

Fig. 4. Principle of Surface Plasmon Resonance Spectroscopy, a label-free detection technique (Brandt & Hoheisel, 2004).

The first commercial instrument was launched in 1990 by Biacore to assay molecular recognition on a planar surface; since that date the sensitivity and handling have been improved and adapted to specific cases making the technique very powerful in a wide range of applications, food or environmental monitoring, detection in medicine for example (Homola, 2003; Karlsson, 2004).

DNA hybridisation to PNA probes, immobilised on a planar gold surface, may be measured by using Surface Plasmon Resonance (SPR). In the latter case, DNA binding to PNA induces a change in the refractive index, proportional to the mass uptake on the chip surface and enabling a real-time monitoring of the hybridisation process (Jensen et al., 1997). A small review of some PNA-based biosensors has been recently published, presenting some examples of biosensors using labels or not, and showing the interest of using these DNA mimics (Brandt & Hoheisel, 2004; Corradini et al., 2004); they report in particular that PNA monomers may be modified by adding a chiral center to enhance their mismatch recognition sensitivity by SPR (Corradini et al., 2004); also, instead of using the direct grafted PNA format, PCR products may be attached to the SPR sensor surface, followed by PNA oligomer hybridisation leading to highly efficient PNA hybridisation; this has been attributed to the better accessibility of PNA probes to the immobilised PCR, compared to that of DNA oligonucleotides (Feriotto et al., 2001).

However, the SPR detection sensitivity often needs to be enhanced by incorporating labels or using a second hybridisation (sandwich format). Using Au Nanoparticles labels, Yao et al. report a very high sensitivity of the SPR technique in DNA hybridisation, down to the femtomolar level (Yao et al., 2006). Another example is reported by Su et al. who describe a method relying on the use of charge neutral peptide nucleic acids as capture probes and polymer-modified DNA as targets: protonated aniline monomers, that do not adsorb on neutral PNA (Fan et al., 2007a), are first adsorbed to the DNA molecules; polymerisation into polyalinine then occurs and, enhanced refractive index changes are observed when this DNA-polyalinine hybridises to PNA (Su et al., 2008); the lowest concentration of DNA, detectable in this way by SPR, was 0.1 pM which is close to that attained by fluorescent methods (Will et al., 1999).

More recently, a Localised Surface Plasmon Resonance (LSPR)-based label-free biosensor utilising gold-capped nanoparticles, modified with DNA probes, was developed. The optical properties of gold nanoparticles, measured from the absorbance strength, are modified upon DNA hybridisation. The LSPR-based biosensor was made of a gold-coated glass substrate on which 100 nm silica nanoparticles were deposited and then capped with gold leading to a full and homogeneous layer of nanoparticles; the SPR absorbance, at ca 537 nm, increased upon increasing the adsorbed molecular layer, e.g. upon DNA binding to PNA probes; this system permitted to reach a limit of detection equal to 0.7 pM target DNA, with a good sequence selectivity (Endo et al., 2005).

Interestingly, the kinetics and affinity constants of the DNA-DNA and PNA-DNA pairings were compared, using chromophore-labeled oligonucleotides and SPR detection; the two systems, where the probes were surface-attached via biotin-avidin linkages, showed similar affinity constants, 2 to 3 x 10^7 M^{-1}, but PNA-DNA binding showed some deviation from the classical Langmuir DNA-DNA model; this was interpreted by a first binding of DNA to uncharged PNA followed by a rearrangement on the surface; this simply underlines, that by using an uncharged oligonucleotide, important changes in the structure/conformation of the duplex may occur and change the kinetics of the hybridisation reaction (Kambhampati et al., 2001).

Surface Plasmon Fluorescence Spectroscopy (SPFS) is another derivative of SPR, which we will not detail in this chapter; let's just mention that this technique was applied to detect PNA-DNA hybridisation and characterise the kinetic parameters of this system. The authors confirm possible structural changes of PNA-DNA duplexes after hybridisation, strongly influenced by the ionic strength of the solution (Liu et al., 2006).

2.2.2 Quartz Crystal Microbalance (QCM)

Quartz Crystal Microbalance (QCM) technique measures, in real time, changes in mass of the surface of a resonating quartz, by monitoring its resonance frequency; it gives information similar to that obtained by SPR, but also, it provides precious data about the kinetics of interaction and about the structure of the adsorbed layer by measuring dissipation energy. Obtaining these complementary sets of information is unique and permits valuable discussions about correlating the reactivity/sensitivity of a sensor to the immobilisation method for example (Höök et al., 1998).

F. Höök et al. developed a QCM-based PNA-DNA sensor, showing the interest of measuring the frequency and dissipation changes simultaneously for studying various ways of immobilising PNA probes (Höök et al., 2001). The authors immobilised PNA probes in two different ways, either directly to the gold quartz via a thiol function, or on an intermediate biotin-avidin layer. Interestingly, responses observed upon DNA hybridisation were different: thiol-PNA forms a rigid structure with essentially no affinity toward complementary DNA, while biotin-PNA, bound to a 2D arrangement of streptavidin, forms a flexible layer with a high affinity to complementary DNA. Note that a single mismatched DNA was also recognised, but to a lesser extent and overall, its binding was reversible conversely to that of the fully complementary oligonucleotide. Eventually, the authors compared the PNA-DNA and DNA-DNA layers, by measuring the changes in frequency and dissipation when binding DNA; it appears that biotin-DNA forms a more expanded layer than biotin-PNA, with very little dissipation change upon DNA hybridisation (see the ΔD = f(Δf) curve, fig. 5); biotin-PNA forms a flexible but less expanded layer, with higher dissipation change upon DNA hybridisation; this difference is obviously related to the interactions between charged or uncharged oligonucleotides.

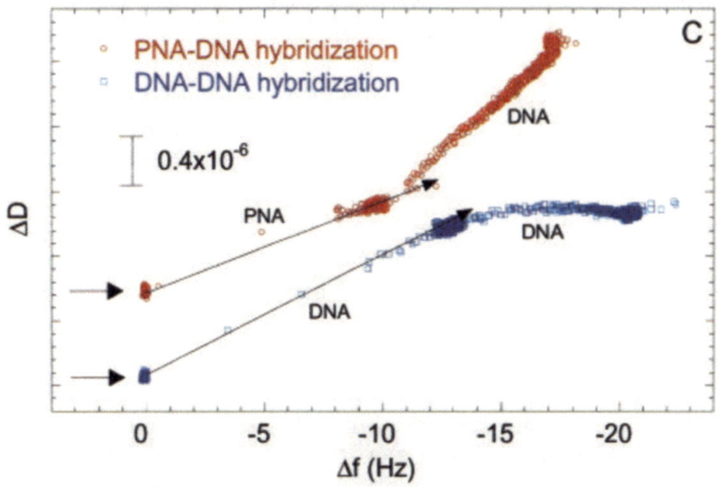

Fig. 5. ΔD versus Δf curves for biotin-DNA and biotin-DNA binding to streptavidin, followed by DNA hybridisation, from (Höök et al., 2001).

The high sensitivity of Quartz Crystal Microbalance was demonstrated by Wang et al. who measured the hybridisation of single-base altered DNA strands, even in the presence of a large excess of single-base mismatch oligonucleotides (Wang et al., 1997a). They estimated the detection limit, in the case of a 15 mer-long probe, around 1 μg/ml.

In a more recent study, QCM measurements were combined to SPR analyses in order to circumvent the problem raised by changes in the refractive index when denaturants, or potential changes, are applied to facilitate single mismatch detection (Lao et al., 2009). When 22-mer probes are involved, hybridisation to both PNA and DNA probes occurs but PNA probes show a higher efficiency for single mismatch discrimination. The authors demonstrate that PNA probes are more stable and efficient in mismatch identification, even when dehybridisation is assisted by potential changes.

Another type of chemistry was applied to immobilise single-stranded DNA molecules at the air-water interface, using cationic Langmuir monolayers (Ramakrishnan et al., 2002; Sastry et al., 2000). Interestingly, the hybridisation of complementary PNA molecules was achieved at this interface, leading to very stable DNA-PNA hybrid monolayers. The PNA-DNA hybridisation was measured by QCM; again, in the case of a single mismatch DNA sequence, no hybridisation with PNA was observed. Note that the stability of these hybrid complexes was investigated by measuring the absorbance as a function of temperature, showing an enhanced stability on the cationic layer; this has been ascribed to the screening of the DNA charges by the monolayer, thus stabilising the duplex. This approach demonstrated first that DNA or PNA may be immobilised and hybridised successfully at an air-water interface and second, the importance of the attachment layer; in the presented case, the cationic monolayers screened the electrostatic interactions and leaves the bases of the DNA molecules well oriented and accessible thus favouring hydrogen bonding of the complementary PNA; this had never been observed in solution.

PNA-DNA interactions have been used to direct the assembly of nanoparticles into macroscopic arrangements. The quantification of the hybridisation efficiency was ensured by fluorescence (Chakrabarti & Klibanov, 2003).

In a very recent study, hybridisation of hepatitis B virus by PNA was detected by QCM with a detection limit of 8.6 pg/L (Yao et al., 2008). This work relied on the immobilisation of PNA probes on a gold quartz using Carruso et al. method, grafting of a thiol on which avidin was chemically bound and then the biotinylated PNA probe (Carruso et al., 1997). Hybridisation with complementary and mismatch sequences was then measured by monitoring the quartz frequency, showing a remarkable mismatch discrimination. The authors underline the paramount importance of the probe immobilisation procedure to ensure low non-specific interaction and high reproducibility. Eventually, the detection sensitivity was improved by coating complementary ssDNA probes with RecA protein, before hybridisation to PNA in the QCM cell.

2.3 Electrochemistry

Electrochemical concepts have also proven to be very useful for sequence-specific biosensing of DNA, because they provide simple, rapid, lable-free and low-cost detection of nucleic acid sequences [Wang et al., 2000; F. Patolsky et al., 1999]. The binding of the surface-confined probe and its complementary target strand is translated into a useful electrical signal. Among the electrochemical methods, the most used is based on redox labels, which generate a signal change upon hybridisation. Of course, the main drawback of these techniques is the need for this redox label to be added in solution, or grafted on DNA strands. To solve this problem, the redox indicator can be covalently grafted onto the electrode. Following this scheme, electrochemical methods like Cyclic Voltametry (CV), Differential Pulse Voltametry (DPV) or Electrochemical Impedance Spectroscopy (EIS) have been successfully used (Reisberg et al., 2008 and ref. in).

Among the electrochemical sensors, we will report on those, which involve PNA immobilised on the electrode surface as a probe for the recognition of the target DNA. The electrical neutrality of the PNA backbone, the adsorption of PNA onto charged carbon or mercury electrodes differs greatly from that of DNA in terms of potential dependence, and surface packing. Therefore, the strong adsorption of PNA, combined with the electroactivity of the nucleobases, can be exploited for developing highly sensitive and selective sensors for measuring trace levels of DNA (Wang et al., 1996).

2.3.1 Potentiometry

The signal measured is the potential difference (voltage) between the working and the reference electrodes. The working electrode's potential depends on the concentration of the analyte in the gas or solution phase. The reference electrode is needed to provide a defined reference potential.

Direct methods rely on the intrinsic electrochemical properties of DNA (the oxidation of purine bases, particularly guanine), or in changes in some of the interfacial properties after hybridisation. The first report in which guanine oxidation chemistry was used for target detection was described by Wang et al., who showed how the chronopotentiometric signal of guanine decreased after incubation of an oligo d[G] modified electrode with a guanine-free target (Wang et al., 1997b). Wang et al. have reported the use of PNA as a recognition probe for the electrochemical detection of the hybridisation event using chronopotentiometric measurements. The method consists of four steps: probe (PNA) immobilisation onto the transducer surface, hybridisation, indicator binding ($Co(phen)_3^{3+}$), and chronopotentiometric transduction (Wang et al., 1996).

A carbon-pasted electrode is in this process bearing the immobilised DNA or PNA probe. The hybridisation experiment was carried out by immersing the electrode into the stirred buffer solution containing a desired target, followed by measurement of signal. The detection limit was of 10 pmol of the 15-mer oligonucleotide target was observed following a 10 min hybridisation. PNA carbon-paste biosensor was used for the detection of specific mutation in the p53 gene, a mutation related to various types of cancer. Challenging, the PNA biosensor with single-base mismatch oligomer resulted in a 3% error, as compared to a 91% error for the DNA recognition (Wang et al. 1997c).

2.3.2 Voltametry

Voltametry is an electrochemical technique in which a controlled potential is applied to an electrode (the working electrode), and any current that results from an electron transfer reaction at the electrode is measured. A potentiostat is used to apply the desired potential to the working electrode, relative to a reference electrode, and to measure the resulting current. While it is possible to perform voltametry with just two electrodes, in practice a third electrode, the auxiliary electrode, is employed in the current measurement system. The potentiostat is designed to prevent any current flow at the reference electrode, which might result in changes to its electrochemical potential (Van Benschoten, 1983). There are different modes of voltametry depending of the information desired. Cyclic Voltametry (CV) is a form of linear sweep voltametry that is carried out at a stationary electrode in a quiet solution, and is an important technique for characterisation of electroactive species. In cyclic voltametry, a solution component is electrolysed (oxidised or reduced) by placing the solution in contact with an electrode surface, and then making that surface sufficiently positive or negative in voltage to force electron transfer.

Voltametry technique has been applied for PNA-DNA detection in several studies. PNA molecules are immobilised as capture probes on a gold substrate. The redox complexes do not interact electrostatically with the PNA probes due to the absence of the anionic phosphate groups on the PNA probes. But after hybridisation, the complex is adsorbed on the DNA backbone, giving a clear hybridisation detection signal in ac voltametry. The process combines the selectivity of the peptide nuclecic acid recognition layer with the sensitivity of ac voltametry.

We describe several examples using complexes as redox markers, and different modes of applying voltametry as a detection technique. Aoki et al. have described the use of mixed monolayers of PNA and 6-mercapto-1-hexanol on gold disk electrodes to detect complementary oligonucleotides at micromolar level by cyclic voltametry. The system relies on the electrostatic repulsion of the diffusing ferrocyanide redox marker, accrued from the hybridisation of the negatively-charge target DNA and the neutral PNA probe. Binding of the complementary oligonucleotide to the PNA probe monolayer increases the negative charge at the surface of the electrode, which results in electrostatic repulsion between the redox marker $[Fe(CN)_6]^{4-/3-}$ in solution and the monolayer, thereby hindering the redox reaction of the maker; this allows the indirect detection of the complementary oligonucleotide (Aoki et al., 2000).

Steichen et al. have reported that the cationic ruthenium complexes ($[Ru(NH_3)^6]^{3+}$), is adsorbed on the DNA backbone only after hybridisation, giving a clear hybridisation detection signal in ac voltametry (Steichen et al., 2007). Furthermore, new method for the PNA-DNA detection has been developed. Ferrocene-containing cationic polythiophene does not bind electroscally to the PNA probes due to the absence of the anionic phosphate groups before hybridisation. After the PNA-DNA hybrid is formed, ferrocene-containing cationic polythiophene interacts electrostatically with the negatively charged phosphate groups and is adsorbed on the DNA backbone, giving a clear hybridisation detection signal in the cyclic voltamograms (qualitative information) and Differential Pulse Voltametry (DPV) (quantitative information). DPV has a much higher current sensitivity and better resolution than cyclic voltametry, because DPV provides a convenient peak shape for quantification, and the compounds, that get oxidized at different potential, will show up as separate peaks if their oxidation potentials are sufficiently different (Adams et Justice, 1997; Fang et al., 2008b). Kerman et al. report on electrochemical biosensor based on PNA for detection of PNA-DNA hybridisation the oxidation signal of guanine at carbon paste electrode detected by using DPV (Kerman et al., 2003).

Square Wave Voltametry (SWV) is a very sensitive and fast technique (voltamograms can be obtained in a few seconds), therefore, very well suited to study DNA hybridisation (Liu et al., 2006). SWV have been used to detect and quantify PNA-DNA hybridisation, based on ferroceno (Fc)-streptavidin conjugates. The quantification of target DNA can be easily obtained on this sensor platform with good stability and reproducibility, and the PNA-DNA affinity constants can be obtained from the redox-labeled streptavidin coupled to the duplex. Another example of detection of the electrochemical changes using SWV, PNA were attached covalently onto a quinone-based electroactive polymer, following changes in flexibility of the PNA probe strand upon hybridisation generates electrochemical changes at the polymer–solution interface. An increase in the peak current of quinone was observed upon hybridisation of probes by the target DNAs, whereas no change is observed with non-complementary sequence. Hybridisation was detected by recording the modification of the redox process of the quinone group, using SWV (Reisberg et al, 2008).

Hashimoto et al. have described the elaboration of electrochemical PNA arrays for the detection of the cancer gene ras; PNA was immobilised on gold electrodes of the array, and by using Linear Sweep Voltammetry (LSV) can provide a quick and convenient method for determining target DNAs specifically and quantitatively, with a detection limit of 10^{-13} M (3 fmol) (Hashimoto, K. & Ishimori, Y. 2001).

The PNA–SAM sensor was tested to differentiate the A2143G point mutation of H. pylori versus the wild-type sequence oligonucleotide, showing a good selectivity and sensitivity. *H. pylori* is recognised as one of the most common pathogens afflicting humans, the presence of the bacterium in the gastric mucosa is associated with chronic active gastritis and is implicated in more severe gastric diseases (Steichen et al., 2007). The detection limit of the complementary DNA oligonucleotide is 80 pM. Currently a hybridisation volume of 20 μl of DNA target is exposed to the PNA–SAM electrode, meaning that 1.6 fmol of the complementary target can be detected. However the use of microelectrodes could significantly improve the detection limit. DPVs detection limit for PNA-DNA hybridisation is 1.0×10^{-8} M on a planar electrode and reproducible results Residual Standard Deviation

(RSD) of 5% was obtained for four repetitive measurements of hybridisation of ss-PNA probe with $4.0x10^{-8}$ M target DNA (Fang et al., 2008).

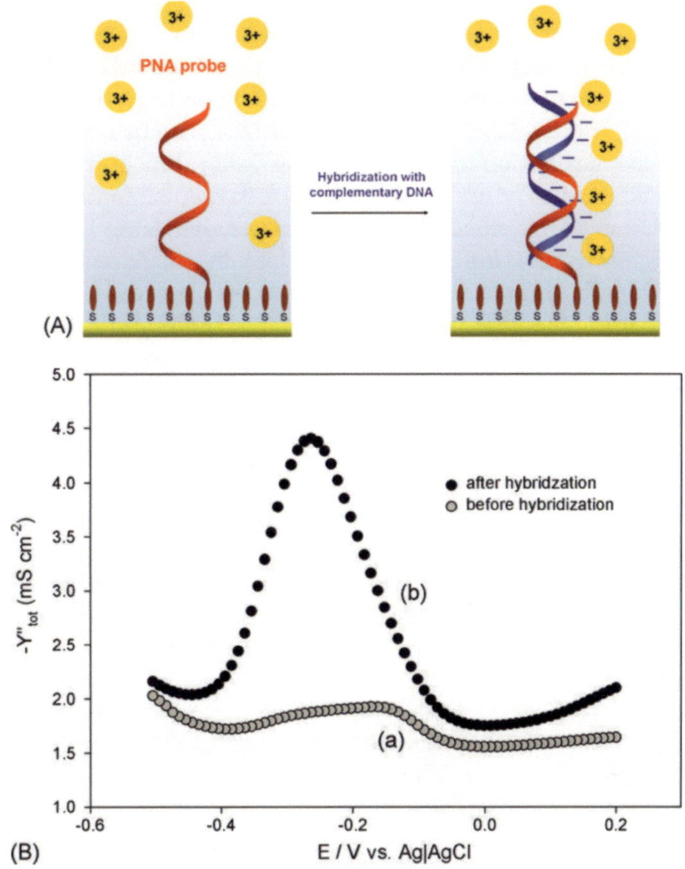

Fig. 6. (A) Schematic representation of the electrostatic DNA hybridisation detection method using $[Ru (NH_3)_6]^{3+}$ as redox markers, and PNA as capture probes on gold. (B) Imaginary admittances of the PNA sensor before (a) and after (b) hybridisation with 1μM complementary DNA (from Steichen et al., 2007).

2.3.3 Electrochemical Impedance Spectroscopy (EIS)

Electrochemical Impedance Spectroscopy (EIS) is an experimental method to characterise electrochemical systems. This technique measures the impedance of a system over a range of frequencies; the frequency response of the system, including the energy storage and dissipation properties, is revealed. Often, EIS reveals information about the reaction mechanism of an electrochemical process: different reaction steps will dominate at certain frequencies, and the frequency response shown by EIS can help identifying the rate limiting step. Among the used electrochemical techniques, electrochemical impedance spectroscopy has been shown very effective and sensitive for the characterisation of biomaterial-functionalised electrodes and biocatalytic transformation at electrode surfaces.

The principle of impedimetric sensing of DNA hybridisation is based on the formation of nucleic acid/DNA complexes at an electrode surface. The resulting negatively charged interface electrostatically repels the negatively charged redox indicator $Fe(CN)_6^{3-/4-}$. The electrostatic repulsion of the redox-active molecules leads to an enhanced charge transfer resistance, R_{ct}. Thus, R_{ct} will increase with the increasing amount of hybridised DNA. Electrochemical impedance spectroscopy was already successfully used for the visualisation of DNA hybridisation. In EIS, the binding of the target strands to surface-immobilised capture probes is indicated by a shift in the impedance spectrum of the modified electrode [Katz et al., 2003]. In addition, label-free detection of DNA can be obtained by interaction of DNA with electrochemically active ligands [Wang 2003]. Liu et al. have studied in situ hybridisation kinetic studies with label-free DNA target oligonucleotides on a mixed monolayer of PNA and mercaptohexanol on Au electrodes using EIS. EIS can be used to follow the in-situ hybridisation kinetics of PNA/DNA by recording the change of R_{ct} with time (Liu et al., 2005). The immobilised PNA probes on the sensor surface are uncharged, and hence, do not affect the charge transfer from the redox indicator $Fe(CN)_6^{3-/4-}$ to the electrode. Once DNA targets hybridise to PNA, the charge density at the sensor surface will be changed, being a probe to monitor the PNA/DNA hybridisation process. This experiment demonstrated for the first time that EIS is a simple and convenient technique for the in-situ kinetic analysis of DNA hybridisation. A single-base mismatch can be directly seen in the kinetic curves. Moreover, the exact association (hybridisation) and dissociation rate constants can be obtained. Thus, the method is comparable to a fluorescence technique (Liu et al., 2005).

Monolayers of cysteine-linked peptide nucleic acid assembled on gold electrodes, were investigated for the sensing of DNA recognition (Degefa et al., 2008). The monolayer was characterised by cyclic voltametry. The electron transfer through the monolayers was investigated using electrochemical impedance spectroscopy in the presence of target DNA and redox marker ions $[Fe(CN)_6]^{3-/4-}$ as hybridisation indicator. The sensing of DNA at the PNA SAMs was also investigated at different concentration of the target DNA. Degefa et al. show that at lower target DNA concentration, a lower charge-transfer resistance, Rct, was observed, and as the concentration was increased the resulting charge-transfer resistance, Rct, increased too. The PNA surface was also studied for the detection of mismatched target DNA, the fully matched DNA resulted in a higher charge transfer resistance, Rct, than that of mismatched DNA target at higher target concentration. The non-complementary nucleic acid showed a much reduced effect at all target concentrations.

Keighley et al. present a detailed EIS-based study of the simultaneous co-immobilisation of thiol-modified PNA probes and mercaptohexanol (MCH) onto gold electrodes, an optimal density exists, corresponding to a maximum in the change of *R*ct for the negatively charged ferri/ferrocyanide redox couple, upon hybridisation with target DNA (Keighley et al., 2008). The optimisation of PNA surface density and the measurement ionic strength are key factors to the success of electrochemical impedance spectroscopy for label-free detection of DNA hybridisation. A detection limit of 25 fmol target is demonstrated. This is likely to be further improved by reduction of the electrode area and sample volume, this would allow reducing the detection limit to 3 amol.

DNA biosensors, especially those based upon detection of the intrinsic negative charge of target DNA, can be greatly improved by the use of uncharged peptide nucleic acid probes. Hybridisation causes an increased electrostatic barrier for the negatively charged ferri/ferrocyanide redox couple, resulting in an increase in charge transfer resistance *R*ct that is measured using electrochemical impedance spectroscopy.

3. Conclusion

PNA, an ingenious DNA mimic, has two main advantages compared to DNA as a probe: first, it has no phosphate ions making the latter unique labels for the presence of DNA; second, its backbone is uncharged permitting a better hybridisation and the use of other matrix molecule or polymer to increase the binding and detection qualities. PNA offers a promising opportunity for highly specific nucleic acid recognition.

In this chapter, we present a quick overview of some surface analysis techniques that have been successfully applied to the detection of PNA-DNA hybridisation. While some surface sensitive techniques are compatible with on line measurements, like all electrochemical techniques, SPR and QCM, some are applied after hybridisation reaction; this is the case of RAIRS, and of course XPS and ToF-SIMS that need vacuum conditions. It is clear from this overview that, whatever the selected detection technique, the way of immobilising the PNA probe is crucial; some gain in sensitivity were observed when the density and accessibility of PNA were controlled. One also saw that playing with the hybridisation of neutral PNA with positively charged DNA offers advantages, like binding nanoparticles, redox indicators or polymerisation of oligomers, that increase the detection sensitivity. Chemical differences in PNA and DNA backbones also provide with marked hybridisation "labels" that have been exploited by the XPS or RAIRS techniques.

Table 1 summarise the techniques, their principle and associated sensitivity from the literature overview. One main observation is that the reported sensitivity values are very much fluctuating and this because researches in the PNA-DNA field are still recent and, for some of them, focussing on the feasibility and technical developments for these rather novel

Technique	Basic Principle	Sensitivity	Reference
SPR	Change in the refractive index upon hybridisation	0.1 pM	(Su et al., 2008)
		0.7 pM	(Endo et al., 2005)
		A few nM	(Liu et al., 2006)
QCM	Change in the resonance frequency of a quartz	8.6pg/L	(Yao et al., 2008)
		5 μM	(Ananthanawat et al., 2009)
		10 μg/mL	(Wang et al., 1997)
		1 μM	(Höök et al., 2001)
SERS	Enhanced electromagnetic field on nanostructured surfaces	1 pM	(Fang et al., 2008)
ToF SIMS	Detection of PO_2^- and PO_3^- fragments		(Arlinghaus & Kwoka, 1997; Brandt et al., 2003)
RAIRS	PO_2^- vibrational frequency	100μM	(Mateo-Marti et al., 2007)
XPS	Phosphate binding energy	100μM	(Mateo-Marti et al., 2007)
EIS	Impedance/frequency response	1 nM	(Keighley et al., 2008)
Potentiometry	Potencial difference (voltage)	10 pM	(Wang et al., 1997c)
Voltametry	current	3 fM	(Hashimoto & Ishimori, 2001)

Table 1. Summary of the techniques, their principle and their associated sensitivity for PNA-DNA hybridisation detection.

techniques in the domain. To our view, more important than sensitivity that very much depends on the measurement conditions and, in some cases, types of labelling, the use of synthetic PNA, instead of DNA, offers a remarkable specificity to a single mismatched oligonucleotides ; this is critical for many gene desease recognition. Let's keep in mind that using this remarkably specific PNA-DNA hybridisation process, is attractive for genetic diagnosis. Work is left to be done to improve the sensitivity, not forgetting that non specific events have to be kept silent.

4. References

Adams, N.R. ; Justice, J.B. Jr. (1997). Voltammetry in the neuroscience : Principles, methods and applications. USA.

Ananthanawat, C., Vilaivan, T., and Hoven, V. P. (2009). Synthesis and immobilization of thiolated pyrrolidinyl peptid nucleic acids on gold-coated piezoelectric quartz crystals for the detection of DNA hybridization. *Sens. Actuat. B* 137, 215-221.

Aoki, H.; Buhlmann, P. and Umezawa, Y. (2000). Electrochemical detection of a one-base mismatch in an oligonucleotide using ion-channel sensors with self-assembled PNA monolayers. *Electroanalysis* 12, 1272-1276.

Arlinghaus, H. F. and e. al. (1997). Analysis of biosensor chips for identification of nucleic acids. *Anal. Chem.* 17, 76-84.

Attard, G. and Barnes, C. (1998) *Surfaces,* Oxford university press, New York.

Brandt, O. and et. al; (2003). PNA microarrays for hybridization of unlabelled DNA samples. *Nucleic Acids Res.* 31, E119.

Brandt, O. and J. D. Hoheisel (2004). Peptide nucleic acids on microarrays and other biosensors. *Trends in Biotechnology* 22, 617-622.

Briones, C., Mateo-Marti, E., Gomez-Rodriguez, C., Parro, V., Roman, E., Martín-Gago, J.A., (2004). Ordered self-assembled monolayers of peptide nucleic acids on gold surfaces with DNA recognition capacity.*Physical Reviews Letters* 93 (20) 208103.

Briones, C., Mateo-Marti, E., Gomez-Rodriguez, C., Parro, V., Roman, E., Martín-Gago, J.A., (2005). structural and functional characterization of self-assembled monolayers of peptides nucleic acids and its interaction with complementary DNA. *Journal of Catalysis A: Chemical* 228, 131-136.

Buetow, K.H., Edmonson, M., MacDonald, R., Clifford, R., Yip, P., Kelley, J., Little, D.P., Strausberg, R., Koester, H., Cantor, C.R., Braun, A. (2001). High-throughput development and characterization of a genomewide collection of gene-based single nucleotide polymorphism markers by chip-based matrix-assisted laser desorption/ionization time-of-flight mass spectrometry. *Proc. Natl. Acad. Sci.* USA 98, 581-584.

Carruso, F., Rodda, E., Furlong, D. N., Niikura, K., and Okahata, Y. (1997). Quartz Crystal Microbalance Study of DNA Immobilization and Hybridization for Nucleic Acid Sensor Development. *Anal. Chem.* 69, 2043-2049.

Casero, E.; Darder, M.; Diaz, D.J.; Pariente, F.; Martin-Gago, J.A.; Abruna, H.; Lorenzo, E. (2003). XPS and AFM characterization of oligonucleotides immobilized on gold substrates. *Langmuir* 19, 6230-6235.

Cattani-Scholz, A. Pedone, D. Dubey, M. Neppl, S. Nickel, B. Feulner, P. Schwartz, J. Abstreiter, G. and tornow, M. (2008). Organophosphonate-based PNA-functionalization of silicon nanowires for label-free DNA detection. *ACS-Nano* 2, 1653-1660.

Cattani-Scholz, A. Pedone, D. Blobner, F. Abstreiter, G. Schwartz, J. Tornow, M. and Andruzzi, L. (2009). PNA-PEG modified silicon platforms as functional bio-interfaces for applications in DNA microarrays and biosensors. *Biomolecules* 10, 489-496.

Chakrabarti, R., and Klibanov, A. M. (2003). Nanocrystals modified PNAs. *J. Am. Chem. Soc.* 125, 12531-12540.

Corradini, R., and et al. (2004). Enhanced recognition of cystic fibrosis W1282X DNA point mutation by chiral pNA probes by a SPR biosensor. *J. of Mol. Recognit.* 17, 76-84.

Demidov, V.V.; Potaman, V.N.; Frank-Kamenetskii, M.D.; Egholm, M.; Buchardt, O., Sonnichsen, S.H.; and Nielsen, P.E. (1994). Stability of peptide nucleic acids in human serum and cellular extracts. *Biochem. Pharmacol.* 48, 1310–1313.

Degefa, T.H.; Kwak, J. (2008). Electrochemical impedance sensing of DNA at PNA self-assembled monolayer. *Journal of Electroanalytical Chemistry* 612, 37-41.

DeRisi J.L., Iyer, V.R., Brown, P.O. (1997). Exploring the metabolic and genetic control of gene expression on a genomic scale. *Science* 278 680-686

Egholm, M., Buchardt, O., Christensen, L., Behrens, C.,. Freier, S.M, Driver, D.A., Berg, R.H., Kim, S.K., Norden, B., Nielsen, P.E. (1993). PNA hybridizes to complementary oligonucleotides obeying the Watson–Crick hydrogen-bonding rules. *Nature* 365, 566-568.

Endo, T., kerman, K., Ngatani, N., Takamura, Y., and E.Tamiya (2005). Label-free detection of peptide nucleic acid-DNA hybridization using localized surface plasmon resonance optical biosensor. *Anal. Chem.* 77, 6976-6984.

Fabris, L., Dante, M., Braun, G., Lee, S. J., Reich, N. O., Moskovits, M., Nguyen, T.-Q., and Bazan, G. C. (2007). A heterogeneous PNA-based SERS Method for DNA Detection. *J. Am. Chem. Soc.* 129, 6086-6087.

Fang, B.; Jiao, S.; Li, M.; Qu, Y.; Ximing, J. (2008). Label-free electrochemical detection of DNA using ferrocene-containing cationic polythiophene and PNA probes on nanogold modified electrodes. *Biosensors and Bioelectronics* 23, 1175-1179.

Fan, Y., Chen, X., Trigg, A. D., Tung, A. D., Kong, J., and Gao, Z. (2007). Detection of MicroRNAs Using Target-Guided Formation of Conducting Polymer Nanowires inNanogaps *J. Am. Chem. Soc.* 29, 5347-5443.

Fang, C., Agarwal, A., Buddharaju, K. D., Khalid, N. M., Salim, S. M., Widjaja, E., and Garland, M. V. (2008). DNA Detection using nanostructured SERS substrates with Rhodamine B as Raman label. *Biosens. & Bioelectr.* 24, 216-221.

Feriotto, G., and al., e. (2001). PNA and biosensors for real time detection of the cystic fibrosis W1282X mutation by SPR. *Lab. invest.* 81, 1415-1427.

Fodor, S.P.A; Read, J.L.; Pirrung, M.C.; Stryer, L.; Lu, A.T.; Solas, D. (1991). Light-directed spatially addressable parallel chemical synthesis. *Science* 251, 767–773.

Hashimoto, K., and Ishimori, Y. (2001). Preliminary Evaluation of electrochemical PNA array for detection of single base mismatch mutations. *Lab Chip* 1, 61-63.

Homola, J. (2003). Present and Future of Surface Plasmon resonance biosensors. *Anal. Bioanal. Chem.* 377, 528-539.

Höök, F., Rodahl, M., Brzezinsli, P., and Kasemo, B. (1998). Energy Dissipation Kinetics for Protein and Antibody-Antigen Adsorption under Shear Oscillation on a Quartz Crystal Microbalance. *Langmuir* 14, 729-734.

Höök, F., Ray, A., Nordén, B., and Kasemo, B. (2001). Characterization of PNA and DNA Immobilization and Subsequent Hybridization with DNA using Accoustic-Shear-Wave Attenuation Measurements. *Langmuir* 17, 8305-8312.

Jensen, K. K., and et al. (1997). Kinetics for hybridization of peptide nucleic acids (PNA) with DNA and RNA studied with the BIAcore technique, . *Biochemistry* 36, 5072-5077.

Kambhampati, D., Nielsen, P. E., and Knoll, W. (2001). Investigating the kinetics of PNA-DNA and PNA-DNA interactions using surface plasmon resonance-enhanced fluorescence spectroscopy. *Biosens. & Bioelectr.* 16, 1109-118.

Karlsson, R. (2004). *J. Mol. Recogn.* 17, 151-161.

Katz, E. and Willner, I. (2003). Probing Biomolecular Interactions at Conductive and Semiconductive Surfaces by Impedance Spectroscopy: Routes to Impedimetric Immunosensors, DNA-Sensors, and Enzyme Biosensors. *Electroanalysis* 15, 913-947.

Kerman, K. Ozkan, D., Kara, P., Erdem, A., Meric, B., Nielsen, P.E., Ozsoz, M., (2003). Label-free bioelectronic detection of point mutation by using peptides nucleic acid probes. *Electroanalysis* 15, 667-670.

Kerman, K., Vestergaard, M., Nagatani, N., Takamura, Y., Tamiya, E. (2006). Electrochemical Genosensor Based on Peptide Nucleic Acid-Mediated PCR and Asymmetric PCR Techniques: Electrostatic Interactions with a Metal Cation. *Anal. Chem.* 78, 2182-2189.

Keighley, S. D., Estrela, P., Li, P., and Migliorato, P. (2008). Optimization of label-free DNA detection with electrochemical impedance spectroscopy using PNA probes. *Biosensors & Bioelectronics* 24, 906-911.

Landegren, U.;. Nilsson, M; Kwok, P.Y. (1998). Reading Bits of Genetic Information: Methods for Single-Nucleotide Polymorphism Analysis. *Genome Res.* 8, 769-776.

Lao, A.I.K., Su, X. et al. (2009). SPR study of DNA hybridization with DNA and PNA probes under stringent conditions. *Biosens. & Bioelectr.* 24, 1717-1722.

Liu, J., Tian, S., Nielsen, P.E., and Knoll, W. (2005). In situ hybridization of PNA/DNA studied label-free by electrochemical impedance spectroscopy *Chem commun*, 23, 2969-2971.

Liu, J.; Tiefenauer, L.; Tian, S.; Nielsen, P.E.; Knoll, W. (2006). PNA-DNA hybridization study using labeled streptavidin by voltammetry and surface plasmon fluorescence spectroscopy. *Analitycal Chemistry* 78, 470-476.

Mateo-Marti, E., Briones, C., Roman, E., Briand, E., Pradier, C.M., Martín-Gago, J.A. (2005). Self-Assembled Monolayers of Peptide Nucleic Acids on Gold Surfaces: A Spectroscopic Study. *Langmuir* 21, 9510-9517.

Mateo-Marti, E., Briones, C., Pradier, C.M., Martín-Gago, J.A. (2007). A DNA biosensor based on Peptide Nucleic Acids on Gold Surfaces. *Biosensors and Bioelectronics* 22, 1926-1932.

Mantsch, H. H., Chapman, D. *Infrared Spectroscopy of Biomolecules*; Wiley-Liss: New York, 1996.

Mikkelsen, S.R. (1996). Electrochemical biosensors for DNA sequence detection. *Electroanalysis* 4, 7-14.

Moulder, J.F., Stickle, W.F., Sobol, P.E. and Bombrn, K.D. *Handbook of X-ray Photoelectron Spectroscopy*, USA, 1992.

Nielsen, P.E., Egholm, M., Berg, R.H., Buchardt, O. (1991). Sequence selective recognition of DNA by strand displacement with a thymine substituted polyamide. *Science* 254, 1497-1500.

Orum, H. ; Nielsen, P.; Jorgensen, M.; Larsson, C.; Stanley, C.; and Koch, T. (1995). Sequence specific purification of nuceic acids by PNA controlled hybrid selection. *Biotechniques* 19, 472-480.

Okahata, Y.; Matsunobu, Y.; Ijiro, K.; Mukae, M.; Murakami, A.; Makino, K. (1992). Hybridization of nucleic acids immobilized on a quartz crystal microbalance *J. Am. Chem. Soc.* 114, 8299-8300.

Patolsky, F., Katz, E., Bardea, A, Willner, I. (1999). Enzyme-Linked Amplified Electrochemical Sensing of Oligonucleotide−DNA Interactions by Means of the Precipitation of an Insoluble Product and Using Impedance Spectroscopy. *Langmuir* 15, 3703-3706.

Petrovykh, D.Y., Kimura-Suda, H., Whitman, Ll.J., and Tarlov, M.J. (2003). Quantitative Analysis and Characterization of DNA Immobilized on Gold. *J. Am. Chem. Soc.* 125, 5219-5226.

Ramakrishnan, V., M.D'Costa, Ganesh, K. N., and Sastry, M. (2002). PNA-DNA Hybridization at the Air-Water Interface in the Presence of Octadecylamine Langmuir Monolayers. *Langmuir* 18, 6307-6311.

Reich E., Goldberg H. I., (1964) *Prog. Nucleic Acid Res. Mol. Biol.*, 3, 183-234

Reisberg, S.; Dang, L.A.; Nguyen, Q.A.; Piro, B.; Noel, V.; Nielsen, P.E.; Le, L.A.; Pham, M.C. (2008). Label-free DNA electrochemical sensor based on a PNA-functionalized conductive polymer. *Talanta* 76, 206-210.

Sastry, M., Ramakrishnan, V., Pattarkine, M., Gole, A., and Ganesh, K. N. (2000). Hybridization of DNA by sequential Immobilization of Oligonucleotides at the Air-Water Interface. *Langmuir* 16, 9142-9146.

Steichen, M.; Decrem, Y.; Godfroid, E.; and Buess-Herman, C. (2007). Electrochemical DNA hybridization detection using peptide nucleic acids and $[Ru(NH_3)_6]^{3+}$ on gold electrodes. *Biosensors and Bioelectronics* 22, 2237-2243.

Su, X., Teh, H. F., Aung, K. M. M., Zong, Y., and Gao, Z. (2008). Femtomol SPR detection of DNA-PNA hybridization with the assistance of DNA-guided polyaniline deposition. *Biosensors & Bioelectronics* 23, 1715-1720.

Ujihara, M., Orbulescu, J. I., T, and Leblanc, R. M. (2005). Film Structures of Poly(Amido Amine) Dendrimers with an Azacrown Core and Long Alkyl Chain Spacers on Water or Ag Nanoparticle Suspension. *Langmuir* 21, 6846-6854.

Van Benschoten, J.J.; Lewis, J.Y.; Heineman, W.R.; Rosten, D.A.; Kissinger, P.T. (1983). Cyclic voltammetry experiment. *J. Chem. Educ.* 60, 772.

Wang, J.; Palecek, E.; Nielsen, P. ;Rivas, G.; Cai, X. ; Shiraishi, H.; Dontha, N.; Luo, D.; Farias, P. (1996). Peptide nucleic acid probes for sequence-specific DNA biosensors. *J.Am.Chem.Soc* 118, 7667-7670.

Wang, J., Nielsen, P. E., Jiang, M., Cai, X., Fernandes, J. R., Grant, D. H., Ozsoz, M., begleter, A., and Mowat, M. (1997 a). Mismatch-Sensitive Hybridization Detection by Peptide nucleic Acids Immobilized on a Quatz Crystal Microbalance. *Anal. Chem.* 69, 5200-5202.

Wang, J.; Rivas, G.; Cai, X.; Palecek, E.; Nielsen, P.E.; Shiraishi, H.; Dontha, N.; Luo, D.; Parrado, C.; Chicharro, M.; Farias, P. A.M.; Valera, F.; Grant, D.; Ozsoz, M. and

Flair, M. (1997 b). DNA electrochemical biosensors for environmental monitoring. A review. *Anal. Chim. Acta* 347, 1-8.

Wang, J.; Rivas, G.; Cai, X.; Chicharro, M.; Parrado, C.; Dontha, N.; Begleiter, A.; Mowat, M.; Palecek, E.; Nielsen, P.E.; (1997 c). Detection of point mutation in the p53 gene using a peptide nucleic acid biosensor. *Anal. Chim. Acta* 344, 111-118.

Wang, J. (1998). DNA biosensors based on peptide nucleic acid (PNA) recognition layers. A review. *Biosensors and Bioelectronics* 13, 757-762.

Wang, S.; Peng, T. Z.; Yang, C. F. (2003). Investigation of the interaction of DNA and actinomycin D by cyclic voltammetry. *J. Electroanal. Chem.* 544, 87-92.

Wang, J. (2000). From DNA biosensors to gene chips. *Nucleic acid Res.* 28, 3011-3016.

Will, G., Kudryashov, E., Duggan, E., Fitzmaurice, D., Buckin, V., Waghone, E., and Mukherjee, E. (1999). Excited state complex formation between 3-aminophthalhydrazide and DNA: a fluorescence quenching reaction. *Spectrochim. Acta Part A: Mol Biomol. Spectrosc.* 55, 2711-2717.

Xu, X. H.; Bard, A. J.(1995). Immobilization and Hybridization of DNA on an Aluminum(III) Alkanebisphosphonate Thin Film with Electrogenerated Chemiluminescent Detection. *J. Am. Chem. Soc.* 117, 2627-2631.

Yao, X., Li, X., Toledo, F., Zurita-Lopez, C., Gutova, M., Momand, J., and Zhou, F. (2006). Sub-attomole oligonucleotide and p53 cDNA determinations via a high-resolution surface plasmon resonance combined with oligonucleotide-capped gold nanoparticle signal ampliWcation. *Anal. Biochem.* 354, 220-228.

Yao, C., Zhu, T., Tang, J., Wu, R., Chen, Q., Chen, M., Zhang, B., Huang, J., and Fu, W. (2008). Hybridization assay of hepatitis B virus by QCM Peptide nucleic acid biosensor. *Biosens. & Bioelectr.* 23, 879-885.

17

Uncoated Quartz Resonator as a Universal Biosensor

Tatiana Yakhno[1], Anatoly Sanin[1], Vyacheslav Kazakov[1], Olga Sanina[1], Christina Vacca[2], Frank Falcione[2], and Vladimir Yakhno[1]
[1]*Institute of Applied Physics of Russian Academy of Sciences,*
[2]*Aria Analytics, Inc.,*
[1]*Russia*
[2]*USA*

1. Introduction

Quartz Crystal Microbalance (QCM) sensors are widely used to perform medical diagnostic testing of biological liquids. These sensors have coatings that selectively bind specific chemicals or structures. This binding affects the acoustic properties of the liquid such as velocity, attenuation and frequency. Based on this approach, rapid detection of fibrinogen and fibrin degradation products was developed (Aizawa et al, 2004); bacteria, immunoglobulins, and C-reactive protein were detected (Muramatsu et al., 1989; Chue et al., 1996); different human blood cells can be detected (Konig, & Gratzel, 1993a; 1993b). Also QCM sensors with special coatings can be used as gas-sensors (Zhou et al., 1994; Lazarova et al., 1996). Uncoated QCM sensors are commonly used for mass measuring in static and dynamic conditions (Gomes, 2001; Yamasaki et al., 2004). The measured frequency shift is proportional to the mass of the deposited film, so the sensor provides thickness data by measuring the film density and acoustic impedance. Another utilization of QCM sensors is measuring viscosity of liquids (Martin & Ricco, 1987).

In the classical QCM sensor technique, the evaporation of solvent is viewed as a significant technical hurdle. We propose a modification of the QCM technique, which takes advantage of this previously undesirable process. The monitoring of a sample (a small 3 µl or 5 µl droplet) as solvent is evaporated provides unique insight into the transitions between physicochemical states of the tested liquid. Increasing the concentrations of solutes as solvent is removed allows probing of a series of states from dilute to concentrated, which may include aggregated, gel, and crystalline states. Using an uncoated quartz resonator as a sensor and measuring the changes of the Acoustic and Mechanical Impedance (AMI) over time, enables detailed monitoring of dynamics of molecular rearrangements in the drying sample droplet. In the proposed method, a single sensor demonstrates, over time, a change in its relative sensitivity to the contributions of different molecules to the measured signal, which is equivalent to using a large array with multiple sensors with unique sensitivity to various molecular components of the tested liquid.

A drop of liquid, drying on a solid substrate, is a natural model of a self-organizing system. There are many variants of the drying processes such as drop volume, environment, substrate properties, and liquid composition (Deegan, 2000; Deegan et al., 2000; Ragoonan & Aksan, 2008; Yakhno, 2008, Yakhno & Yakhno, 2009). Thus, if we control all outer parameters except liquid composition, only this parameter will be responsible for self-organizing processes in the drying drop. Self-organizing processes in drying protein solutions were first reported by E. Rapis (Rapis, 1988). L.V. Savina (Savina, 1999), V.N. Shabalin and S.N. Shatokhina (Shabalin & Shatokhina, 2001) used this phenomenon in medical diagnostics. Morphology of human biological fluids is based on comparing the structure of dry drops of biological fluids of people in normal state to those of people with different diseases. However, such an approach has drawbacks, including the subjective estimate of structures, the difficult formalization of results, and the necessity of using expensive optical equipment and computer software for video-image processing. Moreover, the morphological analysis of dry drops is usually performed only after the complete drying (film water evaporation), which takes no less than two days.

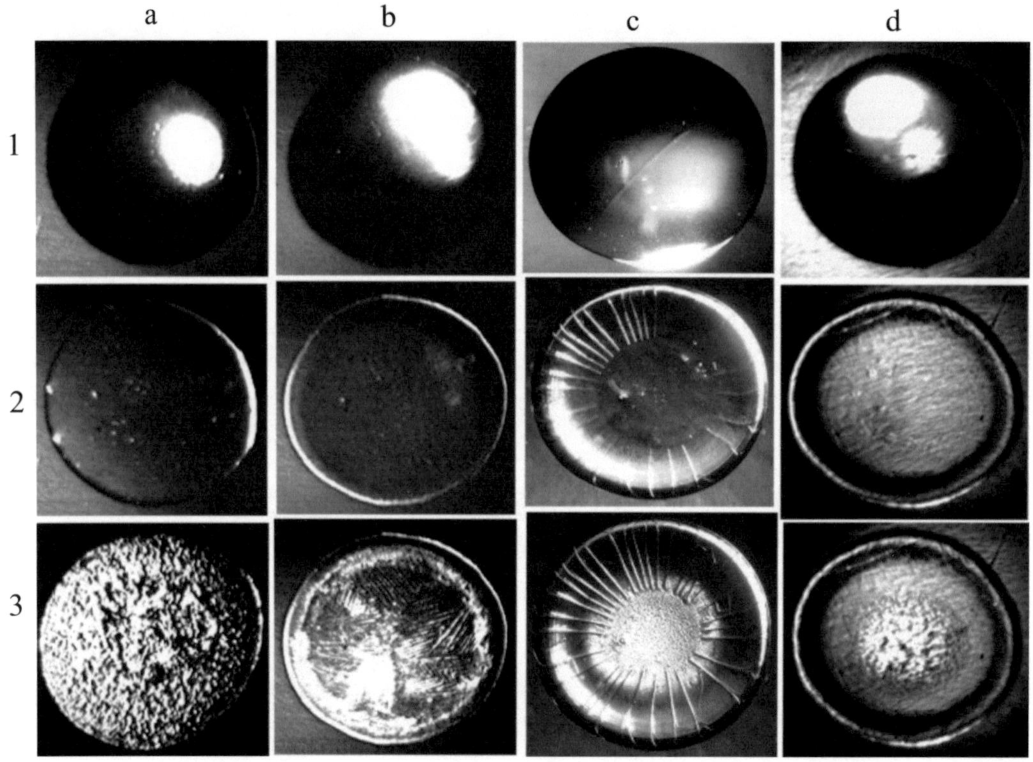

Fig. 1. Phase transitions in drying drops of (a-c) urine, saliva, and blood serum, respectively, of a healthy donor and (d) blood serum of a patient with hepatitis B: (1) beginning of drying; (2) gel matrix formation; (3) salt crystallization into gel (Yakhno et al., 2004).

We showed that, during free water evaporation, it is possible to get diagnostic information not only from morphological features of dried drops, but also from dynamic parameters (Yakhno et al., 2001). It allowed us to shorten the measurement time to 30-40 min, although subsequent treatment of the results was cumbersome. At that time we took photographs of drying drops every minute, made collages of pictures, and measured dynamics of structurization - average velocity, acceleration, and front propagation length from the edge to the center of the drop. In spite of the fact that we got significant difference between donors and patients with different diseases, it was clear, that more efficient way should be developed. Thus, quartz sensor setup was created for registering the dynamics of drop drying process (Yakhno et al., 2002). It is important to note, that the measuring procedure did not visibly disturb the self-organizing processes in drying drops, and they kept the same central symmetry zones as the drops, when dried on a glass substrate. In 2006 A. Killeen and coauthors (Killeen et al., 2006) confirmed the fact that the dynamics of pattern formation created by drying droplets of serum on cover slips differed when comparing normal samples to those containing monoclonal proteins. The authors came to this conclusion by registering the image dynamics in different parts of 1μl serum droplets during drying. Subsequent treatment of these data by special software (Support Vector Machine classifier) also allowed quantitative separation of myeloma and normal serum samples.

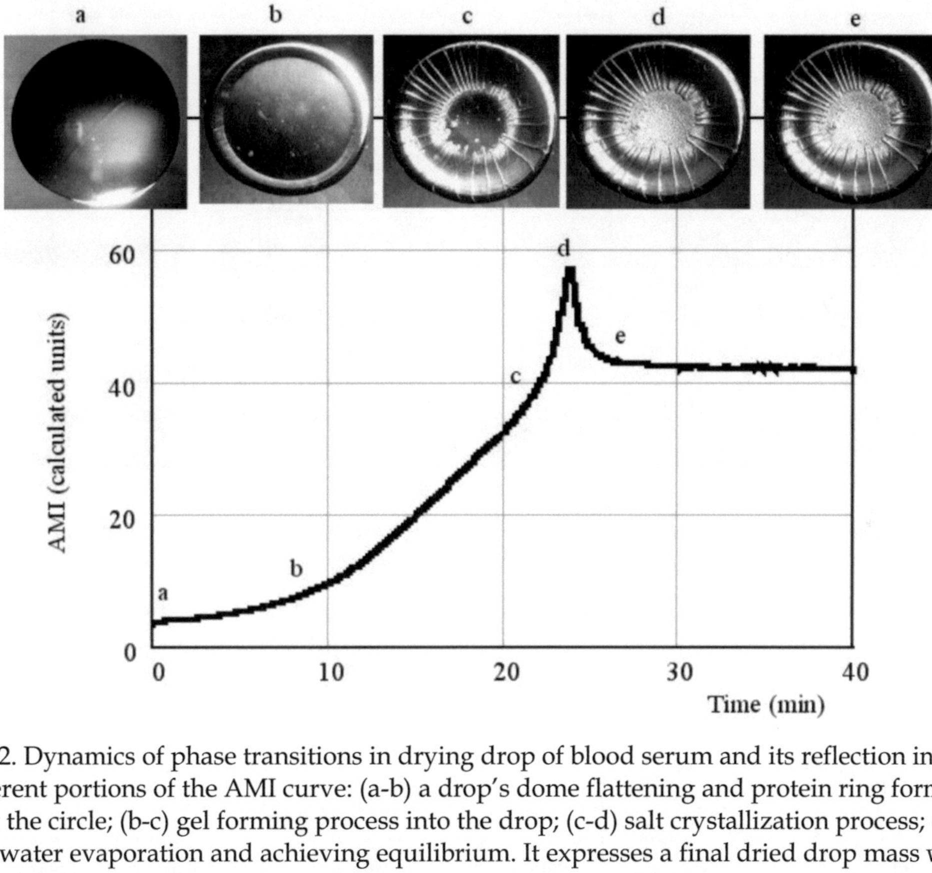

Fig. 2. Dynamics of phase transitions in drying drop of blood serum and its reflection in the different portions of the AMI curve: (a-b) a drop's dome flattening and protein ring forming over the circle; (b-c) gel forming process into the drop; (c-d) salt crystallization process; (d-e) free water evaporation and achieving equilibrium. It expresses a final dried drop mass with film water.

A drop drying process of blood serum begins with phase transitions of proteins, and protein phase perturbations are finished by forming of a gel matrix (Yakhno et al., 2004). The final stage of drop drying involves salt crystallization in the residuals of liquid phase immobilized into gel (Fig. 1). If a drop dries on the surface of a quartz resonator, the drop self-organization is represented by the dynamics of phase transitions that are recorded using variation in the AMI. The kinetics of water evaporation during the phase transitions of salts is determined by physical properties of the gel, thus, it can charachterize liquid as a whole. Also it was established that the dynamics of AMI signal variation corresponds to the sequential stages of structure formation in a drying drop, and can be used for their description (Fig. 2). Thus, a shape of a curve "AMI vs. time" reflects features of drop drying dynamics. Different heuristic algorithms for parameterization the shape of AMI curves were developed. Comparing the dynamics of self-organization in drying drops of blood plasma with the help of these algorithms - Shape Indices (SI) - it was possible to distinguish different diseases on the plane of features (Yakhno et al., 2005).

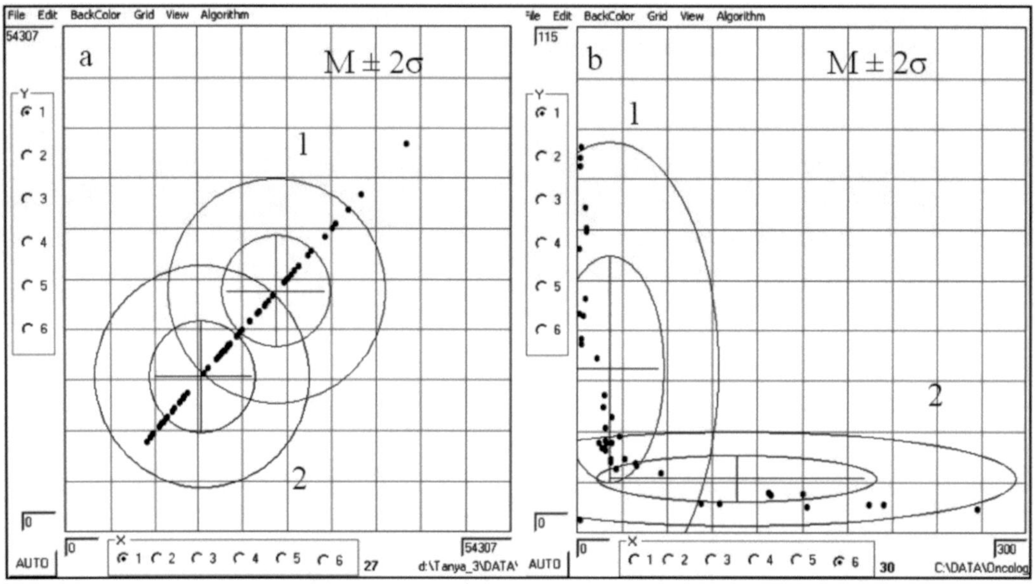

Fig. 3. Distribution of the data of breast cancer women (1) and donors – women of the same age (2) on the plane of features in coordinates of different SIs (M ± 2σ). Blood serum (a) and urine (b) both contain diagnostic information.

The fact is diagnostic information can be extracted not only from serum, but also from urine (Fig. 3). There were shown that sensitivity and specificity for oncology case detection (total) was 76% and 100% respectively. These indices for breast cancer diagnostic were 92% and 86%; for lung cancer diagnostics – 96% and 73%; for paraproteinemia hemoblastosis – 100% and 100%. Furthermore breast cancer and lung cancer could be separated from each other with sensitivity 93% and selectivity 73%. There was also shown good prospects in gestation and threatened abortion diagnostics (Fig. 4). These aptitude tests used a drying drop as a "black box" with very complex processes into it during drying. We come to know the particulars of these processes using model protein and salt water solutions, which mimic human serum (Yakhno et al., 2007a; Yakhno et al., 2007b; Yakhno, 2008). As long as some deseases are accompanied by high level of immunoglobulines, and different levels of fibronectin (Fn) in blood serum (Heil, W. et al., 1999), we would like to see what changes in shape of the AMI curves take place when some of these serum components are added to the Human Serum Albumin (HSA) solution. The aim of this work was to trace some causal relationships, which were responsible for diagnostic data, using model protein-salt solutions of different content and structure.

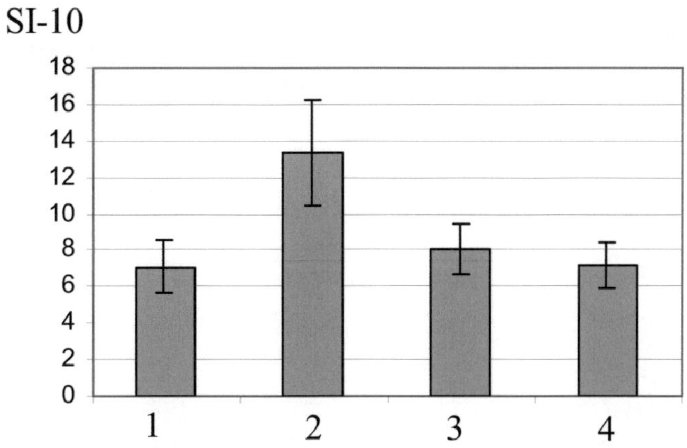

Fig. 4. SI-10 value in women - donors (1), normal pregnancy women (2), pregnancy women with threatened abortion (3), and women after premature birth (4).

2. Methods and materials

2.1 Device description

A drop is dried on the surface of a quartz sensor, while it oscillates in the shear mode. The quartz sensor is a resonator in the form of a rectangular bar of quartz XYS/1°30′ with section 48.0 by 4.8 by 1.0 mm. (Fig. 5). Electrodes on which sinusoidal voltage is fed to excite mechanical oscillations are applied on the upper and bottom plane faces. The resonator is suspended by wire conductors soldered to the bar in the middle. The operating mode is the mode of longitudinal bulk oscillations of the bar, i.e., the mode of compression-decompression oscillations in the direction of the length. The operating frequency of the excitation voltage corresponds to the frequency of the first longitudinal resonance of the bar, i.e., the bar length corresponds to one a half of the length of the longitudinal sound wave in the resonator (60 kHz). In this case, the distribution of the oscillatory velocity amplitude over the plate length has a sinusoidal form with a zero value in the middle of the length. A drop of a liquid under study is placed at the surface on the operation end of the bar, where the oscillatory velocity amplitude of the surface is approximately constant. Part of the area of the electrodes on the operating end of the sensor is removed (Fig. 5) to place the drop directly on the polished surface of a quartz crystal. Shear displacements of all side faces of the bar occur under bulk oscillations in the direction of the length. Under such conditions, the drop is an acoustical (mechanical) load of the resonator for shear oscillations. The AMI is a value of this load. The amplitude of mechanical oscillation is chosen such that to make the minimum disturbance for self-organization processes.

The AMI of a drop is determined from the electric conductance of the resonator operated at a fixed frequency, which is equal to the resonance frequency of the unloaded resonator. For the AMI measurements, we used bridge circuit, which allows cancellation of the static resonator capacitance and provides for an imbalance voltage that is inversely proportional to the modulus of the AMI (Yakhno et al., 2003).

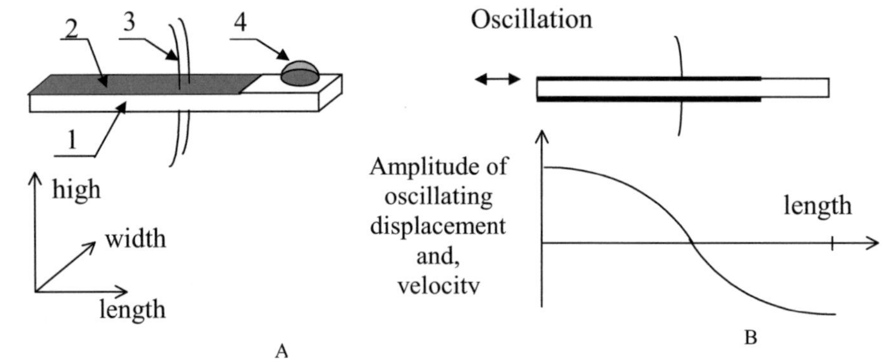

Fig. 5. Design and oscillation mode of a quartz resonator. A is a quartz resonator with a drop of studied liquid, 1 is a quartz plate, 2 is the metallization, 3 is the supporting conductors, and 4 is a drop of studied liquid. B is the distribution of the oscillatory velocity amplitude and longitudinal displacement.

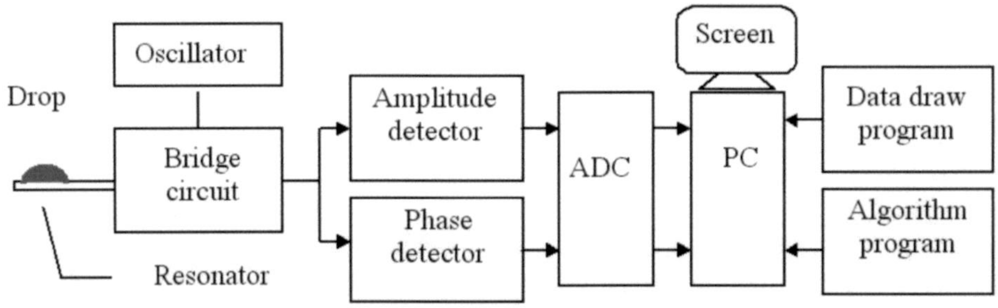

Fig. 6. Block diagram of the device for measuring the AMI dynamics.

A block diagram of the device is shown in Fig. 6. An amplitude detector detects the output voltage of the bridge circuit. Detected signal is fed through an analogue-to-digital converter (ADC) to a personal computer (PC). The drop drying process is displayed on the screen in the form of an amplitude curve corresponding to the modulus of the AMI (Fig. 6). A more detailed description of the device construction and measurement procedure can be seen also in (Yakhno et al., 2003; Yakhno et al., 2005).

Actually, the AMI is a complex value, which is the sum of acoustical and mechanical impedances. Each of them has its own "weight coefficient": H1, H2, H3, and H4. These coefficients and their temporal changes during the drop drying depend on the liquid (its content, structure, etc).

$$\mathrm{AMI} = \mathrm{H1}\,(1 + \mathrm{j})\,\mathrm{S}\sqrt{\pi f \rho \eta} + \mathrm{H2}\,\mathrm{j}\,2\pi f m + \mathrm{H3}\frac{k}{\mathrm{j}\,2\pi f} + \mathrm{H4}\,\mathrm{kfric} \tag{1}$$

where j is an imaginary unit, S is the square of liquid-solid interface, f is the frequency of resonator oscillation, ή is the liquid viscosity, ρ is the liquid density, m is the loading mass; k is the elasticity, and the kfric is the friction coefficient.

At the beginning of drying, when a drop is a liquid, its impedance is proportional to the specific resistance of a shear wave (Mason, 1964):

$$AMI_{beg} = H1\,(1+j)\,S\,\sqrt{\pi f \rho \eta} \quad (2)$$

where AMI_{beg} is the AMI value at the beginning of drying. Usually $\eta \sim 10^{-2}$ Pa · s, and $\rho \sim 10^{3}$ kg/m^{3} for the liquids under study. Under these conditions the height of the drop does not influence the AMI value, because at the set frequency the shear wave penetration depth is approximatelly 10 μ (Mason, 1964). Therefore the beginning of drying is represnted by equation (1) where coefficient H1 = 1, and H2 = H3 = H4 = 0. When drying is complete solid sediments usually adsorb to the quartz plate and the resonator is loaded with the impedance of co-oscillated mass m_{end} of these residuals:

$$AMI_{end} = H2\; j\; 2\pi f m_{end} \quad (3)$$

where AMI_{end} is the AMI value at the end of drying, m_{end} is mass of dried residuals. Therefore at the end of drying process weight coefficient H2 = 1, and other ones H1 = H3 = H4 = 0. Correspondence of AMI level to the equations (2) and (3) at the beginning and the end of drop desiccation was examined experimentally by measuring the real and imaginary parts of electrical conduction of the resonator (or by measuring the real and imaginary parts of AMI). It was shown that the very initial and the final stages of drying can be described by the equations (2) and (3). However such simple situations as "a liquid drop at the beginning" and "a solid mass at the end" are not usual. For example, some liquids have unequal real and imaginary parts of AMI, in contrast with (2), or liquids can have non-zero real parts at the end of drying, in contrast with (3). Registering AMI using share wave mode is a crucial factor for this technology, because it provides a high sensitivity of the AMI level for genesis and growth of new phase structures on the liquid-quartz border, as well as the acoustical and mechanical properties of resultant sediments.

2.2 Liquids under study

Protein-salt solutions were prepared using either lyophilized bovine serum albumin (BSA, 68 kDa) or human serum albumin (HSA, 67 kDa) in distilled water or salt-in-water solutions. Albumins were purchased from Sigma (USA). Salts (NaCl, KCl) were labeled "chemically pure" ("Reaktiv, Inc.", Russia). Other human blood serum proteins were obtained from "IMTEK, Ltd." (Russia): immunoglobulin G (IgG, 150 kDa), immunoglobulin M (IgM, 900 kDa), and Fibronectin (Fn, 420 kDa). All solutions were prepared a day prior to experimentation, refrigerated overnight and allowed to come to room temperature before testing. For morphological analysis, 5 μl drops of test solutions were placed on clean glass slides and air-dried at room conditions for two days. The preparations were examined and photographed using an MBI-3 microscope fitted with a Canon digital camera.

Protein content in human blood serum model solutions varied from 70 g l^{-1} to 86.4 g l^{-1}. This coincides with the normal total protein concentration in human serum (Heil, W., et al., 1999). Every protein mix had a corresponding HSA control solution of the same protein mass (Tab. 1) and was dissolved in physiological NaCl solution (9.0 g l^{-1}). As a nonionic surfactant, we used OP-7 ($O(CH_2CH_2)nCH_2CH_2OH$) (GOST 8433-81, Russia). Every protein variation was tested at least 10 times. All samples under comparison were tested under the same laboratory conditions (T = 18-22°C, P = 740-760 mm Hg, and H = 60-70%). Table 1 below summarizes the protein content of the protein-salt samples.

3. Results and discussion

Typical shapes of the AMI curves of protein-salt solutions and distribution of the data on a plane of features (SI-1 vs. SI-3) are represented at Figure 7. Adding the micro quantity of fibronectin to the HSA salt solution (Tabl. 1) results in left shift of the AMI curve, and changes the geometry of saline peak. As an example of formalization the changes in the shape of the AMI curves we used Shape Index 1 (in calculated units), which is based on the value of averaged derivative of the ascending part of the AMI curve. For every the AMI curve this segment is determined as a time of salt crystallization (Fig. 8, internal brace), which was placed to left (Fig. 8, external brace), so, measuring part of the curve was limited by the angle A, as it is shown at the picture.

№	Protein composition	[Total protein] g l^{-1}	[HSA] g l^{-1}	[Fn] g l^{-1}	[IgG] g l^{-1}	[IgM] g l^{-1}
1	HSA	70	70	-	-	-
2	HSA+Fn	70.4	70	0.4	-	-
3	HSA+Fn+IgG	86.4	70	0.4	16	-
4	HSA (control 1)	86.4	86.4	-	-	-
5	HSA+Fn+IgG+IgM	84.5	70	0.3	12	2.2
6	HSA (control 2)	84.5	84.5	-	-	-

Table 1. Protein Content in Protein-Salt Solutions

Looking at the picture (Fig 1, b,c), we can see that HSA solutions contaning IgG, and IgG+IgM, differ in the shape of the AMI curves from corresponding control solutions that contane only HAS of the same concentrations (Table. 1). It is interesting that adding Fn to HSA leads to decrease in Shape Index 1, whereas replacement of a part of HSA to the same mass of immunoglobulines in solutions leads to increasing in it (Table 2). Fn is the most investigated glycoprotein of intercellular martix (Nikolaev, 1998). It participates in reparation processes in the tissues, forming a net, which works as a skeleton for the cells occupying a wound area. Fibronectin also plays an important role in opsonization of bacteria (Gilot et al., 1999). The decreasing in Shape index 1 after Fn adding in our experiments means that salt crystallization processes in drying drops carryed out more slowly than in drying drops of HSA solution. We believe that this is a result of protein consolidation at the drop-air border due to Fn net formation. Thus, Fn in drying drop can manifest its native function.

Protein solution	Shape index 1 (M±σ)
HSA	12.0±0.1
HSA+Fn	10.9±0.4
HSA+Fn+IgG	16.6±0.8
HSA (control 1)	13.3±0.3
HSA+Fn+IgG+IgM	23.7±1.2
HSA (control 2)	13.4±0.5

Table 2. Shape index value for the AMI curves of protein-salt solutions.

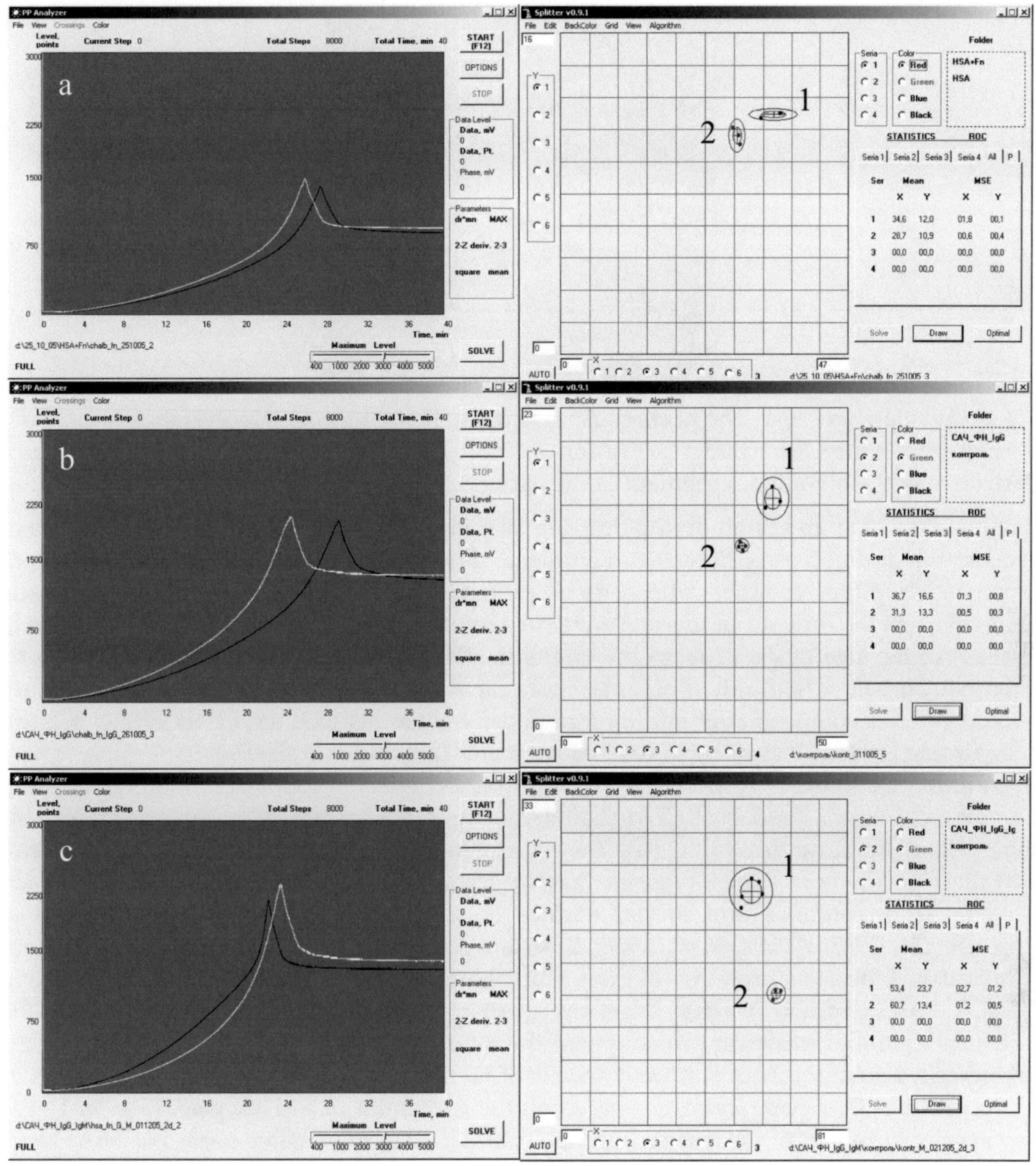

Fig. 7. Comparison of HSA solutions containing various human proteins in each case described in Table 1. Left, for every picture: X-axis is time (min), and Y-axis is AMI (calculated units); (a) HSA+Fn (white) and HSA (black); (b) HSA+Fn+IgG (white) and control 1 (black); (c) HSA+Fn+IgG+IgM (white) and control 2 (black). Right: corresponding data (M ± 2σ) on the plane of features (SI-1/SI-3), M ± 2σ. For every picture 1 is protein mix under study, 2 is its control.

It is known that extension in size of surfactant molecule by one CH_2 - unit, increases its surface energy in 3 - 3.5 times, simultaneously its solubility in water decreases in the same range (Tchukin et al., 2004). Thus, we can dispose serum proteins an accordance with growth their surface activity the following way: HSA - IgG - Fn - IgM. It signifies that

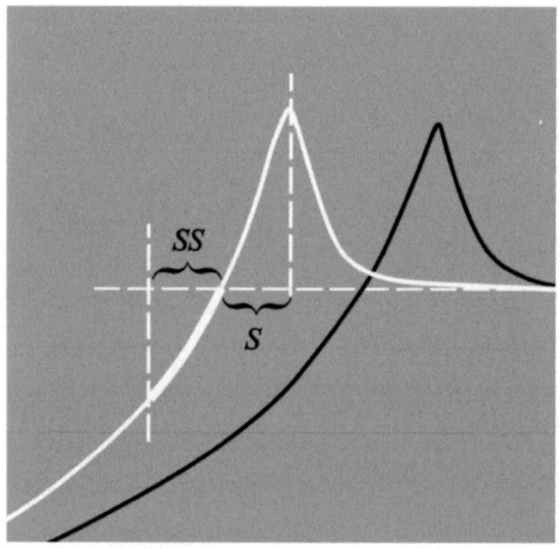

Fig. 8. Calculation of SI-1. The portion „S" is equal with the time of salt crystallization. The portion „SS" is the mirror image of portion „S". SI-1 is calculated using these areas averaged derivative of the highlifhted segment of the curve.

immunoglobulines and Fn in drying drops must occupy the upper position, and act on water evaporation during drying. Because immunoglobulins have no mechanical functions in blood, in drying drop they conduct themselves as proteins with a high surface energy, and settle themselves on the drop-air border, resulting in a lowering of suface tension. This fact leads to increase in the area of the drop on the quartz sensor, and water evaporation becomes more intensive. So, salt crystallization becomes more rapid (SI-1 decreases). The lowring in surface tension of HSA solutions after adding immunoglobulines, as well as rise in surface tension after adding Fn, were shown by direct measurements (Yakhno et al., 2007a).
In addition, we tested BSA solutions (70 g l^{-1}) in either NaCl or KCl water solutions (9 g l^{-1}). The replacement of NaCl by KCl in the BSA solution led to manifest changes in the AMI dynamics as the drop dried (Fig. 9a). These differences are due to Na^+ and K^+ ion features, and their positions in the Hofmeister line, in accordance with their ability to salting-out proteins from solutions and to rise surface tension on the phase boders (Muschol & Rosenberger, 1997; Curtis et al, 1998; Boström et al., 2004). Despite the fact that both solutions had the same protein/salt mass ratio, their initial ionic strength (I) was differerent: I(NaCl) = 0.08, and I(KCl) = 0.06. Thus, the ion charge and size play a significant role in the initialization and developing protein phase transitions in drying drops of protein solutions. Parametrization of the AMI curves by means of SI-6 allows to represent these differences in a digital form. The Shape Index 6 is based on the maximum of the salt peak (Fig 9a, 1), the level of the right part of the curves (Fig. 9a, 2), and geometry of saline peak. For BSA+NaCl SI-6 was equal 514.7±40.4, and for BSA±KCl it was 324.5±19.0.
We extended these experiments, and added to this line 7% BSA water solutions in 0.9% wt divalent clorides: $MgCl_2 \times 6H_2O$ or $CaCl_2 \times 6H_2O$. The results of parametrization is shown on Fig. 10 in coordinates of SI-1. The data were placed in accordance with the Hofmeister series, and were proportional to the surface charge density of the cations (Table 3). Keeping in mind that K+ is a weak chaotrop (K+ binds water more weakly than water binds itself), and the other cations are kosmotrops of different rates (they bind water stronger, than water binds itself), these properties are definded by value of Jones-Dole viscosity B coefficient. It is clear, that in the line from K^+ to Mg^{2+} cation hydrated radius increases due to bound water, it influence viscosity of the solutions (4), and reverberate in dynamical processes during drop drying.

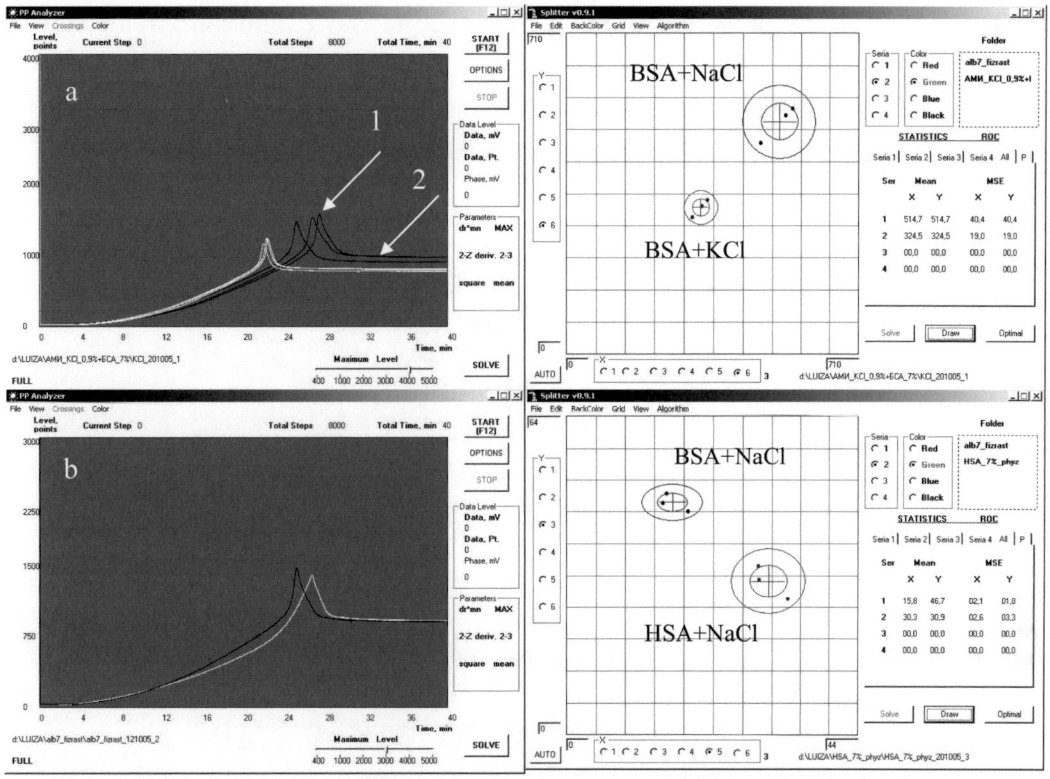

Fig. 9. Comparison of the solutions under study. Left, for both pictures: X-axis is time (min), and Y-axis is AMI (calculated units); (a) NaCl (black) vs. KCl (white) in BSA solution. 1 is maximum height of the salt peak; 2 is the level at which equilibrium is reached. (b) BSA (black) vs. HSA (white) in NaCl solution. Right – distribution of the data on plane of features (M ± 2σ). Above shows SI-6 vs. SI-6; bottom shows SI-3 vs. SI-5.

$$\eta / \eta_0 = 1 + Ac^{1/2} + B \quad (4)$$

η - viscosity of an aqueous salt solution;

η_0 - viscosity of water at the same temperature;

C - concentration;

A - electrostatic term, and

B - a measure of ion-water interactions (Jones-Dole viscosity B coefficient)

The next series of experiments was aimed at tracing differences in drop drying processes when BSA and HSA at one and the same weight concentrations (70 g l^{-1}) were dissolved in NaCl physiological solution (Fig. 9b). We calculated Shape index 1, which was equal 8.7±0.5, and 12.0±0.1 for BSA and HSA solutions, consequently. Also we applied Shape Index 3, which is based on the value of averaged derivative of the descending part of saline peak of the AMI curve from its maximum to the constant the AMI value level. The Shape Index 3 was 46.7±1.8 for BSA, and 11.1±0.6 for HSA solutions. Thus, we can see that in drying drops of HSA salt solution, salt crystalization is a slower process than in BSA salt solution. We suggest that these distinctions are governed by the differences in molecular shape, as well as discharge value and distribution around them (Chang & Bae, 2003). These initial protein features influence the properties of the protein gel and water diffusion throughout the entire drying process.

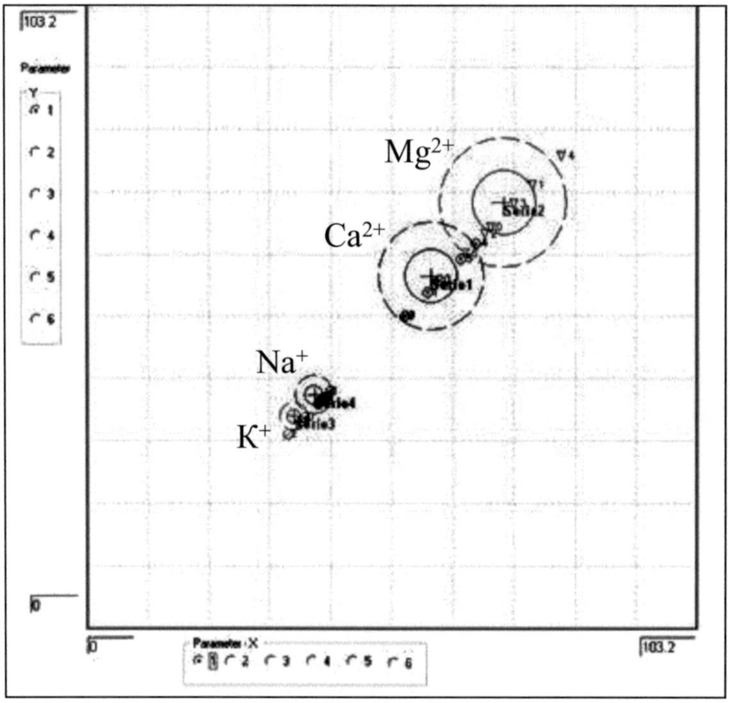

Fig. 10. Distribution on the plane of features 7% BSA solutions in 0.9% different salt-in water solutions in accordance with Hofmeister Series (M ± 2σ) in coordinates SI-1 vs. SI-1.

Cation	Ion Radius (pm)	Surface area of spherical ion (in pm^2)	Surface charge density (Relative value)	B
K^+	138	239.3	0.59	- 0.007
Na^+	102	130.7	1.06	0.086
Ca^{2+}	100	125.7	2.24	0.285
Mg^{2+}	72	65.1	4.3	0.385

Table 3. Some physical-chemical parameters of the cations under study (Collins, 1997).

When a surfactant is added to protein solution, it begins to replace protein from the adsorptive layers, lowering the surface tension of the system (Joos & Serrien, 1999). Ionic and nonionic surfactants have some differences in their action, but their main influence on the solutions is the same (Mackie et al., 2000; Gunninh et al., 2004). The adding nonionic surfactant to BSA salt solution stimulates the dose-dependent left shift of the AMI curves of drying drops (Fig. 11). Our microscopic investigations show that addition of surfactant reduces clustering of colloidal particles and gelation. Most strikingly, the addition of this surfactant systematically reduced the time required for the beginning of NaCl crystallization. The degree of drop cracking intensifies with increase in surfactant concentration. Furthermore, cracks show up earlier in the drop drying process. Gradual decrease of surface energy on the drop-air border eases water diffusion through the adsorbtive layer, and evaporation becomes more intensive. Because water is a plasticizer, its evaporation increases the fragility of the system, and leads the earlier and more intensive cracking of drying drops as the surfactant concentration increases. This dependence becomes apparent when we are looking at the AMI curves.

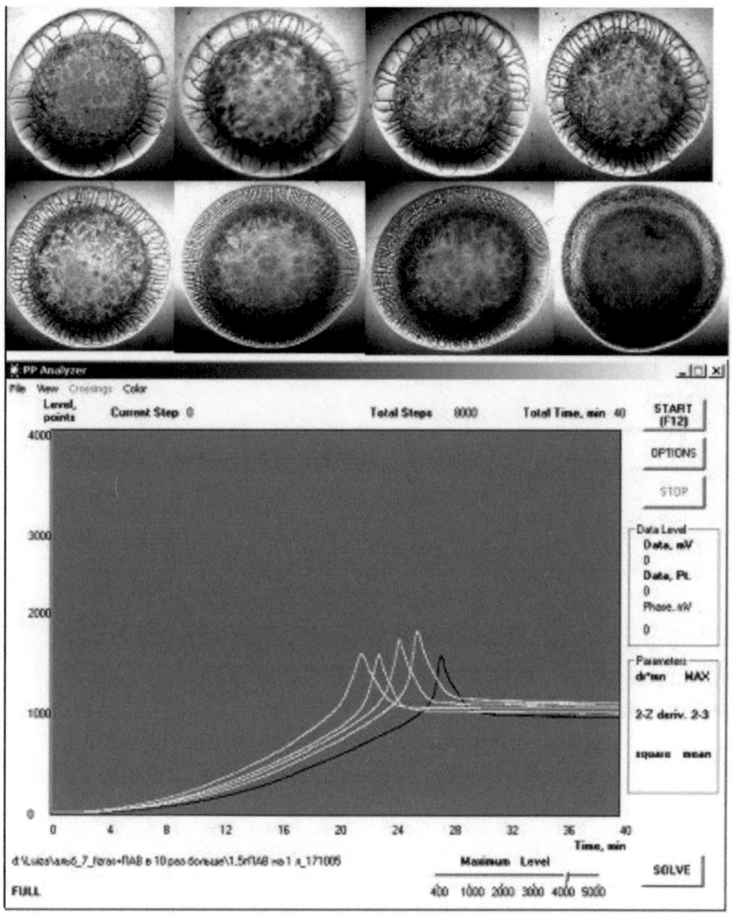

Fig. 11. Microimages (upper line) of dried drops of [BSA] 70 g l^{-1} in [NaCl] 9 g l^{-1} water solution, with adding nonionic surfactant in different concentrations (above), and dynamics of the AMI of the same solutions during drying (below). Surfactant concentration (drops, from left to right): 0,00 g l^{-1}; 0,05 g l^{-1}; 0,10 g l^{-1}; 0,15 g l^{-1}; 0,20 g l^{-1}; 0,50 g l^{-1}; 1,00 g l^{-1}; 2,00 g l^{-1}. Magnification is x10.
AMI curves (bottom line) of drying drops of the same solutions without surfactant (black), and after surfactant adding (white, from right to left): 0,20 g l^{-1}; 0,50 g l^{-1}; 1,00 g l^{-1}; 1,50 g l^{-1}. X-axes is time (min), and Y-axes is the AMI (calculated units).

We also evaluated the effect of a magnetic field on the dynamic processes in drying drops of protein solutions (Fig. 12). The solutions under study were placed in a static magnetic field (400H), and were mixed with a plastic spoon for 10 min. The solutions were then removed from the magnetic field, and underwent a measuring procedure.

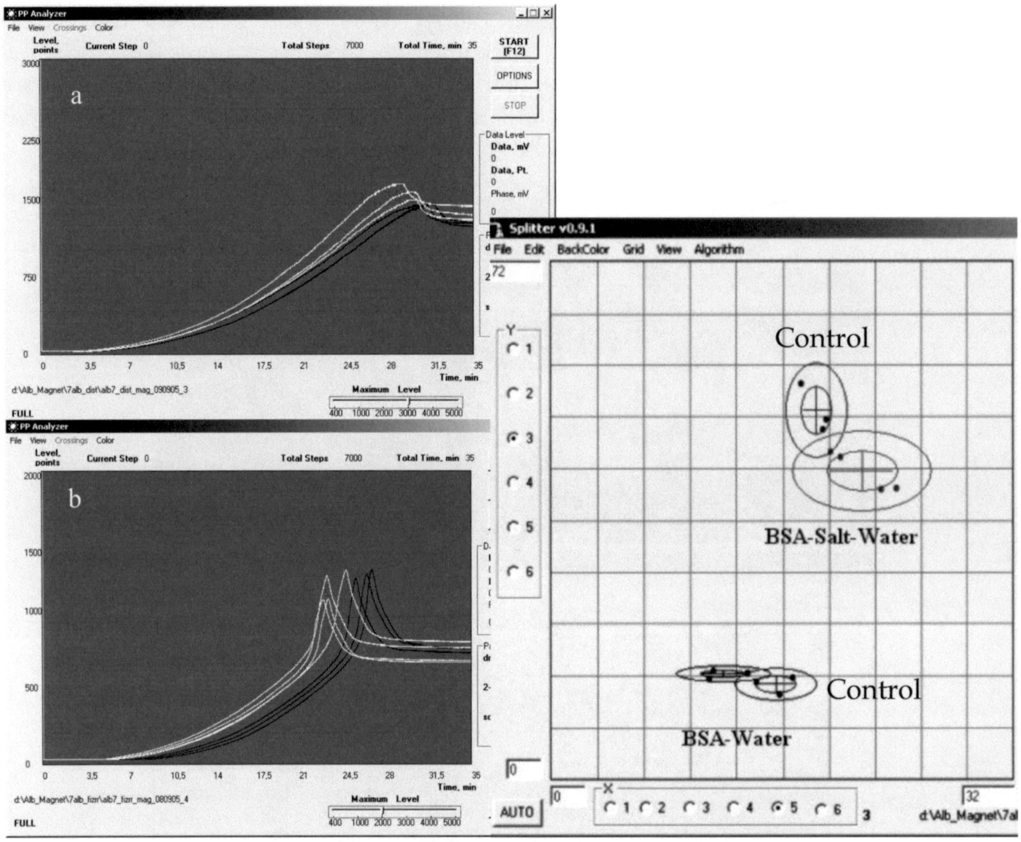

Fig. 12. Influence of magnetic field (400 H) on the dynamic processes in drying drops of protein water solutions: Left (a) 7% BSA in distilled water; (b) 7% BSA in 0.9% NaCl water solution. Black curves - control, white curves - after irradiation. X-axes is time (min), and Y-axes is the AMI (calculated units). Right - data distribution on a plane of features SI-3 vs. SI-5 (M ± 2σ).

Control samples also were mixed 10 min without contact with magnetic field and underwent the same measurement procedure. These results were also compared to our earlier studies (Yakhno et al., 2004) of the effect of UV-irradiation on the 0.5mg/ml carboanhydraze solution in 0.9% NaCl water solution by XeCl excimer laser exposure (λ = 308 nm) (Fig. 13). The extent of the UV-irradiation-induced protein damage was evaluated by fast protein liquid chromatography (FPLC system, Pharmacia Biotech). Before irradiation the protein solution was present in the form of monomers (Fig. 13, a1). Exposure to XeCl excimer laser radiation in a doze of 20 J/m^2 led to the appearance of dimers and molecular fragments (Fig. 13, a2). Upon a tenfold increase in the radiation dose, protein mostly occurred in the form of dimer, trimer, and polymer fractions with a considerable amount of molecular fragmentation (Fig. 13, a3). A change in the state of protein in solution was also indicated by the light-scattering ability of drops within the very first minutes of drying (Fig. 13, b). The drops of solution that were not subjected to irradiation retained a homogenous structure up to the moment of salt crystallization. Irradiation of the protein solution in a dose of 20 J/m^2 led to a significant increase in the light scattering of drying drops as a result

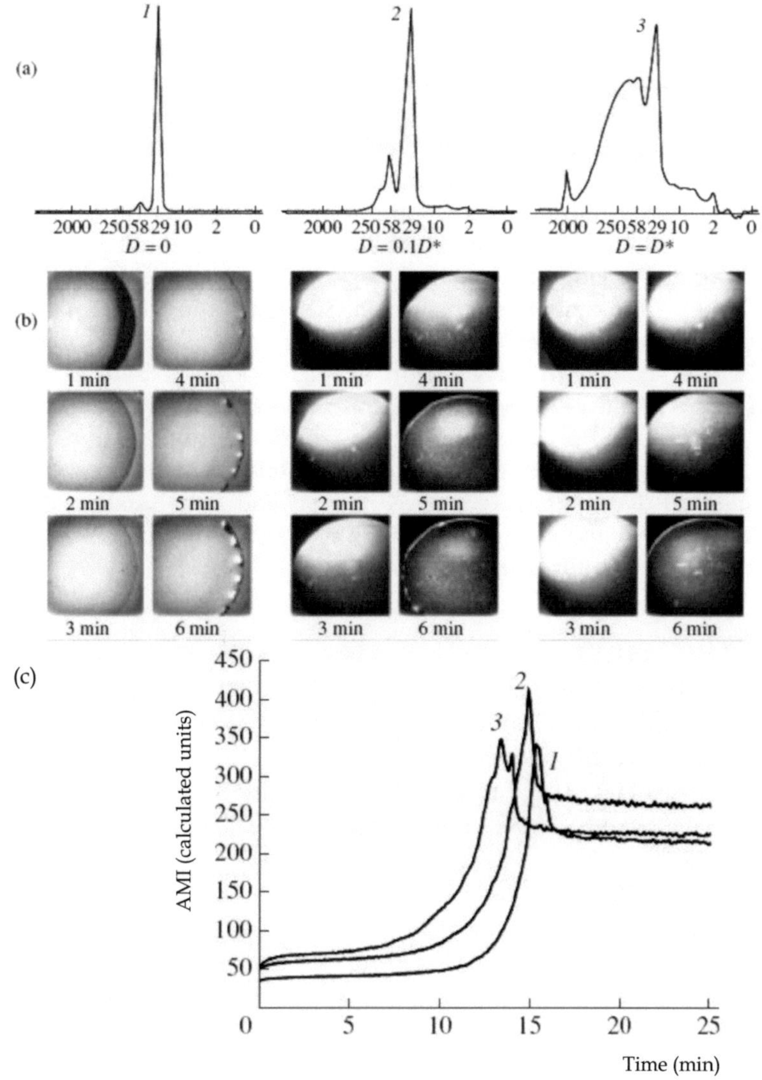

Fig. 13. The action of UV-irradiation on the 0.5 mg/ml carboanhydraze solution in 0.9% NaCl water solution (1) before and (2,3) after irradiation with a dose of 20 and 200 J/m^2, respectively: (a) molecular mass distribution; (b) pattern formation of light scattering during the first six minutes of drops drying. (c) AMI dynamics of the solutions (1) before and (2,3) after UV irradiation in a doze of 20 and 200 J/m^2, respectively.

of protein aggregation, and was accompanied by the formation of a coarse protein matrix with an admixture of protein aggregates (Fig. 13, b2). An increase in the radiation dose to 200 J/m^2 led to very rapid aggregation of the damaged protein: massive aggregates precipitated on the substrate within one minute and did not take part in subsequent events (Fig. 13, b3). Acceleration of the protein aggregation and its precipitation on the quartz crystal surface upon irradiation are manifested by the radiation-dose-dependent leftward shift of the ascending part of the AMI curves (Fig. 13, c).

4. Conclusion

Studies presented here demonstrate the unique use of an uncoated quartz resonator in the diagnostics of multicomponent liquids without detection of their content. This is a new type of analytical instrument, based on nonlinear nonequilibrium processes in drying drops, so-called self-organization. The main feature of this approach is that phase transitions in drying drops were registered and used as the informative parameter. Here every component displayed its physical-chemical properties in the solution, and also their influence the total drying process. Addition of Immunoglobulins and Fn to the solutions demonstared opposite effects on the drying process. These effects can be related to their different native functions in blood. Our methodology also allows generation of numerical differences between solutions that contain different proteins and salts at the same weight concentrations. We showed that the drop drying process is dependent on surfactant concentration, and is sensitive to the action of different external physical factors. In the other words, some of puzzles of a cause-effect chain in informativity of dynamic processes of drying drops were solved. All these data give us grounds to suggest that application of this approach in medical diagnostics, as well as in food and drug quality control should be promising. Further development of the instrumentation is being used to expand our research and develop more applications for medicine and industry.

5. References

Aizawa, H., Kurosawa, S., Tozuka, M., Park J-W, Kobayashi K. (2004). Rapid detection of fibrinogen and fibrin degradation products using smart QSM-sensor. *Sensors and Actuators B,* 2004, 101, 150-154.

Boström M., Williams, D.R.M., Ninham, B.W. (2004) Why the properties of proteins in salt solutions follow a Hofmeister series. *Current Opinion in Colloid and Interface Science,* 2004, 9, 48-52.

Chang, B.H., Bae, Y.C. (2003). Salting-out in the aqueous single-protein solution: the effect of shape factor. *Biophysical. Chemistry,* 2003, 104, 523-533.

Chue, X., Jiang, J., Shen, G., and Yu, R. (1996). Salting-out in the aqueous single-protein solution: the effect of shape factor. *Analytica Chimica Acta,* 1996, 336, 185-193.

Collins, K.D. (1997). Charge density-dependent strength of hydration and biological structure. *Biophysical Journal,* 1997, 72, 65-76.

Curtis, R.A., Prausnitz, J.M., and Blanch, H.W. (1998). Salting-out in the aqueous single-protein solution: the effect of shape factor. *Biotechnology and Bioengineering,* 1998, 57, 11-21.

Deegan, R. D. (2000). Pattern formation in drying drops. *Physical Review E,* 2000, 61 (1), 475-485.

Deegan, R. D., Bakajin, O., Dupont, T. F., Huber, G., Nagel, S.R., and Witten, T.A. (2000). Contact line deposits in an evaporating drop. *Physical Review E,* 2000, 62 (1), 756-765.

Gilot P., Andre P., and Content J. (1999). Listeria monocytogenes Possesses Adhesins for Fibronectin. *Infection and Immunity.* Dec. 1999. 67(12): 6698–6701.

Gomes, M.T.C.R. (2001). Is a quartz crystal really a mass sensor? *Curr. Topics Anal. Chem.,* 2001, 2, 187-193.

Gunning PA, Mackie, AR. Gunning AP, Woodward NC, Wilde PJ & Morris VJ (2004). The effect of surfactant type on surfactant-protein interactions at the air-water interface. *Biomacromolecules,* 2004, 5, 984-991.

Heil, W., Koberstein, R., and Zawta, B. (1999). *Reference ranges for adults and children. Pre-analytical consideration,* Roche Diagnostics GmbH, 1999, Mannheim.

Joos, P., Serrien, G. (1999). The principle of Braun-Le Chatelier at surfaces. *Journal of Colloid and Interface Science,* 1999, 145, 291-294.

Killeen, A., Ossina, N., McGlennen, R.C., Minnerath, S., Borgos, J.,Alexandrov, V., and Sarvazyan, A. (2006). Protein Self-Organization Patterns in Dried Serum Reveal Changes in B-Cell Disorders. *Molecular Diagnostics and Therapy,* 2006, 10, 6, 371-380.

Konig, B., and Gratzel, M. (1993a). Development of piezoelectric immunosensor for detection of human erythrocytes. *Anal. Chim. Acta,*1993, 276, 229-233.

Konig, B., and Gratzel, M. (1993b). Detection of human T-lymphocytes with a piezoelectric immunosensor. *Anal. Chim. Acta,* 1993, 281, 13-18.

Lazarova, V., Spassov, L., Gueorguiev, V., Andreev, S., Malonov, E., Popova, L. (1996). Quartz resonator with SnO_2 thin film as acoustic gas-sensor for NH_3. *Vacuum,* 1996, 47 (12), 1423-1425.

Mackie, A.R., Gunninh, A.P., Wilde, P.J., and Morris, V.J. (2000). The competitive displacement of B-lactoglobulin from the air-water interface by SDS. *Langmuir,* 2000, 16, 8176-8181.

Martin, S.J., and Ricco, A.J. (1987). Acoustic wave viscosity sensor. *Appl. Phys. Lett.,* 1987, 50, 1474-1476.

Mason,W.P. (1964) *Physical Acousics. Principles and methods.* V.1 A, 592, Academic Press, NY&L., 1964.

Muramatsu, H., Tamita, E, Karube, I. (1989). Determination of microbes and immunoglobulins using a piezoelectric biosensor. *Journal of Membrane Science.* 1989, 41, 281-290.

Muschol, M., and Rosenberger, F. (1997). Liquid-liquid phase separation in supersaturated lysozime solutions and associated precipitate formation/crystallization. *Journal of Chemical Physics,* 1997, 107, 1953-1962.

Nikolaev, A.Ya. (1998). *Biological Chemistry,* Medical Informative Agency, 1998, Moscow.

Ragoonanan, V., and Aksan, A. (2008). Heterogenity in dessicated solutions: Implications for biostabilization. *Biophysical Journal,* Match 2008, 94, 2212-2227.

Rapis, E., G. (1988). Well-ordered structure formation during protein film drying. *Pis'ma v Zh.T.Ph.,* 1998, 14, 17, 1560-1565.

Savina, L.V. (1999) *Crystalloscopic structures of blood serum of healthy people and patients.* Soviet Kuban', 1999, Krasnodar [in Russian].

Shabalin, V.N., Shatokhina, S.N. (2001). *Morphology of Biological Fluids,* Khrisostom, 2001, Moscow.

Tchukin, E.D., Pertsov A.V., Amelina E.A. (2004). *Colloid Chemistry,* High School, 2004, Moscow.

Yakhno, T.A., Yakhno, V.G., Levin, G.Ya., Korochkina, O.V., and Buzoverya, M.E. (2001). Dynamics of self-organization processes of biological liquids in the norm state and in some diseases. *Proceedings of the IVth International Conference on Mathematical Modeling,* 2, 265-275, Moscow, 27 June-1 July 2000, STANKIN, Moscow, 2001.

Yakhno, T.A., Yakhno, V.G., Sanin, A.G., and Shmelev, I.I. (2002). Study of the dynamics of phase transitions in liquids of different types by measuring the acoustomechanical impedance of a drying drop. *Biophysics,* 2002, 47, 6, 1101-1105.

Yakhno, T.A., Yakhno, V.G., Sanin, A.G., Sanina, O.A., and Pelyushenko, A.S. (2003). A Method for Liquid Analysis by means of Phase Transitions during drop drying. *Proceedings of SPIE, Bioengineered and Bioinspired Systems,* 5119, 87-99, Maspalomas, Gran Canaria, Spain, 19-21 May 2003, SPIE, Maspalomas.

Yakhno, T.A., Yakhno, V.G., Sanin, A.G., Sanina, O.A., and Pelyushenko, A.S. (2004). Protein and salt: spatiotemporal dynamics of events in a drying drop. *Technical Physics,* 2004, 49, 8, 1055-1063.

Yakhno, T., Yakhno, V., Sanin, A., Egorova, N., Terentiev, I., and Smetanina, V. (2005). The informative-capacity phenomenon of drying drops. Aptitude test in medical diagnostics. *IEEE Engineering in Medicine and Biology Magazine,* 2005, 24, 2, 96-104.

Yakhno, T., Kazakov, V., Sanin, A., Shaposhnikova, O., and Chernov, A. (2007a). Mechanical properties of adsorption layers in solutions of human blood serum proteins: a comparative assessment. *Technical Pphysics,* 2007, 52, 4, 510-512.

Yakhno, T., Sanin, A., Pelyushenko, A., Kazakov, V., Shaposhnikova, O., Chernov, A., Yakhno, V., Vacca, C. ,Falcone, F., Johnson B. (2007b). Uncoated quartz resonator as a universal biosensor. *Biosensors and Bioelectronics,* 2007, 22, 9-10, 2127-2131.

Yakhno T. (2008) Salt-induced protein phase transitions in drying drops. *Journal of Colloid and Interface Science,* 2008, 318, 225-230.

Yakhno, T.A., Yakhno, V.A. (2009) Structural evolution of drying drops of biological fluids (2009) *Technical physics,* 2009, vol. 54, No 8, 1219-1227.

Yamasaki A., Cunha, M.A.S.D.A., Oliveira, J.A.B.P., Duarte, A.C., Gomes, M.T.S.R. (2004). Assessment of copper toxicity using an acoustic wave sensor. *Biosensors and Bioelectronics,* 2004, 19, 1203-1208.

Zhou, R., Vaihinger, S., Geckeler, K.E., Gopel, W. (1994). Reliable CO_2 sensor with silicon-based polymers on quartz microbalance transducers. *Sensors and Actuators B,* 1884, 19, 1-3, 415-420.

18

ALAD (δ-aminolevulinic Acid Dehydratase) as Biosensor for Pb Contamination

Muhsin Konuk, İbrahim Hakkı Ciğerci and Safiye Elif Korcan,
Afyon Kocatepe University, Faculty of Science & Literatures, Biology Department, Afyonkarahisar
Turkey

1. Introduction

Heavy metals are defined as those having a specific density of more than 5 g/cm^3. The main threats to human health are associated with exposure to lead, cadmium, mercury and arsenic (arsenic is a metalloid, but is usually classified as a heavy metal) (Järup 2003). Heavy metals have been used in many different areas for thousands of years. Lead has been used for at least 5000 years, early applications including building materials, pigments for glazing ceramics, and pipes for transporting water. In ancient Rome, lead acetate was used to sweeten old wine, and some Romans might have consumed as much as a gram of lead a day. Mercury was allegedly used by the Romans as a salve to alleviate teething pain in infants, and was later (from the 1300s to the late 1800s) employed as a remedy for syphilis.
Although adverse health effects of heavy metals have been known for a long time, exposure to heavy metals continues and is even increasing in some areas. Since the middle of the 19th century, production of heavy metals increased steeply for more than 100 years, with concomitant emissions to the environment. Emissions of heavy metals to the environment occur *via* a wide range of processes and pathways, including to the air, waters, and soil (Järup 2003).
Lead, mercury, cadmium and arsenic form a significant potential threat to human health, both occupational and environmental (Hu 2000). Over the past few decades, heavy metal contamination of aquatic system has attracted the attention of a number of researchers in all over the world. Many industrial and agricultural processes have contributed to the contamination of fresh water systems thereby causing adverse effects on aquatic biota and human health (Wang 2002, Dautremepuits 2004). The fact that heavy metals cannot be destroyed through biological degradation and have the ability to accumulate in the environment make these toxicants deleterious to the aquatic environment and consequently to humans who depend on aquatic products as sources of food. Heavy metals do mainly accumulate in the tissues of aquatic animals and can be of public health concern to human beings (Kalay 1999, Ashraf 2005).
In fact, there are several heavy metals known to be carcinogens, including arsenic, chromium and nickel. Many of the toxic effects of metals, including carcinogenicity, can be modified by concurrent exposure to other metals. The emphasis now is on testing the effects of mixtures of chemicals to simulate actual environmental conditions. Researches have already demonstrated links between lead and polychlorinated biphenyl exposure and

neurodevelopmental effects. It is now frightened that neurobehavioural and neurodevelopmental deterioration may take place in the next generations (Tang et al. 1999, Winneke et al. 2002, Stein et al. 2002, Yang et al. 2003).

Reports which link autoimmune diseases to environmental factors have appeared in recent literatures (Molina & Ehrenfeld 2003, Dooley & Hogan 2003). In many exposed populations, some individuals are extra sensitive while some extra tolerant. Especially, children are more susceptible to mercury and lead exposures (Needleman et al. 1990). In order to comprehend the basis of these special high or low risk groups, regarding comparative anatomy, physiology, metabolism and genetics, more in depth studies in toxicodynamics and toxicokinetics are needed. It is assumed that state-of-the-art technology where occupational safety, product safety, environmental quality maintenance and accident prevention are in-built under good manufacturing practices. As a result of these studies, conventional problems in occupational toxicology are expected to decrease. Exposure to chemicals already loaded in the environment will still be responsible for delayed effects and indirect exposure. Molecular epidemiology, armed with designed molecular probes and noninvasive diagnostics will become a leading component in risk assessment and health management in future.

2. Lead and lead pollution

Lead (Pb) is one of the most widely used metals in industries and almost in all over the world exposure to Pb continues to be a common problem. Batteries, paints and pigments, plastic, ceramic, secondary foundries and welding are the most important occupational settings. The general population may get exposed to Pb due to food and water contamination, and air pollution caused by industrial emission and fuel containing Pb compounds.

Due to environmental ubiquity and persistence of Pb, its accumulation in organisms and biomass throughout the trophic chain, imply a continuous exposure. This metal can cause mortality in cases of acute poisoning or can indirectly affect the populations by altering reproductive success, behavior, immune response, and physiology in cases of chronic exposure (Mazliah et al. 1989, Burger 1995, Burger & Gochfeld 2000b, Fair & Ricklefs 2002).

Sometimes wild birds might be exposed to very high metal levels, for example, at waste disposal sites or through the ingestion of lead-shot pellets. Such acute poisonings are easily diagnosed, although longer-term effects are difficult to assess. Lead in blood is a good indicator of newly exposure, while chronic exposure can be estimated when concentrations in accumulator tissue(s) are available. Although studies on dead animals provide useful information, ethical, legal, and scientific reasons indicate the need for other types of more easily available samples (feathers, eggs, excrements, regurgitated food, etc), which enable us to estimate exposure conditions (Burger & Gochfeld 2000a, Dauwe et al. 2000). In recent years the usefulness of feathers as a biomarker of heavy metal exposure has been investigated. Results were very satisfying to monitore mercury and lead levels, while contradictory results have been obtained for cadmium (Furness 1993).

In spite of significant reductions in use, most notably in paint production and as a fuel additive, Pb continues to enter the environment primarily by anthropogenic resources, retaining its status as a priority pollutant (USEPA 2006).

As the focus has turned towards remediation concerning to prevent the human exposure, much is still needed in the way of determining appropriate measures to monitor and protect the aquatic environment. Usually, water quality criteria (WQC) continue to rely principally on water hardness (i.e. Ca^{2+}) despite growing evidence that other chemical parameters [e.g. pH, salinity and dissolved organic carbon (DOC)], which may vary greatly on a local basis, also strongly influence Pb toxicity (Macdonald et al. 2002, Grosell et al. 2006).

Efforts to improve WQC for metals have resulted in several toxicity models which designed to encircle the influences of all major water chemistry parameters. The most widely accepted model, the biotic ligand model (BLM), is currently used by the USEPA to set WQC for copper. In core, the BLM is resposible for site-specific water conditions considering the competitive effects from other cations and complexity with organic/inorganic agents that prevent the metal from interacting with the site of toxic action (Paquin et al. 2002).

There has been no demonstrated biological need for Pb. Therefore, its uptake and toxicity is likely mediated through imitating of other cations (Ballatori 2002). The most reasonable candidate is Ca^{2+}. There are strong evidences that Pb acts as a Ca^{2+} antagonist (Busselberg et al. 1991, Rogers & Wood 2004). However, the identification of a specific ligand for Pb remains elusive. As in mammals, the principal effects of chronic Pb exposure to fish are presumably hematological (Hodson et al. 1978), neurological (Davies et al. 1976) and renal (Patel et al. 2006) defects. Some studies have also examined reproduction and behavioral effects (Holcombe et al. 1976, Weber 1993).

These metals and other toxicants are commonly present as mixtures in the environment. Genomic approaches are well suited to locate such problems by filling in where more conventional methods prove insufficient to precise key environmental stressors or elucidate the contributions and additive effects from multiple toxicants. Additionally, microarrays give opportunities not only for establishing the molecular basis of toxicity, but potential for gaining insights into modes of action and higher order effects. Thus, defining toxicant-specific mechanisms that link signature gene transcript profiles to chronic effects would greatly help in monitoring and diagnosing water quality and also prioritizing higher ranked tests in ecological risk assessment. The significance of genomics in this regard was recently referred by the USEPA (Dix et al. 2006).

3. Lead toxicity and δ-ALAD as biosensor for lead toxicity

Pb is a natural component of ecosystems with no known biological role and is highly toxic. Its toxicity originates from its ability to mimic biologically important metals and to produce membrane damage through lipid peroxidation. Most Pb poisoning symptoms are thought to occur by interfering with an essential enzyme, δ-aminolevulinic acid dehydratase (ALAD), the activity of which is markedly inhibited by Pb. This is in total agreement with almost all studies and confirms the toxic effects of Pb for the taxa including bacteria, fishes, amphibians, reptiles, birds, mammals and humanbeings.

A biosensor is a device for the detection of an analyte that combines a biological component with a physicochemical detector component (http://en.wikipedia.org/wiki/Biosensor). It consists of 3 parts:

- The *sensitive biological element* biological material (eg. tissue, microorganisms, organelles, cell receptors, enzymes, antibodies, nucleic acids, etc.), a biologically derived material or biomimic] the sensitive elements can be created by biological engineering.
- the *transducer* or the *detector element* (works in a physicochemical way; optical, piezoelectric, electrochemical, etc.) that transforms the signal resulting from the

interaction of the analyte with the biological element into another signal (i.e., transducers) that can be more easily measured and quantified;

- Associated electronics or signal processors that are primarily responsible for the display of the results in a user-friendly way (Cavalcanti 2008).

An enzyme, an analytical device, can be used as a biosensor. This combines an enzyme with a transducer to produce a signal proportional to target analyte concentration. This signal can result from a change in proton concentration, release or uptake of gases, such as ammonia or oxygen, light emission, absorption or reflectance, heat emission, and so forth, brought about by the reaction catalyzed by the enzyme used. The transducer converts this signal into a measurable response, such as current, potential, temperature change, or absorption of light through electrochemical, thermal, or optical means. This signal can be further amplified, processed, or stored for later analysis. Because of their specificity and catalytic properties, enzymes have found widespread use as sensing elements in biosensors. Since the development of the first enzyme-based sensor by Clark & Lyons (1962), who immobilized glucose oxidase on an oxygen-sensing electrode to measure glucose, there has been an impressive proliferation of applications involving a wide variety of substrates. A variety of the enzymes belonging to classes of oxido-reductases, hydrolases, and lyases have been integrated with different transducers to construct biosensors for applications in health care, veterinary medicine, food industry, environmental monitoring, and defense (Guilbault 1984).

Enzyme biosensors have been widely used in clinical and food analysis, where analytes represent natural substrates of the enzymes employed. At difference, in environmental analysis, pollutants (e.g. pesticides, heavy metals, etc.) are generally detected as monitoring the inhibition of enzymatic activity caused by those toxic materials. The reduced specificity of inhibition phenomenon makes only possible the determination of such parameters, i.e. total concentration of the substances belonging to a certain class. On the other hand, it is expected that biosensor detects only contaminants, which are actually harmful to life.

Enzyme biosensor has got some advantages and same disadvantages. Their advantages are: being more specific than cell based sensors; faster responds due to shorter diffusion a path (no cell walls). Disadvantages: being more expensive to produce; and enzymes are often unstable. Additonally, many enzymes need cofactors for the detection of substances (http://www.rpi.edu/dept/chem-eng/Biotech Environ/BIOSEN/enzbio.htm).

Biosensors for heavy metals have been mainly developed in environmental analysis in water (Evtugyn et al. 1999). As far as enzyme biosensors for heavy metal determination are concerned, a certain number of papers have appeared, reporting the use of different enzymes and biosensor configurations/transducers (Ciucu et al. 2001, Compagnone et al. 1995 and Donlan et al. 1989b, Starodub et al. 1999, Vel Krawczyc et al. 2000, Pirvutoiu et al. 2001, and Dzyadevych et al. 2003). In several cases the inhibition of enzymes by heavy metals is reversible, even if for rapid restoration of enzymatic activity the use of strong ligands, like EDTA, is required.

Most of the heavy metals bind to the sulfhydryl groups, thus inhibiting enzymic activity, disrupting cellular transport and causing changes in protein functions. The toxicity of heavy metals includes the blocking of functional groups of important molecules, e.g. enzymes, polynucleotides, transport systems for essential nutrients and ions, and substitution of essential ions from cellular sites.

During the last decades there was an increasing interest to investigate other sublethal endpoints, especially in relation to those biochemical responses that may be considered as early biosensors of contamination (Huggett et al. 1992) Among them, the inhibition of the enzyme δ-aminolevulinic acid dehydratase (ALAD, E.C. 4.2.1.24) is recognized as a useful biomarker of Pb exposure and effect, both in humans and other animal species (Rand 1995, Timbrell 2000).

Endogenous metals are essential components of many enzyme systems, for instance, δ-aminolevulinate dehydratase (δ-ALAD or called PBGS, EC 4.2.1.24) is a metalloenzyme requiring zinc ions for activity (Jaffe et al. 1995). δ-ALAD catalyses the asymmetric condensation of two aminolevulinic acid (ALA) molecules to form porphobilinogen (PBG) in heme biosynthesis (Gibson et al. 1955) (Figure 1-2) pathway. The pyrrole is common precursor of the tetrapyrrole pigments such as heme, chlorophyll, and cobalamin, corrins, and its biosynthesis pathways are similar in all organisms (Senior et al. 1996, Shoolingin-Jordan 2003). PBGS is very highly conserved in sequence and structure but contains a remarkable phylogenetic variation in metal ion usage for catalytic and allosteric functions

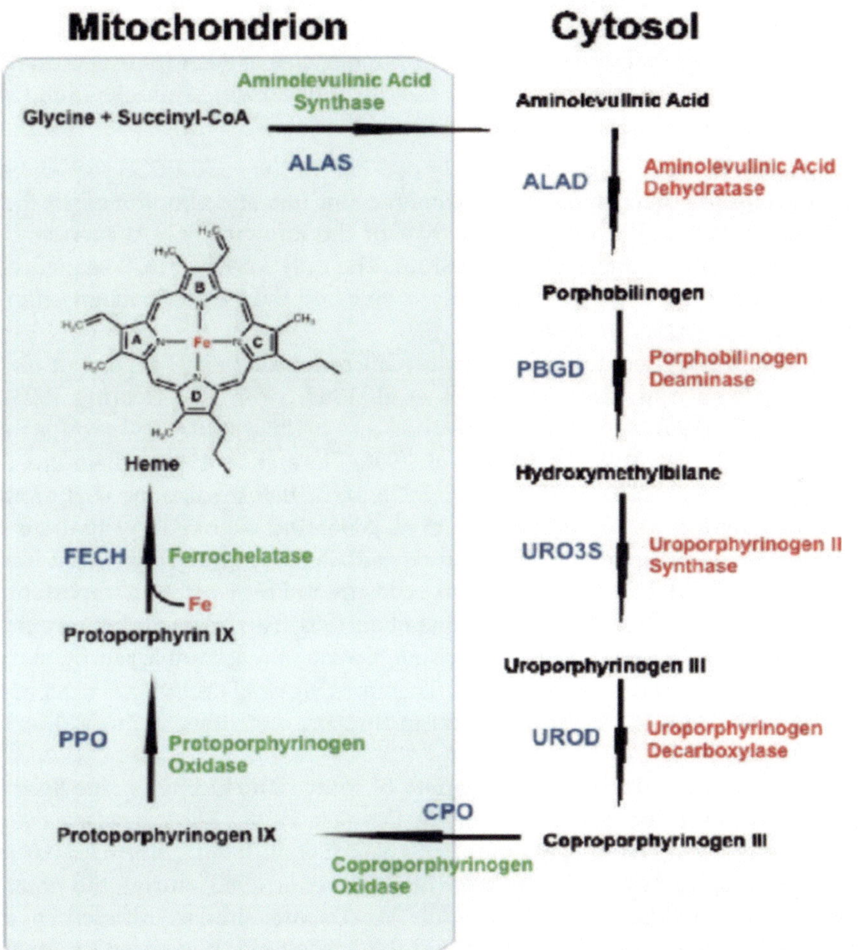

Fig. 1. The heme biosynthetic pathway. Mitochondrial enzymes are depicted in green and cytosolic enzymes in red (Richard et al., 2006).

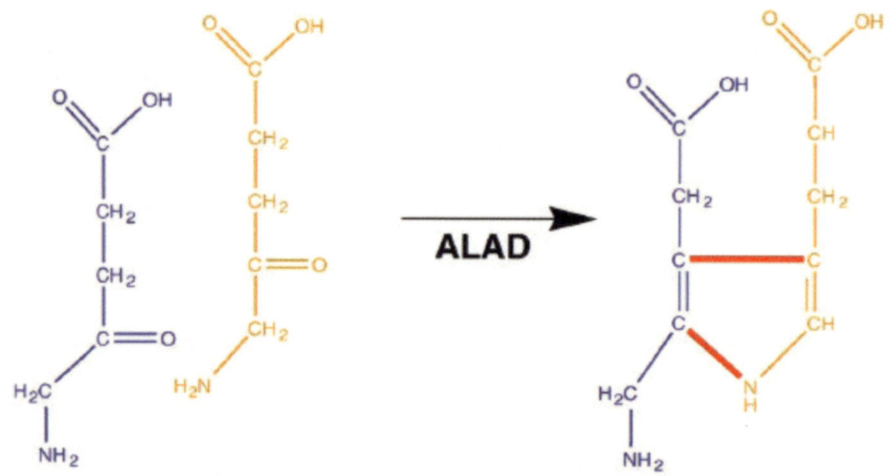

Fig. 2. Synthesis of porphobilinogen (PBG). Two molecules of ALA (blue and orange) are condensed to form PBG, a monopyrrole, by the cytosolic enzyme aminolevulinic acid dehydratase (ALAD) (Richard et al. 2006).

(Jaffe 2000, 2003). As of 2003, approximately one-half of the ~130 PBGS sequences available contained the binding determinants for a catalytic zinc ion, and about one-half did not (Jaffe 2003). On the other hand, approximately 90% of the known PBGS sequences contain the binding determinants for allosteric magnesium. The only known PBGS sequences that lack the binding determinants for both the catalytic zinc and the allosteric magnesium are in the bacterial genus *Rhodobacter* (Jaffe 2003).

δ-ALAD is a sulfhydryl containing enzyme (Gibson et al. 1955, Barnard et al. 1977) and numerous metals such as lead (Rodrigues et al. 1989, 1996, and Goering 1993), mercury (Rocha et al., 1993, 1995), and other compounds that oxidize sulfhydryl groups modified its activity (Emanuelli et al. 1996, Barbosa et al. 1998, Flora et al. 1998). Therefore, δ-ALAD is inhibited by substances that compete with zinc and/or that oxidize the -SH groups (Farina et al. 2002, Nogueira et al. 2003a-b, Santos et al. 2004) and is linked to situations associated with oxidative stress (Folmer et al. 2002, Pande et al. 2001, Pande & Flora 2002, Tandon et al. 2002, Soares et al. 2003). In addition, human exposure to Pb^{2+} causes an important inhibition of blood δ-ALAD (Meredith et al. 1979, Fujita et al. 1981, Pappas et al. 1995, Polo et al. 1995, Pires et al. 2002) and is associated with an intense anemia accompanied by an increase in urinary δ-ALA excretion (Oskarsson 1989). Therefore, δ-ALAD activity is used as one of the most reliable indicators of Pb^{2+} intoxication in humans and other animals (Meredith et al. 1979, Pappas et al. 1995).

ALADs have been purifed from a wide variety of sources, including bovine liver (Gibson et al. 1955), human erythrocytes (Anderson & Desnick 1979), *Rhodopseudomonas capsulatus, Rhodobacter sphaeroides*, (Nandi & Shemin 1973; Nandi et al. 1968), *Escherichia coli* (Spencer & Jordan 1993) and spinach, *Spinacia oleracea* (Liedgens et al. 1983) during the time. Although the fundamental catalytic properties of all ALADs are similar, differences in enzyme primary structure, metal ion requirement and thiol sensitivity have been observed between the various purified enzymes. Metal dependency allows ALADs to be divided into two main categories, the Zn^{2+} -dependent and the Mg^{2+} -dependent dehydratases. The Zn^{2+} -dependent enzymes include the ALADs from mammalian sources, which have 'pH optima' of between 6.3 and 7.1 and have been shown to require Zn^{2+} for maximal catalytic activity (Shemin 1972, Cheh & Neilands 1976). The yeast and *E. coli* enzymes can also be included in this class, requiring Zn^{+2} for activity but with more alkaline pH optima than the animal counterparts: 9.8 for the yeast and 8.5 for the enzyme from *E. coli* (Borralho et al. 1990). The animal, yeast and *E. coli* ALADs have a homo-octameric structure and have thiol groups that are extremely sensitive to oxidation. The oxidation of the thiol groups has been shown to be accompanied by a decrease in catalytic activity and a stoichiometric loss of bound metal ions (Tsukamoto et al. 1979), thereby demonstrating that the cysteine residues are required for Zn^{2+} binding. It has been established that ALADs from this class contain both catalytic and non-catalytic Zn^{+2} (Dent et al. 1990). Techniques such as EXAFS predict that the non-catalytic Zn^{2+} has a tetrahedral co-ordination of at least two and often four cysteine residues. The catalytic Zn^{2+} can be bound in either a tetrahedral or pentaco-ordinate fashion with cysteine, histidine and often water as ligands (Jaffe 1993). The Mg^{2+} -dependent class of dehydratases includes the plant ALADs, which have been reported to have alkaline pH optima of c.a. 8.0-8.5 (Liedgens et al. 1983), but again these values were determined by measurement of an average rate of reaction as described above. They have an absolute dependence on Mg^{2+} as well as subtle differences in their primary structure, especially in the putative metal-binding domains. In addition, some of the plant enzymes seem to be homohexameric and to be less sensitive to oxidation than their animal counterparts; consequently a minor role has been postulated for their thiol groups (Liedgens et al. 1983). This may be due to the fact that the cysteine residues are not involved in metal chelation in the Mg^{2+} -dependent enzymes and their oxidation therefore does not lead to the loss of metal ions. In an attempt to show conclusive differences and/or similarities in the ALADs, a detailed study of the properties of the ALADs from *E. coli*, yeast and pea was conducted. Evidences were presented supporting this hypothesis that the variances in metal binding between the enzymes are a reflection of significant biochemical differences that affect substrate recognition and binding and can therefore be used in the design of specific inhibitors (Senior et al. 1996). It was also revealed that the yeast enzyme, previously assumed to be only Zn^{2+}-binding, is similar to the *E. coli* ALAD in that Mg^{2+} can be substituted at the catalytic site to restore enzyme activity although there is no stimulation of activity. Finally, the crystallization of the yeast ALAD is reported, which will permit the determination of the structure of the enzyme by X-ray diffraction methods.

The yeast ALAD has been overexpressed, purified and found to be a Zn^{2+} -dependent. Mg^{2+}-binding enzyme that is similar in behaviour to, but not identical with, the ALAD from *E. coli*. Comparative studies with the ALADs from three different sources have given an insight into some of the features required for molecular recognition, demonstrating that there are real differences both between and within the different classes of ALADs. These are sufficient to enable the selective inhibition of the enzymes. It will not be possible to rationalize all of the inhibition results collected until the three-dimensional structure of the yeast enzyme has been solved and substantial progress has been made towards this goal with the reported crystallization of the yeast enzyme.

More specific biochemical screening methods are being used by toxicologists such as, protein kinase variants, nitric oxide, interleukin 4 (IL4) and auto-antibodies in plumbism apart from gross changes such as stippling of erythrocytes or inhibition of ALAD (Nag et al. 1996).

Not only δ-ALAD is inhibited but also a number of other enzymes in heme biosynthesis pathway, including coproporphyrinogen oxidase and ferrochelatase are affected by lead.

Inhibitions of ALAD are most profound, and the degree of erythrocyte ALAD inhibition has been used clinically to estimate the degree of Pb poisoning in humans. ALA has neurotoxic activity and may contribute to Pb-induced neurotoxicity (Sithisarankul et al. 1997). At the molecular level, Pb displaces a zinc ion at the metal binding site, not the active site, producing inhibition through a change in the enzyme quaternary structure. ALAD is the second enzyme in the heme biosynthetic pathway, which is cytosolic and non-limiting in heme synthesis in healthy cells. Heme plays important roles in oxygen transport, electron transport systems, detoxification, and transcriptional regulations.
Porphobilinogen is the pyrrole precursor utilized by all living systems for the biosynthesis of tetrapyrroles, including hemes and chlorophylls (Jordan 1991). The ALAD polymorphism has not been established, but it is clear that geographic and strainspecific factors define the distribution of the two recognized ALAD alleles (Fleming et al. 1998). It has also been shown that organisms bred in environments containing high levels of Pb are endowed with multiple copies of the ALAD gene (Bishop et al. 1998).

4. Result

Determination of the blood Pb level alone cannot indicate the toxicity of Pb, since each individual has different degrees of tolerance of Pb (Marcus 1985). As known, atomic absorption spectrophotometry (AAS) or ICP is required for the determination of Pb, and both are expensive. These instruments are available only in specialist laboratories, and can be operated only by a well-trained technician. For these resons same Pb affected enzymes have been employed as biosensors in monitoring Pb toxicity. Among these, ALAD is most popular one, and its results showed good combination with the blood Pb level determined by atomic absorption spectrophotometry or ICP. There are some mathematical equations deviced by several authors to give the Pb concentration by looking at the activity of ALAD (Ogunseitan 1999, Ogunseitan et al. 2000, Korcan et al. 2007, Ciğerci et al. 2008, Konuk et al. 2008).
The expression of ALAD activity gives us a clear indication of the severity of the effect of Pb pollution along the pollution gradient. That is why it is an important biosensor for Pb contamination and pollution. Further studies should be focused on the determination of molecular basis of its effect on ALADs in different organisms and these studies should be strengthened by immobilization studies.

5. References

Anderson, P.M., Desnick, R.J., (1979). Purification and Properties of δ-Aminolevulinic Acid Dehydratase from Human Erythrocytes, J. Biol. Chem., 254, 6924-6930.
Ashraf, W., (2005). Accumulation of heavy metals in kidney and heart tissues of Epinephelus microdon fish from the Arabian Gulf. Environ Monit Assess. 101, 311.
Ballatori, N., (2002). Transport of toxic metals by molecular mimicry. Environ. Health Perspect. 110 (Suppl. 5), 689–694.
Barbosa, N.B.V., Rocha, J.B.T., Zeni, G., Emanuelli, T., Beque, M.C., Braga, A.L., (1998). Effect of organic selenium on δ-aminolevulinate dehydratase from liver, kidney, and brain of adults rats. Toxicol. Appl. Pharmacol. 149, 243–253.
Barnard, G.F., Itoh, R., Hohberger, L.H., Shemin, D., (1977). Mechanism of porphobilinogen synthase—possible role of essential thiol-groups. J. Biol. Chem., 252, 8965–8974.

Bishop, T. R., Miller, M. W., Wang, A., and Dierks, P. M., (1998). Multiple copies of the ALAD gene are located at tle Lvlocus in Mus domesticus mice. Genomics, 48, 221-231.

Borralho, L.M., Ortiz, C.H.D., Panek, A.D. and Mattoon,. J.R. (1990). Purification of Gaminolevulinate dehydratase from genetically engineered yeast. Yeast 6, 319-330.

Burger, J., (1995). A risk assessment for lead in birds. J Toxicol Environ Health 45:369–396.

Burger, J., Gochfeld, M., (2000a). Metals levels in feathers of 12 species of seabirds from Midway Atoll in the northern Pacific Ocean. Sci Total Environ 257:37–52.

Burger, J., Gochfeld, M., (2000b). Effects of lead on birds (Laridae): A review of laboratory and field studies. J Toxicol Environ Health B Crit. Rev. 3(2):59–78.

Busselberg, D., Evans, M.L., Rahmann, H., Carpenter, D.O., (1991). Effects of inorganic and triethyl lead and inorganic mercury on the voltage activated calcium channel of Aplysia neurons. Neurotoxicol., 12, 733–744.

Cavalcanti, A., Shirinzadeh, B., Zhang, M., Kretly, L.C., (2008). "Nanorobot hardware architecture for medical defense". Sensors 8 (5): 2932–2958.

Cheh, A. and Neilands, J. B., (1976). The aminolevulinate dehydratase: Molecular and environmental properties, Struct. Bond., 29, 123–170.

Ciğerci, İ.H., Korcan, S.E., Konuk, M. and Öztürk, S., (2008). Comparison of ALAD activities of Citrobacter and Pseudomonas strains and their usage as biomarker for Pb contamination. Environ. Monitor. Asess., 139(1-3), 41-48.

Ciucu, A., Lupu, A., Pirvutoi, S. and Palleschi, G., (2001). Biosensors for heavy metals determination based on enzyme inhibition. Scientific Bulletin-University "Politehnica" of Bucharest, Series B, Chem. Mater. Sci. 63 (4), pp. 33–44.

Clark, L.C. and Lyons, C., (1962). Electrode systerm for continuous monitoring of cardiovascular surgery Ann. NY Acad. Sci., 102,2945.

Compagnone, D., Palleschi, G., Varallo, G. and Imperiali, P.L., (1995). Amperometric biosensors for the determination of heavy metals In: T. Vo-Dinh, Editors, Proceedings of SPIE, vol. 2504: Environmental Monitoring and Hazardous Waste Site Remediation, pp. 141-152.

Dautremepuits, C., Paris-Palacios, S., Betoulle, S., Vernet, G., (2004). Modulation in hepatic and head kidney parameters of carp (Cyprinus carpio L.) induced by copper and chitosan. Comp. Biochem. Physiol. C Toxicol. Pharmacol., 137, 325-33.

Dauwe, T, Bervoets L., Blust, R., Pinxten, R., Eens, M., (2000). Can excrement and feathers of nestlings songbirds be used as biomonitors for heavy metal pollution? Arch. Environ. Contam. Toxicol., 39:541–546.

Davis, P.H., Goettl, J.P., Sinley, J.R., Smith, N.F., (1976). Acute and chronic toxicity of lead to rainbow trout *Salmo gairdneri*, in hard and soft water. Water Res., 10, 199–206.

Dent, A.J., Beyersmann, D., Block, C. and Hasnain, S.S., (1990). Two different zinc sites in bovine 5-aminolevulinate dehdratase distinguised by EXAFS. Biochemistry, 29, 7822–7828.

Dix, D.J., Gallagher, K., Benson, W.H., Groskinsky, B.L., McClintock, J.T., Dearfield, K.L., Farland, W.H., (2006). A framework for the use of genomics data at the EPA. Nat. Biotechnol., 24, 1108–1111.

Donlan, A. M., Moody, G.J. and Thomas, J.D.R., (1989). The amperometric detection of some enzyme inhibitors, Anal. Proceed. 26, pp. 369–371.

Dooley, M.A., Hogan, S.L., (2003). Environmental epidemiology and risk factors for autoimmune disease. Curr. Opin. Rheumatol., 15, 99–103.

Dzyadevych, V., A.P. Soldatkin, Y.I. Korpan, V.N. Arkhypova, A.V. El'skaya, J. Chovelon, C. Martelet and N. Jaffrezic-Renault, (2003), Biosensors based on enzyme field-effect transistors for determination of some substrates and inhibitors, Anal. Bioanal. Chem., 377, 496–506.

Emanuelli, T., Rocha, J.B.T., Pereira, M.E., Porciuncula, L.O., Morsch, V.M., Martins, A.F., Souza, D.O., (1996). Effect of mercuric chloride intoxication and dimercaprol treatment on aminolevulinate dehydratase from brain, liver and kidney of adult mice. Pharmacol. Toxicol., 79, 138–143.

Evtugyn, G.A., Budnikov, H.C. and Nikolskaya, E.B., (1999). Biosensors for the determination of environmental inhibitors of enzymes, Russ. Chem. Rev., 68, 1041–1064

Fair, J.M., Ricklefs, R.E., (2002). Physiological, growth, and immune responses of Japanese quail chicks to the multiple stressors of immunological challenge and lead shot. Arch. Environ. Contam.Toxicol., 42:77–87.

Farina, M., Barbosa, N.B.V., Nogueira, C.W., Folmer, V., Zeni, G., Andrade, L.H., Braga, L.A., Rocha, J.B.T., (2002). Reaction of diphenyl diselenide with hydrogen peroxide and inhibition of daminolevulinate dehydratase from rat liver and cucumber leaves. Braz. J. Med. Biol. Res., 35, 623–631.

Fleming, D. E. B., Chettle, D. R., Wetmur, J. G., Desnick, R. J.,Robin, J. P., Boulay, D., (1998). Effect of the deltaaminolevulinatedehydratase polymorphism on the accumulationof lead in bone and blood in lead smelterworkers. Environ. Res., 77, 49–61.

Flora, S.J.S., Gubrelay, U., Kannan, G.M., Mathur, R., (1998). Effects of zinc supplementation during chelating agent administration in cadmium intoxication in rats. J. Appl.Toxicol., 18, 357–362.

Folmer, V., Soares, J.C.M., Rocha, J.B.T., (2002). Oxidative stress in mice is dependent on the free glucose content of the diet. Int. J. Biochem. Cell Biol., 34, 1279–1286.

Furness, R.W., (1993). Birds as monitors of pollutants. In: Furness RW, Greenwood JJD (eds) Birds as monitors of environmental change. Chapman & Hall, London, pp 86–143.

Gibson, K.D., Neureberger, A., Scott, J.J., (1955). The purification and properties of delta-aminolevulinic acid dehydratase. Biochem. J., 61, 618–629.

Grosell, M., Gerdes, R., Brix, K.V., (2006). Influence of Ca, humic acid and Ph on lead accumulation and toxicity in the fathead minnow during prolonged water-borne lead exposure. Comp. Biochem. Physiol. C-Toxicol. Pharmacol. 143, 473–483.

Guilbault, G.G., (1984). Analytical Uses of Immobilized Enzymes Marcel Dekker, New York.

Hodson, P.V., Blunt, B.R., Spry, D.J., (1978). Chronic toxicity of water-borne and dietary lead to rainbow trout (*Salmo gairdneri*) in Lake Ontario water. Water Res., 12, 869–878.

Holcombe, G.W., Benoit, D.A., Leonard, E.N., McKim, J.M., (1976). Long-term effects of lead exposure on three generations of brook trout (*Salvelinus fontinalis*). J. Fish. Res. Board Can., 33, 1731–1741.

http://en.wikipedia.org/wiki/Biosensor

http://www.rpi.edu/dept/chem-eng/Biotech Environ/BIOSEN/enzbio.htm

Hu, H., (2000). Exposure to metals. Prim. Care., 2, 983–996.

Huggett, R.J., Kimerle, R.A., Mehrie P.M. and Bergman, H.L., (1992). Biomarkers: Biochemical Physiological and Histological Markers of Anthropogenic Stress, Lewis Publishers, London.

Jaffe, E.K., (2000). The porphobilinogen synthase family of metalloenzymes. Acta Crystallog. D Biol Crystallogr., 56:115–128.

Jaffe, E.K., (2003). An unusual phylogenetic variation in the metal ion binding sites of porphobilinogen synthase. Chem Biol., 10:25–34.

Jaffe, E.K., Ali, S., Mitchell, L.W., Taylor, K.M., Volin, M., Markham, G.D., (1995). Characterization of the role of the stimulatory magnesium of *Escherichia coli* porphobilinogen synthase. Biochem., 34, 244–251.

Järup, L., (2003). Hazards of heavy metal contamination, Brit. Med. Bull., 68:167-182.

Jordan, P. M., (1991). New comprehensive biochemistry.Amsterdam, The Netherlands: Elsevier.

Kalay, M., Ay, P., Canil, M., (1999). Heavy metal concentration in fish tissues from the northeast Meditereansea. Bull Environ. Contam. Toxicol., 63, 673-671.

Konuk, M., Ciğerci, İ.H., Aksan, Ş. and Korcan, S.E., (2008). Isolation and biochemical characterization of δ-aminolevulinic acid dehydratase from *Streptomyces yokosukanensis* ATCC 25520. Appl. Biohem. Microbiol., 44, 356-360.

Korcan, S.E., Ciğerci, İ.H. and Konuk, M., (2007). Screening of δ-Aminolevulinic Acid Dehydratase from Pseudomonas strains as biosensor for Lead and some other metals contamination. Environ. Monitor. Asses., 134, 263-269.

Liedgens, W., C. Lutz, and H. A. W. Schneider., (1983). Molecular properties of 5-aminolevulinic acid dehydratase from *Spinacia oleracea*. Eur. J. Biochem., 135:75-79.

Macdonald, A., Silk, L., Schwartz, M., Playle, R.C., (2002). A lead-gill binding model to predict acute lead toxicity to rainbowtrout (*Oncorhynchus mykiss*). Comp. Biochem. Physiol. C-Toxicol. Pharmacol., 133, 227–242.

Marcus, A.H., (1985). Multicompartment Kinetic Models for Lead: Part1, B one Kinetic and Variable Absorption in Human without exceessive lead exposure. Env. Res., 3,459-479.

Mazliah, J., Barron, S., Bental, E., Reznik, I., (1989). The effect of chronic lead intoxication in mature chickens. Avian Dis., 33:566–570.

Meredith, P.A., Moore, M.R., Goldberg, A., (1979). Erythrocyte ALA dehydratase activity and blood protoporphyrin concentrations as indices of lead exposure and altered haem biosynthesis. Cli. Sci. Mol. Med., 56, 61–69.

Molina, V., Ehrenfeld, M., (2003). Environmental factors in autoimmune diseases, 4–5 February 2003. Durham, NC, USA. Autoimm. Rev., 2, 284–287.

Nag, D., Jaffery, F.N., Viswanathan, P.N., (1996). Clinical and biochemical screening tests for identification of high risk groups. In: Richardson, M.L. (Ed.), Risk Reduction. Chemicals and Energy into the 21st Century. Taylor & Francis, London, UK, pp. 285–302.

Nandi, D.L. and Shemin, D., (1968). Delta-aminolevulinic acid dehydratase of Rhodospeudomonas spheroides II. Association to polymers and dissociation to subunits. J. Biol. Chem., 243, 1231–1235.

Nandi, D.L. and Shemin, D., (1973). ALAD of *Rhodopseudomonas capsulatus*, Arch. Biochem. Biophs., 158, 305-311.

Needleman, H.L., Schell, A., Bellinger, D., Leviton, A., Allred, E.N., (1990). The long-term effects of exposure to low doses of lead in childhood: an 11 year followup report. N. Engl. J. Med. 32, 83–88.

Nogueira, C.W., Borges, V.C., Zeni, G., Rocha, J.B.T., (2003b). Organochalcogens effects on aminolevulinate dehydratase activity from human erythrocytic cells in vitro. Toxicol., 191, 169-178.

Nogueira, C.W., Soares, F.A., Nascimento, P.C., Muller, D., Rocha, J.B.T., (2003a). 2,3-Dimercaptopropane-1-sulfonic acid and meso- 2,3-dimercaptosuccinic acid increase mercury- and cadmiuminduced inhibition of δ-aminolevulinate dehydratase. Toxicol., 184, 85–95.

Ogunseitan, O. A., (1999). Microbial proteins as biomarkers for ecosystem health. In K. Scow, G Fogg, D. Hinton, & M. Johnson (Eds.), Integrated assessment of ecosystem healty (pp. 207-222). Boca Raton, FL: Lewis.

Ogunseitan, O.A., Yang, S. and Ericson, J., (2000). Mikrobial δ-aminolevulinate dehydratase as a biosensor of lead biovailability in contaminated environments. Soil Biol. Biochem., 32, 1899-1906.

Oskarsson, A., (1989). Effects of perinatal treatment with lead and dissulfiram on ALA-D activity in blood, liver and kidney and urinary ALA excretion in rats. Pharm. Toxicol., 64, 344–348.

Pande, M., Flora, S.J.S., (2002). Lead induced oxidative damage and its response to combined administration of α-lipoic acid and succimers in rats. Toxicol., 177, 187–196.

Pande, M., Mehta, A., Pant, B.P., Flora, S.J.S., (2001). Combined administration of a chelating agent and an antioxidant in the prevention and treatment of acute lead intoxication in rats. Environ.Toxicol. Pharmacol., 9, 173–184.

Pappas, J.B., Ahlquist, J.T., Allen, E.M., Banner Jr., W., (1995). Oral dimercaptosuccinic acid and ongoing exposure to lead: effects on heme synthesis and lead distribution in a rat model. Toxicol.Appl. Pharm., 133, 121–129.

Paquin, P.R., Gorsuch, J.W., Apte, S., Batley, G.E., Bowles, K.C., Campbell, P.G., Delos, C.G., Di Toro, D.M., Dwyer, R.L., Galvez, F., Gensemer, R.W., Goss, G.G., Hostrand, C., Janssen, C.R., McGeer, J.C., Naddy, R.B., Playle, R.C., Santore, R.C., Schneider, U., Stubblefield, W.A., Wood, C.M., Wu, K.B., (2002). The biotic ligand model: a historical overview. Comp. Biochem. Physiol. C-Toxicol. Pharmacol., 133, 3–35.

Patel, M., Rogers, J.T., Pane, E.F., Wood, C.M., (2006). Renal responses to acute lead waterborne exposure in the freshwater rainbow trout (*Oncorhynchus mykiss*). Aquat. Toxicol., 80, 362-371.

Pires, J.B., Miekeley, N., Donangelo, C.M., (2002). Calcium supplementation during lactation blunts erythrocyte lead levels and deltaaminolevulinic acid dehydratase zinc-reactivation in women nonexposed to lead and with marginal calcium intakes. Toxicol., 175, 247–255.

Pirvutoiu, I. Surugiu, E.S. Dei, A. Ciucu, V. Magearu and B. Danielsson, (2001), Flow injection analysis of mercury (II) based on enzyme inhibition and thermometric detection, Analyst 126, 1612–1616.

Rand, G.M., (1995). Fundamentals of Aquatic Toxicology: Effects, Environmental Fate and Risk Assessment, Taylor & Francis, London.

Richard, S. A., Phillips, J. D., Kushner, J. P., (2006). Biosynthesis of heme in mammals. Biochim. Biophys. Acta., 1763, 723–736.

Rocha, J.B.T., Freitas, A.J., Marques, M.B., Pereira, M.E., Emanuelli, T., Souza, D.O., (1993). Effects of methylmercury exposure during the second stage of rapid postnatal brain growth on negative geotaxis and on delta-aminolevulinic acid dehydratase of suckling rats. Braz. J.Med. Biol.Res., 26, 1077–1083.

Rocha, J.B.T., Pereira, M.E., Emanuelli, T., Christofari, R.S., Souza, D.O., (1995). Effect of treatment with mercury chloride and lead acetate during the second stage of rapid postnatal brain growth on delta-aminolevulinic acid dehydratase (ALA-D) activity in brain, liver kidney and blood of suckling rats. Toxicol., 100, 27–37.

Rodrigues, A.L., Bellinaso, M.L., Dick, T., (1989). Effect of some metalions on blood and liver delta-aminolevulinate dehydratase of *Pimelodus maculatus* (Pisces, Pimelodidae). Comp. Biochem.Physiol., 94, 65–69.

Rogers, J.T., Wood, C.M., (2004). Characterization of branchial lead-calcium interaction in the freshwater rainbow trout *Oncorhynchus mykiss*. J. Exp. Biol., 207, 813–825.

Santos, F.W., Oro, T., Zeni, G., Rocha, J.B.T., do Nascimento, P.C., Nogueira, C.W., (2004). Cadmium induced testicular damage and its response to administration of succimer and diphenyl diselenide in mice. Toxicol.Lett., 152, 255–263.

Senior, N.M., Brocklehurst, K., Cooper, J.B., Wood, S.P., Erksine, P., Shoolingin- Jordan, P., Thomas, P.G., Warren, M.J., (1996). Comparative studies on the 5- aminolevulinic acid dehydratase from *Pisum sativum, Escherichia coli* and *Saccharomyces cerevisiae*. Biochem J. 320:410-412

Shemin, D., (1972). Aminolevulinic acid dehydratase, Enzymes, 7, 323-337.

Shoolingin-Jordan, P.M., (2003). The biosynthesis of Coproporphyrinogen III. In: Kadish KM, Smith KM and Guilard R. , editor. The Porphyrin Handbook. Vol. 12. Amsterdam, Elsevier Science; pp. 33–74.

Sithisarankul, P., Schwartz, B.S., Lee, B.K., Kalsey, K.T., Strickland, P.T., (1997). Aminolevulinic acid (ALA) dehydratase genotype mediates plasma levels of the neurotoxin, 5-aminolevulinic acid, in lead exposed workers. Am. J. Ind. Med., 32, 15–28.

Soares, J.C.M., Folmer, V., Rocha, J.B.T., (2003). Influence of dietary selenium supplementation and exercise on thiol-containing enzymes in mice. Nutrition 19, 627–632.

Spencer, P., Jordan, P.M., (1993). Purification and characterization of 5-aminolaevulinic acid dehydratase from Escherichia coli and a study of the reactive thiols at the metal-binding domain. Biochem. J., 290, 279-287.

Starodub, N.F., Kanjuk, N.I., Kukla, A.L.,Shirshov and Yu, M., (1999). Multi-enzymatic electrochemical sensor: field measurements and their optimization, Anal. Chim. Acta, 385, pp. 461–466.

Stein, J., Schettler, T., Wallinga, D., Vallenti, M., (2002). In harm's way: toxic threats to child development. J. Dev. Behav. Pediatr. (Suppl. 1), 13–22.

Tandon, S.K., Singh, S., Prasad, S., Srivastava, S., Siddiqui, M.K.J., (2002). Reversal of lead-induced oxidative stress by chelating agent, antioxidant, or their combination in the rat. Environ. Res., 90, 61–66.

Tang, H.W., Huel, G., Compagna, D., Hellier, G., Boissinot, C., Blot, P., (1999). Neurodevelopment evaluation of 9-month old infants exposed to low levels of Pb in vitro: involvement of monoamine neurotransmitters. J. Appl. Toxicol., 19, 167–172.

Timbrell, J.A., (2000). Principles of Biochemical Toxicology, Taylor & Francis, London.

Tsukamoto, I., Yoshinaga, T., Sano, S., (1979). The role of zinc with special reference to the essential thiol groups in delta-aminolevulinic acid dehydratase of bovine liver. Biochim. Biophys. Acta., 12;570(1):167–178.

USEPA, (2006). National RecommendedWater Quality Criteria. Office ofWater, Washington, DC.

Vel Krawczyc, K., Moszczynska, M. and Trojanowicz, M., (2000). Inhibitive determination of mercury and other metal ions by potentiometric urea biosensor, Biosens. Biolectron., 15, pp. 681–691.

Wang, W. X., (2002). Interaction of trace metals and different marine food chains. Mar. Ecol. Prog. Ser. 243, 295-309.

Weber, D.N., (1993). Exposure to sublethal levels of waterborne lead alters reproductive behavior patterns in fathead minnows (*Pimephales promelas*). Neurotoxicol., 14, 347–358.

Winneke, G., Walkowiak, J., Lilienthal, H., (2002). PCB induced neurodevelopmental toxicity in human infants and its potential mediation by endocrine dysfunction. Toxicol., 181–182, 161–165.

Yang, J.H., Derr-Yellin, E.C., Kodavanti, P.R., (2003). Alterations in brain protein kinase c isoforms following developmental exposure to a polychlorinated biphenyl mixture. Brain Res. Mol. Brain Res., 123–135.

19

Bioelectronic Noses Based on Olfactory Receptors

Jasmina Vidic
Institut National de la Recherche Agronomique
France

1. Introduction

The discovery and characterization of the great multigene family encoding olfactory receptors has led the way to both fundamental and biotechnological investigations. Human and animal noses can perceive more than a hundreds of thousands of odorant molecules. Detection of different odors results from the association of the odorant molecules with olfactory receptors, carried by olfactory sensory neurons. Only a subtle difference in the molecular structure of an odorant can lead to pronounced modification in odor quality, due to the complex olfactory coding. These features have made the development of an artificial odor-sensing system, that is the bioelectronic nose challenging for research. Bioelectronic noses may have many potential applications in different fields of food and beverage, cosmetics and environmental monitoring, disease diagnostics…

Several biosensor concepts for odorant detection using different olfactory receptors have been published. Some of them are based on the direct immobilization of the olfactory mucus, or of various whole cells expressing olfactory receptors. Another type of sensors is based on immobilized cellular membrane fractions carrying olfactory receptors. The recognition of the odorant by such olfactory sensing elements can be detected by surface plasmon resonance, quartz crystal microbalance, or by direct electrochemical measurements. Here, a brief overview of different bioelectronic noses will be given.

2. Biolectronic nose development

Odorant detections by terrestrial vertebrates have evolved to meet the numerical and physical challenges since olfactory systems operate over a dynamic range of several orders of stimulus magnitude and can recognize an enormous array of low to medium molecular weight organic molecules. Theoretically, there is no limit to the number and variety of compounds that can be considered odorant and that can be detected by some animal olfactory system. Humans, for example, are thought to be capable of distinguishing more than hundreds of thousands of distinct odor molecules. Subtle alternations in the molecular structure of an odorant can lead to pronounced changes in the perceptive odor. How are the diversity and specificity of olfactory perception accomplished? The detection and discrimination of chemically distinct odorants results from the association of odorous ligands with specific olfactory receptors expressed on the cilia of olfactory neurons that are located in a specialized epithelium in the nose. Olfactory receptors belong to the large super family of G protein coupled receptors (Mombaerts, 2004). The activated receptor interacts with the G protein which mediates the signaling cascade transmission to olfactory bulb, where olfactory signals are processed before reaching cortical structure in the brain (Firestein, 2001). Each olfactory receptor can recognize a range of odorants that share specific molecular characteristics. Their responses can vary along multiple odorant structural dimensions allowing discrimination of odorants with different molecular shapes and sizes, functional groups, charge, hydrophobicity, atomic composition and even concentration. The olfactory system utilizes en encoding mechanism in which a combination of activated olfactory receptors determines the odor quality. Functional analyses of structurally similar receptors that recognize overlapping sets of odorants with distinct ligand specificity and affinity have confirmed this combinatorial receptor code model (Firestein, 2001; Buck, 2004; Mombaerts, 2004).

Sensory evaluation is one of the important parameters for air quality monitoring, quality assessment for food, wine and beverages, as well as for control of many cosmetic and fermentation products. Furthermore, odors can constitute a signature of metabolic stress and diseases (tuberculosis, schizophrenia, diabetes, etc). Odors are associated with drugs and explosives or with domestic and environmental pollutants. Typically, sensory evaluation of odor is performed by a panel of well-trained professionals based upon their sense of smell, taste, experiences and mood. Likewise, trained dogs, rats or bees are employed to detect drugs or explosives. Within the clinical field, trained dogs and rats are also used for detection of some odors associated with different pathologies or with physiological states (Turner & Magan, 2004). Many efforts have been made to replace humans and animals by analytical instrumentations for odorant detection. Unfortunately, current electronic noses have significant limitations in odor detection concerning sensitivity, reliability and selectivity, among others. Typically, artificial electronic noses have as a recognition part metal oxide semiconductors, conduction organic polymers, porphyrins, or calixarenes (Harper, 2001). Their limitations are at the basis of persistent difficulty of this technology to reach essential applications in different areas. One possibility to overcome these limitations is replacing the physical and chemical sensitive elements of electronic noses with natural olfactory receptors. This results in bioelectronic noses. Due to the pharmacological profile of olfactory receptors, bioelectronic noses would provide detection and identification of specific odorants at even very tiny or trace amounts, large operational availability and fast and reliable detection. For instance, traditional electronic noses usually have concentration thresholds up to 0.1 ppb, while animal olfaction displays much lower detection limits down to 10^{-6} ppb, or even lower.

3. Olfactory receptor preparations and their sensor integration

Despite intensive efforts to determine the pharmacological profile and odorant specificities of individual olfactory receptors, until now, response specificities to odorants have been examined in detail only for a few receptors. The main reason of such lack of knowledge is that these studies are difficult to be undertaken in the olfactory epithelium since individual sensory neurons mainly express a single type of olfactory receptor out of several hundreds of olfactory receptor genes in the genome (Mombaerts, 2004). Moreover, there are inherent difficulties associated with the expression of olfactory receptors in heterologous cell lines (Lu et al., 2003; McClintock & Sammeta, 2003), which have enabled the use of recombinant receptors for pharmacological and biophysical studies . In consequence, until now, most bioelectronic noses have been developed for only a few olfactory receptors (rat receptor 17, human OR17-40, *C. elegant* ODR-10, human 2AG1). These receptors served as models to prove the feasibility of the bioelectronic nose concept since their preferential odorant ligand and working concentration ranges are known.

One of the major challenges for achieving the bioelectronic nose are sample preparation and immobilization onto a sensor solid surface. Since they are G protein coupled receptors, olfactory receptors need to stay in their membrane environment to be functional. So, the first bioelectronic nose was based on the direct immobilization of the olfactory cilia, or of various whole cells expressing olfactory receptors. A second type of sensor has been achieved using semi-purified receptor preparations such as membrane fractions carrying them. Such olfactory receptor preparations can be integrated into a sensor either by simple adsorption or by capturing via its specific antibody previously attached to the surface. By the adsorption method, olfactory receptors are bound to the sensor surface indirectly, through the interaction of their surrounding hydrophobic lipids with the substrate. In consequence, the receptor binding site is free and remains accessible for odorants. However, with adsorption, olfactory receptors are immobilized in a random orientation in relation to the sensor surface. In contrast, when the olfactory receptor is poorly expressed in the membrane fraction the second method is more adequate since specific receptor grafting increases receptor surface concentration and ensures its uniform surface orientation.

4. Bioelectronic noses based on whole cells expressing olfactory receptors

In 1999, Wu immobilized a crude bullfrog cilia preparation onto a piezoelectric electrode which served as a signal transducer. Using this biosensor he was able to detect trace levels of various odorants with concentrations fully correlated with the olfactory threshold values of human noses. Similarly, Liu et al., (2006) showed that the bionic designed hybrid system composed of olfactory receptor neurones and olfactory bulb neurones cultivated on the surface of a light-addressable potentiometric sensor can be used as a novel bioelectronic nose. Indeed, this device was sensitive to environmental odor changes.

Wu (1999), also partially fractioned olfactory receptors from the cilia preparation and coated them separately onto the crystal surface. A quartz crystal microbalance was used for detecting the binding of odorant molecules to the olfactory receptors. This method can be successfully applied for odorant detection, since odorant molecules binding to the receptors coated onto the crystal alters the resonance frequency of the crystal. An array made of six sensors consisting of five different cilia fractions was able to rapidly and stably detect responses to different volatile compounds. However, since olfactory receptors in these fractions were separated by gel filtration chromatography with respect only to their molecular weights it was inevitable that each fraction contained a mixture of various receptors.

To apply an olfactory whole-cell biosensor for checking ligand specificity of a particular olfactory receptor, heterologous cells expressing one type of receptor should be employed. For instance, mammalian HEK cells transfected to express rat receptor 17 were coated onto the crystal of a quartz microbalance (Sung et al., 2006). Their stimulation by one of the receptor 17 preferential ligands, octanal, produced strong and dose-dependent sensor responses. This device did not respond to several other odorant non-ligands. This work suggested that bioelectronic noses can be applied for the quantitative measurements of odorants.

Similarly, the same authors heterologously expressed *C. elegans* olfactory receptor ODR-10 in HEK cells and applied the Surface Plasmon Resonance (SPR) technique to characterize molecular interactions (Lee et al., 2006). HEK cells were seeded on the sterilized bare gold sensorchip surface previously treated with poly- lysine to allow their good adherence to the gold substrate. The activation of the transfected cells by the receptor ligand diacetyl induced an increase in the intracellular calcium ions, which subsequently resulted in the SPR signal change. Moreover, the SPR signal increase was proportional to the diacetyl concentration. This cell-based SPR method was proposed to have a potential application in the identification of odorant ligands specific to each olfactory receptor in a real-time manner and without any labeling.

Our team has shown the feasibility of a bioelectronic nose based on whole yeast cells expressing human receptor OR-1740 immobilized onto an interdigitated thin film microelectrode (Marrakchi et al., 2007). When yeast cells attached to the gold microelectrode surface pre-treated with poly-lysine solution were stimulated with the receptor ligand helional it was possible to detect conductiometric changes due to the ionic exchanges resulting from the recognition of the ligand molecule by the olfactory receptor. *S. cerevisiae* yeasts are more convenient than mammalian cells for olfactory receptor expression since they are much cheaper and easier to cultivate. In addition, *S. cerevisiae* has been successfully used for functional expression of many G protein coupled receptors including olfactory receptors (Pausch, 1997, Minic et al., 2005a) which is one of the major difficulties in olfactory sensor development. In addition, yeasts provide a null background for mammalian G protein coupled receptors (Minic et al., 2005a), thus allowing the correct pharmacological characterisation of receptors. Indeed, specificity, selectivity and dose-response to helional obtained with immobilized yeast carrying OR1740 receptor suggested that this conductiometric biosensor preserves the natural receptor characteristics of odorant recognition (Marrakchi et al., 2007).

It should also be noted that modified yeast cells in solution may serve as a biosensor. Functional similarities between the signal transduction cascade of olfactory receptors in mammalian neurons and the pheromonal response pathway in yeasts allows the development of the yeast cell-based biosensor for odorant screening. Such systems are easily adaptable for a high throughput format (Minic et al., 2005a). Upon stimulation of the olfactory receptor by its odorant ligands in yeasts engineered to co-express either rat I7 or human OR 17-40 receptor and the mammalian Gα subunit, an activation of a MAP kinase signaling pathway takes place, which induces the synthesis of a functional reporter luciferase (Minic et al., 2005b). In that way bioluminescence responses are detected upon odorant binding to the receptor. This assay enables the quantitative measurement of receptor activity, or alternately the detection of its odorant ligands. In one previous study yeasts were modified to provide odorant-dependent yeast growth on histidine-deficient or hygromycin-containing medium, respectively (Pajot-Augy et al., 2003; Minic et al., 2005a). Such assays are commonly used by pharmacological laboratories for ligand screenings of non-olfactory G protein coupled receptors. However, luciferase is the more convenient reporter because of its sensitivity, rapidity and easy to perform enzymatic reaction.

Using whole cells as biological recognition elements in bioelectronic noses provides the opportunity to elicit full functional information since it necessarily involves the influence of the cellular signaling cascade on sensor response. Whole cell systems have, thus, possible applications in the fields of pharmacology, cell biology, toxicology and environmental measurements (Keusgen, 2002; Bousse, 1996).

5. Bioelecronic noses based on partially purified olfactory receptors

When analytical information is needed instead of functional information, it is more adequate to use isolated biological molecules as recognition parts in biosensors. This second approach allows developing specific analytical devices for fast routine measurements in many fields of analysis. Moreover, using isolated olfactory receptors instead of whole-cells enables scaling down the biosensors and their convergence with micro- and nano-technologies.

The first requirement to develop such bioelectronic noses is the immobilization of receptors in a manner to preserve their function. As mentioned before, olfactory receptors are extremely hydrophobic and require a lipid or detergent environment to maintain their native conformation and function. Usually membrane receptors are expressed in heterologous cells, solubilized and purified in an adequate detergent before being reconstituted in proteoliposomes and immobilized onto the sensor (Minic et al., 2005c). However, olfactory receptors are poorly expressed in heterologous cells and, so, their purification before reconstitution typically cannot be considered. Consequently, producing lipid vesicles by disturbing the membrane of the cells where receptors have been expressed seems to be a better strategy. In this way, the receptor remains in its native membrane environment which obviates the risk of receptor alternation or activity loss, which may occur when G protein coupled receptors are reconstituted in proteoliposomes.

Sung et al., (2006) coated the surface of a quartz crystal microbalance with crude insoluble membrane extract of *E. coli* expressing the ODR-10 receptor and examined its interactions with various odorant molecules. They showed linear dose-dependent responses of the piezoelectric biosensor upon the membrane extract stimulation with natural receptor ligand diacetyl. Using a similar set-up but with the rat olfactory receptor I7 specifically captured on a quartz microbalance transducer, Rodriguez Segui et al., (2006) explored the first step toward the production of a quartz microbalance olfactory sensor. For this, a self-assembled multilayer was grafted onto the sensor surface. It was composed of a mixed MHDA - Biotinyl PE self-assembled monolayer and a biotin-avidin bridge system which allows binding of biotinylated antibodies. In the final step, the receptor specific biotinylated antibody was used to bind a membrane fraction carrying receptor I7 to the quartz crystal.

In one recent study, the membrane fraction carrying human olfactory receptor 2AG1 was covalently integrated by amino-link to conducting polymer nanotubes functionalized with carboxylic acid (Yoon et al., 2009). Nanotubes were then attached to a microelectrode array to create a field-effect transistor, which generated changes in electrical signal when odorant molecules activated the receptor protein. Through the miniaturization of the sensor, the signal was efficiently transferred to the nanotubes due to the covalent attachment. The bound receptor detected a femtomolar concentration of its natural ligand amyl butyrate. Related esters that differ from the ligand molecule by a single carbon atom (butyl and hexyl butyrates), produced no response at a billion times higher concentration. This good selectivity suggests that the receptors remain in good conformational shape after being grafted which is very promising.

We developed a surface plasmon resonance bioelectronic nose in our laboratory in Jouy-en-Josas. Small membrane fragments (nanosomes), obtained from cells expressing a given olfactory receptor can be easily immobilized on commercial L1 Biacore sensorchips. We demonstrate that olfactory receptors maintain their activity in such membrane fragments (Vidic et al., 2006). Since the surface plasma resonance signal is proportional to the molecular weight of the analyte, low-molecular weight molecules, as the majority of odorants, cannot be detected directly by the Biacore3000 system. To overcome this problem, we took advantage of the presence of G protein in the nanosomes to monitor receptor activation by an odorant, through the departure of the G_α subunit from the preparation (Vidic et al., 2006). The same bell-shaped concentration-dependence responses were obtained as in a whole cells, in terms of threshold concentration and concentration at the maximum, which gives evidence that this receptor functional response in the living cell indeed arises from its own behavior upon odorant stimulation, with no artefactual contribution from the cellular transduction pathway. As assessed by surface plasmon, resonance responses monitoring olfactory receptors efficiently discriminate between odorant ligands and unrelated odorants.

This system can fruitfully serve to evaluate the comparative coupling efficiency of olfactory receptors to various G_a protein subunits, without the interference of cellular contribution (Vidic et al., 2006). Furthermore, this new bioelectronic nose can be applied for the fundamental investigation of molecular mechanisms of olfaction. Indeed, it is assumed that the first event in peripheral olfactory detection involves at least 3 partners: olfactory receptor, odorants and olfactory binding protein (OBP). Whole yeast cell expressing an olfactory receptor cannot be applied for investigation of receptor-OBP interaction because their cell wall impairs OBP penetration. However, a bioelectronic nose based on nanosome expression of a given olfactory receptor was successively applied for characterization of this three-partner reaction (Vidic et al., 2008). Interestingly, such a study showed that the presence of OBP enhanced odorant detection sensitivity of the device.

6. SPOT-NOSED prototype of olfactory nanobiosensor

In 2003, the European project SPOT-NOSED began with the aim to develop nanobiosensors based on single olfactory receptors anchored between nanoelectrodes, in order to mimic the performances of a natural olfactory system. The next step was to create arrays of nanobiosensors that could then increase odorant sensitivity and/or widen the odorant detection spectrum. For this, two model receptors, rat I7 and human OR 17-40, were expressed in *S. cerevisiae* yeast (Minic et al., 2005a). Then, lipidic nanosomes bearing the olfactory receptors were prepared from the yeast. Nanosomes are small vesicles (50-100 nm in diameter). They can be obtained by cell disruption, purification of membrane microsomes and then by size homogenization and miniaturization of microsomes by extensive sonication (Vidic et al., 2006; Casuso et al., 2008). Each of this nanometric vesicular structure was shown to contain one or few receptors of the given type (Casuso et al., 2008; Vidic et al., 2007). The maintenance of nanosome homogeneity in the solution suggested that they can be used as a recognition part in an elementary nanobioelectronic sensor (Casuso et al., 2008; Vidic et al., 2006; Gabriel et al, 2006).

Next, surface plasmon resonance was performed on nanosomes for quantitative evaluation of olfactory receptor responses to odorant stimulation. These tests strongly suggested that olfactory receptors in nanosomes retain their full activity (Vidic et al., 2006) since they discriminated between odorant ligand and unrelated odorants, as previously shown in whole yeast cells with a reporter gene (Vidic et al., 2006; Vidic et al., 2008). This finding led to the use of nanosomes in nanobiosensor fabrication.

Nanoelectrodes were fabricated using conventional photolithography and focused ion beam milling, with sizes in adequation with the nanosomes. In order to optimize nanosome functional immobilization on them, several immobilization methods were checked on mili- and micrometric scale. Functional responses were observed when nanosomes were simply adsorbed on the hydrophobic surface (Hou et al., 2006; Vidic et al., 2006; Benilova et al., 2008; Vidic et al., 2007) or when the receptor was captured by its specific antibody previously grafted to the sensor surface (Hou et al., 2006; Benilova et al., 2008). To further determinate optimal surface orientation of the receptor, various tagged OR17-40 were produced in yeast. The intensity of the specific response was particularly enhanced when nanosomes were captured via an antibody to the tag attached to the receptor C-terminal (Vidic et al., 2007). Strikingly, capturing the OR 1740 receptor via its tag attached to the N-terminus abolished functional responses upon odorant ligand stimulation. This probably originates from steric hindrances to the odorant binding due to the immobilization of the receptor N-terminus.

Thus, in the final device configuration, nanosomes bearing olfactory receptors tagged on their C-terminal were specifically immobilized onto conducting substrates via a self assembled monolayer containing biotinyl groups. Biotinyl groups were used to attach neutravidin and specific anti-tag antibodies to allow receptor specific grafting (Hou et al., 2006; Vidic et al., 2007; Benilova et al., 2008). The process was optimized by microcontact printing, and the anchored nanovesicles were visualized by Atomic Force Microscopy (Vidic et al., 2007, Casuso et al., 2008). Positive and negative elastomeric polydimethylsiloxane stamps were replicated from silicon-based molds elaborated using deep reactive ion etching. Pattering was performed by inking procedures of the stamps after hydrophilization with oxygen plasma in order to ensure correct surface coverage.

Finally a direct electrochemical impedancemetric spectroscopy method can be employed to directly detect electrical changes produced by olfactory receptor conformational change induced by odorant binding (Hou et al., 2006; Benilova et al., 2008; Minic et al., 2006a, Gomila et al., 2006). The same method was successfully employed to characterize each step of electrode functionalization and nanosome grafting. For nano-scale measurements a transimpedance preamplifier suited for low-noise wide-bandwidth measurements was designed and fabricated to be directly connected to the nanoelectrodes. Also, a friendly interface with a specific odorant identification algorithm was developed.

The biolectronic nose prototype developed during the Spot-Nosed project has shown the feasibility of an olfactory nanobioelectrical sensor. Miniaturization of structures allows integration of many sensors into arrays that may mime the animal nose and may be suitable for the screening of natural and chemical odorants as well as their combinatorial libraries.

7. Perspectives

Until now, no commercially available bioelectronic nose based on olfactory receptors has existed but they can be expected in the future thanks to the strong demand and a constant progress made in the field. Feasibility of bioelectronic noses based on olfactory receptors has been demonstrated. The next step is to assemble devices with an autosampler, electronic data acquisition and an odorant identification algorithm. Significant advances in bioelectronic nose fabrication are constantly being made. The development of sensor technology incorporating natural olfactory receptors provides the basis for a bioelectronic nose mimicking the animal olfactory system. Such devices can be used for qualitative and quantitative identification and monitoring of a spectrum of odorants with much higher selectivity and sensibility than the present electronic devices. Thanks to the natural combinatorial olfactory code these new bioelectronic noses should provide a platform for fingerprinting of complex mixture of odorants. I am currently involved in a research project that is developing an olfactory nanobiosensor array based on immobilized nanosomes carring olfactory receptors in order to mimic the animal nose (BOND, European project).

8. References

Benilova, I., Chegel, V.I., Ushenin, Y.V., Vidic, J., Soldatkin, A.P., Martelet, C., Pajot, E., & Jaffrezic-Renault, N. (2008) Stimulation of human olfactory receptor 17-40 with odorants probed by surface plasmon resonance. *European Biophysical Journal,* Jul;37(6), 807-814.

Bousse, L. (1996) Whole cell biosensors. *Sensors Actuators* B34, 270-275.

Buck, L.B. (2004). Olfactory receptors and odor coding in mammals. *Nutritional Review,* Nov;62(11 Pt 2):S184-8; discussion S224-41.

Casuso, I., Pla-Roca, M., Gomila, G., Samitier, J., Minic, J., Persuy, M.-A., Salesse, R. & Edith Pajot-Augy (2008) Immobilization of olfactory receptors onto gold electrodes for electrical biosensor. *Materials Science and Engineering: C,* Jul; 28(5-6), 686-691.

Firestein, S. (2001). How the olfactory system makes sense of scents. *Nature,* Sep 13;413(6852), 211-218.

G. Gomila, I. Casuso, A. Errachid, O. Ruiz, E. Pajot, J. Minic, T. Gorojankina, M.A. Persuy, J. Aioun, R. Salesse, J. Bausells, G. Villanueva, G. Rius, Y. Hou, N. Jaffrezic, C. Pennetta, E. Alfinito, V. Akimov, L. Reggiani, G. Ferrari, et al.(2006) Advances in the production, immobilization, and electrical characterization of olfactory receptors for olfactory nanobiosensor development. *Sensors and Actuators B: Chemical,* 28Jul; *116(1-2), 66-71.*

Harper, W.J. (2001) The strengths and weaknesses of the electronic nose. In: *Headspace Analysis of Food and Flavors: Theory and Practice,* edited by Rouseff & Cadwallader. Kluwer Academic / Plenum Publishers, New York.

Hou, Y., Jaffrezic-Renault, N., Martelet, C., Zhang, A., Minic-Vidic, J., Gorojankina, T., Persuy, M.A., Pajot-Augy, E., Salesse, R., Akimov, V., Reggiani, L., Pennetta, C., Alfinito, E., Ruiz, O., Gomila, G., Samitier, J. & Errachid, A. (2007) A novel detection strategy for odorant molecules based on controlled bioengineering of rat olfactory receptor I7. *Biosensors and Bioelectronics.* Feb 15;22(7), 1550-1555.

Keusgen, M. (2002) Biosensors: new approaches in drug discovery. *Naturwissenschaften.* 89, 433-444.

Lee, J.Y., Ko H.J., Lee, S.H. & Park T.H. (2006) Cell-based measurement of odorant molecules using surface Plasmon resonance, *Enzyme and Microbial Technology*, July3;39(3), 375-380.

Liu, Q., Cai, H., Xu, Y., Li, Y., Li, R. & Wang, P. (2006) Olfactory cell-based biosensor: a first step towards a neurochip of bioelectronic nose. *Biosensors & Bioelectronics*, Aug 15;22(2), 318-322.

Lu, M., Echeverri, F. & Moyer , B.D. (2003) Endoplasmic reticulum retention, degradation, and aggregation of olfactory G-protein coupled receptors.*Traffic*, Jun;4(6), 416-433.

Marrakchi, M., Vidic, J., Jaffrezic-Renault, N., Martelet, C & Pajot-Augy, E. (2007) A new concept of olfactory biosensor based on interdigitated microelectrodes and immobilized yeasts expressing the human receptor OR17-40, *European Biophysical Journal*,. Nov;36(8), 1015-1018.

McClintock, T.S. & Sammeta, N. Trafficking prerogatives of olfactory receptors. *Neuroreport*. Aug 26;14(12), 1547-1552.

Minic, J., Sautel, M., Salesse, R. & Pajot-Augy, E. (2005a) Yeast system as a screening tool for pharmacological assessment of g protein coupled receptors, *Current Medical Chemistry*, Jan;12(8), 961-969.

Minic, J, Persuy, M.A., Godel, E., Aioun, J., Connerton, I., Salesse, R. & Pajot-Augy, E. (2005b) Functional expression of olfactory receptors in yeast and development of a bioassay for odorant screening. *FEBS Journal*, Jan; 272(2,)524-537.

Minic, J., Grosclaude, J., Aioun, J., Persuy, M.A., Gorojankina, T., Salesse, R., Pajot-Augy, E., Hou, Y., Helali, S., Jaffrezic-Renault, N., Bessueille, F., Errachid, A., Gomila, G., Ruiz, O. & Samitier, J. (2005c) Immoblisation of native membrane-bound rhodopsin on biosensor surfaces. *Biochimica and Biophysica Acta*, 1724, 324-332.

Mombaerts, P. (2004). Genes and ligands for odorant, vomeronasal and taste receptors. *Nature Review Neuroscience*, Apr;5(4), 263-278.

Pajot-Augy, E., Crowe, M., Levasseur, G., Salesse, R., Connerton, I. (2003) Engineered yeasts as reporter systems for odorant detection, *Journal of Recepttors and Signal Transduction Researc*, 23(2-3), 155-171.

Pausch, M.H. (1997) G-protein-coupled receptors in Saccharomyces cerevisiae: high-throughput screening assays for drug discovery. *Trends in Biotechnology*. Dec;15(12), 487-494.

Rodríguez Seguí, S., Pla, M., Minic, J., Pajot-Augy, E., Salesse, R., Hou, Y. Jaffrezic-Renault, N., Mills, C.A., Samitier, J., & Errachid, A. Detection of olfactory receptor I7 self assembled multilayer formation and immobilization using a quartz crystal microbalance. *Analytical Letters*, Jul; 39(8), 1735-1745.

Sung, J.H., Ko, H.J. & Park, T.H. (2006) Piezoelectric biosensor using olfactory receptor protein expressed in Escherichia coli. *Biosensensors & Bioelectronics*, Apr15;21(10), 1981-1986.

Turner, A.P. & Magan, N. (2004) Electronic noses and disease diagnostics. *Nature Review Microbiology*, Feb;2(2),161-166.

Vidic, J.M., Grosclaude, J., Persuy, M.A., Aioun, J., Salesse, R. & Pajot-Augy E. (2006) Quantitative assessment of olfactory receptors activity in immobilized nanosomes: a novel concept for bioelectronic nose. *Lab Chip*. Aug; 6(8):1026-1032.

Vidic, J., Pla-Roca, M., Grosclaude, J., Persuy, M.A., Monnerie, R., Caballero, D., Errachid, A., Hou, Y., Jaffrezic-Renault, N., Salesse, R., Pajot-Augy, E. & Samitier, J. (2007) Gold surface functionalization and patterning for specific immobilization of olfactory receptors carried by nanosomes. *Analitical Chemistry*, May; 79(9,)3280-3290.

Vidic, J., Grosclaude, J., Monnerie, R., Persuy, M.A., Badonnel, K., Baly, C., Caillol, M., Briand, L., Salesse, R. & Pajot-Augy, E. (2008) On a chip demonstration of a functional role for Odorant Binding Protein in the preservation of olfactory receptor activity at high odorant concentration. *Lab Chip*, May; 8(5), 678-688.

Yoon, H., Lee, S.H., Kwon, O.S., Song, H.S., Oh, E.H., Park, T.H. & Jang, J. (2009) Polypyrrole nanotubes conjugated with human olfactory receptors: high-performance transducers for FET-type bioelectronic noses. *Angewandte Chemie International Edition*, 48(15), 2755-2758.

Wu, T.Z. (1999) A piezoelectric biosensor as an olfactory receptor for odour detection: electronic nose. Biosensors & Bioelectronics, Jan 1;14(1), 9-18.